Trends in EU Health Care Systems

Trends in EU Health Care Systems

Win de Gooijer

Springer

Win de Gooijer
Silodam 250
1013 AS Amsterdam
The Netherlands
w.j.degooijer@graansilo.nl

ISBN-13: 978-1-4419-2190-1
e-ISBN-10: 0-387-32748-7
e-ISBN-13: 978-0-387-32748-8

Printed on acid-free paper.

9 8 7 6 5 4 3 2 1

springer.com

for Aaltje

Contents

Part Three: Reflections

Foreword

Since the beginning of the 1980s, governments all over the developed world have been engaged in reforming their health care systems and in trying to find ways of coping with the problem of continuously rising costs. Methods aimed at improving the effectiveness and efficiency of health care delivery, shifting the financial burden from public to private financing, as well as reducing the health care infrastructure, are being studied and developed. During the many years that I served on the Board of the Federation of Dutch Health Care Organizations, including as Chairman from 1992 to 1999, I experienced directly the consequences of limiting the financial resources available to health care. It became apparent to me during those years that the social climate regarding health care in the Netherlands was changing. That changing climate can be encapsulated by the word *accountability*. Accountability has come to mean that health care is the business of a range of stakeholders, all of whom want developments to go their way. In short, health care now has multiple owners.

Later, after I had joined the Governing Council of the International Hospital Federation, I found that similar developments could be observed throughout the developed world. These developments are characterized by the decreasing involvement of governments in the financing and delivery of health care. Instead, the market, and with it the price of health care, is increasingly becoming the instrument for coordinating of supply and demand.

The reform of health care systems in most of the countries of the European Union is conditional on providing equal access for all citizens, regardless of their ability to pay. National constitutions, or their equivalents, mandate governments' responsibility in this respect. As a consequence, exemption regulations aimed at protecting vulnerable members of society have been introduced by EU governments which have carried through cost-saving measures. These regulations are meant to uphold the idea of solidarity in health care.

Whether or not EU governments, by applying exemption regulations, have succeeded in living up to their promise of equal access is, in fact, the theme of this book. In order to deal with it, the author has chosen an original approach, by considering health care in the context of the recent developments in the international political economy. Since 1975, that context has been characterized by governments of the developed world withdrawing from the economic process and leaving the production and consumption of goods and services increasingly to the market. As a consequence, inequalities in health care—as in society as a whole—are increasing. The author concludes that, despite the application of exemption regulations, increasing inequalities put the solidarity principle, a mainstay of most EU health care systems, at risk.

The arguments for governments to withdraw from the economic process are twofold. Firstly, it is argued that the phenomenon of globalization forces governments of the developed world to reduce the costs of labor in order for businesses to stay competitive. Secondly, it is argued that a free market economy with the price mechanism as the instrument for coordination, instead of a government interfering in the economic process, better serves to satisfy the needs of individual consumers. As a member of the Dutch Social Economic Council in the 1990s, I was aware that these arguments were applied to many spheres of economic activity. I concluded that these two arguments are far less suitable for application to health care if the principle of equal access is to be realized. Furthermore, according to the author of this book, both arguments are controversial. Societies appear to have more freedom to choose their social arrangements than the international political economy wants us to believe.

After having read the manuscript, I unreservedly recommend the book to politicians, health care policy-makers, insurers, managers, and all those who take equity in health care to heart.

Ton Krol
Former President of the International Hospital Federation

Acknowledgments

I have worked at the CEO management level in health care in the Netherlands for more than 25 years. During those years, I experienced times of plenty, when the sky was the limit, as well as times of want, when I had to think of measures to increase the efficiency and effectiveness of daily operations. Working in health care was an enriching challenge for me, the more so since I also had the honor to serve on several national governing boards. That taught me how closely health care policy is connected to the economy and to politics.

Furthermore, I had the privilege of representing the Federation of Dutch Health Care Organizations in the European Hospital and Health Care Federation (HOPE) for more than 20 years. Because this federation appointed me to the office of President of its Subcommittee on Economics and Planning, I had the opportunity to learn about health care developments in the other countries of the European Union.

During the years when I worked in and for health care, I had the pleasure to meet with experts from the Netherlands and abroad. Many of them have become friends. Knowing that I was working on this book, they not only brought me important information, but they were also prepared to discuss my ideas and to comment on draft versions of the book. Now that the book is finished, it's time to express my gratitude for their kindness.

First of all I want to thank several members of the European Hospital and Health Care Federation to whom I am particularly grateful. They are Kris Schutyser (Belgium), former Secretary-General of HOPE; Brian Edwards (United Kingdom), the president of HOPE, who regularly informed me about publications that could be useful for the manuscript, as did his predecessors Gérard Vincent (France) and Denis Doherty (Ireland). The latter also commented on earlier draft versions of the manuscript. As for other (observer) members of HOPE, it is with pleasure that I thank the Secretary-General, Pascal Garel (France); my successor as President of the Subcommittee on Economics and Planning, Carine Boonen (Belgium); as well as Ursula Fronaschütz (Austria), Anetta Dokova (Bulgaria), György Harmat (Hungary), Willy Heuschen (Belgium), Lars Johansson

(Sweden), Eero Linnako (Finland), Douglas McKenzie (United Kingdom), Isabel Pinto Monteiro (Portugal), Diana Puntule (Latvia), Jeff Schmit (Luxembourg), Martin Staniforth (United Kingdom), and Martin Walger (Germany). They all provided useful information and/or commented on ideas during our meetings. A stimulating commentator, though not a member of HOPE, has been Viljo Rissanen (Finland). Finally, Frank Castles from the University of Edinburgh kindly commented on what I have written about his research in chapter 11.

In addition to these people from other EU countries, I want to thank a number of my fellow Dutch citizens for their comments on the manuscript. They are all involved in health care, either as CEOs of hospitals, or as scientists, governors, or health policy experts. They are Wim Bonhof, Joep Heesters, Bert Hermans, Marieke Koken, Rob Koning, Erik Können, Ton Krol, Ruud Lapré, Wim Meijer, René Peters, and Gery van Veldhoven.

Since the book is rather critical of medical professionalism, I thought it appropriate to ask a number of medical specialists for their comments. In this regard, I am grateful to Jan Beks, Ton van Dam, Hans Huysmans, Chris Plasmans, Piet van Velthoven, and Jelle Vleer for their positive feedback in response to my request.

Moreover, because of my hope that this book will also be read by people who are not involved day to day in the world of health care, I asked some people I respect for their intelligent insights to comment on the manuscript. I am grateful to Heino van Essen, Arie Garstman, Cees de Gooijer, Thijs de Haas, Henk van Zuthem, and Jan Zwemmer for their willingness to do so. The same applies for Gerrit Dijkstra, David Lowery, and Frits van der Meer, colleagues of mine at Leiden University.

Finally, it is with pleasure that I thank Alfred Moest from the library of Statisics Netherlands for delivering important statistical information, Lodewijk Klootwijk for his indispensable support in making my personal computer do what I wanted it to do, and Anne Messer (Australia) for checking my English.

Although all these people deserve my gratitude and respect, it should be clear that the content of the book is my sole responsibility.

Win de Gooijer

Preface

Once, in 2004, I had to collect some medicine. When I entered the local pharmacy, there was an elderly lady standing at the counter, also collecting her medicines. While handing over the parcel, the dispenser's assistant said to her, "That makes €11.30." The elderly lady answered, "But this is included in my health insurance. I didn't pay for it last time!" To which the assistant replied, "Yes, that's true, but since the first of January, it is no longer included." The elderly lady replied, "But I don't have the money to pay for it myself!" And then she left, without the medicines she needed.

On 18 June 2005, the British newspaper *The Times* informed its readers of a 32-year-old female victim of a road accident, who, after having been referred by her general practitioner, was told she would have to wait 80 weeks for a brain scan in a London hospital. However, the hospital's letter containing this message also offered a solution. A handwritten note on the letter said, "If you want to go privately, call 0845 60 80 991 for prices." This telephone number referred to the hospital's "self-pay" private clinic, where the procedure could been done in two weeks for £983.[1]

Now, if you live in one of the countries of the European Union,[2] think back 25 years and ask yourself if it would have been possible to hear or read messages like these in your country in those days. I would guess that your answer would be negative, because it was characteristic of health care systems in many EU countries in those days to provide equal access for all citizens, according to need. Ability to pay was not an issue. Those systems were based on notions about solidarity with the vulnerable citizens in society. They were the foundation for the establishment of EU welfare states in a time when we thought that society was manageable, and that governments were able to look after their citizens from the cradle to the grave.

As for health care, these notions were believed to be so important that all countries of the European Union included provisions about their governments' responsibility for their citizens' health in their constitutional laws. Moreover, because they intended to take solidarity in health care matters seriously, the countries of the EU took legal measures to this end during the 1960s and 1970s.

At present, however, there is reason to worry about whether the countries of the European Union still sufficiently live up to their notions of solidarity in health care. The examples given above illustrate that ability to pay *is* an issue these days, that the principle of equal access *is* losing meaning, and that a market for health care *is* emerging. This is becoming increasingly clear from the growing number of uninsured people, the limitations on collectively financed coverage packages, rising personal contributions, an ever-more-favorable environment for preferential treatment, and the shifting of responsibilities from governments to other social actors through privatization and deregulation.

These health care developments are part of a broader change in the policies of the international political economy. This change started in about 1975. Central to it are two arguments—one economic and one ideological. First of all, the economic argument assumes that the phenomenon of globalization will lead to a worldwide interconnectedness, which, in turn, will make it increasingly difficult for governments to control developments at the national level. Globalization will rule the world and will force employers in the global economy to reduce the costs of labor as much as possible in order to stay competitive. "There's no alternative," in Thatcher's words. Secondly, the ideological argument, captured by the term *neo-liberalism*, argues that the ultimate objective of any economic order should be to satisfy the needs of individual consumers through an optimal market economy, with the price mechanism as the instrument for coordination, instead of having the government as the central planning institution. Neo-liberals want to limit the role of governments, because governments are believed to impede the pursuit of personal objectives. Thus Reagan said, "get government of our backs," so that personal initiative could get a chance. In combination, these arguments are the leading principles in the present-day international political economy. As a consequence, governments from all over the developed world, including those of the European Union, are withdrawing from the economic process, leaving things increasingly to the market. In this (re)turning to the market, the idea of the welfare state is being reconsidered, resulting in stricter eligibility criteria for social security, decreasing levels of welfare benefits, and people being increasingly left to their own devices. In short, since 1975, the social context of the developed world has been changing. The effect is an increasing number of victims, people who have lost in the market game or who did not even get the chance to play that game.

Health care is no exception to this changing social context, particularly when we consider acute care. However, the problem is that, due to their constitutional obligations, governments cannot simply decide to leave health care to the market. Moreover, they know very well that good-quality health care is very important to their citizens. They also know that citizens who can afford to do so are prepared to pay for it. Finally, they know that solidarity in access to health care is a broadly supported principle in the countries of the developed world. These facts ensure that the introduction of a market for health care is almost by definition a delicate matter, since policies in this respect may easily be at odds with the solidarity principle. As a consequence, reform policies regarding health care in EU countries are not characterized by "grand designs," but by taking small steps of incremental change, by trial and error, and sometimes even by a "ready–fire–aim" approach, trying out some reform idea and seeing what happens.

Meanwhile, these policies increasingly demonstrate that governments are frenetically trying to hold on to their promises of equal access. Moreover, these promises are translated into huge bureaucracies with manifold regulations, including patchworks to exclude the vulnerable members of society from cost-containment measures. As a consequence, health care in several EU countries seems to have become a matter of bookkeeping. This would not be a problem if solidarity were maintained. But it is not. The examples given above illustrate that, despite the frenetic attempts by governments to uphold the foundations of their health care systems, there is something going fundamentally wrong with solidarity in health care. And there is more. The huge bureaucracies that have been set up and the many regulations that have flooded the world of health care to enable governments to control these developments have also limited the managerial scope of health care managers. Although these managers are expected to perform as entrepreneurs, the primacy of politics in health care increasingly turns them into figureheads.

The ultimate consequence of the reform measures in health care may be that it will no longer be justifiable to describe health care systems in EU countries as an expression of solidarity between citizens. I will argue in this book that EU countries are on their way to that situation. Reviewing the aggregate of reform measures in health care over recent decades presents a disturbing picture of decreasing equal access; of underconsumption for financial reasons by vulnerable groups in society; and, in general, of emerging "two-class" health care systems. On the one hand, we see a growing for-profit market in health care. On the other hand, coverage packages are being reduced to safety nets. In short, EU health care systems are no exception to the general trend of increasing inequalities in society. In reaction to this development, one can take two positions. One can either accept the present trend of decreasing solidarity in health care as an inevitable effect of the arguments that rule the international political economy, or one can attempt to verify the veracity of these arguments. I have chosen to do the latter.

By doing so, I deal with the developments in health care systems in EU countries in the context of the international political economy. I take this approach because discussing developments in health care systems is rather meaningless if the political context is excluded. That political context itself is also changing, in the sense that developments in health care systems are no longer exclusively determined by politics at the national level. Increasingly, politics at the international or global level have implications for national health care systems. To my knowledge, such an approach to the developments in health care systems is new. Although there is plentiful information available on health care reforms in EU countries, the descriptions are mostly limited to detailed and dated information over a certain period of time, about a given number of countries. In those cases, an introductory or summary chapter serves to connect the information presented. I have adopted an EU-wide integrated approach that focuses on the *trends* in health care systems, based on a cross-section of health care reforms in EU countries since the 1980s. After all, in health care trends live longer than facts.

This approach has consequences for the structure of the book. First of all, the present-day international political economy has to be described. That is what the first part of the book is about. The first chapter starts with a description of the analytical context. Central to this context is the most important question that any economic order (or country) has to deal with, namely: "Who decides on the production and consumption of goods and services?" To answer this question, the German economist Walter Eucken distinguished between two theoretical extremes.[3] According to him, these decisions can in theory be left either completely to the market, or completely to the government. The reality of economic orders, however, is always a mixture of these two extremes; i.e., there is always more or less government involvement in the economic process. Between the two extremes one can think of a straight line, which I call a continuum, and one can situate any actual national economic order somewhere on that line at a given moment in time. But a few things should be kept in mind. First of all, economic orders in Eucken's days were mainly national in scope. At present, however, decision-making regarding the production and consumption of goods and services is increasingly influenced by circumstances and agreements beyond the national level. Secondly, one has to realise that the economic order is a dynamic phenomenon. Countries may move along the continuum from left to right or vice versa, i.e., they may choose, through democratic means, for more or less government involvement in the economic process. Regarding this, it is tempting to compare the history of the international political economy since the beginning of the twentieth century with a swinging pendulum, with economic orders moving along the continuum from left to right and vice versa. Since 1975, the countries of the Western world, including EU countries, have clearly been moving in a direction where the market is the (more) determining factor for the economic process. And, of course, such a movement has its supporters and opponents. In democracies, both try to influence decision-making regarding movements along the continuum. That is the topic of the second chapter. Promoters, particularly corporate business, want the market economy to be increasingly liberalized, which would facilitate their competition in a global economy. In contrast, opponents, comprising a variety of (non-) institutional organizations and movements, want to maintain or increase government control of the economic process. On balance, it seems as if promoters of the market economy determine the course of things in the present-day international political economy. In general, EU governments follow their previously mentioned arguments. These arguments are dealt with in the third chapter. Here, it is important to mention that these arguments receive impetus from a new morality that has as its point of departure the view that rational individuals, out of self-interest, only pursue the maximization of their personal utility. Since 1975, the neo-liberal view, combined with this new morality, provides the *leitmotif* for policies of various political leaders in the Western world. In particular, Reagan and Thatcher acquired a certain reputation in this regard. As a consequence, Keynesian economics, which had dominated politics in the developed world for decades, appeared to be losing its relevance in the course of the 1970s. The idea that the shortcomings of the market system should be corrected through selective government interventions and that the state has an interest in effective social welfare was replaced by a new course, which was meant to restore the stimuli for an entrepreneurial spirit. The effects of this new approach on the arrangements of society are brought together in the fourth chapter. It shows a new trend in the development of economic orders of the Western world. To this new trend belong increasing inequalities, worsening labor terms and conditions, insecurity (in particular for low-skilled workers), down-sizing, et cetera. All EU countries are following this trend.

The second part of the book deals with the implications of the changing social context for health care systems in EU countries. Here, the focal question of the book could be re-specified by focusing on health care goods and services. However, conceptual and practical dilemmas make an answer to the question, "Who are the ones to decide on the production and consumption of health care goods and services?" a complicated matter. This is the topic of the fifth chapter. As for the conceptual dilemmas, the idea that health care in EU countries is "a symbol of democratic rights and citizenship"[4] refers to ideological preferences that economic orders have to take into account. These preferences make the introduction of market principles in health care controversial. Moreover, there are several practical dilemmas that influence decision-making. The many interested parties in health care, for example, make it very difficult for governments in democracies to carry through fundamental changes, particularly when these changes have to do with restrictions. Furthermore, the aging of the population adds extra problems for governments that want to introduce market-style mechanisms in health care. Finally, developments in health care may involve ethical problems, not only regarding moral judgements, but also in relation to the solidarity principle.

The developments in health care are to a considerable extent determined by the immanent dynamics of the health care process. These dynamics make health care a very difficult matter to control in any democratic economic order. To explain these dynamics, I define health care as a complex and dynamic process of continuous innovation, i.e., of constantly changing new combinations of science, technology, organization, politics, economics, and (medical) culture. An analysis of the six elements of this definition, which is the topic of the sixth chapter, leads to the conclusion that governments in democracies have only limited power to control developments in health care. In fact, the only effective instrument they have is finance.

According to the Maastricht Treaty of 1992, health care in EU countries is subject to the subsidiarity principle, which means that each member state is free to choose its own organizational and financial arrangements. In chapter seven, however, I argue that as a consequence of an ongoing economic integration at the EU level, the subsidiarity principle with regard to health care is slowly being eroded. Although policy lines from Brussels, political considerations, and rulings of the European Court of Justice will not result in a universal EU health care system, I argue that there will be a certain convergence regarding the financial and quality aspects of health care. It is not unlikely that European Commission will take the lead in this respect.

Chapters eight and nine deal with movements along the continuum regarding health care. Although a considerable number of innovations in health care date back to the Second World War or immediately thereafter, the quantitative analysis in these chapters is divided into two periods since 1960, because there is hardly any useful aggregated quantitative or qualitative information available from dates prior to that year. The first period is 1960–1980, which I have labeled as the time of "investing in health care." This was the time when health care organizations changed from closed systems into open ones. But it was also the time when the combined influence of technological, scientific, organizational, political, and economic change led to the creation of the "health industry." Finally, it was the time when it was thought that a good health care system, equally accessible to all citizens, would contribute to making the world a better place. In regard to this last point, the experiences of the Second World War particularly inspired the American government to create a favorable environment for (further) developments in health care. As a result, the funding of scientific medical research soared, the number of doctors increased tremendously, medical specialization took off, and accessibility to all was embedded in legal arrangements. In short, those were "the glory days of [American] medicine,"[5] during which money was no problem and the medical establishment, much admired by the public at large, determined the course of events. Consequently, expenditure increased substantially, often in double digits on an annual basis. Taking advantage of a period of strong economic growth, many EU countries followed the Americans from around the beginning of the 1960s. What is most characteristic of this period is that developments in health care were unrestrained. Critical questions were seldom asked, and planning was hardly an issue. In general, during this period governments approved the developments from the sidelines, letting things go instead of controlling.

Around the beginning of the 1980s, governments started to realize that things had to be turned around. As a consequence, from this period onward, EU health care systems were subjected to reforms. These reforms were many. They are brought together in the ninth chapter in a cross-sectional matrix around four themes, which have been worked out with some examples. The first theme is accountability, referring to the fact that health care professionals, health care institutions, and health care insurers have had to accept that the external environment has started to interfere in their business. Legal regulations regarding the quality of care and (legal) measures directed at empowering patients are examples. Organizational reforms, the second theme, may have followed from deliberate changes in (political) views on how health care policy and health care delivery should be designed. Reforms like these may be initiated by health care professionals or institutions, or they may be enforced by insurers or patients. They may be motivated by arguments like cost containment, effectiveness, efficiency, quality improvement, workload, or task performance. Policies of decentralization and deregulation, as well as the creation of internal markets for health care and private initiatives, are examples. The third theme is rationing and priority-setting. One of the objectives was for the public at large to start to realize that the production and consumption of health care goods and services is not as self-evident as people have come to believe. In several EU countries, public campaigns were established in order to convey the message that health care goods and services are also subject to scarcity. Further examples of rationing and priority-setting include testing new medical opportunities through technology assessment, providing health care along the lines of protocols, as well as (deliberately creating) waiting lists. The fourth theme is cost-containment, elaborated with policy examples regarding pharmaceuticals, cost-sharing, and the financing of hospitals. As during the period of investing in health care, so also reform measures in health care were to a considerable extent American-led. Because of this, chapters eight and nine also provide American examples.

As previously discussed, the ninth chapter provides a cross-sectional outline of health care reforms in EU countries. It shows that, in health care, EU countries are also moving to the right side of the continuum, thus choosing for the market. An important question following from this policy is whether governments, while moving to the right side of the continuum, have succeeded in achieving the threefold objectives of their reform measures, i.e., improving quality, containing costs, and maintaining equal access. The tenth chapter has been written to address this question. As for quality, it has to be observed that, despite all the time and money that have been spent on the different aspects of health care, we simply do not know if this has contributed to higher-quality outcomes. Regarding cost containment, the period from 1980 to 2000 can be labeled as the time of "cleaning up the mess." After all, it is not too difficult for governments to do something about cost control after years of neglect. The result is that the "organizational slack"[6] of the world of health care has been skimmed off. What also has been achieved is that health care providers have started to think about the efficiency and effectiveness of their actions. But whether governments are really capable of controlling health care costs, while maintaining equal access, still has to be proven. After all, controlling presupposes the ability to steer and to direct future developments. With an innovative sector like health care, governments have only limited powers to do so. There are already disturbing examples to illustrate that, due to the reform measures, the idea of equal access according to need has been damaged, and that ability to pay has become an issue. In this respect, the present climate of the international political economy, with its dogmatic focus on the market as the only alternative, will make things even worse. This raises the question whether EU countries can still rightfully maintain that their health care systems are based on the principle of solidarity between their citizens. Admittedly, the idea of solidarity cannot be caught in mathematical equations. Nevertheless, the least one can say is that the trend of the developments is negative, which puts the foundations of EU health care systems at risk.

Therefore, the final part of the book is a reflection on its first part. This reflection starts in chapter eleven with a reconsideration of the changing social context. In this regard, the reader is reminded that there is no right or wrong answer to the question of which side of the continuum is preferable. Choosing a position on that continuum is a matter of normative economics. Such a choice implies taking a personal position regarding the desirable arrangements in society. In this regard, I believe that the countries of the developed world, as they are moving toward the market, have reached a position where social cohesion is dangerously threatened. Admittedly, this is a rather pessimistic perspective. But it is a perspective that follows from the assumptions that underlie the present-day international political economy. Critically reviewing these assumptions may thus result in a change of mind. Consequently, in the eleventh chapter, I will examine the strength of the arguments addressed in the third chapter. In this respect, chapter 11 shows, first of all, that people are not so focused on individually maximizing their utility as public choice theory wants us to believe. It also shows that present-day neo-liberalism neglects what Adam Smith in his days intended "liberalism" to mean, and that despite all the talk about globalization, trade appears to be very much concentrated in trading blocs with geographically contiguous countries. The challenges facing the developed world, therefore, do not result from a globalising economy, but from domestic developments like rising inequalities, the need for flexibility, and the demand for essential public services. To put it differently, it is not the economy that rules, but the ideology. To deal with these issues is more difficult than dealing with the global economy. Globalization offers no motive to reduce the costs of labor because there is no convincing correlation, so far, between economic growth and spending on social security. The EU countries appear to have more freedom to choose their social arrangements than ideas on globalization suggest. Here, an enlarged EU offers opportunities in the longer term. If the "old" countries of the EU are willing to invest sufficiently in the new member states, particularly the former transition countries, the EU could become a very strong economy, which does not have to go along with American views on the world, and which can uphold its historical sense of taking care of the needy in society, including the basis of solidarity of its health care systems. However, turning away from the present course of the international political economy is conditional in this respect. The all-time low interest of EU citizens in politics and the functioning of democracy is an important obstacle to change. People feel misled, cheated, unimportant to the ruling elite, et cetera.[7] It will take convincing and reliable political leadership to restore an interest in democratic procedures, as well as confidence in the rulers. Convincing and reliable political leadership may also contribute to restoring a climate of trust among the stakeholders in health care. In this respect, the final chapter presents some ideas on health care management from the perspectives of governments, medical specialists, and top managers in hospitals. At first glance, the reader may find this chapter to be a stranger amidst the other chapters. However, my personal experience as a manager of health care organizations for many years was an important motivation to write it. I experienced the "good times" and the "bad times," and although I enjoyed working in health care till the age of retirement, by that date I had become convinced that management in health care had come to mean trying to shape your entrepreneurial ideas in an over-bureaucratized environment characterized by mistrust and a hardening of viewpoints. Changing that situation, and giving room for entrepreneurship, will certainly have a positive influence on the image of health care as a professional field. It will also stimulate efficiency and effectiveness and, through that, contribute to upholding the solidarity principle that EU countries claim is the mainstay of their health care systems. Therefore, it is legitimate to pay (relatively limited) attention to some managerial aspects regarding health care.

In the end, however, the meaning of the concept of solidarity is determined by what kind of society we want. To complete the book, a brief epilogue will address this question.

About the Author

Win de Gooijer is Professor in the Department of Public Policy at Leiden University, Netherlands, where he teaches a course on Health Care Systems in an International Perspective. He has also created and organized a professional management course for health care administrators and insurers from the former communist countries, which joined the European Union in 2004. De Gooijer holds degrees in teaching, economics and law from the Free University of Amsterdam, and he received his Ph.D. in 1976 from the Technical University of Enschede, the Netherlands. He has spent over 25 years in the health care industry, as general manager of a psychiatric hospital and later, as CEO of a foundation for care of the elderly. During his career in health care he served on several governing and advisory boards in the Netherlands and the European Union.

For twenty years he represented the Federation of Dutch Health Care Organizations in the European Hospital and Health Care Federation (HOPE), spending many years as the President of its Subcommittee on Economics and Planning. He has published many articles in national and international health care journals, and presented papers on health care during congresses all over the world.

1
Moving Along a Continuum

Writing about the future of health care systems, or about their past, is rather meaningless if the social context is left out.[1] That social context, i.e., the complexity of cultural, economic, and political aspects which, in combination, condition the practical operation of health care systems, is constantly subject to change. Consequently, health care systems are also constantly subject to change.

Changes in the cultural patterns of a country may influence the way health care delivery is organized; worsening or improving economic conditions of a country may affect its health care system's organizational slack, and changes in a country's political constellation may alter a government's interference with its health care system.

To study each and every single change in health care systems, however, is also rather meaningless, particularly in the context of the European Union. Comparing health care systems this way would yield a number of facts, but this information would be outdated as soon as it was collected. Nevertheless, observing successive single changes in health care systems over a longer period of time may well reveal certain trends in their development. These trends are worth studying.

There have been times that health care systems as we know them now did not exist. The Middle Ages was such a time. In the specific social context of those days, looking after those who needed care was mainly the business of religious congregations. As far as "governments," i.e., those in power, were concerned, they were not only motivated by reasons of compassion, but also by self-interest. After all, cholera did not choose between rich and poor, nobility and peasants.[2]

Health care systems as such—that is, specially designed infrastructures that deal with health care—date back to the beginning of the eighteenth century. From then on, these systems gradually became an essential element of government interference with the arrangements of society.

At present, governments everywhere are involved in health care systems, albeit in different ways and to differing degrees.

Also at present, the social context of health care systems is changing. This started around the beginning of the 1980s. Since then, the sequence of changes in health care systems has resulted in a new trend which, contrary to the prior two decades, is characterized by withdrawing governments who leave the health care process increasingly to the market.

Regardless of whether one approves of this trend, it is reconditioning the practical operation of health care systems. That reconditioning may have unintended consequences regarding the basic values of solidarity and equity on which the health care systems in the countries of the European Union were founded.

In order to understand and to explain the present developments in health care systems, we need to analyze their social context. That is what this first chapter of the book is about. Furthermore, if one does not appreciate these present developments, an analysis of the current social context may be of help in considering alternative approaches.

Those readers who are daily involved in health care may believe such an analysis to be unnecessary. They may be inclined, therefore, to skip this first chapter. They should realize, however, that health care, economics, and politics are very much intertwined in society. The reasoning in this respect is very simple. If there is no money, there is nothing one can do. And if there is no political will, promoters of a sound health care system will expend their energy to no avail. The United States, for example, spends roughly 13.6% of its GDP on health care. Nevertheless, 44 million Americans have no health insurance coverage at all.[3] This suggests that the United States lacks the political will necessary to make health care accessible to all American citizens. In contrast, the countries of the European Union[4] spend considerably less on health care, but have nevertheless far fewer citizens going around uninsured. Here, obviously, there is the political will to make health care accessible for all. In both situations the social context is decisive. Therefore, it cannot be ignored.

Central to the following analysis of the present social context of health care systems is the concept of the economic order, i.e., the organizational structure of national economies, or alternately countries or societies. I will argue that policy decision-making in national economies is increasingly influenced by circumstances, events, ideologies, and institutions beyond the level of national economic orders. I will outline these influences and examine their effects on society. All in all, the first chapter presents a schematic outlook on the current international political economy, which in my view will have consequences for the future of European health care systems. Therefore, this chapter is an overture to this expected future.

For the sake of those readers who are daily involved in health care but not familiar with political economy, I have tried to present the following analysis in a not too extensive but readable way. In order to avoid an ill-founded argument, however, the analysis refers to an extensive literature list, for those who are interested, at the end of the book.

1.1 The Dynamics of the Economic Order

The objective of this section is to establish a framework for the rest of the book. It deals with decision-making on the macro-level of democratic economic orders, in particular the balance between, on the one hand, private initiatives pursued by individuals, private organizations, and interest groups, and, on the other hand, government interference in the economic process. It is also addresses the development of economic orders and asks whether this may have consequences for the future.

1.1.1 The Analytical Context

Because of the fact that any economy's production capacity is limited by technical knowledge and by the availability of (natural) resources, every society has to make choices regarding the production and consumption of goods and services. The twentieth century produced some great economists who, in one way or another, dealt with this problem of decision-making, notably John Maynard Keynes, Paul Samuelson, Friedrich Von Hayek, and Walter Eucken. Although their terminologies and points of departure differed, these economists were all interested in the way a society decides on the *what*, the *how*, and the *for whom* of the production and consumption of goods and services. And although they put their reflections on paper more than half a century ago, "these three fundamental questions of economic organization [. . .] are as crucial today as they were at the dawn of human civilization."[5] In fact, they are questions for all times.[6]

The *what* refers to, for instance, the choice between consumer goods and investment goods; the *how* can, for example, relate to generating electricity from coal or from wind mills; and the *for whom* includes distribution matters, such as income and accessibility in health care. The reality of economic orders shows that the process of decision-making in respect of the *what*, the *how*, and the *for whom* always involves government interference in the economic process. And since this involvement may vary within and between societies, the number of economic orders is, in fact, unlimited.

It is to Eucken's credit to have brought some structure to the complexity of economic orders by distinguishing between two opposite basic types, or analytical constructions (*Grundformen*). He has distinguished between, on the one hand, an economic order where every aspect of decision-making regarding the *what*, the *how*, and the *for whom* of the production and consumption of goods and services is left completely to a central government (*Zentralgeleitete Wirtschaft*).[7] That central government is the only planning institution. It designs the plans, it commands their execution, and it inspects the results. This economic order is ruled by command and control, in which individual freedom is limited and bureaucracy is inevitable.

Eucken's second basic type, on the other hand, is an economic order in which decision-making regarding the *what*, the *how*, and the *for whom* is left completely to the market (*Verkehrswirtschaft*). Here, every member of society makes his or her own plans and bears personal responsibility for their execution and adjustment. Coordination of all the individual plans comes about through the use of the price mechanism,[8] instead of an established bureaucracy. It is assumed that individual freedom will be optimized through voluntary exchange.[9]

Eucken's basic types (*Idealtypen*) are a formalization of reality. If this were not the case, an economic order in which every aspect of decision-making regarding the production and consumption of goods and services was left to the market would result in a society where the idea of the "survival of the fittest" would be the leading principle. On the other hand, an economic order where these aspects were left completely to a central government would result in a society of slaves, with that government in the position of "the fittest to survive."

The reality of economic orders, however, is always a mix of decision-making through the market and through a (central) government. Consequently, one can think of an imaginary line connecting the two extremes. I call this line a continuum, i.e., a line between the two extremes, and argue that any actual economic order can be situated somewhere along this continuum. In the extreme situation of an economic order where the answers to questions about the *what*, the *how*, and the *for whom* result merely from private initiative and responsibility, with the price mechanism as the coordinating instrument, we have a complete market economy. In the other extreme situation, we have a complete command economy where answering these same questions is solely a matter of government initiative and responsibility.[10] These two extremes can be illustrated by drawing a simple line, with private initiative symbolized by a capital P at the right end, and a commanding government symbolized by a capital G at the left end.

G ———————————— **P**

As discussed, any economic order, society, or country can be situated somewhere along this continuum. Those positioned on the left side experience relatively more government interference in the economic process than those on the right side, where market operation is more decisive. To be concrete: it would be reasonable to situate the United States more to the right side of the continuum, whereas China's position would be more to the left side.

A country's position on the continuum is not permanent, however. On the contrary, countries are constantly on the move from left to right along the continuum, and vice versa, for the simple reason that people are constantly on the move. Consequently, the economic order is a dynamic phenomenon.

This chapter of the book is about moving along the continuum, from left to right, and vice versa, i.e., decreasing or increasing government interference in the economic process. In doing so, my particular focus is on the consequences of a government's withdrawing from the economic process with regard to a particular aspect of the political culture of the countries of the European Union. For these countries, this culture is "deeply imbued with a sense of general duty to aid the needy."[11] More specifically, the subject matter of the book is whether leaving the answers on the *what*, the *how*, and the *for whom* increasingly to the market will negatively influence this sense of general duty to aid the needy.

This general sense of duty refers to "a [somehow] very European principle"[12] which is captured by the term *solidarity*. This refers to solidarity between the rich and the poor, the sick and the healthy, the young and the old. Solidarity is a generic term, however.[13] There is no "one size fits all." Its content differs from country to country and is determined by economic conditions, by cultural and moral values,[14] and by political constellations.[15] In short, solidarity is determined by aspects which, separately and in combination, are subject to change.[16]

Solidarity is organized in systems of social security. Why? Because in the countries of the European Union, systems of social security are believed to be the cement that holds society together.[17] In other words, systems of social security are instrumental for maintaining social cohesion in society. Thus, a logical question is, How much cement does a society need to prevent it from falling apart? Or, how far one can reform systems of social security without endangering social cohesion? One can argue about this, which explains why the interpretation of the solidarity principle has been the subject of ongoing dispute throughout the history of European civilization. In the course of that history, "the struggle between individuating and integrating forces has been the core battleground of politics."[18] This history, furthermore, is characterized by continuously changing combinations of self-interest and solidarity. Moving along the continuum in the direction of P may alter this combination to the detriment of solidarity.[19]

As discussed, the economic order is a dynamic phenomenon. One of the relevant dynamics, in this regard, is the development of economic orders. In this respect, it is common to distinguish between the successive stages of development from a natural economy, via a monetary economy, to a credit economy. Or, alternately, from a household economy that is succeeded by, respectively, a city economy, a regional economy, and a national economy. The underlying assumption of such an approach is that a higher form of economic order results from a gradual transition from a lower one.[20]

Since Eucken first published his ideas, the world has changed fundamentally, with science and technology being the most important boosters. Kahn and Wiener's 1967 list of 100 predicted technical innovations, which they expected to be realized in the course of the 20th century, has been achieved to about 95%.[21] The developed world has become ever richer, and its citizens substantially older. Human endeavor in one part of the globe may now have consequences for people living in far away places. All corners of the world have become interrelated. Today, "each nation is like a big corporation, competing in the global market place," thus former United States President Clinton.[22] Competition between countries and continents, therefore, would be similar to that of corporations.

Thus it seems that we have reached a new stage in the development of the economic order. The sequence could now be described as natural economy—city economy—national economy—European economy—global economy.[23] And, of course, this development has consequences for decision-making processes at the national level regarding the answers to the questions on the *what*, the *how*, and the *for whom* of the production and consumption of goods and services. In many cases, these answers are no longer a country's own business, because they may have consequences for other countries. In such cases, decision-making must rise from the level of the nation state to a higher level. Consequently, the members of the European Union must satisfy the directives from Brussels, which, in turn, may impose adjustments on their domestic institutional structures,[24] if rulings of the European Court of Justice force them to do so.[25] Furthermore, through the United Nations and its institutions, like the Security Council, the World Bank, the International Monetary Fund, the World Trade Organization, and the World Health Organization, we now have established global platforms for regulating peace and trade, for stabilizing global finance, supporting developing countries, tackling health disasters and protecting the environment.[26] As a consequence, decision-making within national economic orders has to take the outside world into account, more than ever. In other words, we have, at least partly, to adjust decision-making on the *what*, the *how*, and the *for whom* at the national level to a growing global economic order. This has various consequences.

First of all, there is the question of complexity, which is naturally followed by the problem of manageability. Are we capable of dealing with problems resulting from a global economic order? Is it possible to substantiate the modern concept of global governance? Secondly, there is the question of identity. Do we want to stay our own boss, or are we willing to transfer powers of decision-making to the detriment of the nation state? And, related to this, how do we cope with the little smouldering fires of separatism that already exist?

Finally, we have to ask ourselves whether it is possible to run an economic order beyond the level of the national economy in a democratic way.

1.1.2 A Swinging Pendulum

There is no right or wrong answer to the question of which side of the continuum is preferable. Indeed, history has produced two great philosophers, Marx and Smith, who take opposing views in this regard.[27] The choice between left and right is a matter of normative economics, because it involves ethical and value judgements. What do we want different levels of welfare to be? Should we tighten the criteria for eligibility to welfare benefits? Should health care be equally accessible to all citizens, or do we accept preferential treatment? To what level do we believe that inequalities in income can be justified? Should education beyond a certain level be free of charge for each citizen? These are all examples of questions that cannot be answered on the basis of an economic analysis. They require political debate.[28] Decisions reached via political debate reflect a more general feeling of what society should look like.

Since the times of Marx and Smith, the relationship between market forces and government responsibility has been a regular topic of discussion. Beginning in the 1930s, during the Great Depression when disappointment with market processes was widespread, scholars started to think about how governments could supplant the price system and yet allocate goods and services without losing the efficiency of the market. Both issues were pertinent, because the preceding economic freedom and limited government involvement had left "the evils that remained [. . .] all the more prominent and evoked a widespread desire to do something about them."[29] As a result, models of a "planned" economy of "market socialism" and the idea of a "welfare function" in society became prominent (Lange, Bergson, Arrow, Samuelson) and spread throughout Western Europe in the 1950s.[30] This transition to a "planned" economy, however, did not occur overnight, and was itself unplanned. Instead, it was the end result of many ad hoc measures through which governments had already corrected and conditioned market forces. In other words, state intervention preceded state planning.[31]

Around the same time, Keynes' ideas on counter-balancing shortfalls in private investment in the market economy through counter-cyclical governmental policies directed at creating effective demand became accepted by many governments of the Western world, particularly after the Second World War.[32] This led to a long period of Keynesian economics. During this period, government was pointedly present in the economic process, not only by the application of Keynesian economics, but also due to new concerns about the efficiency of the market, such as externalities (pollution) and economies of scale.[33] In addition to this, the provision of public goods (that is, creating the welfare state) became the subject of government regulation. Consequently, this was the time when large bureaucracies were established which were thought to be necessary for the execution of an increasing number of government tasks.[34]

The reversal started around the beginning of the 1970s, when Von Hayek's 1944 message to "The Socialists of All Parties" that government interference with the economic process would result in "A Road to Serfdom" was renewed in 1972. The proposed new economic policy was labeled "neo-liberalism."[35] Neo-liberals favor a laissez-faire economic policy that is embedded in a solid judicial framework. On the one had, such a framework favors the functioning of the price mechanism in a market economy, while on the other hand, it prevents the development of power positions by employers as well as by laborers. Furthermore, neo-liberals pay attention to the relationship between economic and political institutions in society. To them, it is not sufficient for liberal ideas to be enshrined in a society's constitution. The entire system of law must also be in line with these ideas. In contrast to the rigid ideas of the old liberals, neo-liberals consider that a close bond between the state and its system of law must replace the old liberals' repudiation of government interference in the economic process. Government interference should be directed at systematically optimizing the efficiency of a market economy through legal arrangements, with the price mechanism as the instrument for coordination.

A well-known supporter of neo-liberal ideas in the 1970s was Milton Friedman. Friedman launched a fiftieth anniversary edition of Von Hayek's message,[36] and Friedman's book *Free to Choose* was sufficiently convincing that both President Reagan and Prime Minister Thatcher drastically changed political course from the beginning of the 1980s. That course can be summarized in four features: (a) a market economy that is as free as possible, (b) a limited role for the government, (c) privatization and deregulation, and (d) members of society who are individually responsible for the pursuit of their personal objectives.

At present, political leaders of the developed world seem to be in search of a more balanced path, which they call "the third way."[37] This present-day politics has a meaningful advantage when compared to the ideas of the neoliberal scholars. These scholars promoted optimizing the price mechanism, which remained the instrument of coordination in a free market economy. Present-day governments of the developed world, however, aim to maintain social cohesion as an additional objective. The combination of these two objectives makes politics a delicate affair. Delicate, because politics is now directed at determining the minimum role of government in the economic process (or, alternately, establishing the maximum freedom of a market economy) in such a way that social cohesion persists and capitalism remains "inclusive."[38] The rhetoric accompanying these politics is captured by terms like "the stakeholder society," "opportunity," "responsibility," "community," "empowerment," and "people first."

By 1999, center–left governments had been elected in most countries of the European Union. One would therefore expect to have seen some results of this new approach by now. Instead, so far, the "third way" mainly appears to be wishful thinking, since there is barely any meat on the rhetorical bones. According to Galbraith, therefore, the practice of the third way still stands for a capitalist democracy for the fortunate.[39]

It is tempting to look at the movement from the left side to the right side of the continuum, and vice versa, from the perspective of a swinging pendulum.

The first swing, then, would be one from right to left, reminding us of the prosperous times of the "roaring" 1920s, which came to an end with the Great Depression of 1929. This depression was not only caused by speculation on the stock market, but also by the greatly uneven distribution of wealth during the 1920s. Wealth was unbalanced between the rich and the middle class, between industry and agriculture, and between the United States and Europe. This created an unstable economy.[40] However, the policy of the then United States President, Calvin Coolidge, was that government should interfere as little as possible in the economic process, which was completely in line with the rigid form of liberalism of those days.

This attitude began to change in 1933 with Roosevelt's New Deal, which provided for minimum wages and prices and support for the farmers (followed by a second New Deal in 1935–1936). Government interference in the economic process, therefore,[41] increased after the Second World War with the application of Keynesian economics and the establishment of the welfare state.[42]

The swing to the left came to an end in the 1970s, when government came to be seen as an impediment to sound economic development and individual freedom. One government after another shifted to the right side of the continuum, a process which is still ongoing. Neo-liberal politics began to rule government, and there is opposition to Keynesian economics and state socialism. The new political mantras stipulate personal responsibility of citizens, deregulation, and privatization. It is the time of the "Hayekian imperative: the need to trim back overdeveloped welfare states." It is the time of restoring fiscal balance, reducing costs for corporate business, eliminating rigidities in labor markets, and loosening bureaucratic trammels.[43] It is the time of what Stiglitz calls "the roaring nineties" when the "seeds of destruction" were sowed.[44]

Taking the pendulum view and a more-or-less comparable time span, we might have expected to see government back in business again by the end of the current decade. However, with the unexpected fall of communism (the Berlin Wall coming down in 1989), there seems to be no other side of the continuum for the pendulum to swing to. Market socialism, with its all-embracing ideas of planning and the manageability of the economic order, has failed.[45] Great economists from the left side of the continuum like Klein and Samuelson, both winners of the Nobel Prize for economics, have been pushed aside.[46] They have been replaced by, ironically, Nobel Prize–winning economists from the right side of the continuum, like Von Hayek and Friedman, both champions of the free market.

Does the fall of communism mean that we may expect economic orders to stand still on the continuum? Or, in the words of Fukuyama, have we reached the end of history, now that liberal democratic capitalism has been demonstrated to be the only legitimate source of authority in the modern world? This is, indeed, what neo-liberals like to believe. Fukuyama, however, is rather subtle in this respect. He warns that people have the desire to be recognized as equal to others, which is the missing link between a liberal economy and liberal politics. Such recognition is a matter of human dignity.[47] From this perspective, one may consider the unemployment of people who want to work as a failure to recognize their usefulness to society, which harms their dignity, because self-respect is probably the most important primary human good.[48] Citizens' dissatisfaction with neo-liberal democratic capitalism may encourage them to restart history. Actually, Fukuyama sends a serious message here. In fact, he warns us to be very careful about cutting back the welfare state on our way to the right side of the continuum, because this may harm the dignity of people who cannot share the benefits of neo-liberal capitalism.[49] And Fukuyama is certainly not alone in this respect. Scholars like Galbraith, Reich, Albert, Thurow, Peterson, Handy, Dawson, and many others[50] penetratingly warn governments that, apart from moral objections, cutting back the welfare state, which is "one of the greatest achievements of our civilization,"[51] may cause increasing tensions in society. History would be restarted if these tensions reached such a magnitude that they could no longer considered to be a "problem of" but a "contradiction to" the system.[52] Consequently, cutting back the welfare state is a delicate matter. Cutting too much would result in what Galbraith calls an extraordinary, cruel, and dangerous "naked capitalism." To him, therefore, it is wise to make capitalism socially and politically acceptable by correcting it socially.[53] Such a correction would involve ending the present-day's "people-disconnected capitalism," which has been shown to be insensitive to personal and community-based concerns.[54] In this respect, while moving to the right side of the continuum, one has to realise that social security is an important "peace formula" of the welfare state,[55] because "a society of extremes is a breeding ground for forced repression, demagoguery, and tyranny, and quite contrary to the pursuit of welfare."[56] This is exactly what Handy meant when he wrote that "with the unexpected end of the communist dream, capitalism is now its own worst enemy."[57] Therefore, neo-liberal democratic capitalism will have to prove that, while moving to the right side of the continuum, it is able to maintain a fair and just society on the basis of individual freedom. The triumph of capitalism in 1989 has raised the question about "the guts and heart of a liberal society," in Berman's words.[58] If liberal capitalism is not shown to have these qualities, Fukuyama's prediction of "The End of History" may be as premature as was Bell's prediction of "The End of Ideology" in 1959.[59]

In this respect, present-day neo-liberal capitalism might take to heart the lessons that have clearly been understood by the political leaders of the Asian "tigers": South Korea, Taiwan, Thailand, Malaysia, and Singapore. In response to the threat of communism (South Korea from the North, Taiwan from China, Thailand from Vietnam and Cambodia), these leaders, while pursuing economic growth, explicitly aimed to create greater social equality, not by direct income transfers, but by overcoming obstacles to individual's economic achievements. Land reform and land redistribution, universal education, increased employment opportunities, as well as the provision of low-cost housing were among the instruments these political leaders used. They realized that, in accordance with several empirical studies, economic growth tends to be faster in a more equitable environment.[60]

1.1.3 A Framework for Decision-Making

Thus far, we have established two things: First, regarding decision-making on the *what*, the *how*, and the *for whom* of the production and consumption of goods and services, the government plays a more or less important role in the economic order. Second, within any specific economic order, as it moves along the continuum, the role of government may change over the course of time. But we do not know yet how decision-making works. This section will fill this gap.

The argument here is limited to those economic orders which are positioned relatively more to the right of the continuum, i.e., private-enterprise market economies in which every individual (in principle) makes his or her own plans, bearing personal responsibility for their execution or adjustment, and where the price mechanism is the instrument for coordination. These are the economic orders of Western democracies, where, nevertheless, governments have interfered so much in so many domains of economic life that "private enterprise" no longer means "free enterprise."[61] In fact, all private businesses in developed welfare states have been subjected to state control to varying degrees, as Myrdal has established.[62] This particularly occurred during the third quarter of the twentieth century, which, in turn, found expression in ever larger public budgets.[63]

Within this limitation, the focus of this book is mainly on the national economies of the countries of the European Union. In these national economies, government interference mainly occurs indirectly and after the fact, instead of directly and preventively. Consequently, governments' actions in these national economies are limited to conditioning and correcting, while in principle governments are tolerating.[64] Implicitly this means that in Western democracies it is assumed that private enterprise is rooted in some kind of natural sense of responsibility.[65]

Finally, when speaking of democracies, one has to take into account that the countries of the European Union can differ enormously from each other.[66] This book is not a study of democracy, however.[67] Therefore, we can limit ourselves to the fact that, despite the many differences, democracy is the binding principle of the countries of the European Union: i.e., they function in a specific constitutional and procedural framework, which is founded on the democratic ideals of freedom, equality, and sovereignty of the people; and at the same time, this framework permits these ideals to be in open competition with other objectives of society.[68] All countries having such a framework are thus democracies. How they organize the realization of their democratic ideals is of secondary importance.

With this in mind, we can craft a framework for decision-making regarding the *what*, the *how*, and the *for whom* of the production and consumption of goods and services in democracies, keeping in mind that reality may differ in specific circumstances.

As said previously, governments always play a role in the economic process. As for the exertion of government influence in Western democracies regarding decision-making on the *what*, the *how*, and the *for whom* of the production and consumption of goods and services, one can distinguish between different categories of policy instruments.[69]

First of all, governments have global instruments through which they can influence the economic climate in general terms. These instruments may be monetary (discount policy, cash reserve policy), budgetary (fiscal policy, public spending), or they may be functional arrangements (competition policy, wage control).

Secondly, governments have specific instruments, encompassing a large range of government activities which can be classified as (a) policies to stimulate economic growth, like improving the physical infrastructure, subsidizing scientific research and fiscal deductions policies; (b) instruments for specific sectors, like industrial policy directed at the allocation of production factors over different sectors of economic activity (agriculture, transport, the self-employed);[70] (c) legal instruments through which governments can intervene in production processes by orders or prohibitions; and (d) instruments that work through the price mechanism, like levies and subsidies.

Finally, there is a residual group of instruments, like government bonuses on investments, government policies directed at the development of specific regions, or selective investment arrangements.

Government interference in economic life does not happen in a vacuum, since all Western democracies have established a more or less balanced social-economic infrastructure in order to reach agreement on not only what the objectives of their economic order should be, but also on how these objectives should be achieved. Here, the confrontation between interest groups in parliamentary democracies is paramount. In this respect, it is essential that there be formal mechanisms for citizens in democracies, by participating in interest groups and by taking part in elections, to determine both the objectives of the economic order and the organizational structure to achieve them. A complicating factor, however, is social pluralism, which means that new autonomous interest groups are regularly established that have objectives that may conflict with the objectives of other interest groups. For example, the objectives of employers and employees are not always aligned. The same applies to the relation between consumer organizations and producers of consumer goods. Finally, one can think of high-paid workers versus low-paid ones, of corporate business versus small enterprises, et cetera. In short, social-pluralistic democracies encompass so many differing interests that pessimists could easily conclude that society is held in the grasp of conflicts.[71] In social-pluralistic democracies, these differences become manifest in a relatively large number of political parties. They may differ in viewpoints, in objectives, in strategy, or in all three respects.

Interest groups try to find support for their viewpoints with political parties, or they become political parties themselves. Also, interest groups can use instruments to achieve their objectives. For example, businesses use advertising as an instrument, and unions can strike. Apart from this, there is the phenomenon of extra-parliamentary action.

Interest groups also try to influence movement along the continuum. Supporters of an as-free-as-possible market will pursue decreasing government interference in the economic process. Adversaries of a too-free market economy will pursue the opposite. International competition among producers, for example, may induce corporate business to demand a reduction in the costs of labor. Those who want to maintain an existing system of social security, financed to a large degree through corporate taxation, will be opposed to such a reduction. Producers will want as much freedom as possible in the arrangements of their production processes. Opponents, in this respect, demand attention for possible negative externalities, like pollution.

However, social pluralism in open and mature democracies, like the countries of the European Union, leads to a fragmentation of society, which is characterized by the constantly differing demands of interest groups. Because of this, some characterize these democracies as "interest-group-democracies," with all interest groups throwing their demands into the country's garbage can, so to speak, and leaving the government to sort out the mess. In such democracies, it is difficult for governments to direct social developments and to execute policies. Consequently, by definition, governments in mature democracies are rather weak.[72] In the words of Kalma, one ascribes power to governments, which they do not have and which in democratic societies they even cannot have.[73]

Interest groups meet on what is called the institutional level of the economic order. This refers to a complicated and carefully established framework of (representative) contacts between interest groups. On this institutional level, one exchanges views and ideas, one negotiates, one compromises, and one tries to make coalitions, in order to come to a common agreement through which the relations between interest groups can be regulated. Such an infrastructure is a reflection of social-pluralistic democracy.[74]

In this respect, it is common to distinguish between two types of social-economic infrastructures. The first is the so-called Rhine model, which exists in countries like the Netherlands, Scandinavia, Italy, and Germany. In all these countries, labor unions and management share power, while governments provide welfare through a safety net of pensions, education, and health benefits.[75] The Rhine model is a consensual form of "non-majoritarian" negotiated democracy.

The other social-economic infrastructure is a confrontational "winner-takes-all" style of "majoritarian" liberal democracy, known as the Anglo-Saxon, or Anglo-American, model.[76] It refers to the present British and American relations among employers, unions, and governments. Here, there is more scope for free-market capitalism, subordination of the state bureaucracy to the economy, and a looser state-provided safety net.[77] The difference between the two models is immediately evident in the following diagram.[78]

Rhine Model	Anglo-American Model
Stakeholders	Shareholders
Decision-making by consultation	Decision-making by a principal
Long-term orientation	Short-term orientation
Collective objectives	Individual objectives
Norms and values result from debate	Norms and values imposed by authorities

Essential for social-pluralistic democracies is that the objectives of the economic order and the organizational structure to achieve them can change in response to changes in political constellations. This might be considered a disadvantage for the continuity of established policies. However, the reality is that these changes will evolve gradually, though in times of elections politicians are inclined to promise drastically alternative ways. Usually, changes occur rather incrementally.[79] For example, if one compared the objectives of the so-called Atlantic societies of the 1950s with those of the 1970s, one would discover that full employment, a reasonable growth of wealth, a sound balance of payment, a stable price level, and a fair distribution of income[80] have continuously headed the list of objectives to be achieved.[81] Thanks to the publication of Meadows' report for the Club of Rome in the early 1970s,[82] two further objectives have been added to this list since 1975: care for the environment and the responsible use of natural resources. Foreign aid also became an objective. These objectives are still valid today. However, it would not be surprising if present-day research regarding the objectives of the economic order reveals two more objectives, namely, (a) inflation control and (b) safety of individual citizens' living environment.

Finally, some remarks should be made regarding the objectives of the economic order of social-pluralistic democracies.

Firstly, the complexity of decision-making on the macro-level of social-pluralistic democracies causes the objectives of the economic order to be formulated in rather global terms.

Secondly, one has to take into account that each of the objectives of the economic order are themselves elastic, which means that in practice results may be relative. For example, a number of 100,000 unemployed people is a rather modest figure, if one was previously used to 300,000.

Thirdly, the objectives of the economic order are not of equal importance. For example, research from 1976 has shown that the ranking of objectives may change in accordance with the needs of a specific moment—and this can happen very quickly. The oil crises of 1973 and 1979 underlined the importance of natural resources for our economic order, which is directed at economic growth; and caring for the environment and combating inflation remained a priority only as long as there were no significant impediments to achieving full employment.[83]

Fourthly, emphasis on the pursuit of objectives may differ between countries, depending on their experiences. In the United Kingdom, for instance, given the unemployment level of the 1930s, full employment was of relatively more importance than the other objectives. For West Germany, given the runaway inflation of the 1920s, price control received relatively more emphasis.[84]

Finally, it has to be considered that if democracies are more social-pluralistic, political decision-making in general will be characterized by taking small steps, with little room for "grand designs." In contrast, if democracies are less social-pluralistic, governments can act more easily in accordance with their own views. In Becker's words, they will be more governmentally effective.[85]

One separate point must be made, because it has a significant influence on the framework approach. The framework is based on a state-centric view of democracy, which refers to a state–society relationship which, apart from state-centrism, is characterized by institutional insulation and homogeneity, state sovereignty and superiority, as well as a focus on constitutional arrangements. The state, in this view, is the undisputed locus of power, which can enforce the political will of the dominant political constituency.[86] However, due to the emergence of economic orders beyond the state level, as well as increasing complaints regarding the functioning of democracies, this relationship is changing. In this respect, Pierre and Guy Peters distinguish between three scenarios of shifting political power: (a) downward to regions and localities, (b) upward to trans-national organizations, and (c) outward toward institutions operating at arm's length from the state. Together, these scenarios link the political system with its environment, thus covering the whole range of relationships and institutions which are involved in the process of governing.[87] Since the final quarter of the twentieth century, it has become common to use the term *governance* for this linkage. Any further developments in this regard will certainly have consequences for the way the central state is expected to give direction to society. Firstly, one will expect a shift from input control to output or outcome control. Secondly, it may be expected that the central state will become increasingly dependent on other actors in society, whereas, thirdly, the central state will be expected to cope with a bureaucracy that is perceived to be rigid, expensive, and inefficient.[88] Broadly defined, in a governance perspective the state will derive its strength more from coordinating public and private resources than from relying on legal and constitutional powers. In other words, the state's "powers over" are replaced by "powers to."[89] This does not necessarily mean that the power of the state will weaken. Its power will change from something derived from legal and constitutional strength into something which is contextual and entrepreneurial.[90]

As discussed, this changing state–society relationship also influences decision-making beyond the level of national economic orders. In this respect, Marks et al. argue that "states no longer serve as the exclusive nexus between domestic politics and international relations."[91] Instead, multi-level governance at, for example, the level of the European Union, is emerging, with national governmental control becoming diluted by activities of supranational and subnational actors.[92]

1.2 Movement at the National Level

During the 1999 annual national debate on health care in the Netherlands, one of the participants, a former minister of economic affairs, argued that the Dutch health care system was about to burst. Considerations of international and even global competition had made it too expensive. Therefore, he argued that collective financing of the system should be wound back. The most sensible alternative would be a universal but limited basic package, financed through income-related premiums, with the rest left to the market. And, of course, this alternative would have to provide safeguards for the vulnerable in society.

This minister represented a population of only 16 million people. But all the same he could have spoken for his (then) fourteen colleagues from the European Union, i.e., for 375 million people.[93] Those ministers would have had a point, since figures illustrate that the countries of the European Union perform relatively poorly in the globalizing economy.[94] Why is this so?

It is increasingly assumed that this poor performance is the result of the differences in the way the countries of the European Union, on the one hand, and the United States, on the other, have organized their societies. As noted above, European political culture is deeply imbued with a sense of a general duty to aid the needy—far more so than in the United States. Therefore, these differences between the United States and the countries of the European Union resound in their specific interpretations of the concept of solidarity. I will not go into the historical interpretations of this concept, but will limit myself to the time when this imbued sense of duty to aid the needy became particularly expressed in the creation of what we call the welfare state,[95] i.e., the establishment of a mature social security system[96] that can best be understood as "a subsection of the public sector, concerned with redistribution [via social security and social assistance] and the provision of those social goods which have a strong redistributive element, like health care and education."[97] Although the countries of the European Union differ in timing and scope in this respect, the beginning of this particular interpretation of the solidarity concept can roughly be positioned to have started after the Second World War.[98] From that time on, the countries of the European Union pointedly started to move to the left side of the continuum.

1.2.1 Developing the Welfare State[99]

After the Second World War, and particularly stimulated by a period of strong economic growth which started in the beginning of the 1960s, two new imperatives were added to the notion of civilization in the wealthier countries of the European Union. The first was that economic and social policy came to be seen as interrelated. The second was that social policy became a collective good and not something intended only for the poorer members of society.[100] In the current time, however, both imperatives, and especially the second one, are increasingly challenged. People protest because they feel that their social and political rights have been injured. This has everything to do with moving to the left and to the right on the continuum, i.e., the establishment and the reform of the welfare state in national economies. In both respects, I follow Geleijnse et al., who distinguish four phases of the welfare state. To them, the first phase, being the *foundation* of the welfare state, lasted until around the beginning of the Second World War. In many countries of the European Union, this foundation included legal arrangements on matters such as industrial injuries, invalidity, pensions, sick leave, et cetera. The second or *extension* phase started at the end of the Second World War and took about 30 years. During this phase, social security was extended by legal arrangements on matters such as child benefits, unemployment, disability pensions, and provisions for widows and orphans. It was also the phase during which "government sectors expanded inexorably, fiscal conditions deteriorated, stagnation grew endemic, labor was too expensive and inflexible, and an excess of taxation and regulation stifled entrepreneurship." It was a time of "Eurosclerosis," i.e., "the combination of democracy, statism, welfarism and inflation."[101] The third phase involved *restructuring* social security systems. It lasted some 15 years, from around 1975 to 1990. During this phase, the focus was on economizing through, among other things, limiting eligibility criteria to benefits, reducing the level of employee insurance, and decoupling the relation between wages and benefits. The final phase, which started around the beginning of the 1990s, is still running. To some, this is an unstable transition phase, during which we are moving away from a paternalistic welfare state to a more mature phase of independent and individually responsible citizens.[102] It is a phase of fundamental reforms to the systems of social security through, for instance, other methods of financing and paying benefits, the introduction of new personal risks and a re-allocation of responsibilities between governments and social partners.[103] My focus is on the final three phases.

We start with the extension phase, i.e., the creation of the welfare state, during which the pendulum swings to the left side of the continuum, caused by increasing government interference in the economic process. This phase can be symbolized as follows:

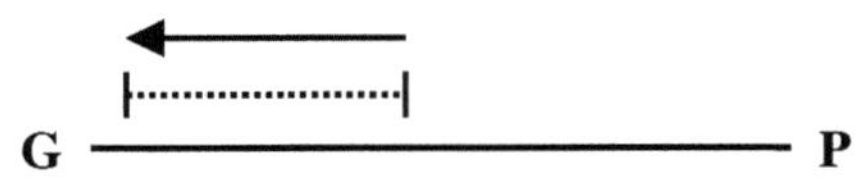

Several aspects have been added to the continuum line we first saw in section 1.1.1. The dotted line, first of all, illustrates that systems of social security are positioned on the left side of the continuum. The dots also symbolize that social security systems differ from country to country. Each dot can be seen as a specific national welfare state economy. The more that economy is situated on the left side of the continuum, the more extensive its welfare state will be and, consequently, the more intense its government interference with the economic process. The direction of the arrow illustrates the development in the second phase described by Geleijnse et al., in which countries extend the content and reach of their social security system. This is particularly true since half-way through the third quarter of the twentieth century. During this time, based on a long period of economic growth that started around the beginning of the 1960s, many countries of the European Union substantially invested the results of this prosperity in creating a welfare state. It is only since that time that the term *welfare state* came into use.

The third quarter of the twentieth century was a time of widespread belief in the manageability of society and of expectations that the economic "pie" would grow indefinitely, providing increasing benefits and wealth for everyone. Western societies did not have an eye for the storm clouds that, halfway through the 1960s, were already gathering on the horizon (such as decreasing demand, a slowdown in economic growth, and cheap competition from countries like Japan).[104] Instead, as indicated before, it was assumed that society could be managed, and governments of most European Union countries were expected to do so and to look after their citizens from the cradle to the grave.[105] This dream was cruelly disturbed by the oil crisis of 1973, which, for instance, led the then Dutch Prime Minister to sigh that things would never again be as they were. But things could not be changed overnight. It took a second oil crisis in 1979 and a new economic phenomenon, called stagflation,[106] to really wake up.

At about the same time, i.e., from 1975, the third phase, reforming the welfare state, was on the agenda of each government of the European Union. This was based on the argument that globalizing forces demanded a more flexible market economy. It involved a period of around 15 years of adjustments, mostly within the existing structures. As discussed above, this phase was followed by the still-ongoing process of more fundamental reforms to social security systems.

This book is not about how all the separate countries of the European Union dealt with the developments during the four phases. Instead, it is about trends that emerged during the third and fourth phases. These trends were directed at a new combination of self-interest and solidarity. This new combination can be illustrated by adding a second arrow to the continuum line, which symbolizes the pendulum swinging to the right because of decreasing government interference in the economic process.

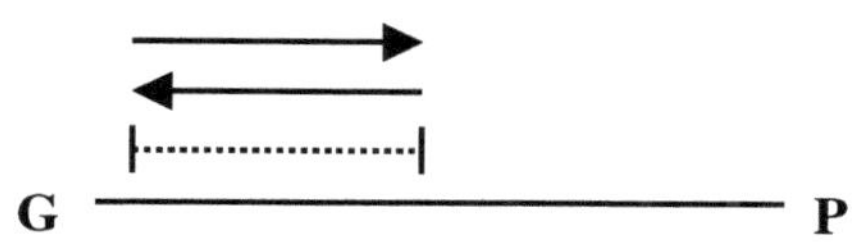

Though the trends are the same, there are important differences in the way the Rhine-model countries and the Anglo-Saxon countries have implemented their reform policies, trying to create more flexibility and to improve their competitiveness in a globalizing economy. To the Rhine-model countries, social pacts among the government, employers, and trade unions were instrumental in carrying through reforms in the welfare state. Reforms were agreed through a revival of neo-corporatist practices on the national as well as on the corporate level.[107] All in all, in Rhine-model countries, reforming the welfare state was a process of negotiated change through neo-corporatist practices that promoted "internal" labor market flexibility. The Anglo-American countries, however, favored a regime of "external" flexibility, advocating the reduction of non-wage labor costs, the cutting of unemployment benefits, more wage differentiation, and looser worker protections.[108] Instead of neo-corporatist practices, the Anglo-American approach was a state-led imposition of market-based labor reforms. These were first initiated by Prime Minister Thatcher, who opted to impose reforms from above through a strong, authoritative state, bringing an end to the "clubbable consensus" by making use of her "elected dictatorship."[109]

Creating the welfare state demanded money. In a system based on solidarity, this implied a redistribution of tax revenues or premiums to those in need. The following table shows the redistribution (expenditure) and financing (revenue) for two periods of 15 years for the United States, the countries of the European Union, and Japan. The first period, 1960–1985, covers the extension phase with the pendulum swinging to the left. The second period, 1985–2000, is the reform phase with the pendulum swinging to the right.[110]

Government Expenditure and Revenue as a % of GDP

	1960[111]		1985		2000[112]	
Continent	Exp.	Rev.	Exp.	Rev.	Exp.	Rev.
USA	27.0	26.3	36.7	31.1	30.1	31.6
European Union	28.2	28.5	51.6	45.7	43.0	43.8
Japan	18.3	20.7	32.7	31.2	36.8	29.4

The table shows that in 1985, particularly in the United States and the countries of the European Union, expenditure and revenue were considerably out of balance. Therefore, the United States and the European Union had every reason in 1985 to economize, with balancing governments' accounts being the obvious primary objective. After all, deficit financing without intervention would increasingly expose governments to a slippery slope, because national debts would increase.

The figures for the year 2000 illustrate the success of the reform policies. Consequently, the United States and the European Union have succeeded in balancing expenditure and revenue again, which was substantially aided by strong economic growth at the end of the millennium.

Mission completed, one would assume, were it not for the fact that from around 1975, both an ideological argument (neo-liberalism) and an economic argument (globalization) came into fashion, which favored the reduction of public spending. As for the latter argument, which implicitly refers to international competitive power, the countries of the European Union have an additional handicap, since their level of public spending, which was already 40.6% higher than that of the United States in 1985, increased to 42.9% in 2000. It should also be taken into account that the balanced budgets at the end of the millennium were not simply the result of reform policies; this was also caused by the strong economic growth of that period. After all, it is easier to settle one's debts if income increases.[113] Consequently, problems became serious again when, in 2002, the next recession started. Moreover, the countries of the European Union have to live up to a Union-wide agreement not to let their national budget deficits exceed 3%. Several member states used this agreement to carry out severe austerity measures.[114] Altogether, welfare states experience a threefold problem: (a) balancing the books in a way that takes account of agreements at the European level, (b) a globalizing economy with its consequent pressure on labor costs, and (c) the ideology of neo-liberalism, which rejects concluding collective arrangements in national economic orders. In times of recession, these problems particularly touch upon the fundamentals of welfare states.

Globalization has, for many years, presented an economic argument for European employer organizations to keep the costs of labor, an important source of finance of social security, as low as possible, because this would enhance their global competitive position. This seems to be a valid argument for European employer organizations, because labor, particularly in the Rhine-model countries of the European Union, is twice as expensive as in the United States and Japan.[115] In addition to this, EU workers have fewer working hours per year.[116] Moreover, they enjoy longer paid holidays and a more generous social security system than their colleagues in the United States and Japan, whereas, furthermore, the intra-European differences are considerable.[117] For example, a few years ago, the corporate tax burden was 60% in Germany and almost 52% in France, but had meanwhile decreased to 45% in the United States. Altogether, in terms of taxes, social security, pension benefits, and contributions to health insurance, Europe spent 41% of GDP in the mid-1990s, compared to 30% in the United States and Japan.[118] Currently, state-funded pension schemes alone consume 21% of government spending across the European Union. By contrast, the U.S. Social Security system consumes no more than 4.8% of GDP.[119] Therefore, it seems sensible not to exclude further pressure by employer organizations to reduce labor costs. I will come back to this point in chapter eleven.

All in all, reforming the welfare state is more than balancing the books. Were reforming only a matter of balancing the books, we could have stopped the still-ongoing process of fundamental reforms in 2000, taking into account that a certain level of economic growth is necessary for maintaining existing levels of social security. However, this did not happen, because reforming the welfare state is also about a new combination of self-interest and solidarity, the ideological argument.

In this respect, Komter et al. rightfully observe that the industrial crisis of the 1970s, together with a rapid increase in unemployment, also created a crisis for the welfare state. However, Komter et al. argue that this was not only caused by financial circumstances. They argue that it also had to do with the legitimacy of the idea of the welfare state and the confidence that citizens could have in this idea. After all, the welfare state that was expected to bring security and stability in times of economic recession, demonstrably failed to do so when it was needed, for the simple reason that, in times of recession, the state's financial resources are also under pressure. Consequently, in times of recession, welfare benefits are under pressure. To Offe, this refers to a structural contradiction inherent in the genes of the welfare state.[120] This contradiction is that the welfare state, which provides incomes and services as citizens' rights, "is itself highly dependent upon the prosperity and continued profitability of the economy."[121] Additionally, to Komter et al., the crisis of the welfare state also has to do with a cultural contradiction. To them, the fact that private enterprise has to provide the financial means for an organized collective solidarity is a remarkable product of liberalized and socialist principles, and is too abstract an institution to generate much loyalty. The pendulum cannot swing to the left and to the right at the same time. This cultural contradiction can also cause fraud and limit citizens' knowledge of their rights and obligations regarding welfare benefits. Together with the large-scale bureaucratic government organization necessary to execute and finance the welfare state, this almost automatically reproduces the differing interests and cultures within the welfare state. The answer to this is a withdrawing government that leaves social security increasingly to the market.[122]

Now, if one questions the legitimacy of the welfare state and argues that it has a structural contradiction in its genes, one must also question why it was established in the first place. It is not sufficient to answer this question simply by reference to the strong economic growth that started in the beginning of the 1960s. After all, the benefits of economic growth do not necessarily have to result in policies of a more equal redistribution between the members of society, as present times demonstrate. It seems more plausible, in this respect, to refer to worldwide politics during the Cold War. Like the Marshall Plan, the establishment of the welfare state also helped to prevent the spread of communism to Western Europe. It should not be forgotten that, during the Cold War, several countries of the European Union had strong communist political parties, which were supported by the Soviet Union. In this political climate, American outlet malls were readily compared to empty Russian shop shelves—but not only to illustrate that the citizens of the West had easy access to consumer goods. The point was that those Western shopping malls also stood for freedom and democracy, whereas the empty Russian shelves were metaphors for control and oppression.[123] In short, establishing the welfare state, which contributed to making the West a showpiece of capitalism during the Cold War, was a very strong weapon in the fight against communism. Now, with communism defeated, the welfare state may indeed appear to be a too abstract institution to generate much loyalty.[124] I will come back to this point in chapter eleven.

1.2.2 Privatization and Deregulation

A withdrawing government leaves unaddressed the fact that citizens expect their government to provide social security and public goods because they are used to these things. Both have become essential arrangements in the countries of the European Union. Their citizens will not be sufficiently sensitive to the argument that the crisis of the welfare state also involves a cultural contradiction. Nor will they be sensitive to the argument that globalization forces governments to carry through changes in the existing social security arrangements, even if many citizens already experience increasing inequalities in society in a personal way. People who are used to the benefits of the welfare state will pose structural resistance to reform because their desire for protection has become "intrinsically linked to democracy."[125]

Nevertheless, globalization seems to deliver the economic argument for privatization and deregulation. One can wonder, however, if this is the real reason. In this respect, Castells characterizes changes in the existing social security arrangements as "a recapitalization of capitalism," i.e., a revaluation of the way society organizes the production and consumption of goods and services. Deregulation and privatization are the key words for this revaluation.[126] Mainly, it is this revaluation that has caused the present problems of what Luttwak calls "turbo-capitalism" with its "societally disruptive structural change in jobs, firms, industries and localities." These are problems, which, combined with a peculiar phase of technological progress, have been brought about by government deregulation and privatization. To him, globalization has played a minor role here.[127] Therefore, authors like Castells and Lutwak in fact hold the view that it is not globalization but the ideology of neo-liberalism, which is the decisive argument for privatization and deregulation.[128]

Through privatization and deregulation, governments withdraw from the economic process, causing the pendulum to swing to the right side of the continuum and assuming that this will increase efficiency and effectiveness. And, indeed, many examples can be given in support of this.[129]

Nevertheless, one can have doubts about the real effects of deregulation and privatization. Research by Feigenbaum et al. is interesting in this regard. Because, based on a study of the privatization process in four Western countries, they conclude that much of what is sold as privatization appears to be government entrepreneurship dressed up in different clothes.[130] For instance, the privatization of public utility corporations in the United Kingdom, the forerunner of privatizations, soon led to the establishment of so-called "regulatory agencies" to restrain the increases in prices of gas, water, and electricity in favor of shareholders and overpaid managers.[131] And in some cases, regulatory agencies have grown into organizations of hundreds of people.[132] Given these adjustment measures, one may therefore argue that the role of government has changed, but not disappeared. Government is no longer the manager, but the "referee, setting the rules of the game."[133]

This last point refers to another aspect of the privatization of public services, which is that privatization, through abuses and malfunctioning, may weaken the democratic operation of the national economic order. After all, privatization means that public and transparent government power, subjected to democratic control, is shifted to the private sector, which has limited accountability to the public at large. To Barber, the consequence of such a shift is that the power of democratic control moves into the hands of private elites, which will not let themselves be controlled or restrained.[134] Also, as noted above, abuses would considerably discredit the privatization hype if they were widely known. Apart from this, one also has to answer the question whether these privatizations have improved the service level. In many cases, this cannot be maintained.

1.2.3 Participation in Decision-Making

The 1990s saw several protests against intended reductions in public spending.[135] Apparently, not everybody agrees with cuts to public spending. There are numerous relevant questions regarding the functioning of democracy in this respect: Is democracy alive? Are citizens really heard by those in power? And do ordinary citizens really influence decision-making regarding movement along the continuum? This section attempts to provide a preliminary answer, which consists of two elements. First of all, we will consider the working of social-economic infrastructures, like the Dutch "polder model," in daily practice. Secondly, we will consider the interest of individual citizens to take part in political decision-making.

Social-economic infrastructures like the Dutch "polder model" exist for the purposes of reaching agreement on the question of what a fair society should look like. In fact, these infrastructures are instrumental to the task of defining where exactly on the continuum a national economy wants to be. In this respect, a distinction between the Rhine model and the Anglo-American model was previously made. The social-market Rhine model is typical for many countries of the European continent. This neo-corporatist model, however, is more than sharing power among labor unions, corporate management, and the government through time-consuming negotiations and procedures. It is also a cultural model,[136] which can be found in multi-colored variations from the south of Spain to the north of Finland. One might say that it is in the genes of the citizens of the European continent.

According to various scholars, this model should be cherished. In reality, however, it is increasingly coming under pressure. Michael Porter has even suggested that it be put out for the dustman.[137] Many scholars blame the phenomenon of globalization for this development. Globalization demands flexible and quick adjustments in global competitive relations. In this climate of global business, corporations should not be hindered by time-consuming neo-corporatist procedures of consultation or government interference. Such scholars see a need, therefore, to liberalize the neo-corporatist relations. However, some ambiguity can be observed here. On the one hand, in line with the prevailing ideas of liberalization, governments are withdrawing from the economic process. On the other hand, features of government interference in the political process have become stronger.[138] Governments seem to be purposely restoring the primacy of politics. In this respect, circumstances may differ between the countries of the European Union. Consultation at the institutional level in Scandinavian countries and the Netherlands seems to have decreased. Germany lags behind, whereas the French government appears to be favoring more consultation, while at the same time maintaining its leading role in the economic process.[139] These observations boil down to the conclusion that the Anglo-American model is slowly taking the lead in the social-economic infrastructures of democracies of the developed world.

Although the criticism regarding the Rhine model may be partly true, it should not be forgotten that globalization may cause conflicts about what a fair society should look like. In Rodrik's terms, "since trade policy almost always has redistributive consequences (among sectors, income groups and individuals), one cannot produce a principled defence of free trade without confronting the question of fairness and legitimacy of the practices that generate these consequences."[140] Moreover, it should be kept in mind that a sound and solid social-economic infrastructure is an important factor for the location of businesses.[141] Multinational corporations base their decisions to locate themselves in a certain country on considerably more than the wage level.[142] Therefore, it is wise to be careful if one wants to restructure in this way.

As for the interests of individual citizens in political decision-making, there seems to be something fundamentally wrong in the relationship between politicians and the public. In this respect, a 1993 survey conducted for the European Commission found that 55% of the voters were unhappy about the functioning of democracy in their country.[143] Figures since then give no reason to be more optimistic now.[144] Though democracy presupposes the sovereignty of the people, reality seems to be different.[145] Why is this so? There are five arguments in this respect.

Firstly, it is argued that politics has subordinated the well-being of citizens to the interests of corporate business.[146] Because of this, politics itself has been subordinated to corporate business as a consequence of deliberate corporate globalization policies, which are intended "to deprive national politics of its power."[147] As a result, governments are no longer capable of controlling market operations. Moreover, "governments no longer act to conceive or defend the common good."[148] To a certain extent, one can even say that corporate business buys politics.[149] As an example: candidates for the American federal elections in 2000 managed to raise $2.73 billion for their campaigns.[150] Similar developments can be observed in the countries of the European Union, not so much in financial terms, but in influence-peddling schemes.[151] Opinions and facts like these leave politics, and with that the state, rather powerless. It seems as if corporations "have gained additional scope for action and power beyond the political system."[152]

A second argument is that politics in the Western world has itself changed. Deakin uses the term "*one vision democracy*" here, which means that there is no longer a difference between the political left and right.[153] Apparently, ideology and conviction about how society should look like are considered to be elements of a disappearing world.[154] Consequently, the old dispute between left and right "has exhausted its capacity to clarify issues and to provide a reliable map of reality," according to Lasch.[155] In other words, "the left has sold out."[156] As a result, some countries have essentially become one-party countries,[157] where political cartels have elicited ideological dullness[158] and where politicians are mainly preoccupied with (political) system control.[159]

In line with this, one wonders if this colorlessness of politics may have consequences for the idea of representative democracy.[160] These consequences might be that representative democracy will be replaced by systems of managing people[161] with all the Kafka-like consequences this would imply.[162]

Thirdly, it may be that politicians are losing the citizens' respect because, firstly, they demonstrate that they are not able to run the country.[163] Secondly, politicians may lose the citizens' respect because of political and party corruption. For example, in addition to the scandals of 1991 that brought down the Italian system, similar revelations have emerged of political and financial corruption in the 1990s among governments in Belgium, France, Spain, Austria, and Germany.[164] This leads Phillips to conclude that there is "a moral convergence to match the contagion of market-driven philosophy."[165] A final reason why citizens may no longer respect the political trade could be the regular occurrences of deception, or at least the smell of it.[166]

Fourthly, but speculatively, it may also be that the citizens of the developed world have come to believe that politics does not matter anymore, not only because politicians seem no longer trustworthy, but also because they demonstrate not to be capable of protecting their citizens against insecurity and crime.[167] Comparable opinions seem to exist among young people in the former communist countries of Eastern Europe.[168]

Finally, and also speculatively, it may be that the citizens of Europe have developed an attitude of not needing politics anymore. After all, within the European Union, many citizens enjoy a rather prosperous life. They can go their own way. They neglect or are not interested in the fact that, despite the enormous growth of wealth over the past decades, its distribution over the population has become ever more unequal, resulting in an increasing number of fellow-citizens who do not share in the increasing wealth.[169] In short, there is a growing split in society between the "haves" and the "have-nots." The latter do not need politics anymore because they feel betrayed. They are a breeding ground for extreme right-wing parties. People may vote for such parties because they feel that they are ignored by the political establishment.[170]

As for the final two arguments, the question remains whether they are an expression of true human characteristics, or whether they must be seen as a consequence of the slackness of governments to do something about the things that really matter to people, i.e., justice, fairness, safety, and so on.

Nonetheless, because of these arguments, politics has become an ever more fading brand that people find increasingly difficult to recognize. As formulated by the Commission on Global Governance, "governments have suffered an erosion in their authority."[171] Restoring that authority is the first requirement if politics is to win back the people. For as long as politics does not succeed in doing this, people will not win back politics.[172] Winning back politics may be promoted if politicians realize that differences in political colors are essential for the very existence of politics.[173]

1.3 Movement at the European Level

The preceding sections dealt with decision-making regarding movement along the continuum within the context of national economic orders. Within that context, the aftermath of the Second World War made a mixed economy attainable at the level of the national state. That nation state controlled its borders, which made it possible for nations to have national fiscal, monetary, regulatory, social, and developmental policies. These policies included macro-economic management, social contracts between industry and unionized labor, supervision and regulation of financial institutions, the use of banks as engines of national development, subsidized strategies for economic development, and so on.[174] However, by adding the European economy to the sequence of economic orders, as I did in section 1.1.1, I meant to indicate that it is not consistent with today's economic reality to limit the line of reasoning to the level of national economies. Nations as well as interest groups have lost some of their macro-economic leverage because of international developments.[175] Consequently, states can no longer be sovereign in the traditional sense of the word. For both physical and ideational reasons, "a state cannot in contemporary globalizing circumstances exercise ultimate, comprehensive, absolute and singular rule over a country and its foreign relations. State sovereignty depends on territorialism, where all events occur at fixed locations: either within territorial jurisdictions or at designated points across tightly patrolled borders. The end of territorialism has therefore brought the end of sovereignty."[176] Consequently, territorialism must be complemented with "supra-territoriality."[177] Because of all these changes, decision-making regarding movement along the continuum on the *what*, the *how*, and the *for whom* of the production and consumption of goods and services may also be influenced by events, developments, or strategies beyond the level of national economies. It is reasonable, therefore, to deal with the possibilities of upward supra-territorial shifts of regulatory competences, i.e., transferring sovereignty to a higher level of government. This means that we have to identify relevant players on the international scene from the perspective of their power to influence decision-making with respect to movement along the continuum. In order to do so, this section will address the phenomenon of the European Union.

1.3.1 The European Union: A Delicate Endeavor

In line with what has been said in section 1.1.1 on the stages of development of economic orders, it should not be assumed that the "European state" is the consequence of a straightforward evolution from the city-state, via the absolute state, to the modern nation-state. On the contrary, quite apart from the diversity in physical characteristics and economic structures between the member states,[178] the European Union is "a patchwork of different cultures, religions, languages, and views."[179] Its history is characterized by many conflicts and struggles, resulting in many regressions instead of a neat evolutionary progression.[180] The European Union, therefore, is not the result of a gradual transition to a higher form of economic order. It is an economic order which has been deliberately designed.[181] It is also an economic order which is continuously in a state of incubation. Therefore, the European Union is a fact as well as a dynamic process, of which the final profundity is hard to predict.[182] The EU is an enthusiastic civilization ideal, a "multi-interpretable open-ended concept" (author's translation).[183] Nobody knows, however, whether in the end, the European Union will be present as a firm and solid next step in the sequence of economic orders. The possibility of regression, or (further) "differential integration"[184] cannot be excluded. However, I will not deal with this possibility here.[185] My starting point is optimistic in that I assume that European politicians demonstrate the necessary leadership to solve integration problems, be it only for the fact that the disintegration of the European Union would cause many difficulties and disadvantages for the member states.[186] Furthermore, because "there is no clear political mechanism for aggregating European opinions,"[187] I take it for a fact that, despite the existence of supranational European institutions like the European Central Bank and the European Court of Justice, the sovereign member states of the European Union will continue to play an important role in the further shaping of economic integration and cooperation. The European Union, therefore, is a negotiated[188] addition to the nation-state. It does not replace the latter.[189] I accept, therefore, that the European Union will have to live with a chasm between two kinds of policies—policies regarding an ongoing unification, integration, and enhanced cooperation on the one hand, and policies which remain with the sovereign states on the other.[190] This makes further European integration a delicate endeavor, demanding patience and a willingness to compromise, resulting in decisions which can be considered as "peace treaties" between competing member states.[191] With all this in mind, I will in the remainder of this section focus on the consequences which ongoing European integration and cooperation may have for individual member states regarding the position they want to have on the continuum, including the consequences of enlargement of the European Union.

1.3.2 Economic Integration and Cooperation

The fact that Europe has a Single Market at last is not only the result of the initiatives of the European Commission, the rulings of the European Court of Justice, and the leadership of politicians like Jacques Delors[192] in striving for the aforementioned objectives of unification, integration, and enhanced cooperation. It is also, if not primarily, based on the threat of competition from the United States and the Far East, as well as a growing consensus among governments of the member states on the topic of deregulation.[193] To a certain extent, "global competitive pressures have [. . .] acted as an external catalyst for integration, forcing EU countries to investigate the potential benefits to be had from pooling their resources."[194] Therefore, the economic argument of globalization, as well as the ideological argument of neo-liberalism, are also unrestrictedly applicable to the level of the European Union.

The threat of globalization not only seems to be the guiding principle for daily policy practice of member-states' governments. It is also instrumental to a common European competition policy. Against this background, some see the Single Market as essentially nothing more than a defensive construction on behalf of the European population to prevent Europe from becoming a colony of the Americans and the Asians.[195]

Apparently, the European Commission took the competitive threat from the other two regions seriously. It promoted growth, competition, and employment as explicit objectives during the five-year period following the completion of the internal market program. Determined to make up for the arrears, during the Lisbon Summit of 2000, the political leaders of the European Union robustly declared it their ambition to make the European Union "the most competitive and dynamic knowledge-based economy in the world by 2010, capable of sustainable economic growth, with more and better jobs and greater social cohesion."[196] The pillars of this new policy were market liberalization, deregulation, and a restructuring of collective solidarity mechanisms. Consequently, competition policy at the level of the European Union implied a move to the right side of the continuum.

In pursuing this new policy, the European Union's political scene was, of course, strongly supported by European employer organizations. Even stronger, the necessity to defend the interests of the citizens of Europe in a globalizing economy led to a closer cooperation between "Brussels" and European industry.[197] Altogether, "spurred on by the competitive challenge posed by the USA, Japan and other East Asian economies, EC states sought refuge in collective action rather than stand-alone policies. The 'common external threat' inevitably served to deepen the spirit of unity amongst most of the EC's political and business partners."[198]

The Single Market, whether or not seen as a defensive construction, can play a meaningful role in a globalizing economy. But it is not enough. Equally important is the creation of a European currency, along with the establishment of a European Central Bank, if only for the fact that adopting the same currency has a positive effect on trade between countries and thus on economic growth.[199] Both have been achieved, but with a consequential loss of sovereignty for the member states. The introduction of the Euro, for instance, implied that member states could no longer make use of monetary policy instruments like re- and devaluation.[200] Introduction of the Euro, together with the start of the European Central Bank, also entailed the establishment of a common monetary policy for the entire Euro area. In this respect, it is important to note that the European Central Bank was deliberately not connected to the European political scene.[201] This made it possible for the bank to pursue its own preference for a "sound money" policy, i.e., price stability. For such a policy to succeed, fiscal discipline was necessary, as well as radical neo-liberal reforms to labor markets and welfare states. Neo-liberal reforms in the latter two contexts would mean "unemployment benefits at such a level and duration that they act as an incentive to seek work; as much freedom as possible for employers to 'hire and fire'; minimal restrictions on working hours; reduction of trade-union influence over wage-setting and work organization; avoidance of minimum-wage legislation; and reduction of taxes and regulations that make employers reluctant to create jobs."[202] In short, pursuing its own preferences implied that the European Central Bank became a member of the "hegemonic bloc"[203] of neo-liberalists in the international political economy, leaving less room for national policy makers in matters like interest policy and public spending,[204] because the introduction of the Euro and the establishment of the European Central Bank caused the "denationalisation of money."[205]

Now that the Single Market, the Euro, and the European Central Bank exist, the question is whether this is sufficient to enable Europe to play the game of global competition. One can reasonably argue that it is not. George Soros, for instance, a known "financial wizard" in the international financial and political world, argues that the establishment of a European market and a European currency is not sufficient, because in the longer term a common market and a common currency cannot do without a common fiscal policy, "including some kind of centralised tax collection or tax redistribution."[206] There are even those who propose the establishment of a European minimum rate of corporate taxation, in the longer term followed by a "European business tax."[207]

Therefore, it is reasonable to assume that, in the framework of global competitive power, the Single Market and the Euro will be followed by some form of common fiscal policy. Even now, the member states' freedom to carry out independent fiscal policies is restricted by the Stability and Growth Pact.[208] A harmonized fiscal policy at the level of the European Union would, for instance, remove the existing tax competition between member states.[209]

Nevertheless, regarding tax harmonization, a lot of work still has to be done. This work will be complicated, not only because harmonization of taxation is subject to unanimity voting at the level of the European Union, but also because the member states have largely differing interests.[210] As a consequence of these differences, there is not (yet) a sense of solidarity in fiscal policy, which is "one of the key gaps in legitimacy" of the European Union.[211] One may take it for a fact, therefore, that the harmonisation of fiscal policies will also proceed slowly.[212]

1.3.3 Social Policy Objectives

In accordance with the principle of subsidiarity established by the Maastricht Treaty, social policy objectives are member states' own concern. Because of this, the countries of the European Union find themselves in a situation where, due to ongoing economic integration, they must conform to European Union agreements regarding economic objectives, while at the same time they remain their own masters in dealing with social-policy objectives. One wonders if these two positions can coexist in the longer term. Present policy at the European level does not make that a feasible proposition.[213]

The problem with the principle of subsidiarity is that economic objectives are closely interrelated with social objectives. The delicate relation between the two is reflected, for instance, in the outcomes of the two summits of 2000. In addition to the aforementioned statement of the European Union's political leaders during the Lisbon Summit (in section 1.3.2 above), the Nice Summit of December 2000 referred to the Community Charter of Fundamental Social Rights of December 1989 and claimed that the European Union "is built on common and inseparable principles of human dignity, freedom, equality and solidarity" while "putting the individual at the centre of its activities."[214] How the two declarations could be combined remained unclear.

This interrelatedness of economic and social policy objectives, combined with the principle of subsidiarity, produces at least two ambiguities. The first is that attempts to achieve a European social policy have, so far, not progressed much beyond directives from Brussels regarding the labor market and rulings of the European Court of Justice regarding safety and health in the workplace. In fact, these directives were more conditioning to competition policy than they were expressions of social policy.[215] The second ambiguity is that, because of the interrelatedness of economic and social policy objectives,[216] it is very difficult "to exclude social issues" from the European Union agenda.[217] Apart from these ambiguities, there are considerable differences between the member states in the way they have shaped and financed their welfare state.[218] Because of this, it will take decades before there can be some kind of European social policy, if feasible at all.[219]

Given the huge differences in the size and financing of the European welfare states, it is understandable that, for the time being, the European Union is limited to "market making,"[220] taking into account competition policy only. Therefore, in order to improve the (assumed) relatively poor economic performance of the European Union on the global market (section 1.2 above), a new balance between an improved competitive climate for European businesses, while maintaining social cohesion, has to be found. This new balance has to deliver an acceptable trade-off between economic stability and efficiency on the one hand, and the "flanking policies"[221] of social justice on the other.[222] However, the political reality of the European Union is that the latter policies are increasingly subordinated to the economic objectives of creating a more advantageous business environment. As for the latter, deregulation, liberalization, and transferring the tax burden from businesses to individuals, i.e., moving to the right side of the continuum, are instrumental. In line with this, European competition policy has become increasingly characterized by the pressure of employers to reduce the costs of labor. From their point of view, they will do everything to push European Union economic policy in a liberal direction of non-intervention.[223] They are interested in the European "polder model," the Social Dialogue, as long as this results in non-binding agreements.[224] Consequently, the danger is that the European Union, in implementing a defensive strategy in a globalizing economy, will increasingly look like the United States and will further reduce its welfare state arrangements, leaving these arrangements increasingly to the market.[225] In the longer term, harmonization of taxation is the heart of social policy, because most welfare states of the European Union are financed on the basis of taxation policy. Therefore, harmonization of taxation policy will probably lead to a harmonization of social standards of the member states. Therefore, "social policy may thus become a new object of integration."[226] In this respect, it is worth mentioning that Article III-103 of the draft European Constitution assumes that the functioning of the European internal market will promote a harmonization of social security systems.[227] We may only hope that this harmonization will not result in a policy of finding the lowest common denominator.[228] In this respect, two elements have to be considered. Firstly, though decreasing, corporate taxation still is an important source of finance for social security. Corporations will not be interested in a social policy that does not (further) decrease their financial burden. Secondly, as noted above, and particularly with respect to social policy, there are huge differences in the way the member states have shaped their welfare states. It is not unreasonable to assume that in the framework of a social policy for the European Union, the more extensive welfare states will have to implement reductions to the benefit of less extensive welfare states, if only because, for the sake of a continuously politically stable European Union, social differences between the member states should not be too large.[229] This demands, however, political decision-making at the level of the European Union regarding social integration, because the existing divergence between European Union welfare states makes "automatic harmonization" a rather unrealistic proposition.[230]

1.3.4 Enlargement

In 2004, no less than ten new countries joined the European Union, thus increasing the European population by 20%. Enlargement had never been so ambitious. Not only are the new entrants relatively low-income countries, most of which are former socialist or transition economies,[231] but also, the number and diversity of member states after the latest enlargement has increased to such an extent that institutional reform of the European Union is inevitable.[232] Besides, there is the problem of finance.[233] Enlargement has resulted in an even more unbalanced relationship between contributors to the European Union budget and beneficiaries under that budget. A further financial redistribution to the East of Europe will probably increase the pressures on the welfare states of the European Union.[234] Consequently, the most recent enlargement has brought about the "problem of how to address the commitment to income redistribution."[235] European citizens may fear that enlargement "will not bring anything because the newcomers from the East can only benefit at the expense of the present members" (author's translation).[236] Because of this, individual governments and the European Commission will have to explain the "historic necessity"[237] of enlargement to the European citizens. They will have to make it clear that a financial redistribution to the East of Europe will be advantageous to all in the longer term.[238] In other words, they will have to explain that enlargement of the Union is an investment in the future of Europe. A future that, according to Thurow, "can build something that no one else can build—by far the world's biggest, most self-sufficient market [of] 850 to 900 million people."[239] (Apparently, Thurow saw no reason to include possible developments in China when he made this statement in 1993.)

So far, governments of the member states and the European Union have been very slow in selling this future to the European citizens. Though commitments have been made to the new entrants, political leaders "have neither tried to explain to their own electorates why enlargement is necessary, nor where and how they themselves will need to adapt."[240] This may explain why the disinterest of the electorate at the national level can also be observed at the level of the European Union.[241] It should be realized, however, that European citizens, feeling uninformed and unable to influence the direction of integration, may cause a democratic deficit.[242] Therefore, political leaders will have to engage in political tours de force in order to maintain social stability in Europe since, according to Myrdal, the welfare state is a narrow-minded and irrational nationalistic phenomenon.[243] Regarding this, a major point for decision-making is the question of whether the West of the European Union will help the East from a perspective of geopolitical realism, solely based on the interests of the original member states, or from a perspective of an open-society idealism, taking into account the interests of all the citizens of an enlarged Europe.[244]

1.4 Movement at the Global Level

The upward shift of regulatory competencies from the member states to the higher economic order of the European Union implies the transfer of sovereignty from member states to the regional supra-state "government" of "Brussels." Once member states have reached agreement on items to be shifted, they have to live up to the consequences for their national economies. These consequences limit their sovereignty.

1.4.1 On Global Governance

Upward shifting of regulatory competencies to a trans-world level is a completely different affair, because there is no global economic order, or world government, to which sovereignty can be transferred. A world government presupposes the existence of "a central public authority legislating for humanity,"[245] and the world does not have such an authority. It never will.[246] In the absence of a world government, therefore, the concept of global governance refers to "a process of political co-ordination among governments, intergovernmental and trans-national agencies (both public and private) [including multinational corporations and non-governmental organizations]. It works towards common purposes or collectively agreed objectives, through making or implementing global or trans-national rules and managing trans-border problems."[247] It is a pluralistic multi-layered system for co-operation and consultation for the purposes of reaching agreement on rules, norms, and policies regarding a whole range of global issues that affect every single participant. The environment, human rights, labor conditions, the global financial architecture, global drug trade, the preservation of wildlife and many other topics of international reach, are items of global governance. However, despite much talking in many global platforms[248] on these topics, global governance is a process of noncommittal engagement, because there is no transfer of sovereignty. Participants who do not agree with the outcomes of negotiations can easily pull out. Consequently, there is no formal global authority with the power to decide on movement along the continuum at the global level. This can have devastating effects, as can be illustrated with many examples.[249] Several ideas have been launched to change this global reality. Some expect that a solution will emerge from narrowing the gap between governments and citizens. Others believe that "future stability requires that a carefully crafted balance be struck, nationally and internationally, between the freedom of markets and the provision of public goods."[250] Finally there are those who warn that "pro-globalization policies must be accompanied by strong structural and redistributive measures."[251] In fact, the latter two points are an appeal to be careful in dismantling of the welfare state, as well as a warning not to let social inequality in society grow too large. In other words, these points are a call to avoid going too far to the right side of the continuum. How this could be achieved in practice remains unclear, however. After all, the problem remains that there is no global authority with the powers to decide.[252]

1.4.2 Global Institutions

Although we do not have a government to decide on global issues, we do have globally operating institutions like the International Monetary Fund (IMF), the World Bank and the World Trade Organization (WTO).[253] It is impossible to consider these institutions in isolation, because their comings and goings are closely tied up with foreign policy, especially American foreign policy.[254] As for the IMF and the World Bank, it is largely believed that these institutions do not do what they were established for, namely, the promotion of global stability by helping developing countries and, subsequently, the so-called transition countries of Eastern Europe, to achieve stability and growth.[255] Instead, they interpret their task as one of demanding structural adjustment policies, which are "overt in their demands for governments to cut social spending and privatise resources in exchange for loans."[256] In fact, they carry out their activities in developing countries from the neo-liberal perspective.[257] Consequently, to the IMF and the World Bank, social security is not a public good and therefore not governments' business.[258] Furthermore, in the neo-liberal logic of these organizations, a social safety net does not play a socially integrating role. Moreover, based on the same neo-liberal market fundamentalism, both institutions demand that countries in need not only introduce democracy[259] but also speedily liberate their financial markets and adopt privatization, because they believe that self-regulating markets work perfectly, whereas governments never do.[260] With this self-invented interpretation of their task, the IMF and the World Bank, strongly supported by the American Department of the Treasury, pursue the interests of the financial community of the developed world. This explains why they lend money to countries in financial crisis on the condition of strict structural adjustment programs that force governments to reduce public spending and make the local economy safer for foreign investments. Both institutions fail to take account of a country's specific circumstances or acute problems, thus leaving, more often than not, already-poor people even worse off. They simply translate their task into the role of a referee imposing neo-classical economic theory as a "one size fits all"[261] remedy, which can be illustrated with many examples.[262] However, some hope for change has emerged recently, because the World Bank Development Report of 1997 finally recognized that there cannot be a sound economic development without a modern and effective state.[263] Moreover, World Bank president James Wolfensohn admitted in the spring of 1999 that "at the level of the people the system isn't working," by which he meant that it does not provide a better material life for most citizens of the world.[264] Recent examples, however, do not give us reasons to be optimistic in this respect.[265]

It is legitimate, for that matter, to ask how institutions like the IMF and the World Bank can expect debtor countries to introduce democracy, while they themselves are hardly subjected to democratic control.[266] The IMF only reports to the ministries of finance and the central banks of the governments of the world. Thus, it has been able to escape from public accountability, which is standard in modern democracies. Scholte holds the view that although trans-world agencies like the IMF readily preach democracy to others, "they have inadequately applied the strictures to themselves," which leads him to conclude that "the democratic record of supra-state regulatory agencies has been decidedly poor. On the whole, regional and trans-world regimes have proved to be little more accessible, representative and accountable than colonial empires in a previous era of (territorial) world politics."[267] According to Stiglitz, therefore, the time has come to evaluate the IMF's performance democratically and to check whether its programmes indeed contribute to promoting growth and decreasing poverty.[268] In short, it is time for international institutions like the IMF and the World Bank to become transparent. This lack of transparency is the reason why an increasing number of people are protesting about the way they interpret their task.

Like the IMF and the World Bank, the WTO is also criticized for the way it operates. Although it is a legitimate world organization, it has very quickly turned into "an exclusive tool of commerce."[269] In this capacity, it could permit the interests of the developed world to prevail, such that the developing world would not benefit from the WTO, environmental damage caused by free trade would hardly be of concern to the WTO, and labor terms would not be the WTO's business.[270] As discussed, it has been argued that the WTO's activities have contributed mainly to the developed world. To Pilger, therefore, opening up underdeveloped countries to free trade and competitiveness is "a current euphemism for plunder."[271]

In addition, the WTO is hardly subjected to democratic control. It can easily pursue its own neo-liberal (American) preferences by considering each nation's choices in public health, the environment and public services solely in the light of trade rules, thus ensuring that trade takes precedence over all other aspects of public policy.[272] In this respect, Gates observes that "the WTO is not about democracies regulating free trade; it's about regulating democracies so they don't interfere with trade."[273] Furthermore, Palast has delivered information which shows that WTO circles have even been planning to overrule individual nations' parliamentary and regulatory decisions.[274] If only half of Palast's information is true, it is urgently necessary to reconnect the WTO, together with the IMF and the World Bank, with the voters by (a) doing away with the culture of secrecy; (b) increasing accountability, which is not limited to governments, and (c) involving the public.[275] In this respect, forcing the WTO to include the human rights conventions passed by the United Nations, including the Human Rights Charter, in its regulations on international free trade, would be a first step in the right direction.[276]

1.5 Summary

Any economic order involves a certain mix of private initiatives and government interference in the economic process regarding decision-making on the *what*, the *how,* and the *for whom* of the production and consumption of goods and services. By reasoning in analytical constructions, we perceive two extremes: on the one hand, decision-making can be left completely to the government; and on the other hand, decision-making can be left completely to the market. This results in a continuum between the two extremes. Every real economic order or national economy can be positioned somewhere on this continuum. That position is not permanent, because countries are always moving along the continuum from left to right and vice versa. Therefore, the economic order is a dynamic phenomenon.

Moving along the continuum from left to right (and vice versa) may affect the quality of one of the many elements that hold society together, i.e., solidarity among its members. Social security systems are an expression of that solidarity. They are instrumental to social cohesion. Reforming those systems, in the sense of limiting their reach, may endanger that cohesion.

In broad historical terms, it is common to distinguish between stages of development of economic orders, where a higher economic order is the result of a gradual transition from a lower order. The sequence of the household economy, followed by the city economy, the regional economy, and the national economy, is one such distinction. However, in modern times, increasing information and communication have made all corners of the world interrelated. Moreover, the consequences of economic activities may not be restricted to the level of the national economy. Therefore, there is reason to extend the sequence of economic orders with two new stages: the European economic order and the global one. The first is materializing in the European Union, the second in the increasing attention for the subject of global governance. As a consequence of these two new phases, decision-making on the *what*, the *how,* and the *for whom* of the production and consumption of goods and services may increasingly be lifted to a supranational level. Also, decision-making about whether to move to the right or to the left side of the continuum may no longer be exclusively a national economy's business.

The choice of whether to move to the left or to the right side of the continuum, i.e., increasing government interference in the economic process or increasing use of the market, is a matter of normative economics, because it involves ethical and value judgments. Using the metaphor of a swinging pendulum, by and large, the past hundred years shows a swing to the left side of the continuum after the Great Depression of the 1930s. This swing came to an end around halfway through the 1970s and was replaced by a swing to the right side. Since then, leaving things increasingly to the market through privatization and deregulation, has become the order of the day. Cutting back the welfare state is part of this. The label that is used for this swing to the right is "neo-liberalism," which I will return to in the third chapter. In terms of the swinging pendulum, and taking a comparable time span, one would assume that around the end of the current decade, a new swing to the left of the continuum would begin. However, since market-socialism with its all-embracing ideas of planning and the manageability of the economic order has failed and communism almost being defeated, there is no obvious left side for the pendulum to swing to. Consequently, cutting back the welfare state is a delicate matter; cutting back too much may increase tensions in society. Therefore, present-day liberal democratic capitalism may prove to be its own worst enemy if it is not able to maintain a fair and just society on the basis of individual freedom. In this respect, politicians are searching for a "third way." So far, this mainly appears to be wishful thinking, since there is barely any flesh on the rhetorical bones.

In the countries of the European Union, decision-making on what a fair and just society should look like takes place within a specific constitutional and procedural framework, which is founded on the democratic ideals of freedom, equality, and sovereignty of the people. In this context, these countries have all established a more-or-less balanced social-economic infrastructure in order to reach agreement on what the objectives should be and how they should be achieved. Such an infrastructure is a reflection of social-pluralistic democracy. The different interest groups meet at the institutional level of society. This refers to a complicated and carefully established framework of (representative) contacts between interest groups. On this institutional level, one exchanges views and ideas, one negotiates, one compromises and one tries to make coalitions in order to reach a certain common agreement through which the relations between interest groups are regulated.

Due to the emergence of economic orders beyond the level of national economies, as well as dissatisfaction with the functioning of democracies, the state-centric view of democracy is increasingly coming under pressure. Alternatives of shifting political power, upward, downward, or outward are seriously being considered.

2
Promoting and Opposing the Market

As discussed, government interference in the economic process does not happen in a vacuum, but within the context of a more or less balanced social-economic infrastructure that has been established to enable agreement on the objectives that the economic order should try to achieve and how this should be done. Furthermore, the concept of social pluralism was introduced as a factor that complicates the process of reaching acceptable results, because the interests of different groupings in society are not always aligned. Employers and employees, for example, do not necessarily have equal interests. Comparable differences can exist between manufacturers of consumer products and consumer organizations, and so on. All these interest groups want their own objectives to be pursued. To this end, they try to influence the decision-making process regarding the *what*, the *how*, and the *for whom* of the production and consumption of goods and services by promoting or opposing the market economy. They can do this by trying to find support for their viewpoints with political parties, or they can become political parties themselves. Like governments, interest groups can also use instruments to achieve their objectives. These instruments can be acceptable—like advertising by businesses or a strike by labor unions—or unacceptable, like blackmail and bribery. Moreover, interest groups can try to influence the decision-making process regarding the *what*, the *how*, and the *for whom* of the production and consumption of goods and services through the phenomenon of extra-parliamentary action. They can do this at state, supra-state, and global levels.

In short, it is essential to the sovereignty of the people that democracies permit individuals or groups of citizens, and organizations and institutions, to try to influence the moves along the continuum. Analyzing these attempts may give an insight into who, *in fact*, are the ones who decide on the *what*, the *how*, and the *for whom* of the production and consumption of goods and services.[1] At the same time, this implies that there is a difference between the formal design of democracies and their everyday reality.[2]

Regarding the analysis on which side to move to on the continuum, I distinguish between two main groups: those who try to influence the process of political decision-making, be it at national or international level, by promoting the market economy; i.e., they want society to move to the right side of the continuum. Apart from the relevant political parties, corporate business is the main player in this respect. On the other hand, there are those who, for different reasons, oppose the market economy. Besides the fact that, here too, several political parties are involved, one can distinguish between a number of differing interest groups that prefer to restrain the market; i.e., they want movements to the right side of the continuum to be, at minimum, politically controlled.

2.1 Promoting the Market

Rightly or wrongly, it is assumed that corporate business is a powerful force in national economies and beyond. It is even thought that politicians have subordinated the well-being of citizens to the interests of corporate business, and that it is no longer politics that controls corporate business, but corporate business which tells politicians what to do. In this respect, quite a number of scholars argue that corporate business has taken over the course of developments in the world. To give a few examples, Saul speaks of "a coup d'état in slow motion";[3] Hertz wrote of "the silent take over";[4] and to Kaplan, "world government" refers "to the increasingly dense ganglia of international corporations and markets that are becoming the unseen arbiters of power in many countries."[5] It is even assumed that corporate business controls universities and, through that, has "corrupted our higher education."[6] In short, corporate business and, for that matter, Wall Street, are running the world.[7] However, there are two relevant questions here: Is this true? And, if so, is this wrong?

2.1.1 The Power of Corporate Business

As for the first question, there are several confirming facts. Since the mid-1980s, multinational corporations have controlled 50% of the world's manufacturing and two-thirds of its trade.[8] Since the turn of the century, the hundred biggest multinational corporations control about 20% of foreign direct investments worldwide; out of the hundred biggest economic entities in the world, 51 are corporations and only 49 are nation states. The turnover of General Motors and Ford is bigger than the African GDP south of the Sahara; the assets of IBM, BP, and General Electric outrank the economies of most small countries; in 1998 Exxon-Mobil was as big as the Saudi Arabian economy; Bill Gates and Paul Allen, cofounders of Microsoft, together with Warren Buffet from Berkshire-Hathaway, had a net worth in 1999 that was larger than the combined GDP of the 41 poorest nations with their 550 million people, whereas revenues from Wal-Mart, in the United States, exceed those of most countries in Middle and Eastern Europe.[9]

Meanwhile, through mergers and acquisitions, corporations become bigger and bigger. Recent mergers (Vodafone/Mannesmann, Smith Kline Beecham/Glaxo Wellcome, et cetera), while paling the ones from the 1980s,[10] have continued the overall trend. In this respect, Freidheim predicts, as a first wave, that mega-corporations and immense cross-border alliances will soon dominate not only telecommunications and aerospace, but also the automobile industry, banking, energy, commercial aviation, pharmaceuticals, accounting, primary metals, and computer hardware and software. This first wave will be followed by a second wave of companies in biotechnology, textiles, chemicals, paper, wood products, and food.[11] In short, there will be conglomerates for almost every item of production.

Arguments like these make it hard to deny that corporate business holds enormous power. It can create employment and it can take it away. It can invest in impoverished areas or it can choose not to do so. In short, corporate business can act at will, so it seems. And since it is a rather anonymous entity, corporate business lacks accountability and often operates without controls.[12] Is this wrong? Objectivity demands that we admit that not everything corporate business undertakes is wrong. It can and does create employment, it builds schools, and it shows responsibility in health care for its employees in underdeveloped countries.[13] Nevertheless, many examples could be given of deceit, irresponsibility, and fraud by individual firms. The problem with corporate business has to do with the functioning of democracies and with the essential reason behind the existence of corporate business: making a profit.

To begin with the latter, poor societies create a poor business climate. Corporate business needs enduring societies to protect its own survival. Therefore, it invests in social activities and in social justice. But these investments will never be its core business. The only motive for corporate business to do so is that these activities create the conditions to realize its first and foremost motive; return on investment.[14] The return-on-investment motive also compels corporate business to take working conditions and environmental circumstances less seriously if the political environment allows it to do so.[15] In Hertz's words, "corporate business can do good only as long as it is able to prove that this helps making money" (author's translation).[16]

Meanwhile, multinational companies are increasingly under pressure to adopt "corporate social responsibility." In this respect, the United Nations' Secretary-General has proposed a Global Compact among business, governments, NGOs, and the United Nations to raise social standards across the world.[17] Nevertheless, making a profit stays paramount—an observation that is completely in line with, for instance, the position of European employer organisations, which stipulate that their contributions to the financing of the welfare state hamper their competitive power and thereby have a negative effect on their profit potential. Through this argument, corporate business appears to be successful in achieving considerable tax reductions.[18]

Despite the call for corporate social responsibility, the trend of corporate business behavior is quite the opposite. As an example: in 1957, American corporations still provided 45% of local tax revenues in the United States, a figure that had dropped to around 16% by 1987. All in all, American corporate taxation fell by 26% over the final quarter of the past century. In the 1950s, 27% of American government income resulted from corporate taxation. At present it is less than 10%.[19] Recent information illustrates that, next to the ongoing pressure to reduce the costs of labor for reasons of competitive power, new ways to avoid paying taxes have been found. For example, in order to attract employment, governments may grant corporate business substantial tax reductions or even exempt companies from taxation completely. Corporations may receive land for free or be allowed to skimp on working conditions.[20] In this respect, Moore uses the term "ADC" (Aid to Dependent Corporations), which totals some $170 billion a year in "tax-funded federal handouts."[21] All in all, the main task of governments seems to be to offer attractive conditions for corporate business.[22] Tax abatements, for instance, became a widespread strategy in various American states. By the 1990s, it had more or less become a custom for corporations to demand economic concessions from cities and states, threatening to relocate their business elsewhere.[23] In 1995, a total of 44 out of the 82 biggest American companies did not pay the standard 33% corporate tax rate. Of those companies, 14 did not pay taxes at all, whereas more than 8% of those companies, including General Motors, successfully reclaimed millions of tax dollars. In a second category, i.e., companies with assets of over $250 million, 1,279 did not pay taxes because they claimed to have no income in 1995. According to *Forbes* magazine, tax evasion costs American society $10 billion per year.[24]

The United States may be an extreme example, but its development is representative for the model of a flexible labor market that European Union governments and employer organizations are also pursuing. In Germany, for instance, corporate business contributed 13% of total tax revenue in 1997, dropping from 25% in 1980 and 35% in 1960.[25] In the same country, a group of corporations that included the Deutsche Bank, BMW, and Daimler-Benz blocked an attempt by the minister of finance to increase corporate taxation by threatening to invest abroad instead of in Germany.[26] In the United Kingdom, Chancellor Brown's first budget included a reduction in corporate taxation.[27] The social consequences of this development are the same as in the United States.[28]

As for democracy, it seems as if corporate business can do whatever it deems fit. Apparently, there is no institution that can hold corporate business responsible for its comings and goings, not even politics. Regarding this, Self argues that "the most fundamental problem posed by the global economy is the lack of political accountability for its operations. There are as yet no international agencies strong enough or impartial enough to correct the gross instabilities and inequalities of the global economy."[29] Therefore, Hertz predicts the death of democracy if governments do not learn their lessons from the past, if they are not prepared to look for solutions, if they are not capable of opposing the pressure from corporate business if the market mechanism fails, or if the profit motive conflicts with public interest. If they fail in these matters, governments "sign their own execution" (author's translation).[30] If this would happen, we would live in a world where corporate business is the master,where the law is subordinated to the market, and where voting is something of the past.[31]

Speaking of corporate business, one cannot exclude their relocations to low-wage countries. In this respect, a recent German study shows that, whether it is consumer electronics companies, the oil industry, pharmaceutical companies, food products industries, manufacturers of toys, sportswear or financial businesses, they all appear to be involved in pollution, child labor, and abuse of human rights. And if we add to this the fact that corporate business often opposes the establishment of labor unions in underdeveloped countries,[32] we have every reason to be very critical of the way corporations are behaving in those countries.[33]

In this respect, the reprehensible practices of corporate business mainly take place in the so-called Export Processing Zones (EPZs) of underdeveloped countries.[34] At around the turn of the century, there were some 850 EPZs in place worldwide.[35] The most important criterion for the establishment of these zones seems to be the wage level. EPZs, employing many women, because "they endure poverty well,"[36] seem to be outbidding each other in this respect.[37] A World Bank report of 1999 reveals that women are better able to adjust, to "swallow their pride," and to accept whatever job is available in order to care for their families.[38] Working conditions in many of these EPZs are said to be inhumane. Klein speaks of caged factories, surrounded by gates, watchtowers, and soldiers "to keep the highly subsidised products from leaking out and the union organizers from getting in."[39] Facts like these make "free trade" a rather cynical term; all the more so, since it was discovered in the mid-1990s that slave-labor camps and Victorian-style sweatshops also existed in Los Angeles textile factories and in lower Manhattan.[40]

As for child labor, a recent report of the International Labour Office reveals that, worldwide, one in eight children between 5 and 17 years old are exposed to "serious forms of child labour which threaten their mental, physical and moral well-being" (author's translation).[41] This is despite the fact that children's entitlements have been included in the global human rights regime through the Convention on the Rights of the Child, adopted by the General Assembly of the United Nations in 1989 and immediately ratified by 190 UN member states. According to UNICEF, this convention is "the most universally embraced human rights instrument in history." Nevertheless, due to a lack of resources, enforcement powers are limited.[42]

2.1.2 Consumerism

A market economy needs consumers. Because of this, "breeding consumerism"[43] through advertising or other instruments of product promotion is an important tool for manufacturers.[44] According to the figures, manufacturers seem to realize this very well, because advertising has become a big business. World expenditure on product promotion increased from $7.4 billion in 1950 to $312.3 billion in 1993. In 1998, over €350 billion was spent on advertising by brand leaders alone.[45] In the United States, advertising through electronic mass media increased from $270 billion to $358 billion in the mid-1990s.[46] In just four years, the cost of a 30-second TV ad soared from $180,000 to $478,000,[47] and 1,500 advertisements were screened daily on American television around the turn of the century.[48]

Many needs are the result of creating a commodity culture.[49] Klein published a revealing study in 2001 showing how subtly but profoundly people are brainwashed to have Coca Cola, Nike, Gap, Tommy Hilfiger, and many other brand names permanently imprinted in their minds.[50] Consequently, advertising is a normal part of American educational institutions. All major beverage manufacturers have agreements with schools and colleges, which contributes nicely to an increasing turnover of their products.[51] Even teaching materials are subjected to sponsorship, showing an increase of 1,875% since the 1990s.[52] Young children are a special target in advertising.[53] All major advertising agencies and marketing firms have a children's division, if only because market research has found that little children often recognize a brand logo before they recognize their own name.[54] Market researchers even organize focus groups of children of two or three years old.[55] In addition to this, private schools in the United States organize school trips to shopping malls in order to teach their pupils how to shop. These trips are paid for by retail chains, which, through this policy, are breeding "mall rats."[56] In 1998, United States marketing experts even discovered one-year-old children as a new focus group. Moreover, due to a scarcity of financial resources, schools become easy prey for entrepreneurs. The American Channel One, for example, bribes school officials with TV monitors in exchange for delivering the school audience to advertisers.[57]

One further point should be made. Breeding consumerism will work only as long as there is sufficient and effective demand. Krugman points to the fact that, over the past decades, "there has been a steady drift in emphasis in economic thinking away from the demand side to the supply side of the economy."[58] However, keeping demand adequate in order to make use of the economy's capacity has become the world's central problem. To Krugman, the different financial crises that the world experienced recently all involved the problem of creating sufficient demand.[59] Tackling these crises could be interpreted as a correction to the idea of free markets. Therefore, "in a world where there is often not enough demand to go around, the case for free markets is a hard case to make."[60]

2.2 Opposing the Market

The methods used by corporate business in favor of moving to the right side of the continuum are not uncontested. On the contrary, there is increasing opposition to the activities of corporate business. Labor unions, which in a globalizing economy see the labor terms and working conditions of their members threatened, want governments to take protective measures.[61] NGOs and anti-globalist movements expose the abusive behavior of corporations in the developing and underdeveloped world. The church may strike a warning note, and individual scientists commit their concerns regarding policies of moving to the right side of the continuum to paper. In order to bring some structure to this variety of market opponents, I distinguish in this section between, on the one hand, opposing institutions—such as (1) the unions, (2), the church, and (3) non-governmental organisations—and on the other hand, loosely or unorganized movements and groups that endeavor to oppose or counterbalance movements to the right side of the continuum. Here the focus will be on (1) anti-globalists, (2) the power of consumers, (3) critical views on economic growth, and (4) civil society. Each of these matters will be addressed in turn.[62]

2.2.1 *Institutional Opposition*

1. The Unions

As for the role of unions in the decision-making process regarding movements along the continuum, it should be kept in mind that, all over the Western world, the recognition of trade unions as legitimate bargaining agencies in democratic economic orders has been, not the result of economic determinism, but the final outcome of a long period of physical and legal repression of workers, who tried to improve their fate by fighting for social justice.[63] One may conclude, therefore, that governments did not wholeheartedly welcome the unions as new social partners with legitimate interests in the economic process, co-determining whether the economic order should move to the right or to the left side of the continuum. Governments perceived it to be their first responsibility to protect the freedom of the marketplace and the sanctity of the individual contract of employment. Unions were considered to be a threat to both. Because of this, the initial answer to unionization was suppression, or at least containment. In the terms of this book, governments were not prepared to permit developments away from the right side of the continuum. It was questionable, however, whether governments could maintain this reluctance, because these were also times of regular social unrest in the United States as well as in the countries of the European Union, with many workers striking and communism spreading. Therefore, while choosing to make the best of it, governments of the countries of the European Union changed their policies with respect to unionization from about 1875, which found expression in the legalized removal of obstacles to unionization.[64] Altogether, it seems defensible to argue that the emergence and legitimization of unionization has been the reluctantly accepted but inevitable consequence of the natural course of things.

Despite all the initial difficulties, unionized labor cooperated internationally,[65] becoming a firm element of the social-economic infrastructure of national economic orders in the countries of the European Union by the 1960s and co-deciding the moves along the continuum. Consequently, the unions co-determined the design of the welfare state, especially regarding protective measures related to work and working conditions. One can even argue that the social-security arrangements of the welfare state would not have been realized if there had not been a strong union movement. All in all, one can safely argue that the apex of unions' influence in the economic process started in the 1960s. It lasted until the beginning of the 1980s. During this period, a considerable percentage of all wage earners and salaried employees had joined the unions' ranks.[66]

However, there is reason to suspect that, from the beginning of the 1980s, unions' influence in the social-economic infrastructure waned, and with it their power of co-decision regarding movement along the continuum.[67] Here, Friedman's neo-liberal views were influential, particularly in the United States. To him, unions represent a superfluity in the labor market, because in a competitive labor market the worker "is protected from his employer by the existence of other employers for whom he can go to work, [whereas] an employer is protected from exploitation by his employees by the existence of other workers whom he can hire."[68] Since ideas like these are increasingly receiving support in several countries, "unions are very much on the defensive."[69] Furthermore, there is (again) proof of anti-union practices, particularly in the United States.[70] Consequently, the degree of unionization is decreasing: in the United States, it dropped from 30% in 1973 to 9.6% in 2000;[71] in Great Britain, it dropped from 53% in the beginning of the 1980s to 31% in 1995;[72] in the Netherlands, it dropped from 38% in 1980 to 24% in 2002.[73] On the whole, union density for the countries of the European Union decreased from 40% in 1980 to 30% in 1995.[74]

Does decreasing membership mean that unions have less influence in the social-economic infrastructure? And does this, in turn, mean that they have a lesser say in the decision-making process regarding movement along the continuum? For several reasons, the answers to these questions should be given in measured terms.

First of all, union membership in absolute figures is still considerable, a fact which cannot be denied in democracies.

Secondly, decreasing union membership around the turn of the century may have been caused by the increasing prosperity of that time, which may have led potential union members to conclude that they did not need unions to protect their job security and labor terms. This attitude may change in times of recession.

Thirdly, international comparative research covering 80,000 persons from 40 countries has shown that the role of unions in the social-economic infrastructure is also highly appreciated by non-union members.[75] Apparently, unions are seen as an important part of the social fabric of society, sponsoring, for example, community-service projects and acting as agents of the employee voice within the workplace. Unions, therefore, "nourish solidarity values as a counterweight to market values."[76]

Finally, unions may have such a strong position in the social-economic infrastructure that membership figures no longer matter.[77] The Netherlands and Germany, for example, both had low union membership in 1995 (26% and 29%, respectively), but it is unlikely that unions will play a minor role in the social-economic infrastructure of these countries in the near future. On the contrary, though membership is decreasing worldwide, in the industrialized world, unions are still an important player in social-economic spheres, countervailing the interests of corporate business and, if necessary, governments.[78] It remains to be seen, however, whether this will continue to persist in the further shaping of an economic order than at the level of the European Union and in a globalizing economy. In this respect, conflicting interests among unions of different countries may play a negative role.[79]

2. The Church

In the words of Kuttner, "the church is, of course, the longest-running counterweight to the dogmas of a pure market." Thomas Aquinas's teachings were meant to make clear to people that the economy was not solely a matter of individual transactions, but an organic whole. From this it followed that the self-interest of individuals had to be tempered by concern for the community.[80] For the purposes of this book, however, it is not necessary thoroughly to consider ecclesiastical history since Thomas Aquinas. Suffice it to say that, for centuries, the church has been a very important, if not a determining, factor in society.[81] "The Church was regarded, not as a society, but as society itself," said Tawney.[82] This changed during the times of the Renaissance and the Great Discoveries, with the rise of natural science and its promise of intellectual clarity, with the expansion of trade, and with the rise of new classes to political power. It led to a contraction of the social territory within which religion was conceived to run. During these times, "religion has been converted from the keystone which holds together the social edifice into a department within it, and the idea of a rule of right was replaced by economic expediency as the arbiter of policy and the criterion of conduct."[83] Consequently, the church was no longer society itself. Instead, secular and religious aspects of life were seen as parallel and independent provinces, "governed by different laws, judged by different standards and amenable to different authorities."[84] This change of position was reinforced during the second half of the eighteenth century, when several technological innovations and experiments made it possible to use mechanical power for production purposes. Consequently, productive capacity increased enormously, causing the Industrial Revolution, the origin of modern industry, with large-scale production in factories. Large-scale production needed sufficient manual labor, which, in turn, induced many people from the countryside to move to the industrial centers, seduced by the promise of making a living. Industrialization, therefore, caused urbanization, which, in turn, caused modern social problems of poorly paid people living in miserable circumstances in unhealthy quarters of vastly growing cities.

Although Tawney may be right that, between the Reformation and the Restoration, religious aspects came to be seen as an independent province of life, religion nevertheless was very influential in determining the characteristics of the emerging capitalism in those days. In this respect, Weber argues that during those days, branches of Protestant religions, in particular the Puritans (Calvinism, Methodism, Pietism, and Baptism), separated capitalistic enterprise from the pursuit of profit as such. Instead, making a profit became part of a *calling*, i.e., a combination of capital accumulation with a positively frugal life-style in a "this-worldly asceticism."[85] This implied that the religious valuation of unceasing, systematic work in a worldly calling was the highest means to asceticism, and at the same time was the surest and most evident proof of rebirth and genuine faith. In combination, these delivered the most powerful conceivable lever for the expansion of that attitude toward life. This, to Weber, is *the spirit of capitalism*.[86]

The origin of the Industrial Revolution had consequences for the role of the church. No longer was she in control of the course of events in society. Instead, she had to react to the excesses that were brought about by the free-market economy, which set the conditions of market operation. No longer was it sufficient for the church to preach the gospel, and for the priest to visit his rural flock. On the contrary, the intentions of the gospel needed to become a living daily practice. For the church, this meant that from its religious faith, it had to rise against poverty, exploitation, and detestable working conditions, including child labor and extremely long working hours in an inhumane factory environment, and so on. In short, the Industrial Revolution produced profound changes in the pastoral needs of society. And, indeed, the eighteenth century revealed several examples of individual servants of the church who climbed the barricades for a vastly increasing number of industrial workers, or who tried to bring about changes by publishing theological textbooks.

The church as an institution, however, is a different matter. The Industrial Revolution was already a fact for more than hundred years when, in 1891, the Roman Catholic encyclical letter, *Rerum Novarum*, was published, on the one hand as an indictment of the miserable living conditions of the working class and unrestrained competition and the accumulation of social and financial power in the hands of a few industrialists, and on the other hand, as a plea for decent remuneration for the working class as a matter of justice.[87] Reactions like these also appeared from the Protestant side. In this respect, four months after the publication of *Rerum Novarum*, a Dutch Protestant leader labeled the nineteenth century a "sick century" because it had degraded labor into a market commodity. Because of this, he believed, the working class experienced hardships that were sometimes even worse than those experienced by slaves in ancient times.[88]

It remains typical, however, that it took more than 100 years of industrial revolution for churches to react officially to the course of events in society. After all, a feeling of compassion for the poor and oppressed, followed by acting on their behalf, dates back to the beginnings of Christianity. This suggests that there must have been another reason for this delayed official reaction. This reason may have been the emergence of social movements that were not connected to the church. Marxism and socialism, with their associated ideas of class struggle, also gained ground among members of the working class, which resulted in the establishment of socialist labor unions. This might have caused the church to lose its hold over a considerable portion of its supporters. *Rerum Novarum*, however, rejected the idea of class struggle, because religion commanded respect for legal authorities. Therefore, the idea that workers could strike to improve their living conditions was rejected. Furthermore, socialist unions were believed to be a threat to the Roman Catholic faith. Therefore, as a counterweight, the establishment of Roman Catholic labor unions was promoted. Comparable developments were encouraged within Protestant circles of society.[89]

Though it may be that the initial official reactions of the church were inspired by a mixture of Christian compassion and fear of losing grip on society, the fact is that, since 1891, the church has regularly spoken out against the excesses of a free-market economy. In his encyclical letter of 1931, in addition to introducing the principle of subsidiarity, Pope Pius XI reminded the owners of property of the duties which ownership carried, rejecting too much individualism in economic life. In 1963, in *Pacem in Terris*, Pope John XXIII spoke of the right to work, to enjoy safe working conditions, to own property, and to earn a just wage. Two years later, with the encyclical letter *Gaudium et Spes*, this list was extended to economic rights which should guarantee a "truly human life," including unions, employment, working conditions, shelter, food, and education. Furthermore, with *Laborem Exercens* (1981), *Sollicitudo Rei Socialis* (1987), and *Centensimus Annus* (1991), Pope John Paul II stressed the importance of an inclusive society, incorporating the unemployed and the poor. Finally, the so-called liberation theology in South America, which opposes the alliance of conservative landowners and powerful multinational corporations, should also be mentioned.[90]

Comparable messages have been delivered by Protestant Christians. Matters like poverty, unemployment, and the responsibilities of employers and employees were regularly discussed in numerous congresses of the Christian-Democrats in the Netherlands, whereas in Great Britain the writings of Temple and Tawney were influential. Meanwhile, comments of the church on the free-market economy also started to include concerns regarding ecology. Pope John Paul II issued his first document on the subject in 1990. Furthermore, the same Pope, announcing the Jubilee Year 2000 with his *Incarnationis Mysterium* of November 1998, clearly referred to the miserable working conditions in underdeveloped countries when he wrote that "humanity is confronted with new forms of slavery, which are more subtle than those of the past, causing the word 'freedom' to be a meaningless term" (author's translation).[91]

In the context of this book, however, the decisive question is whether at present the church is capable of effectively influencing free-market operations. Two points should be mentioned here: Firstly, it is difficult to escape the impression that, in many countries of the developed world, the church is increasingly losing its grip on societal developments. Here, secularization has not yet come to an end. Secondly, in more recent years, neo-liberals have sought to defend free-market operations by a religious justification of capitalism.[92] All in all, there are not many reasons to be optimistic about the role of the church today as an institution capable of restraining the free-market economy. It is not very likely, therefore, that the church will be capable of opposing movements to the right side of the continuum. This might change, however, if politicians of the European Union take seriously their intention to have transparent and regular dialogues with the church, as laid down in Article I-51 of the draft Constitution of the European Union.[93] It might also change if, as in almost every other part of the world, a resurgence of religion also gets underway in EU countries,[94] provided such a resurgence will not be used as a justification of present-day capitalism.

3. Non-Governmental Organizations

Many NGOs are very active in matters of international environmental policies and human rights. They appear to be able to mobilize many people, and they have regular success in their attempts to change policies (apartheid, Brent Spar, whale fishing, et cetera). Their role in the international arena seems to be accepted. In 1990, most of the major United Nations institutions had established a department for liaison with NGOs.[95] Their existence is recognized by international political organizations in that they are, formally or informally, consulted, and sometimes even participate, in the drawing up of international treaties. We also see that they are increasingly involved in official development assistance (ODA) programs.[96] Although these developments demonstrate that NGOs are increasingly integrated in public policy implementation, there is no common agreement on the question of whether they also have *political* influence. There is little academic research regarding this point. Most of the publications are not much more than "yes" or "no" opinions of the authors, without proof or scientific argumentation. However, a study by Arts is of assistance in this respect. On the basis of several case studies regarding the United Nation's Framework Convention on Climate Change and the United Nation's Environment Programme Convention on Biological Diversity, he concludes that (1) NGOs make some difference in global treaty formulation and implementation (although certainly not in all cases); (2) NGOs' political influence is mainly dependent on their own expertise, on the attitude and conduct of (like-minded) states, on the substance of current environmental regimes, and on the nature of intergovernmental negotiations; (3) NGOs may increase their political influence, mainly by professionalizing their lobbying and advocacy in political arenas and through organizing moderate protest outside.[97] If NGOs would take these lessons to heart, they might, in the longer term, be able indirectly to influence the decision-making process regarding movements along the continuum. Pilger, however, holds the view that NGOs have already drawn too close to governments through funding and their tax-exempt charitable status. Through this, NGOs may increasingly serve to neutralize and de-radicalize movements for real change.[98] We find this confirmed by Neale, who points to the fact that NGOs that work in developing countries get most of their money from Western governments. These NGOs could find themselves in a situation of calling the tune of those who pay the piper. Here, Amnesty International and Greenpeace are exceptions among the larger NGOs.[99] It may be that, because of their independence from politics, they have regular success with their attempts to bring about alternative corporate policies. One may wonder, for example, if Shell would have chosen another solution regarding the Brent Spar affair were it not for Greenpeace's success in mobilizing consumers to effect change. And it remains to be seen if Heineken and ABN AMRO would have withdrawn from Burma without Amnesty International's information campaign regarding the oppression of the country's military regime.[100]

2.2.2 Non-organized Opposition

1. Anti-Globalists

Anti-globalists hold radical protests against things like worldwide poverty, abuse of human rights, child labor, pollution, global free trade, consumerism, et cetera. During their first World Social Forum in 2001 in Porto Alegre, Brazil, organized at the same time that the World Economic Forum met again in Davos, they opposed the negative effects of globalization and the practices of institutions like the IMF, the World Bank, and the WTO. Anti-globalists are known to disturb the regular meetings of these institutions. This is not because they are against globalization as such, but because, to them, globalization is an uncontrolled phenomenon with very negative effects for democracy, working conditions, the well-being of large numbers of people, and the preservation of our natural environment.[101] To them, globalization is treating the planet "as one vast commercial domain, where no rules or restrictions apply, and goods are exchanged with no heed for social, ethical, or environmental values. It's the hegemonic market, intent on devouring everything."[102]

One may not always agree with the methods anti-globalists use, but the increasing frequency of their demonstrations, seen for instance in Seattle, Madrid, Genoa, Prague, and Washington, D.C., and their successful mobilization activities through the internet have resulted in the ironic fact that, inspite of the media-imposed "anti-globalization" label, this movement has turned globalization into a living reality.[103] Besides, it is too simple just to label anti-globalists as agitators. After all, firstly, there is reason to disagree with the intentions of the IMF, the World Bank, and WTO if one observes, as in the first chapter, the outcomes of their policies. Secondly, we do pollute the environment.[104] Thirdly, there is every reason to be critical of the consequences of the dealings of agribusiness, the agrochemical industry, and the pharmaceutical firms in the field of genetically modified organisms.[105] Finally, there is abuse of human rights in many places in the world, and there is child labor.[106]

For that matter, it should be taken into account that, apart from a minority of firebrands, the majority of participants in the aforementioned demonstrations were respectable people who claimed their democratic right to oppose these abuses. And they are met with sympathy from many people on the sidelines. The Genoa protests, for example, were supported by over 60% of citizens in Germany, Greece, and France.[107]

There is another method of protest, thanks to what Friedman calls "internet activism." Its success can be illustrated with several examples.[108] The internet "has created new venues of and for collective resistance transcending national borders,"[109] which means that it has the power to mobilize people worldwide including influencing their voting behavior. I agree that things are going slowly because anti-globalists face an "uphill battle."[110] Nevertheless, there is some progress. It is very difficult for governments to monitor this kind of collective resistance, which, of course, is only open to those who have access to computers, modems, and the internet.[111] Meanwhile, global issues have stimulated the creation of a number of worldwide associations whose members use the internet in the interest of global ecology.[112]

The advantage anti-globalists have is that they urge people to take part in protests against developments that the greater majority of people worldwide do not agree with: increasing inequality, child labor, pollution, and so on. However, the number of protesters is still relatively small, so that their actual influence in changing the course of developments is rather limited. The internet, however, is a promising tool for mobilizing people to oppose the worship of the market as the most efficient way to coordinate human activities.[113]

2. The Power of Consumers

For a start, it should be realized that there is growing opposition to consumerism. People are, for example, rediscovering the benefits of healthy food,[114] cheap own-label products are making a comeback, and the number of Americans sticking to well-known brands is decreasing.[115] Ritzer calls these developments the first signs of "de-McDonaldization."[116] And, not unimportantly, ethics also plays a role in this changing consumer behavior.[117] This is an illustration of what Leadbeater calls people's "self-knowing," which makes them critical in their attitude toward the brands they enjoy. Through their individual self-rule, they, and not corporate marketing departments, are in charge of creating their own identity.[118]

The idea of a general convergence of global cultures assumes that aspects of global culture are accepted equally and uncritically worldwide. However, as demonstrated by the anthropologist Hannerz, for instance, global culture is not only consumed but, in accordance with specific contextual characteristics, also transformed.[119]

The power of consumers can be very effective. Next to the previously mentioned examples of Brent Spar, Heineken, and ABNAMRO, consumers, together with large shareholders, brought about a remuneration adjustment of the newly appointed CEO of Ahold in the Netherlands in 2003, and in the same year the chairman of the New York Stock Exchange was forced to withdraw for reasons of excessive remuneration. Hertz, therefore, is wrong when she argues that "consumer campaigns lack the legality of democratically enforced protests and, therefore, can easily be opposed by corporate business" (author's translation).[120] Firstly, she is wrong because the right to protest by way of extra-parliamentary action is an essential characteristic of democracies. Secondly, she is wrong because the aforementioned examples demonstrate that corporate opposition to consumer protests can be in vain.

The internet, again, is becoming an ever-more important instrument to express consumers' opposition to the present interpretation of the market economy. Via e-mail and thousands of homepages, meetings are organized, strategies discussed, and companies exposed as unscrupulous, while organizations like the Adbusters fight the consumption sickness by parodying well-known advertising campaigns. Others expose concrete abuses through professional research.[121] All these actions are about "X-raying the commodity culture" with the objective of "commodity defetishization."[122] The continuing spread of the internet may, in the longer term, develop into an effective means to counter the usual seller-centric marketing methods. These will, according to Mitchell, be replaced by buyer-centric methods, which will force producers to take customers' wishes ever more seriously. The internet will create a world of informed, sophisticated, sceptical, and even cynical consumers.[123] In making their purchasing decisions, these consumers will also take into account companies' behavior.

They will weigh the working conditions, for example, or their pollution policies. Consequently, customers will increasingly determine how consumer goods are produced.[124] Through the internet, customers will increasingly "talk to companies" via their websites. Illustrative, in this respect, is the fact that in 1993 Cisco Systems' call centers were dealing with 4,000 telephone calls a month from customers, a number which had increased to 950,000 five years later.[125]

Therefore, in terms of the continuum approach in this book, a reversal from seller-centric to buyer-centric marketing could redress the negative aspects of a globalizing economy, thus influencing movement along the continuum.

3. Critical Views on Economic Growth

For a long time, various authors have paid attention to the negative consequences of economic growth. A well-known example is J. K. Galbraith, who in 1958 launched a social commentary on wealth and inequality in the United States with his book *The Affluent Society*.[126] Ten years later, E. J. Mishan warned the readers of his book, *The Costs of Economic Growth*, against the tyranny of the dominant belief in growth.[127] Both publications have become part of the classic economic literature. The reason that critical views on economic growth are included in this book is because there is a generally accepted method of measuring economic growth. In this respect, there is no difference between an economic order that is mainly market-led and one where the government is the decisive factor. Both share the same interpretation of the concept of economic growth. China and the United States are examples. For both types of economic orders, the critics argue that the standard calculation methods regarding the concept of growth and GDP do not take into account the necessary "internalization of externalities,"[128] like pollution and resource depletion. However, for several decades, this interpretation has been contested among the critics themselves, who can be divided into several groups.

First, there are those who argue that "we are consuming the earth's resources beyond its sustainable capacities of renewal, thus running down that capacity over time," while at the same time calling this consumption "income."[129] Therefore, they maintain that economics and ecology should be combined in a scientific "trans-discipline" of "ecological economics" directed at sustainable development. Many organizations worldwide, like the Institute of Ecological Economics in Stockholm and the Environmental Economics Institute of the University of London, promote this approach.[130] These standard-bearers have achieved a certain degree of political consciousness in most developed countries, which has found expression in environmental legislation, though with considerable differences regarding legal regulations and their enforcement. All in all, critics of the first group hold the view that the industrialized world is fooling itself, since it includes in GDP not only the costs of pollution and the exhaustion of natural resources, but also the costs of crime and rising inequality. To them, the present interpretation of the concept of economic growth is "the triumph of the cash economy." It is a triumph of quantity over quality and thus part of a "collective hallucination," according to Sachs.[131] In order to come to a correct calculation, the costs of externalities should be subtracted from GDP so that a Genuine Progress Indicator (GPI),[132] or an Index of Sustainable Economic Welfare (ISEW),[133] remains.[134]

The second group comprises, economists like the Nobel Prize laureate A. Sen, who distinguish between growth and development. They criticize the fact that progress in the developed world is identified with growth of GDP, the increase of personal wealth, and technological innovation. Instead, to them, these aspects should be valued as a means to enlarge the freedoms of the members of society. These individual freedoms are also determined by factors like social and economic benefits and political and civil rights. In this view, development demands the elimination of important impediments to freedom, like poverty and tyranny; deficient economic opportunities and social provisions; neglect of necessary public facilities; and intolerance by oppressive regimes.[135] Instead of valuing economic growth as an objective in itself, governments should try to improve the quality of live and the freedoms we enjoy.[136] Consequently, to economists like Sen, social security is a necessary safety net to prevent people from falling into poverty and starvation, caused by a lack of economic freedom.[137]

Thirdly, there are those who want to bring an end to the dominating belief in quantitative economic growth altogether. Their viewpoint is that the subsystem of economics should no longer take its own expansion as the central objective of society but, instead, should play a supportive role amidst other subsystems.[138] If we apply this point of view to the care sectors of society, this would lead to a reversal of the demand for higher productivity in those sectors so that they could escape from reductions and cut-backs in expenditure, a demand which, because of the so-called Baumol effect, is unrealistic anyway.[139] Such a reversal would imply that the productive sectors of the economy would have to adjust to the needs of a caring society. Consequently, the economy would have to stay within the limits of what society interprets to be necessary care when determining investment and income policy, as well as productivity objectives.[140]

Finally, we have those who criticize the interpretation of the concept of scarcity in Western society. When, in 1969, a Dutch scholar contested this idea in his inauguration lecture, almost every economist in the Netherlands excoriated him.[141] There is no reason to assume that this would be different now. However, one must wonder if there really is so much wrong in criticizing the idea of scarcity in the majority of the Western world. What about a real shortage of consumer goods if, around the turn of the century, out of 525,000 new products launched in Europe within a period of 13 months, no less than 90% failed? What about real scarcity if, also around the turn of the century, packaged goods companies in the United States were spending $2 billion per year on product launches, development costs not included? What about scarcity, given the fact that, in 1975, a typical American supermarket sold 5,000 lines of products, a number that has grown to 35,000 today?[142]

Thus, we have four groups of critics concerned with the interpretation of the concept of economic growth. In terms of the approach in this book, all of these critics want market operations to be conditioned and controlled. Consequently, they want governments to interfere in the economic process to the benefit of non-economic objectives, including global sustainability in the longer term.

4. Civil Society

In political circles, it is believed that reforming the welfare state, which is thought to be necessary in order for countries to remain competitive in a globalizing economy, will be accompanied by the restoration of informal self-help mechanisms. This would be brought about by voluntary work or philanthropy by members of the "civil society," i.e., the area of association and action independent of the state and the market in which citizens can organize to pursue purposes that are important to them, individually and collectively, thus creating "social capital," which comprises things like "participation in the local community, feelings of trust and safety, social connections within the neighbourhood and among friends and family, a tolerance of diversity, and valuing life and work connections."[143] Civil-society actors include charitable societies, churches, neighborhood organizations, social clubs, civil rights lobbies, parent–teacher associations, unions, trade associations, and many other agencies.[144] These actors mobilize resources by appealing to cultural values and social purposes. Contrary to the private interests of business life and governments' pursuit of public interests, their actions are directed at the needs of social groups in society, particularly those groups which are hurt most by the dismantling of welfare state arrangements.[145] Mainly in the developing countries of Asia, Africa, and Latin America, voluntary associations have emerged with the intention to solve local problems by providing services that are needed. In addition to this, they press for better government.

However, voluntary work is also on the increase in the developed world, thus becoming an ever more important element of the welfare state. Some politicians call it the "lubricant" of society.[146] Clearly, some aspects of the welfare state, like care for the elderly and home care, would have very big problems if there were no volunteers to assist the professionals in daily care delivery in many countries of the European Union. If all these unpaid caring services were valued in financial terms, they would have a considerably positive impact on GDP.[147] It makes some sense, therefore, that the Independent Commission on Population and Quality of Life seeks "to redefine work in a broad sense that encompasses both employment and unpaid activities benefiting society as a whole."[148]

When moving to the right side of the continuum, i.e., leaving things increasingly to the market, voluntary work may to a certain extent be considered a substitute for legal welfare state arrangements. But it is an unstable factor.[149] One cannot count on it, and it is limited in scope.[150] All in all, one has to conclude that the influential power of civil society regarding movement along the continuum is limited to the voting behavior of the individual participants. Moreover, despite the noble intentions of volunteers, it is difficult to prevent a certain amount of condescension connected to their work. This is work that, according to Galbraith, fits in "the doctrine that if the horse is amply fed with oats, some will pass through to the road for the sparrows."[151]

2.3 Summary

As argued in the first chapter, it is legitimate for interest groups outside the political structures to try to influence how a society moves along the continuum, i.e., pursuing more or less government interference in the economic process. This topic was the subject of this second chapter. As the first step in this analysis, I distinguished between promoters and opponents. Promoters are those who want the market economy to be increasingly liberalized. Opponents want the opposite, through government control of the economic process.

As for the promoters, corporate business is the most important interest group. Many authors argue that it has considerable power to influence the course of events in a free-market economy. There are even those who believe that corporate business has overruled politics. Consequently, an increasingly liberal free-market economy will be inescapable. To achieve its objectives, corporate business has every interest in maintaining and extending a supply economy. Advertizing, even directed at very young children, to breed consumerism, is instrumental to that.

The methods used by corporate business to achieve its objectives are not uncontested. From different perspectives, opponents try to counterbalance the objectives of corporate business. They want governments to control the free-market economy. Here, unionized labor plays a role. Unions have contributed considerably to the establishment of the welfare state. However, since the 1980s, the unions' influence over movements along the continuum seems to be decreasing. Nevertheless, they remain an important factor in the social-economic infrastructure of democracies at the national level. At the international and global level, however, the influence of unionized labor seems to be less relevant.

Non-governmental organizations and the so-called anti-globalists can also be considered opponents. Their opposition to the dealings of corporate business is attracting more and more attention, not in the least because their protests are proving to be increasingly successful. The same applies for consumers.

As for the church, it has a long history of dominance regarding the development of society. The Industrial Revolution was very important in shaping the role of the church, since it produced a lot of misery for working people in free-market economies. Though many individual clergymen expressed their concern about the lot of the workers, it took more than 100 years of industrial revolution before the church, as a social institution, took a stand. The encyclical letter *Rerum Novarum* marked a turning point. Since then, the church, Roman Catholic as well as Protestant, have spoken out regularly on social developments. It is doubtful, however, if at present the church is able to influence the free-market economy effectively.

A specific way to try to influence present-day free market operations is to promote alternative interpretations of the concept of economic growth. If these alternative precepts were followed, negative consequences like increasing inequality and pollution would be subtracted when determining economic growth.

Finally, there are those who believe that the withdrawal of governments from the economic process will automatically be compensated for by developments in "civil society." Thus, a free-market economy will induce a revival of informal cooperation. It is a perilous undertaking, however, to make social developments dependent on the good will of citizens.

3
The Arguments

As indicated in the first chapter, in the United States and within the European Union, a balance between expenditure and revenue for financing the welfare state had been reached by about 2000. Strong economic growth at the end of the millennium was helpful in this respect. This, however, did not prevent governments from continuing to reform their welfare states. The fourth phase of fundamental reforms to systems of social security through the introduction of other methods of financing and paying benefits and the re-allocation of responsibilities between governments and social partners is still underway. To explain this phenomenon, I examine two arguments that are used by governments from 1975 onward to legitimize their continued pursuit of this new goal, i.e., reducing public spending. These arguments, one economic (that is, globalization) and one ideological[1] (that is, new dogmas), are the subject of this chapter.

3.1 On Globalization

The economic argument justifying reduced public spending is that global competition forces employers to reduce the costs of labor, which are an important source of funding for social security.

During the period 1960–1985, the term *globalization* was not yet the buzzword it is at present. These days, however, it is generally accepted that, in a globalizing economy, the costs of a country's social security system can weaken its competitive position. Whether one reads government policy documents,[2] the viewpoints of advisory bodies,[3] pamphlets of political parties,[4] or documents of the European Union,[5] the policies of both the United States and the European Union are very much the same, and they share the same motivation, namely, that the costs of social security are a burden to corporate business in a global economy. Apparently, we have to accept, in the words of former United States President Clinton, that nations, i.e., national economies, are like big corporations, competing in a global marketplace.[6] Consequently, the global market will determine the way that national economies can organize their societies. The global market will dictate the content of the solidarity principle. Apparently, the global market has taken the lead.

Over the past ten years, the phenomenon of globalization has been the subject of countless puplications. The result is a variety of incompatible opinions and ideas.[7] Trawling through this mound of literature makes it clear that "the only consensus about globalization is that it is contested."[8] Opinions differ as to how to define the phenomenon, its origins,[9] and the way it should be analyzed.[10] I will not go into all these matters but will instead limit myself to describing a range of views on how the phenomenon of "accelerated globalization"[11] should be appreciated. This type of globalization started around 1975. Since then, the spread of "supra-territoriality" (see section 1.3) has been caused primarily by the co-dependent influence of rationalism as the dominant knowledge framework; by capitalism and the drive for surplus accumulation; by technological innovations in communications and data processing; and by regulation facilitating technical and procedural standardization, the liberalization of cross-border movements of money, investments, goods, and services, the guarantees of property rights for global capital, and the legalization of global organizations and activities. It is a time of the "greatest increase in the number, variety, intensity, institutionalization, awareness and impact of supra-territorial phenomena."[12] It is also a time in which globalization has shown unprecedented characteristics, which have been summarized by Legrain as follows: (1) the sheer size of globalization is impressive; until around 1980, it was limited to Europe, the United States, and Asian countries like Japan, South Korea, Thailand, Hong Kong, Taiwan, and Singapore, covering roughly a quarter of the world population. (2) Globalization has accelerated, thanks to developments in transport and communications. (3) World trade is at record highs, being 25% of world GDP in 2000 compared to 8% in 1950. (4) The range of traded products is bigger than ever before, because nowadays services like telecommunications, insurance, software, and finance are also globally traded. (5) Foreign direct investment increased tremendously from $50 billion in 1985 to $1,3 trillion in 2000. (6) Multinationals have become very important; most of world trade is between subsidiaries of individual companies. (7) Nowadays, manufacturing and production are dispersed around the world, with each step in the production process performed where it can be done in the cheapest way. (8) International financial flows have increased beyond human imagination; starting at around $10 billion a day in the early 1970s, currency dealers now trade around $1.2 trillion a day.[13] Summarized, these aspects suggest that globalization refers to the multitude of interconnections between societies that shape the present world system. Globalization describes "the process through which events, decisions and activities in a certain part of the world may cause important consequences for individuals and societies in other parts of the world."[14]

As to the question of how to interpret globalization, Gilpin distinguishes between three differing views.[15]

Firstly, he refers to the communitarian perspective, which is promoted by environmentalists, human-rights advocates, and others who want the world order to be more just, environmentally sound, and egalitarian. They denounce globalization "for foisting a brutal capitalist tyranny, imperialist exploitation, and environmental degradation upon the peoples of the world."[16] Among them there are those who fear the unrivalled power of big financial and industrial corporations who can decide the fate of millions of people.[17] These anti-globalists stipulate the negative effects of globalization, like (a) growing social differences, not only caused by polarization within and between countries, but also worldwide; (b) the leveling down of wages, labor conditions, and social security; and (c) the subsequent erosion of democracy.[18] The French author Viviane Forrester is a good example of an anti-globalist. In her opinion, globalization has become a religious conviction that has resulted in a growing concentration of power in multinational corporations that only pursue the interests of their shareholders, while mercilessly playing poker with laborers all over the world. Governments appear to be incapable of influencing this development. Vehemently, Forrester denounces the ultraliberal philosophy, which is only about money, profits, and the stock market and for which social interests do not count. That philosophy legitimizes unregulated competition, resulting in slavery in the Third World, underpayment in the West, and devastation of the natural environment. To Forrester, globalization refers to a new political system that does not show its true colors. It is a system that ignores those who should control it.[19] And she is not alone. Critics like Klein, Hertz, Cameron, Lubbers, Ehrenreich, Abrams, and Franks (interestingly, all are female authors) are cast in the same mold.[20]

Secondly, there are those who look at globalization from the free market perspective. Many adherents of this view are economists, business leaders, and politicians. They are opposed to strict regulation of the world economy. They believe that a free-as-possible market will increase efficiency in the use of the world's scarce resources. Moreover, these supporters of globalization believe that a free market will strengthen commercial and other bonds among democratic market-oriented societies, thus promoting world peace. In short, to the defenders of the free market, globalization is a blessing. It is "part of the natural evolutionary process. [...] It goes hand in hand with the progress of humanity, something which history tells no one can stand in the way of."[21] Contrary to the views expressed by opponents of globalization, supporters of globalization like Leadbeater hold the view that the critics' pessimism is overdone and self-fulfilling.[22] To him, radical anti-globalists "are latter-day heirs to the traditions of socialism: a romantic response to a world disenchanted by capitalism and a natural world subordinated to technology."[23] Anti-globalists, according to Leadbeater, have long passed the point of realism. "It has become a chronic condition, invariably overdone, morally self-righteous and often just wrong."[24] Nevertheless, he agrees with the anti-globalists that the modern world has some features that need to be reformed, especially inequality and environmental degradation. But to him, reducing global poverty, inequality, poor health, and hunger is best addressed by creating a more integrated and more equitable economy. To achieve this, the global agenda must move on from markets and finance to global governance and social programs. For Leadbeater, this is a condition of the success of globalization or, in other words, for globalization "to be seen as legitimate, world poverty has to be further reduced and dramatically; corporations will have to acknowledge their wider social responsibilities for health, education and the environment as part of the process of economic development from which they benefit; international institutions will have to give greater voice to poorer developing nations; those nations will have to be helped by public and private investments to better equip them to take advantage of international trade; markets in the north will have to be further opened to exporters from the south. It is a big agenda but one that we are now embarked upon."[25] This last point precisely indicates the difference between the optimistic Leadbeater and the pessimistic anti-globalists. Leadbeater may be accused of wishful thinking. His argumentation contains too many "ifs" and "buts." He rightfully accuses the pessimistic anti-globalists of exaggeration at some points. He is also right that innovation and creativity, thanks to technological developments, can be of help in making the world a better place. But that is not today's global reality.[26]

Like Leadbeater, Legrain is also an optimist. To him, it is time to move the debate about globalization forward and focus on the question of what kind of globalization we want. He assumes that we are still free to determine our future through the power of elected governments. Furthermore, according to Legrain, we can pick out the bits of globalization we like and do away with the things we do not like. We can do both: "Our challenge is to grasp the opportunities that globalization offers, while taking the sting out of its threats."[27] Few aspects of globalization are inevitable if there is a will to stop them. Although this sounds wonderful, reality is different. Though Legrain may be right when he argues that globalization and social spending can be complementary,[28] the policies pursued in practice by, for instance, the IMF and the World Bank, are different.[29] Though he may be right that people who need to be equipped with new skills to find another job should meanwhile be protected by a decent welfare system,[30] reality is different. Though he may be right that people in low-paid jobs should be subsidised so that they can have a decent life,[31] reality is different. Though he may be right that society should maintain a generous welfare system so that the least fortunate do not fall by the wayside,[32] reality is different. In short, Legrain's views suffer from shortcomings comparable to those of Leadbeater: too many "ifs" and "buts." Nevertheless, his summaries are more concrete. To him, (1) globalization is primarily a political choice, not an inevitable fate; (2) globalization benefits rich countries as well as poor ones; and (3) though the effects of globalization may look ugly, things are better than they were before.[33] He concludes, "All sorts of things are wrong with the world, but globalization is overwhelmingly a force for good."[34] Both of these optimistic authors acknowledge implicitly that there is something wrong with the way free-market globalization is shaping today's world.

Finally, there are those who represent the populist or nationalist perspective. They blame globalization for growing economic inequality, high unemployment levels, the demise of the welfare state, the destruction of national cultures and national political autonomy, illegal immigration, and increasing crime. Supporters of this view can be found, according to Gilpin, within unionized labor, among business leaders facing competition from imports, and among economic nationalists. They want restrictions on free trade as well as on the investment activities of foreign multinational businesses.

Apart from the fact that it is difficult to distinguish precisely between populists and communitarians, Gilpin's approach needs to be rounded out with several other views on globalization.

Firstly, there are those who think that all the fuss about globalization is overdone. Michael Porter, for instance, holds the view that it is not globalization but the national environment which determines a corporation's competitive advantage.[35] Furthermore, Ruigrok and Van Tulder conclude that the worldwide operational activities of the 100 biggest corporations are rather limited,[36] whereas the OECD argues that competition does not, to a large extent, come from low-wage countries, but from trade within and between OECD countries.[37] The reality of international relations appears to be a reflection of regional activities. In line with this, Hirst and Thompson claim that the world economy is not really global but centerd in Europe, Japan, and the United States. They present data on trade, foreign direct investment,[38] and financial flows that show that globalization is concentrated in the developed countries.[39] In 1994, these three regions together produced 87% of the total world manufacturing output and generated 80% of world merchandise export, rising from 76% and 71% (respectively) in 1980.[40]

Meanwhile, it would be unwise to deny the dynamics of our daily environment. These dynamics show that there is indeed something going on; for instance, there is an increasing number of possible business locations, especially in the countries of Eastern Europe after the collapse of communism in 1990.[41] Despite the fact that the domestic market produces the major part of a country's gross domestic product, these dynamics cause the dominant segments and corporations, the so-called "strategic cores" of all economies, to be closely interrelated with the world market. Their fate is a function of their performance on that market.[42] For them, the nationality of corporations is irrelevant in a "borderless world."[43]

Secondly, and contrary to those who assume that globalization is primarily a trade-driven phenomenon,[44] people like Thomas Friedman, for instance, hold the view that globalization is mainly technology driven, with the internet playing an important role. Starting with 200 internet connections in 1981, we saw an increase to 300,000 in 1990, 50,000,000 in 1999,[45] 140,000,000 in 2000[46] to over 1 billion connections in 2006[47]. In 2000, there were already 2.8 million Web sites with a total of 800 million pages.[48] These technological developments, combined with the fact that, since the end of the Cold War, there has been no major ideological alternative to free-market capitalism, have resulted in a global democratization of technology, finance, and information. The internet, according to Friedman, is becoming "the turbocharged engine that drives globalization forward."[49] This is an engine that can easily be used by everyone who wants to do so. There is no exclusivity in this matter. Countries who take part in this type of democratization are joining the "electronic herd," which is symbolized by the omnipresence of McDonald's, KFC, Nike, and other world brands. Countries who oppose this development will lag behind in the creation of wealth.[50]

Thirdly, there are those who focus on the cultural aspects of globalization. One example is Huntington's work, *The Clash of Civilizations*.[51] This clash may have emerged because globalization forces completely different cultures to meet, whether they like it or not. In this respect, Barber concludes that "caught between Babel and Disneyland, the planet is falling precipitously apart and coming reluctantly together at the very same moment."[52] To him, there are two possible future scenarios. The first is a "retribalization of large swaths of humankind by war and bloodshed." It is a scenario of *jihad* against interdependence, against cooperation, against technology, against modernity, et cetera. In short, it is a scenario directed at combating Friedman's electronic herd. In line with this, Huntington assumes that "the dangerous clashes of the future are likely to arise from the interaction of Western arrogance, Islamic intolerance, and Sinic assertiveness."[53] To him, the revival of non-Western religions is not a rejection of modernity, but a rejection "of the West and of the secular, relativistic, degenerate culture associated with the West." It is a rejection of "Westoxification" by non-Western societies.[54] Similarly, Fukuyama holds the view that the present revival of Islamic fundamentalism is partly caused by the fact that liberal Western values are experienced as a threat by traditional Islamic societies.[55]

Barber's other scenario is completely in line with Friedman's idea of the electronic herd, "pressing nations into one homogenous global theme park, one McWorld, tied together by communications, information, entertainment and commerce."[56] In other words, "*jihad* pursues a bloody politics of identity; McWorld, a bloodless economics of profit."[57]

Whatever the different views regarding the concept of globalization, they all refer to a increasing worldwide interconnectedness. More and more, national and regional economies are linked through trade, financial flows, and foreign investments, with technological progress, particularly in the field of communications, and the liberalization of capital flows as important engines for growth. Since 1975, these engines for growth have accelerated the globalization process and have contributed to hyper-competition.[58] Despite the many differing opinions being proffered, however, daily experience would seem to support only one interpretation: that globalization forces corporate business to reduce the costs of labor in a globalizing economy. This view is supported by politicians at national and international levels. It is an attitude of helplessness, of "there's nothing one can do." Consequently, global forces are thought to be inescapably beyond political control. Globalization, therefore, rules the world.[59]

3.2 New Dogmas

In section 1.2, I showed that, around 2000, the United States and the countries of the European Union appeared to have succeeded once again in balancing their accounts with respect of social security. Nevertheless, since that time, for ideological and economic reasons, fundamental changes regarding systems of social security have continued at a rapid pace. The preceding section dealt with the phenomenon of globalization. The present section will elaborate two further aspects that have together contributed to a change in the outlook of the economic order of the developed world. In subsection 3.2.1, I will deal with neo-liberal views on the economic order in more detail.[60] In subsection 3.2.2, attention will be paid to a new morality, the so-called theory of "public choice." In combination, these two attitudes are the foundation of the present-day international political economy of the developed world, which is characterized by a move to the right side of the continuum.

3.2.1 Neo-Liberal Views on the Economic Order

According to neo-liberals, the ultimate objective of the economic order is to satisfy the needs of individual consumers in the best possible way. All other objectives are expected to be subordinate to that. As for the preferred economic order to achieve this ultimate objective, neo-liberals choose a free market economy, with the price mechanism as the instrument for coordination, instead of a government as the central planning institution. The preferred market economy, however, needs complementary and corrective measures in order to achieve its ultimate objective. This is a matter of political economy. Therefore, some understanding of the instrumental neo-liberal objectives for society, as well as the way these objectives could be achieved, may shed some light on neo-liberal views of the economic order. In this respect, one can distinguish between two types of instrumental neo-liberal objectives, namely, (1) those which are directly *related to the economic order*; and (2) those which are particularly *related to the economic process.*

To the first type belong, first of all, instruments which assist the *optimal allocation of the means of production*. This optimal allocation can be achieved by promoting *perfect competition*, *coordination*, and the *international division of labor*, as well as by *labor and capital mobility*. Pursuing perfect competition not only requires governments to take actions against phenomena like oligopoly, monopoly, cartels, and trusts, because they impede equality of opportunity, but it also requires governments to oversee the administration and coordination of activities regarding territorial and other natural resources, as well as environmental planning.[61] As for the international division of labor, neo-liberals support the free movement of goods, services, capital, and labor. To them, labor mobility can be increased with help from employment agencies, as well as through continuous education and retraining. Neo-liberals favor subsidizing these activities, because this creates equal opportunities. Because very high labor mobility would be incompatible with neo-liberals' need to prevent people from proletarianization and "massafication," capital mobility is also a neo-liberal objective. Capital mobility could be increased through corrections to company legislation and taxation.[62]

A second and very important instrumental neo-liberal objective that is directly related to the functioning of the economic order is *price stability.* To neo-liberals, a sound monetary system is essential to the free play of price-making forces. Over-investment, caused by the creation of money by federal banks, should be prevented.[63]

Furthermore, neo-liberals realize that a free market economy requires complementary and corrective measures that are also directly related to an optimal functioning of the economic order. Here, instrumental neo-liberal objectives are the *provision of collective needs,* the *equalization of individual and social costs, alterations in the distribution of incomes and wealth, prioritizing specific branches of industry, expansion of production, full employment*, as well as *controlling the size and composition of the population.*[64] In the framework of this book, it is important to mention that, to neo-liberals, one of the tasks of governments regarding collective needs is to supply the goods that the market cannot or can only sub-optimally deliver, like transport facilities, defence, health care and education.[65] However, here too the market is paramount. Market sub-optimality regarding social security, for example, is an argument for neo-liberals to establish compulsory social insurance systems. Such systems, however, should stipulate personal responsibility and be as much as possible in accordance with a free market economy.

As for the second type of instrumental objectives, neo-liberals realize that a free market economy as such is no guarantee that the objectives of the economic order will be achieved. For this, it is necessary to make use of instruments of political economy. These instruments are *related to the economic process*. Neo-liberals distinguish between five categories: (1) *instruments that affect the institutional framework of the economic order;* (2) *the exchange rate;* (3) *monetary instruments;* (4) *financial instruments;* and (5) *direct controls.*

To the first category belong, first of all, the *fundamentals of the economic order.* Neo-liberals oppose, for example, the nationalization of the means of production, as well as statutory industrial organizations and worker participation beyond the level of the individual company. These activities are believed to hinder the solution of coordination problems in a free-market economy, because they may impede the optimal functioning of the price mechanism.[66] Also belonging to the first category is the idea of *free competition*. For this, free access to the market, private ownership, and freedom of contract are essential. Free competition should not take place at the expense of suppliers, creditors, laborers, the treasury, and shareholders. Furthermore, free competition should be governed by a very strict law of obligations, and agreements directed at collectively influencing the market should be forbidden.[67]

As a rule, neo-liberals are promoters of free unionization. They acknowledge the right to strike as long as this does not impede the freedom of others. Therefore, neo-liberals favor measures to prevent unions from having too much power. To them, unemployment is caused to a large degree by the way the labor market is organized. The performance of the unions has caused a downward rigidity of wages and labor immobility. In turn, wage rigidity is caused by unemployment benefits, making it possible for unions to demand excessive wage increases. The resulting (further) unemployment is not their business. That problem has to be solved by employers and the government, according to neo-liberals.

As for the exchange rate, monetary and financial measures, as well as direct controls, it is sufficient to say that neo-liberals want these matters to be organized in such a way that each and every influence that disturbs the economic process will be excluded or corrected. The international money system should function as automatically as possible, be based on the market economy, and be directed at the improvement of the international division of labor. Though direct controls are not favored in neo-liberal circles, it is accepted that they could be applied in special circumstances.

Considering the objectives of the economic order and the instruments neo-liberals want to deploy in the economic process, it should be kept in mind that neo-liberals acknowledge that their ideas on perfect competition are rather theoretical. To them, the perfect market is an ideal construction, worthy to be pursued. Thus, neo-liberalists admit the more-or-less utopian character of their approach.[68]

The realization of their convictions, however, meets two important problems. First of all, there must be the political will to change the economic order. Secondly, their wish to implement neo-liberal ideas may be defeated by inevitable historical and technical irregularities. The two problems together imply that neo-liberals do not take into account the dynamics of the economic order. Consequently, they do not have clear answers on how to counter those problems, and to the extent that they think they do have answers, there is much disagreement. Neo-liberalism, however, is an open system, directed at changing the economic order by trial and error. This may lead to changes in the objectives of the economic order, as well as to attempts to try adjustments or other instruments for interference in the economic process. Only in this way can the functioning of the economic order be improved.[69]

Neo-liberalism, therefore, appears to suffer from the same shortcomings that market socialism and welfare economics suffered from after the Second World War (section 1.1.2). And the reasons are the same: the shortcomings are caused by the dynamics of the economic order. Happily, these dynamics make it impossible to capture life even in complicated equations with very many unknowns. The information age has not changed this.

In reaction to the dynamics of the economic order, politics has two options. One is carefully coping with these shortcomings by adjusting and correcting. The other is maintaining the chosen course. Choosing the second option turns theories of the economic order into dogmas. That is what has happened with Adam Smith's original ideas. It led to misery for many people. That is what has happened with market socialism. It delivered a huge bureaucracy and neglected the advantages of private initiative for the development of the economic order. That is what is happening now with neo-liberal politics, bringing misery for an increasing number of people again.

Indeed, in contrast to the ideas of scholars like Hayek, Eucken, Robbins, and others, neo-liberalism has become a dogma, i.e., an unshakable belief that is no longer subject to debate. Consequently, neo-liberalism has developed into a number of linked-up slogans, summarized by Palast as "cut government, cut the budgets and bureaucracies and the rules they make; privatise just about everything; deregulate currency and capital markets, free the banks to speculate in currency and shift capital across borders. But don't stop there. Open every nation's industry to foreign trade, eliminate those stodgy old tariffs and welcome foreign ownership without limit; wipe away national border barriers to commerce; let the market set prices on everything from electricity to water; and let the arbitrageurs direct our investments. Then haul those old government bureaucracies to the guillotine: cut public pensions, cut welfare, cut subsidies; let politics shrink and let the market-place guide us."[70] These are slogans, indeed, but to a substantial extent they are also today's reality. Of course, this is partly a reaction to the bureaucratic excesses of the third quarter of the 20th century. But I believe there is more to it. Present politics is also imbued with the spirit of the new times. I call this spirit the new morality.

3.2.2 The Theory of Public Choice

As I said in the first chapter, solidarity is believed to be the cement of society. Without it, a society cannot exist. Because of this, the history of Western civilization is not only an expression of continuously changing combinations of self-interest and solidarity, it is also a history of relational tensions between individuals and society, due to fundamental changes in social structures and frames of reference. Many years ago, these changing social structures were the subject of study and research by scholars like Durkheim, Weber, and Marx.[71] Like in their days, today there is a growing interest regarding (a lack of) cohesion in society. And, just as it was then, this is happening in a time of fundamentally changing social structures.[72]

One might argue that the final quarter of the 20th century, like the times of Durkheim, Weber, and Marx, saw the beginning of another change in the character of society. More specifically, the beginning of the "information age" meant that individuals were no longer embedded in society, were no longer subjected to social control, and instead simply pursued their self-interest (Durkheim). Again, we see a more subjective individual and a more abstract society (Weber). And, like Marx, we could become pessimistic if we were to analyze the way we organise our production processes to exploit low-skilled workers. We clearly live in times where changing attitudes have their influence on the way people who live in the same society relate to each other. I call this the new morality, or a new dogma, which has as its point of departure that rational people, out of self-interest, only pursue the maximization of personal utility.[73]

In literature, this is called the theory of "public choice." This theory can be defined as "the economic study of non-market decision-making, or simply the application of economics to political science."[74] From the viewpoint of economics, the subject matters of this theory are the state, voting behavior, party politics, and bureaucracy.

The theory largely developed as a separate field after 1950, in reaction to the ideas on the effectiveness of models of "market socialism," which assumed that governments could supplant the price mechanism and allocate goods as efficiently as markets do (Buchanan, Tullock, Olsen, Downs, etc.). As I mentioned in section 1.1.2, supporters of market socialism held the view that state intervention in the economic process was needed to avoid the inefficient shortfalls of private investment and to correct the distributional inequities created by the market. Keynesian economics rests on this view. Although the prosperity of the years after the Second World War reduced concerns about unemployment and distributional issues, concerns about market efficiency remained strong among economists, which led to numerous publications on the conditions necessary for efficient market allocation, against the background of ideas on public goods, externalities, and economies of scale. The market was thought to fail to achieve a

Pareto-optimum if these conditions were not met, which, in turn, provided a rationale for the existence of the state. Consequently, the state exists as an alternative to the market to provide public goods and to neutralize externalities. Also, according to the theory of public choice, the production of public goods should be dealt with in the same way as the production of private goods, which entails (1) behavioral assumptions similar to those that apply in general economics (rational, utilitarian individuals); (2) depicting preference revelation as an analog to the market (voters engage in exchange, voting is a way in which individuals reveal their demand schedules); and (3) asking the same questions asked in price theory (is there equilibrium, is it stable, is it Pareto-efficient?).[75] However, as I will argue in chapter eleven, the reality is not as simple and depressing as the theory of public choice assumes.

The economic model for the proponents of public choice is that of the neo-liberal market of perfect competition. Equilibrium in that market is the result of voluntary exchanges between individuals who are pursuing their own interests. Shifts in that equilibrium are a consequence of efficient allocation. This also applies to labor, which is considered a commodity that responds primarily to market signals. If supply is abundant, its price will go down, and vice versa. Governments should not interfere in this market by embedding it in social arrangements, because that would hamper perfect competition. Consequently, relocating production to low-wage countries is only a matter of allocation efficiency or structural adjustment policy. Markets develop naturally and inevitably. They are self-regulating allocation mechanisms.[76] The proponents of public choice use this idealized model when they list the characteristics of political action, including the bureaucratic apparatus associated with such action. Thus, voters become consumers; political parties become companies that put competing services and tax proposals on the market in exchange for votes, political propaganda becomes advertising; and government institutions are public services that are dependent on political support to cover their costs. In this philosophy, the market is a completely neutral place where people meet as strangers who are interested only in buying or selling.[77] In other words, the proponents of public choice regard the political system as a market of supply and demand for "public goods," i.e., everything that is put forward by a political rather than a market process, including "transfer payments" which ensue from social security.[78] In this view, political connections become a commodity that can be sold on the market.[79] Thus, nowadays aspiring politicians "market their personalities rather than their beliefs or platforms, relying on a growing number of political consultants for promotional assistance." Also, "the well-marketed politician has less need of a political party."[80]

These same proponents of the theory of public choice have also launched an attack on bureaucracy, in particular since it adversely deviates from the real market in lacking both a profit motive as well as a competitive drive.[81] Therefore, they allege that the growth of bureaucracy is entirely bound up with the self-interest of civil servants in terms of salary, esteem, and influence, all culminating in budget maximizing. In this respect, former United States President Reagan is known for his ideological credo, "Get government off our backs!"[82]

3.2.3 The Two Dogmas Combined

As indicated in the preface, since 1975, the ideas of the proponents of the theory of public choice have, in particular, provided the explicit or implicit *leitmotif* for the policies of various political leaders in the Western world. Reagan and Thatcher were the main world leaders who adhered to this doctrine. After coming into office in 1981, the French President Mitterand was an exception to this rule, until he faced a strong right-wing opposition in the National Assembly after the elections of 1986.[83] Though less pronounced, this also applies to the governments of Australia, New Zealand, and the Netherlands, the last of which invented the "no nonsense" policy. The ideology of the Keynesian welfare state, which had dominated politics in the West until the late 1970s, appeared to be losing its relevance. Instead, combating the shortcomings in the functioning of the market system through selective government interventions and the state's interest in effective social welfare disappeared. The new course was to restore the stimuli for an entrepreneurial spirit.

In the United States, the inauguration of President Reagan in 1980 was a milestone for this restoration. From that point onward, the policy of the American federal government became "the political translation of a new morality, specially designed for the winners, the rich and the do-gooders."[84] There were six basic elements to this new morality.

First of all, the new morality favored tax reduction, in particular for the highest income brackets, so that the prosperous would be induced to make greater efforts in taking initiative and in investments.[85] The second element was that expenditure on defense had to be increased to combat communism effectively, which led to Reagan doubling the Pentagon budget in four years,[86] causing a gigantically increasing budget deficit.

The third element was the elimination of poverty from the public conscience. This element was based on the idea that supporting the poor did no good to their personal development and their sense of enterprise.[87] Following his advisors, Reagan described federal support for the poor as a wasteful and destructive form of socialism which encouraged immoral behavior.[88] This moral element provided a legal basis for reducing expenditure on social security in order to provide a partial solution to the budget deficit. The concept of social justice was rejected as untrue, "as an illusory ideal which triggered an endless growth of the state and led to wasteful schemes of redistribution to placate particular interests."[89] Consequently, unemployment benefits, training courses, food stamps, child nutrition, and rent subsidies became the subject of budget reductions.[90] Reagan and his advisors operated some 25 years ago. Recently, however, people like Dinesh D'Souza have appeared, espousing the same principles proclaiming that markets work so efficiently that the declining economic and social condition of minority groups must be the result of their "inherent inferiority."[91]

The fourth element of the new morality is the simple observation that the government cannot be the answer to all problems, because regulation and a helping hand from the state "were destroying the essence of an enterprise culture."[92] Less government intervention was indicated, therefore.

Breaking the power of the trade unions, the fifth element, was intended to contribute to ending the micro-economic pressure of wages on prices. To establish this trend, Reagan fired 11,400 air traffic control workers on 5 August 1981.[93]

Finally, the new morality involved an alternative monetary policy, the sixth element. By making it more difficult for companies to borrow money by increasing interest rates, employers would have to turn down wage claims in order to survive.[94]

This new morality was a fertile breeding ground for the present neo-liberal version of capitalism. It is a form of capitalism that seeks to limit government interference in the economic process as much as possible. Competitive self-seeking and the quest for profit are "the queen of virtues."[95] This new morality recommends deregulation and privatization of state utilities. It wants governments to stop protectionism, and it champions free trade. Governments should leave as many things as possible to the market, because the market is the primary institution in human affairs. And since human behavior is, at its core, materialist and utilitarian, moral values and cultural norms are derived from economic orientation.[96] In fact, national defense could be the only exception. Detention could be left to private enterprise. The same applies for water and electricity supplies, garbage collection, public transport, education, and health care. In short, these are all the neo-liberal slogans mentioned before.

What were the effects of this new morality? Apart from exacerbating income inequalities, for which figures will be delivered in the next chapter, the following information from the Reagan period is illustrative.

Of all the developed countries, America had the highest crime rate, the highest use of drugs, and the lowest inoculation rate. America was 22nd on the world list for infant mortality. On average, the vaccination figures were 40% lower than in other industrialized countries. Teenagers accounted for 10% of all pregnancies. One in five American children lived below the poverty line. In 1987, 12 million children were not insured against medical expenses, which was a rise of 14% since 1981.[97] Despite the fact that 81% of Americans considered health care to be a right and not a privilege,[98] many Americans were not insured or were underinsured against the costs of health care, and government expenditure on health care was 41% below that in any other OECD country.[99]

In implementing the new morality, Reagan found a British collaborator in Margaret Thatcher. During her government, capital gains tax, which had been as high as 98% under Labor governments, fell to 40%. The gap between rich and poor during her regime had never been as great since 1945. After the Conservatives came to power in 1979, the purchasing power of the richest 10% of Britons increased by no less than 50%. In contrast, the poorest 10% fell back by 17%. As a result, the number of Britons dependent on income support increased from 7 million in 1979 to 11 million in 1993.[100] In short, under Thatcher, the United Kingdom became a society in which "inequality is legitimate and welfare policies are subordinate to economic ends." This "two nations" effect was increasingly evident not only in the polarization of income but also in the provision of services.[101] Regarding the latter, the development of the NHS since Thatcher is a good example.

The new morality, which Phillips calls social Darwinism,[102] has, after the United States and the United Kingdom, also gained ground on the European continent.

According to an article in a British newspaper, *The Mail on Sunday*, the highest-paid 10% of the populations of the United Kingdom, France, and Germany together earned on average 3.5 times more than the lowest-paid 10% in 1995. Even more important is the fact that this gap grew over the years.[103] For the Netherlands, the average disposable income of the 20% least prosperous citizens fell by 10% in real terms between 1983 and 1991. In contrast, the average disposable income of the 20% most prosperous households grew by 12.5% over the same period. In 1980, the average income of the unemployed was 60% of that of the employed. In 1989, it was 40%. Finally, in 1989 the richest 10% of Dutch households had more than eight times as much to spend than the poorest 10%. In 1991, this was 11 times as much.[104] During this period, the trend was no different in other European countries. The overall tendency has been for the differences to increase, with the associated element that this increase appears to be accelerating.[105] As a result, on the European continent, the number of poor people is growing. In an official document of the European Commission of 1994, the number of poor people in the European Union was estimated at 50 million, which is around 15% of the population.[106]

3.3 Summary

This chapter dealt with two arguments that together constitute the driving force behind the present-day international political economy. The first argument is an economic argument that assumes that global competitive relations force employers to reduce their costs of labor as much as possible. Therefore, a reduction in public spending is inescapable. This argument pressures welfare states to shrink.

In addition to this there is an ideological argument that combines the two dogmas of neo-liberalism and individualization. This further legitimizes the pressure to shrink.

Since around 1975, initiated by Reagan and Thatcher, these arguments have provided the explicit or implicit *leitmotif* for the policies of political leaders of the Western world. Characteristic for these policies is declining government interference in the economic process, leaving that process, through deregulation and privatization, increasingly to the market. As a result, an increasing number of people do not share in the overall increase in wealth.

4
The Effects

The preceding chapter dealt with two factors that are decisive for a political economy moving to the right side of the continuum. In both cases, the market is assumed to be the most efficient instrument for the pursuit of individual wealth. It is with a certain euphoria that Western political leaders claim the success of this market.

For example, in his final State of the Union address, former United States President Clinton proudly declared that the United States was in its longest period of strong economic growth in history, and Al Gore tried to boost his election campaign by stating the fact that eight years of the Clinton administration had resulted in job growth of millions. The question is, however, at what expense was this "growthmanship"[1] realized? The answer is clear: at the expense of labor conditions. Examples include decreasing wages, longer working weeks, "one day contracts,"[2] and "moonlighting,"[3] lost social security benefits for employees, and massive redundancies caused by downsizing. In chapter three, I provided some trend-setting examples from around the beginning of the final quarter of the 20th century. The present chapter is an update of this trend and deals with increasing inequalities, worsening labor conditions in the developed world (in particular for low-skilled workers), and with top managers who are nicely rewarded for squeezing their workers for the short-term benefit of shareholders. In addition, this chapter addresses changing worldwide relations, as well as the consequences these relations have on labor in the information age. All of this is set against the background of a globalizing economy. I apologize in advance for the many figures I present in this chapter. They are, however, necessary to illustrate that, in my view, political economy in the developed world is moving dangerously far to the right side of the continuum.

4.1 Increasing Inequalities

Increasing crime and social disorder, the decay of family life and kinship as a source of social cohesion, and decreasing confidence in politics are, according to Fukuyama, characteristic of "the great disruption" of Western society. For an explanation he refers, among other things, to the increasingly unequal distribution of incomes and the growing poverty for many people worldwide, combined with increasing wealth for the few.[4]

There is an enormous body of factual information available on this topic. For years now, many scholars have been publishing arguments about the dangers for democracy that are hidden in these developments.[5] So far, however, this has not resulted in a noticeable change of policy. On the contrary, it seems as if we have been dealing with a new normality since the beginning of the final quarter of the 20th century. During the period 1977–1990, the average income of the poorest 20% of Americans declined by 5%, whereas the most prosperous 20% grew by 9%. For family incomes, these figures were minus 7% and plus 15%, respectively. In 1980, the lowest-paid 20% of American taxpayers paid 8.5% of their income in federal taxes. Ten years later the figure was 9.7%, a relative increase of 15%. In the same period, the tax burden of the top 20% fell from 27.3% to 25.8%, a relative decrease of more than 5%.[6] Around the turn of the century, 40% of American children lived on or below the very narrowly defined official poverty line of $16,400 per year for a family of four,[7] whereas in 2001 one out of nine Americans did not know if he or she would have a meal the next day.[8] More recent figures published by Phillips reveal that, since the 1980s, things have worsened. The after-tax income of the lowest 20% of American households decreased by 12% over the period 1977–1999, whereas the top 20% enjoyed an increase of 38.3%. Also, successive tax cuts in 1995, 1997, and 1999 favored people in the highest income brackets.[9] According to the Auditor's Office, tax assessments for Americans with an annual income under $25,000 doubled over the past decades, whereas those earning more than $100,000 saw a taxation decrease of 25%.[10] In addition to this, the top 20% of American households controls more than half of all American wealth.[11] The top 1% was actually 119.7% better-off.[12] Meanwhile, the 400 richest Americans increased their average net worth from $230 million in 1982 to $2.6 billion in 1999.[13] All in all, despite Clinton's talk of "a third way," Phillips rightfully concludes that the United States, the country of equal opportunity, has become the country with the highest levels of inequality[14]; a country "with the industrial world's biggest fortunes and its largest rich-poor gap." This is a situation that, according to Phillips, Americans will have to start thinking about.[15] The facts reveal that the United States is in a process of decreasing social cohesion between its citizens. Etzioni uses the term "downsizing society" here,[16] with consequences like increasing deprivation, insecurity, fear, pessimism, and anger.

On the other hand, one can observe "oligarchic wealth,"[17] being shaped in the United States in "gated communities" for the rich elites with their own private schools and private security organizations.[18] These gated communities have grown in numbers from 1,000 in the early sixties to 80,000 in the mid-1980s, with further dramatic increases in the 1990s.[19] At present, around 16% of the American population live in these gated communities.[20]

To Lasch, these elites have climbed the social ladder and pulled the ladder up after them.[21] They "live in a little world of their own, far removed from the everyday concerns of ordinary men and women."[22] They are mobile people with an increasingly global outlook who refuse to accept limits or ties to nation and place. Increasingly "opting out of American life,"[23] they isolate themselves in their networks and enclaves. They abandon the middle class, divide the nation, and betray the idea of a democracy for all citizens. Leadbeater compares them with an officer class that no longer recognizes its responsibilities to the ranks.[24] They may even refuse to pay local taxes for things like public trash collection, snow removal, or street lighting since these are included in their gated community dues.[25] They are a new class of royalty "with the traditional benefits of royalty, and there is almost no way they can lose."[26] The other side of the coin is that, around 2000, the FBI estimated the costs of burglary and robbery in the United States at $3.8 billion per year. In the final quarter of the 20th century, more than 1,000 new prisons were built in the United States. Around the start of the new millennium, the country had some two million prisoners,[27] which represents a considerable and cheap workforce, producing around $9 billion in products. Consequently, thanks to this, corporate business could downsize another 400,000 jobs.[28]

Gated communities, for that matter, are not an exclusively American phenomenon. In this respect, Klein reveals that security firms do their biggest business in cities where the gap between the rich and the poor is greatest. In Johannesburg, Sao Paulo, and New Delhi, to give just a few examples, selling iron gates, armored cars, and elaborate alarm systems and renting out armies of private guards is big business. Brazilians appear to spend $4.5 billion a year on private security, and police officers are outnumbered by private armed cops by almost four to one. South Africa's annual private security spending is three times as much as the government can spend on affordable housing.[29]

4.2 Working Poor

The United States has been transformed into a society with a growinging "underclass" of 12 million[30] "working poor," where the low-skilled have become "the Epsilons of our New Brave World."[31] According to Hertz, 20% of those employed earn wages that are below the official poverty line.[32] But since these "working poor" do have jobs, they are not counted in the unemployment statistics. These same statistics also do not include Thurow's "missing men," some 5.8 million in 1996. Had they been counted in the unemployment statistics, true unemployment would have been around 14%. There are even those who calculate an unemployment figure of 35% because they include 70 million healthy adults who are not actively seeking a job.[33] In 2000, the American Department of Labor admitted that if part-timers wanting to work more and those wanting a job but lacking the necessary transport or child care were included, the unemployment level would have been twice the official 5.5 million.[34] Finally, Moore mentions that, on average, there were 400,000 new unemployed people each month during 2000, with hundreds of companies announcing mass redundancies.[35]

Consequently, the American labor statistics look misleadingly bright.[36] There are even those who, like Kelly, argue that these statistics are deliberately distorted and misinterpreted to serve the interests of the well-off and people in power.[37] All in all, the United States has become a "winner-take-all-society"[38] with sharp expressions of cynicism.

Research by the American Management Association shows that, of 720 "newly-downsized companies," 30% rehired their employees on new labor terms, which almost always meant that they were no longer insured against the costs of sickness. Regarding this, figures from the American Bureau of Labor Statistics reveal that in 1996, only 26% of employees in the lowest 10% income range had health coverage provided by their companies, declining from 49% in 1986.[39] For the lowest 20% of the income scale, these figures were 41% in 1980 and 32% by the end of the 20th century.[40] Moreover, these employees no longer enjoyed other benefits they had been entitled to before they were fired.[41] As an example: in 1985, 70% of unemployed Americans had access to unemployment benefits, a figure which had decreased to 39% in 2000.[42] Between 1982 and 1996, two things, health coverage and employee benefits, which had been "a great equalizer," instead became part of "the architecture of polarization."[43] This polarization was reinforced by different tax reforms in the 1980s and 1990s, reforms that favored the higher income classes and corporate business. In order to compensate for this taxation policy, payroll taxes for social security and Medicare had to be increased, which hit the lower and middle-income classes especially hard.[44] Altogether, not only decreasing wages, but also the fact that employees had to pay taxes, medical payments, social security levies, and interest payments, led the economist Hyman to create a New Misery Index. This index shows that the total costs of these burdens increased from 24% of personal income in 1960 to 43% in the 1990s.[45] All in all, the purchasing power of the 80% of Americans who do not belong to the highest income bracket is now lower than it was 30 years ago, when Nixon left the White House, despite the fact that labor productivity increased by a third over the same period.[46] No wonder, then, that the personal debts of many Americans grew dramatically over the past 20 years[47] to 120% of personal income by mid-2001.[48] Personal bankruptcies totaled 1.3 million in 1999, whereas household debts rose from 58% in 1973 to an estimated 85% in 1998.[49] Consequently, an increasing number of American families find themselves in a precarious situation. During the period 1995–1999 alone, the number of personal bankruptcies increased by 70%.[50] This may explain to a large extent why the number of working American women with children under six increased from 19% in 1960 to 64% in 1995.[51] Anyway, it seems hard to maintain that this increased labor participation is only a matter of emancipation. If one reads Ehrenreich's story, based on experiences acquired when she worked undercover in low-wage America, terms like oppression, despair, or neglect would be more appropriate.[52] It appears that low-wage workers, which account for 30% of employed American people, are paid only about half of the $14 an hour which, according to the American Economic Policy Institute, would constitute a "living wage." As a consequence, these people have only a 1 in 97 chance of finding a single-room apartment that they can afford to rent.[53] In addition to this, they have to endure degrading and criminal behavior from employers.[54] Thankfully, these depressing facts are somewhat counterbalanced by the fact that, around the turn of the century, some 40 cities and counties in 17 American states had enacted living-wage ordinances,[55] a welcome illustration that there is a difference between Washington/Wall Street and America as a whole.

Apart from the fact that the number of American single-parent families doubled over the past 30 years, labor participation has everything to do with the need to prop up family incomes, especially since the late 1970s when husbands' paychecks began to decline.[56] The weekly earnings of these working poor are simply not enough to satisfy the basic human needs of sufficient nutrition and clothing. In this respect, a survey conducted by the United States Conference of Mayors in 2000 reveals the disturbing fact that 67% of adults requesting emergency food aid are people with a job.[57] Meanwhile, American food banks, of which the state of Washington alone has 300, are increasingly busy,[58] if only because of the fact that, out of 14 million people who were entitled to social security, 10 million lost their benefits during the Clinton years.[59] This precarious situation may explain why the American Department of Labor recorded 20,000 violations of the child labor laws in 1992, twice as many as in 1980.[60] It may also explain why 44 million Americans read and write at the level of a nine-year old child; i.e., they are functionally illiterate.[61] And, finally, it may also explain the fact that the number of American prisoners, of which the large majority left school prematurely,[62] increased from one to two million during the Clinton administration,[63] which leads to a ratio of one prisoner to every 143 Americans, compared to around one to 1,000 for the countries of Europe.[64] At present, an American black boy born in 2001 has a one in three chance of being imprisoned.[65] All this is because global competition demands that the costs of labor be kept as low as possible. Globalization and marginalization appear to be interconnected, with the former driving the latter.[66]

4.3 Downsizing Pays

Downsizing became part of the culture of American corporate business during the past few decades. It is no longer an answer to temporary business cycles but has become "a way of life".[67] It has turned work into a commodity, and it has changed the labor market into a product market.[68] Over the period 1980–1993, the number of jobs at the top 500 American corporations declined from 15.9 million to 11.5 million as a consequence of downsizing.[69] For all American corporations, the numbers vary from a low count of 13 million downsized workers to three times that amount over the same period.[70] This downsizing happens repeatedly within the same corporations. Therefore, Saul rightfully uses the term "corporate anorexia."[71] It is no wonder that American corporate business is accused of behaving like "corporate killers."[72] Apparently, their sole responsibility, pushed by the United States Shareholders' Association of 1986,[73] is to increase value for shareholders. In fact, downsizing, rightsizing, restructuring, reengineering,[74] deselecting, or any other fashionable term for firing[75] is frequently used for short-term stock manipulation. Maintaining employment is not the business of corporations. This unscrupulous attitude caused one in twelve American workers to be laid off during the period 1993–1995, a figure which increased to one in eight during the following three-year period.[76]

Meanwhile, top managers who succeed in carrying through massive layoffs are rewarded beyond imagination, receiving, in addition to their enormous salaries, millions of dollars in stock options.[77] Indeed, "the stock market is rewarding job killers."[78] And these job killers, assisted by accountants, who have changed from watchdogs into lap dogs,[79] do not hesitate to "cook up the books"[80] in order to present rosier corporate results,[81] if only because they have invested in companies they audited.[82] Meanwhile, figures demonstrate a growing divergence between the pay of workers and CEOs. In 1988, CEOs earned 93 times the hourly wages of production workers, a number that soared to 419 in 1999[83] and 531 in 2000.[84]

Although the circumstances of European CEOs are not as absurd as their American colleagues (as far as I know), the tendencies are the same. Politicians, be they American or European, do not seem capable of intervening. Meanwhile, this extravagant remunerations and huge extras were not enough to prevent some CEOs from cheating the public by manipulating financial figures, as recent arrests in the United States have demonstrated. The most well known example is Enron (which had been elected by Fortune magazine as the most innovative company for five consecutive years starting in 1996[85]), whose CEO and other top executives were "falsifying records, concealing company debts, misleading analysts, reporting nonexistent profits, avoiding taxes, creating a cutthroat, no-questions-asked working environment."[86] According to Moore, corporate fraud costs Americans nearly $200 billion a year.[87]

4.4 Not in Europe?

To start with, similar things happen in the United Kingdom. There, too, we see decreasing real wages; longer working weeks for those who (still) have a job; and, in particular, "zero-hours working," which refers to employees who are ready to work but who have to wait unpaid at home, waiting for a call from their employer.[88] There too, we see a depressing world beyond the official statistics, where figures are magically adjusted.[89] There too, people are labeled as "economically inactive" instead of "unemployed" if they refuse to be registered as such because they feel this to be too demoralizing.[90] In 1992, their number was estimated to be two million.[91] There too, many people live in poverty; in 1996 this constituted a quarter of the adult British population, twice the 1979 figure,[92] and the number of children living in poverty has tripled over the past three decades.[93] With Labour back in government since 1997, things have hardly changed. Though the introduction of a minimum wage was supposed to "end the scandal of poverty pay,"[94] it appears to be no more than "a political stitch-up, designed to deliver a manifesto pledge by old Labour and the unions."[95] All these facts together led Pilger to conclude that "the Blairites have become the political wing of the City of London and the British multinational corporations."[96] Chancellor Brown's first budget, which included a reduction in corporate taxation, was even harsher for ordinary British people than any of the Tories' budgets in the previous 18 years.[97] In short, Blair's policy is in sharp contrast with what he promised before he got elected. In other words, it is "organised hypocrisy."[98] Finally, the United Kingdom also has its share of overpaid managers. Over the past decade, the salaries of British top managers increased by 92% from £301,000 to £579,000 per year, which was twice the average wage increase experienced by other workers in Great Britain. In addition, five years ago, maximum bonuses were limited to around 50% of the yearly salary. Now, 50% of top managers award themselves with bonuses of 100%. However, there is hardly any relation between the increase in salaries and bonuses and corporate performance.[99]

Similar developments can be observed in other countries of the European Union. France, for instance, with 7.5% of its population living below the poverty line,[100] had 140,000 unemployed people in 1998 who refused to be registered as such for the same reasons as their British colleagues. In France too, it has become normal for wages and labor conditions of newly hired employees to be worse than those of their predecessors.[101]

As for Germany, this country had nearly 5 million registered unemployed people in the summer of 1997, and 7 million people lived "in the shadow of prosperity."[102]

Hoogerwerf describes widening income gaps for the Netherlands.[103] In 2005, the Netherlands had 250,000 "working poor" and more than 600,000 people living below the poverty line. Furthermore, around the same time, The Hague distributed 700 food parcels daily, and almost 30% of minimum wage-earners said that they were not able to get by.[104]

Comparable developments were evident in Portugal. The applicant countries of the European Union show similar trends. In Hungary in 2000, the top-earning 10% of the population made 7.5 times the income of the lowest 10%, an increase of 4.5 times in the first half of the 1980s.[105] In

Bulgaria 60% of the population live below the poverty line.[106] Finally, reports of the European Union and the OECD confirm these developments.[107]

Meanwhile, downsizing is also a normal practice throughout the European Union.[108] And in the European Union, the motive for these mass redundancies is also to create value for the shareholders and nothing else. The same motive has made redundancies an integral part of business dynamics.[109] That we are dealing with a worldwide phenomenon in this regard is evident from the fact that, at the close of 1999, Nissan, NEC, and Sony announced lay-offs 21,000, 15,000, and 17,000 respectively.[110] Finally, there are also several examples that show that cheating by CEOs is not limited to the United States. The CEO from Ahold in the Netherlands, as well as the leaders of the Italian Parmalat corporation, are European examples.

4.5 Asymmetric Employment Relations

Neo-liberal market ideas regarding a globalizing economy not only have consequences for work and pay in the developed world, as described in the preceding sections. They may also deliver incentives to make use of asymmetric labor relations with respect to the worldwide exchange of goods, services, and capital. Highly skilled professionals can easily sell their knowledge and capacities in places where there is more demand for them or where they are paid better.[111] For low-skilled workers, these opportunities are considerably fewer.[112] The elasticity of demand, then, for low-skilled labor decreases in a globalizing economy, resulting in an increasing pressure on wages, employment security, and working conditions.

Problems regarding the elasticity of demand for low-skilled labor might be countered by education and training; that is, by measures that increase labor productivity. So far, this productivity gives us a comparative competitive advantage, so that low-wage countries are not yet threatening. Capital-intensive production and high-skilled labor still offer sufficient compensation.[113] However, one has to take into account the dialectics of progress in this respect.[114] In addition, the benefits of education and training are not unlimited.[115] Moreover, it is questionable whether the labor market is capable of absorbing low-skilled laborers, after education and training, into more highly skilled jobs.[116]

Meanwhile, the phenomenon of the elasticity of demand is also manifest at the level of highly skilled jobs. Because of the democratization of technology, India, for instance, "is rapidly becoming the back office of the world,"[117] with around 50,000 Indians employed in this way in 2000.[118] Futhermore, companies located in Bangalore and Bombay have become important contractors for the production of software for companies all over the world. The highly skilled Indian engineers and computer specialists, however, earn only 20% of the salaries that are paid for comparable work in the United States. Consequently, Indian software exports, mainly to the United States, jumped from $1 billion in 1995 to $5 billion in 2000 and are expected to rise to $50 billion in ten years,[119] and it is predicted that, in a few years, "hundreds of thousands of Indian and Chinese technicians, programmers and software engineers will be working for American corporations over the Internet."[120] Developments like these led a high-ranking American business officer to conclude that "we don't have any protected domains anymore" since, according to *Business Week*, the global economy delivers "an increasingly better balance of skills in the world."[121] Consequently, skill no longer means job security.[122]

It is not unreasonable to assume that these developments will continue in a liberalized free-trade economy. As a result, the remuneration of labor will "tend to play an important benchmark role for the rest of the economy," whereas one has also to consider that, due to its rapid diffusion, technical knowledge is not "an enduring source of advantage."[123] Therefore, as Peter Drucker rightfully observes, it is of utmost importance for governments of the European Union to realize that "knowledge-workers' productivity is the biggest of the 21st-century management challenges. In the developed countries it is their first survival requirement. In no other way can the developed countries hope to maintain themselves, let alone to maintain their leadership and their standards of living."[124]

4.6 Work in the Third Millennium

Predicting the future is always a risky affair. In the 1970s, Toffler and Gorz confidently foretold that, around the end of the millennium, we would all be working less and enjoying more leisure time, while work would become less important to self-definition and personal identity.[125] Reality appears to be different. Many people, especially those who are low-skilled, have more leisure time but do not enjoy it, either because they cannot afford it financially, or because they would rather have a job but cannot find one. Another category of people could afford leisure time financially but do not have the time for it, since these are people who are too busy with their self-definition and the search for personal identity.[126]

With all this in mind, we have to consider that we just entered the "third industrial revolution," a new episode in history during which human labor for the production of goods and services will increasingly be replaced by machines. The lay-offs mentioned previously are largely a consequence of this development. According to Rifkin, we are on our way to an "automated future," where, especially for industrial production, we will enter a "near-workerless" era in the first decades of the 21st century.[127] During these decades, the disappearance of labor as the key factor of production is going to emerge as the critical "unfinished business of capitalist society."[128] In this respect, a transformation from industrial labor to the services sector has been evident for years already.[129] To some, however, this transformation to a service society offers only temporary solutions. Consequently, unused labor will become the dominant reality for the coming era, which will demand the utmost of each civilized society to prevent social disintegration.[130]

There also are, however, optimistic views on this trend. To Reich, for example, the world has just entered the New Economy or the "Age of the Terrific Deal," by which he means that the major effect of the new communication, transportation, and information technologies will be a change in the terms of competition. It will reduce the advantages of large-scale production, and it will reward entrepreneurs who are able to improve products and services quickly and who invent new ones that will delight consumers even more. This "Age of the Terrific Deal" will be characterized by an increasing importance of innovation to the economy.[131] Competition will be "the mother of invention."[132] It will be the time of an increased rate of technological innovations, of broadly applicable new technologies with shortened processes and product life-cycles.[133] Therefore, there will be a constant need for creative innovators.[134] Those who do not have the talents for this New Economy will lose ground and remain unemployed, unless they are qualified to find jobs in other domains like health, entertainment, beauty, intellectual stimulation, contact, family well-being, and financial security.[135] However, the weak point in Reich's reasoning is that he assumes that those who do not have the talents necessary in the New Economy will be qualified to find a job in one of the domains he mentions. This is rather unlikely, firstly, for quality reasons, since not everyone is suited for jobs in sectors such as beauty, intellectual stimulation, health, or entertainment. Secondly, for quantitative reasons, because the New Economy is also a fast economy; and, due to technological progress, it is growing ever faster.[136] This speed forces businesses to adjust immediately to rapidly changing competitive conditions. In order to stay competitive in the volatile environment of the New Economy, "organizations have to turn all fixed costs into variable costs that rise and fall according to the choices buyers make."[137] Consequently, apart from the question of whether the New Economy will be able to absorb all those who have become redundant in the old economy, the notion of a "steady" job is coming to an end.[138] If only some of these prophecies come true, this will have an enormous impact on the way we are used to defining employment and the way we relate to work and working conditions.

Frank distinguishes between three types of workers, bringing them together in three concentric circles. First of all, there will be workers who represent the irreducible core staff. They represent the inner circle, and they perform the key roles. They have to be available around the clock. For them, the new technology has reinforced the pressures associated with work. Work reaches them by fax, mobile phone, and modern, while pagers follow them everywhere.[139] They work 60 hours a week or more, but they do not have the time to enjoy the fact that they are paid extremely well. For them, "in the acquisitive society, leisure became the casualty of prosperity."[140] The next group of workers are freelancers and contract providers who perform functions that have been contracted out. They represent the middle circle and perform as "Me & Co.," selling themselves as portfolio workers or as service providers on the market.[141] They are self-employed people, who are able to apply the latest knowledge and skills creatively. They are the "key players" in the coming knowledge economy. They are the symbols of what Evans and Wurster call "the deconstruction of the labour market."[142] According to Leadbeater, their number is growing, especially in the advanced economies. This might lead to a situation where a significant share of the workforce will become akin to independent contractors. These contractors do not sell themselves to a company; instead, they sell a service, an outcome, or a capability. Consequently, their relations with employers will become increasingly market-based.[143] Consequently also, this will mean the end of capitalism as we know it, because it will make redundant employment agreements that allow managers to issue instructions and to observe and to monitor staff. People who work in this knowledge economy are people that use their judgement, skills and creativity as personal assets that are, to a certain extent, beyond the control of employers. By their very nature, assets like these are difficult to control. Consequently, knowledge and learning, which underpin the new labor, will cause a corrosion of traditional capitalistic forms of organization that are based on employment agreements.[144] Organizations in the new economy will be determined by a management culture in which flexibility, a flat organizational structure, and confidence are the central characteristics.[145]

The third type, at the outer edge of Frank's circle, are the interchangeable casual, freelance, temporary workers who are taken on if and when needed. People in this category, though willing to work, have to live with disappointment and insecurity. Based on the booming business of temporary work agencies, their number is growing. Frank's distinction is in line with Hutton, who speaks of the "thirty, thirty, forty" society, meaning that 30% of the population lives on the edge of existence, another 30% have jobs, but nevertheless have a marginalized existence due to poor remuneration and uncertain employment conditions, whereas 40% occupy demanding but well-paid positions.[146]

4.7 Summary

This chapter addresses the effects of the pendulum's swinging to the right side of the continuum, i.e., freedom of the market and less government interference in the economic process in an increasingly worldwide economic order. Under the banners of neo-liberal economics and a new individualistic morality, the globalizing economy, hardly controlled by governments, is blamed for decreasing social cohesion throughout the developed world. Worldwide competition is assumed inevitably to force corporate business to decrease the costs of labor and to dismantle working conditions. On the one hand, the effects include increasing inequalities, resulting in large numbers of workers who are either downsized or who have to accept deteriorating labor terms and insecure labor conditions. The proper word for this development is flexibility. It leaves many people behind, because they are either unemployed or they earn wages that make them "working poor." On the other hand, there is a corporate business elite awarded a level of remuneration that is beyond imagination. There even appears to be a positive correlation between the corporate elite's success in downsizing and its remuneration. As a result, the United States in particular is becoming a society of "haves" and "have-nots," with the first increasingly living in gated communities, and the latter increasingly deprived. In this respect, the difference between the United States and the countries of the European Union is only a matter of degree, because neoliberalism, translated into practical policy slogans, and the new individualistic morality have also prevailed there.

Unless a change of policy is carried out, there is no reason to be optimistic about the foreseeable future, because a worldwide free exchange of goods and capital makes employment relations asymmetrical. Even now, low-skilled workers experience the disadvantages of this asymmetry. When, in the near future, the service sector can no longer absorb unemployed low-skilled workers, social problems will become very serious. Later, asymmetric labor relations will also have consequences for higher-skilled workers. The much-cheered "new economy" will not deliver a way out in this respect.

However, taking an optimistic, and probably not unrealistic, view, one might consider asymmetry in labor relations, particularly in comparison with the Asian economies, to be of a temporary nature, although probably having a several-decade horizon. The argument here would be that strong economic growth in countries like China and South Korea will induce an upward pressure on labor terms in those countries. In the longer term, therefore, we could experience a new equalization of labor conditions.

Part Two
Consequences for Health Care Systems

5 Health Care and the Economic Order

As presented in the first chapter, the economic order is a dynamic phenomenon with governments alternately moving to the left or to the right side of a continuum between two theoretical extremes. Since 1975, the governments of the countries of the European Union have pursued policies of moving to the right side of the continuum, increasingly giving power to the market, based on economic arguments (globalization) as well as on ideological arguments (neo-liberalism and the theory of "public choice"). These policies also affect the production and consumption of health care goods and services. This is the theme of the second part of this book.

However, the problem with health care is that the choice between state and market raises conceptual and practical dilemmas.[1] As for the conceptual problems, it must be realized that, within the countries of the European Union, there is a broad consensus regarding solidarity in health care. Solidarity is assumed to be "a way of life," "a sense of non-calculating co-operation based on identification with a common cause,"[2] which in fact dates back centuries.[3] Health care is not the same as any other public good. It is "a symbol of democratic rights and citizenship."[4] In the countries of the European Union, it reflects, therefore, the ideological preferences of society.[5] This is already impeding the introduction of the market principle.[6] On the practical side, one has to take into account the fact that real markets require real prices, which would make health care extremely expensive. Because of these dilemmas, the introduction of market principles to health care is controversial, particularly because it may be to the disadvantage of vulnerable members of society.

The first section of the present chapter will examine these practical dilemmas and address the feasibility of a market for health care. In the second section I will argue that, due to the large number of parties interested in the health care process, it is very difficult for democratic governments to implement fundamental changes to health care policies, in particular when these changes impose restrictions. Thirdly, governments that want to introduce a market in health care will, nevertheless, have to live up to their constitutional obligations. This is the theme of the third section. The fourth section deals with the aging of the population, which exacerbates problems for governments that want to introduce market-style mechanisms in health care. Finally, I will discuss ethical aspects in the development in health care. Governments cannot stay out of the debates that ethical matters in health care may raise in society. These debates not only raise moral questions of "bad" or "good," but also take into account the consequences that ethical issues may have for the solidarity principle.

As an introductory remark, it should first be made clear that this book is about health care *systems*, and not about health. It deals, therefore, with the infrastructure that national economies have established to solve citizens' health problems, either through short-term intervention or through long-term, or even life-long, assistance. Of course, I do realize that a population's health is determined by many conditions other than health care. Nutrition, exposure to violence, environmental pollutants, genetic factors, and sanitation, for example, are important determinants of people's health. So are life-style characteristics like smoking or drinking too much. Moreover, research has shown a correlation between, for example, life expectancy and measures that influence social status, like income, education, occupation, and residence.[7] Taking all these conditioning factors together, we might say, with Wilkinson, that the role of medical and clinical services, and in a larger sense the role of health care systems, is "to pick up the pieces."[8] These services contribute only between 10% and 25% of measured health status in society.[9] Nevertheless, they consume by far the largest portion of available finances. Therefore, the focus of this book is on picking up the pieces, while realizing that the number of pieces to be picked up can be influenced considerably by the many other determinants of health. In this respect, it is meaningful that governments show a (modestly) growing interest in health impact assessment applied to non-health-sector policies, like transport, housing, agriculture, and the environment.[10] But despite all these initiatives, health inequalities "appear to persist over time, in spite of policies aimed at promoting equal access and combating social exclusion."[11]

Secondly, within the framework of this book, there is no need to give a complete history of health care systems. It is sufficient to conclude that, for centuries, the governments of national economies had very little to do with health care. This was, as argued in the first chapter, to a large extent the domain of religious congregations.[12] In so far as "governments," i.e., the wealthy and powerful, did something about health care, this was motivated by arguments of charity and/or self-interest. Health care systems in the sense of infrastructures which were deliberately established by governments to tackle health problems hardly existed in those days. For the purposes of this book, I rely on the distinction of the four phases of the welfare state made by Geleijnse et al[13] (see 1.2.1). My focus is particularly on the three latter phases, i.e., the extension phase from the end of the Second World War to around the beginning of the 1980s, the phase of restructuring that took about ten years from 1980 to 1990, and, finally, from 1990 on, the still-ongoing phase of fundamental reforms to health care systems. For the message that this book intents to deliver, the final two phases are so important that they will be the subject of two separate chapters.

5.1 A Market for Health Care?

In principle, Eucken's theory about the economic order also applies to specific sectors of society. In line with the topic of this book, this means that the problem of decision-making regarding health care should answer the question, "Who are the ones to decide on the *what*, the *how*, and the *for whom* of the production and consumption of *health care* goods and services?" Again, reasoning in extremes, one could decide to leave the answer to this question completely to the market or completely to the government. But, again, that is theory. The reality is that governments always play a role in the process of producing and delivering health care goods and services. That role may be more or less extensive, thus resulting in changing positions of national health care systems along the continuum. And that role, too, is flexible. It depends on political constellations, on moral and cultural aspects, and on macro-economic conditions. In other words, also with regard to health care, societies move along the continuum. Furthermore, health care is also subject to the dynamics of the economic order. Consequently, decision-making regarding movement along the continuum is not necessarily limited to developments within national economic orders. Supra-territorial economic orders, like the European Union, or policies of global institutions, may affect the decision-making process.

It should also be noted with regard to health care goods and services that there is no right or wrong answer to the question of which side of the continuum is preferable. Such an answer involves ethical and value judgements and is, therefore, a matter of normative economics.

An ardent champion of an as-free-as-possible market for health care is Milton Friedman. To him, the countries of the industrialized world have reached such a level of wealth that the majority of their citizens have sufficient financial means to behave as consumers in such a market. Providers of health care goods and services in that market should be able to look after themselves. They should not be dependent on public financing or social insurance money but should, instead, compete for consumers' preferences regarding the majority of health care items.[14] In short, Friedman favors a drastic commercialization of health care.

On the other hand, there are those who ardently oppose a market for health care. To them, health care is not a range of commodities but a social right for each citizen. They advocate the curbing of profit seeking in health care through government intervention and collective financing.

I will argue that the governments of the countries of the European Union initially started to move to the left side of the continuum, particularly after the beginning of the 1960s (chapter eight). However, from around the 1980s, a reverse trend started, toward a health care market (chapter nine).

In line with what has been said before, governments in Western democracies exert influence regarding the production and consumption of health care goods and services. The instruments that governments use are (broadly) similar to those mentioned in the first chapter.

Governments can influence the health care process in *general terms* by, for example, policies of de-collectivization, which transfer the solution of health care problems to the market, or, in contrast, they can include all health care needs in a collective financial scheme. They can use *financial instruments* by, for example, introducing systems of budgeting, imposing budget cuttings, or introducing calculation methods such as diagnostic-related groups. Governments may apply *functional regulations* like the British idea of the fund-holding practitioner, or introducing competition between hospitals, or, like the Dutch, making the insurer the conductor of the health care process. Governments can also introduce *specific instruments* like, for example, the French government, which around the turn of the century decided to establish 300 geriatric units in acute-care hospitals over the next five years, or like the Dutch government, which around the same time decided to reduce the capacity of homes for the elderly. Furthermore, governments may use instruments that are based on *legislation,* or which work via the *price mechanism.* Cost-sharing and co-payments regarding the costs of health care and subsidies for the vulnerable people in society are examples of the latter. Finally, there is a *residual group* of instruments like grants for medical research or selective investment arrangements like, for example, making combating HIV/Aids a focal point of health care policy.

Governmental decision-making regarding the use of instruments to influence the health care process does not happen in a vacuum, because at the institutional level of the economic order, all Western democracies have established a more or less balanced social-economic infrastructure that enables agreements to be reached about health care policies, i.e., the objectives of their health care systems and the way to achieve them.[15] In this respect, it is important to note that health care has very many interest groups which may easily pursue very differing, or even conflicting, objectives. The objectives of all those involved in the health care process are so diverse that one may safely compare the health care field with a large number of frogs, all jumping out of a wheelbarrow in different directions. Therefore, reaching general agreement on health care policies at the level of the national economic order is hardly possible, in particular if these policies are directed at restrictions on the supply side.[16] In these circumstances, governments in democracies continuously have to negotiate and compromise with the parties involved. Although different interest groups may not, as such, have many opportunities to influence health care policies, they appear to have considerable power to obstruct, particularly if they combine their opposition. Moreover, apart from the formal social-economic infrastructure, one has to take into account the influence that is exerted by extra-parliamentary actions. In this regard from the 1980s on, when governments started to economize on their health care systems, it is difficult to find a single year in which one or more European Union governments[17] did not have to deal with strikes by health care interest groups. For example, doctors went on strike in Finland and Portugal, nursing staff did so in Sweden and France, physiotherapists did so in the Netherlands and Ireland, and so on. Almost each and every country of the European Union had its share of strikes during this time. And, most importantly, patients or their relatives also took the streets, quite often finding a willing ear among politicians. As a consequence, governments that wanted to reform their health care systems had to realize that there is not much scope for "grand designs," particularly if social pluralism is widespread.[18] Consequently, decision-making regarding health care policy is, in general, characterized by incrementalism—taking small steps, one at a time.[19] Moving to the right side of the continuum in health care, and leaving things increasingly to the market, is therefore a slow process.

Over the past ten years, however, one can observe a new trend that is characterized by governments' restoring the primacy of politics to health care, bypassing interested parties in the field.[20] As an example: in the 1990s, the federal government of Germany imposed a calculation system for hospitals, almost without consulting the German hospital association. Similarly, the Dutch government rearranged the composition of its advisory bodies for health care in such a way that providers and insurers are no longer represented in the respective boards of governors, thus limiting the scope of the corporatist model that the Dutch were used to. In Belgium, employers stopped participating in the annual budget negotiations in 2002, believing that the government's intervention in health care operational matters had superseded the traditional corporatist model.[21] To date, however, this new trend has not yet led to the implementation of "grand designs." Changes in health care policies in democracies remain characterized by incrementalism. After all, there will always be another election. And governments that want to remain in power cannot afford to lose too much public support as a result of their policies. Nevertheless, governments have taken the lead.[22]

However, it is not only the wheelbarrow with frogs which requires governments in democracies to limit their interventions to incremental policies. The fact that governments have already taken the lead by restoring the primacy of politics indicates that there is more to it. This has everything to do with the uncertainties surrounding the policies of moving to the right side of the continuum. These uncertainties flow from the fact that health care systems of the countries of the European Union are based on social values like solidarity and equity, i.e., health care should be delivered according to need, not ability to pay. This involves solidarity in health care between rich and poor, young and old, and sick and healthy. This sense of "a general duty to aid the needy" (see section 1.1.1) certainly includes the idea that health care should be accessible to all citizens. Research easily produces figures showing that around 90% of all citizens are in favor of this idea.[23] Moreover, over the course of time, people in developed countries have become ever more attached to good health and health care as a priority in life. Research from the Netherlands has shown that, good health has become by far the most important thing in life, bypassing both religion and marriage over the past forty years.[24] Consequently, carrying out changes, if needed, in the way people are used to receiving their health care is a very delicate affair, particularly when it comes to the financial aspects. Governments in democracies that want to introduce a market in health care, thus moving to the right side of the continuum, will therefore have to deal constantly with uncertainties regarding the interpretation and feasibility of the market principle. Can there be a market for health care? And if so, which health care items could be subjected to that principle?

In answering these questions, it must be noted that the neo-liberal market of perfect competition as promoted by the adherents of the theory of public choice[25] does not exist in health care, for the simple reason that the five crucial assumptions (together) of such a health care market do not hold true for any market.[26]

First of all, consumption of most health care items cannot be planned in the same way as one can plan the purchase of commodities like a car or a pair of shoes. The need for health care interventions is mostly unexpected. Moreover, health care intervention may prove to be too costly to be affordable. That's what health care insurance is for. One does not plan to have a heart transplant in two years, but one can plan to have a face lift in three years. For most health care items, however, the assumption that customers have *certainty* does not hold.

Secondly, a free health care market does not account for *externalities*, positively or negatively. On the one hand, vaccination may prevent a need for treatment. On the other hand, treating patients with tuberculosis may prevent other people from being infected.

Thirdly, people may feel sick without knowing what is wrong with their health. And if they do know, they may very well not know what type of treatment they ought to buy in the market for their recovery. Because of this, sick people seek the advice of experts like general practitioners or medical specialists. Therefore, consumers lack the *perfect knowledge* which is assumed in neo-liberal ideas about the perfect market.

Fourthly, and this is connected to the consumer's lack of perfect knowledge, providers are able to influence health care consumption considerably out of *self-interest*. As an example: health care systems based on a fee-for-service may incite providers to overproduction, because this will increase their income.

Finally, ideas on perfect markets assume that very many (including small) providers would be able to enter the health care market and would compete on price only, which would lead to minimal costs for consumers. This also does not hold, since those who would like to enter the market need a license to do so. Licensing, therefore, can be used as an instrument to *control the supply side*, thus possibly exerting an upward pressure on prices. The health care market, therefore, is like any other market: it is imperfect. The assumed ideal conditions do not exist.

Apart from these (economic) assumptions regarding perfect market conditions, there are serious doubts that "normal" people really do want health care to be subject to market principles; they may regretfully accept that it is just one of those things in life that there are always people who, for financial reasons, cannot play the market game. Even in the United States, a country with a relatively extensive health care market, market principles are not sacrosanct. American health care providers, deliberately setting aside market principles, have a long history of charity care. Although there are no hard figures available, it has been estimated that, even in the 1930s, at least 50% of American hospitalized patients paid no professional fees.[27] Admittedly, these patients were (also) interesting teaching material for academic medical centers, but treating them free of charge was characteristic for the "service-maximizers, not profit-maximizers" that these centers were in those days.[28] Although this attitude changed fundamentally with the introduction of Medicare and Medicaid in 1965,[29] charity care in the United States remains considerable. In 1981, $10 billion in charitable donations supplemented the tax-paid health care programs. Furthermore, it has been estimated that, around the beginning of the 1990s, 10% of physicians' services were uncompensated,[30] whereas between 1980 and 1991, unpaid hospital medical services grew 37% faster than total hospital spending on an annual basis. Finally, in 1991, American hospitals and physicians provided $25 billion in care for uninsured patients.[31] Much of this free care is of similar quality to the services delivered to those who do pay, including the use of expensive technology. Apparently, when it comes to health care, there are intricate mechanisms of redistribution which, in fact, eliminate market principles. This should be kept in mind when noting the fact that today there are some 45 million Americans without health insurance.[32]

The fact that markets are imperfect does not, by itself, automatically require governments to intervene. Instead, this depends on the degree of imperfection that economic orders believe to be acceptable. Here, it is important to realize that social values like solidarity and equity in health care are valued so highly that all countries of the European Union have formulations in their constitutions to underline governments' responsibilities to their citizens in this respect. That responsibility forces governments to counter market failures in health care.[33] The more that market fails, the more extensive government intervention will have to be. One of the peculiarities of health care is that, overall, its characteristics lead to market failure on all the aforementioned crucial assumptions. In the framework of this book, however, it is sufficient to deal only with the characteristics of risk and uncertainty regarding health.[34]

Risk and uncertainty regarding the occurrence of illness have led to the development of health care insurance markets, because (most) people are risk-averse. They want to prevent the possibility of having to face a heavy financial burden as a consequence of becoming ill. The very existence of health care insurance markets may, in turn, deliver small or insubstantial economies of scale if the market contains many competing insurance companies. On the other hand, a large monopoly insurer may exploit the insured. An alternative policy could be to have a public monopoly, collecting the financial means for health care through general taxation. Governments must make this choice, taking account of the limitation that their citizens must have equal access to the health care provisions.[35] Whether this is guaranteed by governments acting as health care providers, or by health care insurance markets conditioned by government regulation, is of secondary importance.

The existence of health care insurance markets may furthermore lead to "moral hazard," i.e., excess demand from consumers and/or providers. As for consumer moral hazard, this may take the form of over-consumption or a change in consumers' attitude, resulting from the fact that being insured reduces the costs of treatment at the point of consumption. This reflects an attitude that "We paid for it (through taxation or premiums), so we are entitled to everything!" Governments may counter consumer moral hazard by introducing cost-sharing methods for medical treatment or by excluding specific health care items from the coverage package.[36] Measures like these fit with a policy of moving to the right side of the continuum. However, such a policy may negatively affect solidarity and equity if people do not have sufficient financial means. Therefore, we see that governments that introduce measures like these quite often link them to exemptions for specific members of society (vulnerable, low-income, et cetera). These exemptions illustrate the delicacy that surrounds the movement of a health care policy to the right side of the continuum. As for providers' moral hazard, I have already referred to the fee-for-service system, which may lead to "supplier-induced demand." Governments may counter this type of moral hazard by budgeting medical output, or by introducing a method of degression in tariffs.[37] The Dutch government adopted the latter method as a policy measure applyed to medical specialists in hospitals in the mid-1980s. Budgeting medical output, however, may result in waiting lists, which, in turn, may lead to preferential treatment, thus undermining the principle of equity. A second type of provider moral hazard results from a lack of cost-awareness. Recent ideas on benchmarking providers' performance may be of help in this respect. I will return to this topic later.

Finally, the existence of health care insurance markets may lead to adverse selection, resulting from an asymmetry of information between the insured and the insurer. In order to prevent financial losses, insurers may be inclined to attract young and healthy clients, an approach known as "cream-skimming." Such insurers are not interested in old or handicapped people, since these clients would surely not provide a profit. In a society where solidarity between sick and healthy people, old and young, and rich and poor is believed to be a mainstay of social cohesion, governments, therefore, have to regulate health care insurance markets so that cream-skimming can be prevented.

All in all, moving to the right side of the continuum by introducing the market principle to health care systems is a delicate matter, because health care violates all the premises of an efficient free market. This explains not only incremental decision-making, but also the trial-and-error behavior governments have demonstrated from the beginning of their attempts to reform their health care systems. Two examples may illustrate this point.

Firstly, Margaret Thatcher was the first to introduce the idea of competition between British hospitals. This resulted in the "financial meltdown" of several hospital trusts, because they had to keep their heads above water in a market of irresponsible downward price competition.[38] Tony Blair, still in the opposition in those days, argued against these kinds of reforms for several reasons. To him, the Thatcher policies in health care were based on a blind ideological confidence that the market was the most efficient instrument to get "value for money." The language of the Thatcher reforms—competition, business cases, purchasers and marketing—concealed the real intentions of commercialization and privatization.[39] However, Blair agreed that "worldwide experience over the decades has shown clearly that a centralized state-financed health system tends to be cheaper than one based on private spending or insurance."[40] Nevertheless, once he was in office, though he substituted co-operation for competition and rearranged fundholders into primary care groups, it took years before change occurred in the NHS. In short, for a long time, New Labour's health policy was "characterized more by continuity than by revolution."[41]

Secondly, in the mid-1990s, the Dutch government excluded dental care for people over 18 years old from the coverage package, thereby intending to save 450 million Dutch guilders annually. The affected people had to take additional private insurance to cover these costs. One year later, however, it was argued that elderly people in the Netherlands, living only on an old age benefit, could not afford to pay the additional premium. So, dental care for the elderly (mostly false teeth) was returned to the coverage package, thus reducing the intended savings from 450 to 300 million Dutch guilders.

The problem with moving to the right side of the continuum in health care is that such a policy is very difficult to match with notions of solidarity and equity. Saltman rightfully commented already ten years ago that "thus far, no one has succeeded in structuring a competition-based market on the finance side of their system for their entire population while still retaining a commitment to universal access to equal services. The only convincing evidence to suggest that a satisfactory 'universal' finance-side is possible exists in the realm of economic theory rather than in real-world practice."[42] There is no reason to assume that things are different now.

Consequently, governments intending to move to the right side of the continuum would do better to accept Lipsey and Lancaster's "General Theory of the Second Best," which was promulgated some 40 years ago. This theory holds that, when a specific market is considerably out of line with a pure market, thus yielding outcomes which are not "optimal" in market terms, "attempts to make it more market-like in some, but not all, respects will have indeterminate results for economic efficiency—and sometimes perverse ones."[43] Therefore, as long as governments want to uphold solidarity in health care, they have to accept "second-best" markets, adapting second-best forms of accountability like professional norms, government supervision, regulation, and subsidies. The second-best market is captured in terms like quasi-market, internal market, public competition, and provider market.[44] This is a better approach, because "the hapless attempt to get incrementally closer to the 'first-best' state of a pure free market—in an arena like health care, where price signals are necessarily distorted—may lead to third-best outcomes."[45]

A pure market for health care, with prices resulting from equilibrium between demand and supply, is therefore unrealistic for the greater majority of health care items. Nonetheless, this implies that one can think of exceptions. Here, the central question is what we define as "health care." Let me give some examples. One can argue that a woman who wants a facelift is seeking an aesthetic intervention, not health care. Likewise, one can argue that a man who wants to get rid of his flap-ears is seeking an aesthetic intervention, not health care. But what if both persons claim to be very depressed because of their looks and find a psychiatrist who is willing to support them? And what about a woman who, after a mastectomy, has reconstructive breast surgery, which is defined as a health care intervention? Finally, there is in vitro fertilization (IVF). Is that a health care item?[46] Here, the answer is uncertain. The Dutch, for example, had fully included IVF in the coverage package for many years. Since 2004, however, a person's first use of IVF has become the consumer's private business. In contrast, the Belgians, who originally did not include IVF in their coverage package, have since 2004 included it completely. In France, infertility treatment has, to date, been completely left out of the benefit package,[47] whereas in the United Kingdom, different health authorities, for different reasons, include or exclude these services from the coverage package.[48] All in all, even for the more "disputable" interventions, it is not entirely obvious whether they should be defined as matters of health care.

All these characteristics explain why policy-making with regard to health care reforms, directed at the introduction of market principles, is "essentially remedial, and focuses on small changes to existing policies rather than considering future major policies."[49] Given the attachment to solidarity and equity, governments hardly have any other options.

However, an interesting point is whether the many years of slowly moving toward the market by pursuing incremental reform policies have eroded the solidarity principle that is the basis for health care systems of the countries of the European Union. After all, taking a few small reform steps each year may appear innocuous, but the cumulative effect of doing so for many years may lead one to conclude that we are slowly dismantling the solidarity principle.[50] I will return to this topic in chapter ten.

Finally, it should be mentioned that governments not only try to introduce market principles, albeit incrementally, into the relation between consumers and providers in health care. They also try to do this by introducing elements of competition between providers and between insurers, as well as in their mutual relations. Schut, however, rightfully observes that "in health services and health insurance markets, unregulated competition will not generate an efficient resource allocation due to the presence of pervasive and biased uncertainties."[51] Therefore, governments will have to counter these uncertainties (antitrust policies, adverse selection, market control by the medical profession, et cetera) by regulating these markets, while at the same time upholding the solidarity principle. Only then can competition in health care be in the public interest.[52] The reality, however, is that government regulations in many countries of the European Union have become so intense and, consequently, entrepreneurial freedom has become so limited, that, so far, competition in health care is mainly a slogan.

Altogether, the picture one gets of governments slowly moving to the right side of the continuum since around the beginning of the 1980s is one of policy-makers contortedly trying to combine the principle of solidarity with a market in health care.[53] This policy has resulted in suffocating regulations and bureaucracies. Meanwhile, the costs of health care are still increasing and will further increase due to, among other things, an aging population and medical-technological developments. An obvious question, following from this conclusion, is whether governments are on the right track. I will come back to this question at the end of the book.

5.2 A Wheelbarrow With Frogs

The large number of parties interested in health care who all want health care policy to develop their way, and who all propose arguments and instruments for trying to achieve this, has induced some people to declare that health care is the archetype of political organization.[54] And, indeed, it is difficult to think of other politically debated social activities that are characterized by as many differing and even conflicting interests as health care. In democracies, this tremendously large number of interest groups tries to influence health care policy, pursuing their specific interests which, by them, are deemed more important than the interests of other parties involved in the health care process. They may do so by trying to convince other parties involved in health care of the value they add to the health of the population; they may strike; they may incite their clients; they may discredit or even blackmail other parties. This makes it almost impossible for governments to design a clear policy line and to follow that line consistently. Speaking about the German situation, Deppe maintains that the country's health care system is particularly resistant to governmental change and steering because of its entrenched internal power relations (*verkrusteten Machtstrukturen*).[55] Because of this, as previously discussed, health care policy practice is a matter of incrementalism, with governments trying to carry through changes by taking small steps, which may subsequently be undone. This is a "ready-fire-aim" approach.[56]

The degree of social-pluralism also plays a role. If governments have to take into account a relatively large number of political parties, there will be no room for "grand designs." Carrying out policy changes in these circumstances will be more difficult. Less social-pluralistic democracies can, in principle, be more governmentally effective. Margaret Thatcher, for example, as Prime Minister in a two-party ruling system, firmly initiated changes to the British National Health Service. However, she only dared to start this process of change after being in office for ten years, because she feared that the reform of the NHS was "too sensitive a topic to expose to the electorate."[57] After all, in democracies, there will always be elections again.

In order to illustrate the complexity of health care policy at the macro-level in social-pluralistic democracies, I distinguish five main categories. They are all related to each other, on either a permanent or an incidental basis. Together, these relations make health care a tangled mess that cannot easily be untangled.

The first main category is health care *providers*. Within this category, one can distinguish between health care institutions and health care professionals. As for the institutions, there are those where patients are cured and those where patients are taken care of. As for the institutions where people are cured, there are hospitals, which can be classified as acute or general hospitals, university hospitals, periphery hospitals, and specialized hospitals (cancer treatment, maternity, ophthalmology, military, and so on). These hospitals may be publicly or privately owned. They may work for-profit or not-for-profit. They may or may not be involved in the training of specialists. These hospitals, in turn, may have a Roman Catholic, a Protestant, a Jewish, a Humanistic, or other denomination. Among institutions where people are taken care of, we count psychiatric hospitals, institutions for the mentally retarded, nursing homes, homes for the elderly, and rehabilitation centers. Psychiatric hospitals, in turn, may be classified according to criteria like age (special clinics for the treatment of children) or type of disorder (alcohol and drug abuse, forensic treatment). Comparable distinctions exist for institutions for the mentally retarded. Nursing homes may specialize in the rehabilitation of elderly people or in geriatrics, or they may combine these types of care. And again, all these long-term care institutions may or may not have a religious denomination, they may or may not be engaged in the training of staff, they may be publicly or privately owned, and they may work for-profit or not-for-profit.

Things get even more complicated if we consider health care professionals. First of all, there is a whole range of professionals working in ambulatory settings, like the general practitioner, the dentist, the physiotherapist, the psychologist, the speech therapist, and the social worker. They may have their own individual practice or work in health centers with other professionals. In health care institutions, we may have more than 25 medical specialties (surgeons, internists, orthopaedists, ophthalmologists, neurosurgeons, lung specialists, dental surgeons, thorax surgeons, and so on). The United Kingdom has more than fifty specialties, whereas in the United States, by 1975 the American Medical Association had already recognized 76 specialties.[58] These medical specialists may be self-employed, employed, or a combination of self-employed/employed, working inside or outside the hospital, on their own, or together with colleagues in a group practice. They may or may not be involved in the training of future specialists.

All these (types of) health care providers have their own organized interest groups, trying to pressure or lobby governments to have developments go their way. They may, in line with what has been said in the first chapter, try to form opportunistic coalitions with other interest groups.

The second main category is health care *insurers*. They may be social insurers, which are not-for-profit; or insurers which are for-profit and therefore focus on the better-off in society; or they may deal with both types of insured people. Insurers may try to cover a whole population, or focus only on a certain category of citizens (civil servants, workers in health care, teachers, and so on). Insurers may differentiate their coverage packages (e.g., excluding coverage items, personal risks), their premiums, or their reimbursement systems. Insurers may only be involved in health care or may treat health care insurance as part of a more extended portfolio. Health care insurers also have their own organized interest groups, trying to pressure or lobby governments to have the developments go their way.

The third main category is *industry*. Health care is a very important market for industry, where pharmaceuticals and medical devices, from small instruments and materials to expensive high technology, are the eye-catching elements. In 1999, the European market for technological devices in health care totalled €40 billion, which is around 6% of European expenditure on health care. For the world market for medical devices, the estimated growth in 2001 and 2002 was between 5% and 8%.[59] Surely, industry, through scientific and technological research, has contributed considerably to the improvements in health care over the past half-century. It will continue to do so.

Since, in the Western world, the production of goods and services is a matter of private initiative, based on the profit motive of entrepreneurs, industry is not interested in restricting the health care market. Government regulations regarding the use of high technology, for example, which almost all European countries have, are not in the interests of industry, which understandably is interested in a quick return on investments. Because national markets may be too small for industry, its pressure and lobby activities to influence the health care market are very much directed at political levels beyond the level of national economies.

Other ways for industry to create a market are, first of all, bypassing governments through direct contacts with health care providers, making them interested in new opportunities. Secondly, developments in the medical field may be induced by research grants from industry. An example, is the fact that in the late 1980s, a Dutch university hospital received a donation of two million Dutch guilders for cancer research from a research fund of an American pharmaceutical company that totaled more than 200 million guilders. This phenomenon of contract research has been a normal part of health care for a very long time. It may become more important as hospitals and universities encounter increasing governmental budget constraints. Thirdly, since the fall of communism, the countries of Eastern Europe have become a very interesting market. Although these countries hardly have the financial means to set up a health care system in conformity with present-day technological standards, they nevertheless make use of high-technology equipment, like CT-scanners and MRIs. Hospitals in Eastern Europe may receive this equipment for free or at give-away prices. Finally, if governments from Eastern European countries are unable or do not want to supply the money for high technology investments, industry may conclude contracts with health care insurers to set up diagnostic/therapeutic centers like MRI units or hemodialysis facilities, as has happened, for example, in Hungary. Indeed, industry takes a long-term view.

The fourth main category is *patients*. With a bit of exaggeration, one could say that every patient has his or her own interest group. We have unions or foundations for heart patients, lung patients, kidney patients, schizophrenic patients, Alzheimer patients, rheumatic patients, and so on. In the beginning of the 1980s the Netherlands, for example, already had over 400 patient organizations.[60] Patients, or clients, have become an important factor in health care, executing strategies directed at improving, supplementing, or replacing actual health care policy, or they may protest against (aspects) of that policy. Patient organizations may successfully function as pressure groups, assisted by lawyers who take their needs to heart. Quite often they find a willing ear among politicians, which may lead to considerable government contributions to their finances. It is even assumed that, in line with some types of divide-and-rule politics, governments have deliberately encouraged patient organizations to grow and professionalize in order to act effectively as a countervailing power in their relationships with medical specialists.[61] Moreover, social insurers and individuals, through contributions and donations, may support their activities.[62] In addition to the fact that patients' organizations have strengthened their influence at the macro-level of social-pluralistic democracies, it should also be kept in mind that, at the level of health care delivery and insurance they have, whether or not through legal arrangements, reinforced their position considerably.

The fifth main category is the *government.* In fact, governments in social-pluralistic democracies function as the melting pot for the many differing wishes that the other main categories may have. It is impossible for governments to distill from this melting pot a health care policy that is acceptable for all parties involved. Moreover, governments have to take into account the wishes of other levels of government. Within national economies, this includes the county or municipal level. Within the international context, national economic orders also have to satisfy agreements at the level of the European Union. Further, although health care policy within a national economic order is mainly determined by the department of health, it is considerably influenced by other governmental departments, like economic affairs, the environment, social affairs and education. In addition to this, regarding health care policy, health departments are advised by advisory bodies which may operate more or less independently.

Altogether, we have a rather messy diversity of interest groups in health care. They do not have equal power to influence developments, but they may combine their activities. Additionally, interest groups may, on their own or in combination with other parties, be able to obstruct a policy they do not agree with considerably, thus demonstrating their reluctance to go beyond their own parochial concerns.[63] In order to illustrate this diversity, I have brought the main categories and their mutual relations together in the following diagram.

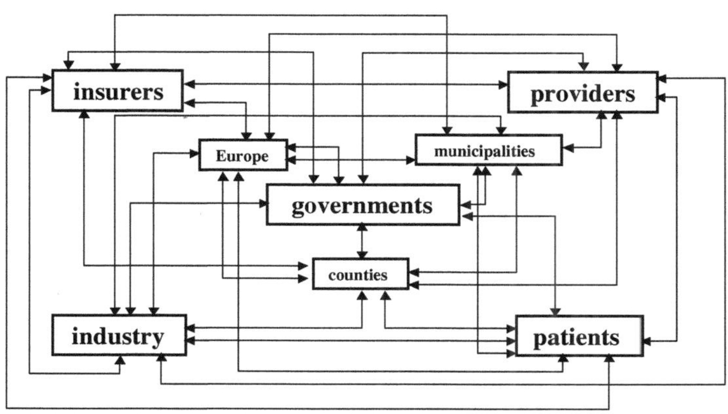

With some good will, one could say that this diagram delivers a rather clear arrangement of the relations between the main categories. Had I included, however, the separate elements of the main categories (for example, the different leagues of medical specialists also play their role), the diagram would have become an inextricable Gordian knot. Moreover, within a main category interests may differ considerably. As an example: the American

Medical Association strongly opposed the Clinton reform proposals of 1994. Nevertheless, these proposals were supported by many other medical associations.[64] As a further illustration, the reader should be informed that French nursing is represented by 60 to 120 organizations,[65] all with their own ideas on health care policy.

More meaningful, however, is which of the main categories governments particularly have to take into account when establishing health care policy. Here, industry and insurers are subject, among other things, to regulations about their performance and competition. Provided that governments can resist industry's "technology push," industry's market performance can be relatively easily controlled and corrected by legal means.

Providers and patients are another matter. They can and do function as pressure groups if health care policy is not to their liking. Moreover, while pressuring governments to devise health care policy in accordance with their wishes, they can very often confidently rely on public support. A few examples may illustrate this point.

Around the beginning of 1970s, the Dutch government was unwilling to provide the money for the purchase of heart-lung machines, which were necessary to perform open-heart surgery. Thanks to the pressure exerted by the union of heart patients, air bridges were set up to London, Houston, and Geneva. Meanwhile, open-heart surgery had become a normal procedure in many nearby countries, but not yet in the Netherlands. This lasted until 1972, when the then president of the union of heart patients, together with 150 members and a coffin, occupied the parliamentary building. Due to the media attention this action received, the government gave in. Within a few weeks, the money necessary for investing in the machines became available.

An example for France is the introduction of the lithotripter.[66] Here, a urology professor from Paris played an important role. He was so convinced of the added value of the new machine that he exerted pressure on the French Ministry of Health to be allowed to buy this piece of high technology. He organized press conferences during which he explained the new technique and, together with his colleagues, incited patients to write letters of complaint to the Director-General of the ministry. After a while, here, too, the government gave in.

In the United Kingdom, the first lithotripter was installed in a private clinic.[67] Although an NHS hospital received the second one, it was financed with private money. Proposed research that would compare the advantages of operating or using the lithotripter was rejected by the urologists. Furthermore, when the government of the United Kingdom wanted the diffusion of CT scanners to occur according to a phased plan, this appeared to be of limited use, since philanthropic donations interfered. For example, a hospital in the city of Liverpool that was not on the phased plan is said to have received the device as a donation from The Beatles. (Liverpool happens to be the band's native city.)

Finally, an example of blackmailing is evident in the story of the first heart transplant in the Netherlands.[68] Since this is a very expensive intervention, it is on the list of expensive procedures, which means that hospitals need special governmental permission to perform them. In 1984, however, the university clinics of Leiden and Rotterdam took the Dutch government by surprise by simply announcing that they had together performed the first heart transplant in the Netherlands without having permission. This caused a lot of fuss, with special debates in parliament. It resulted in the agreement that the two university clinics were permitted to perform 25 such interventions a year, with an intended evaluation after two years. In 1986, however, the reality was that the university clinics of Utrecht and Groningen were also allowed to perform the procedure, and the evaluation was limited to the medical protocol. Officially, the number of operations allowed remained 25, but in reality over 40 had already been performed. In retrospect, the initially firm behavior of the government appears to have been a joke.[69] Heart transplants for Dutch patients had already been done for some years. However, these patients were referred to clinics in the United Kingdom or Belgium, sometimes accompanied by Dutch surgeons. Each of these transplants was performed with government permission. Consequently, the Dutch government paid for them, including the costs of aftercare in the Netherlands.

The examples given in this section raise another important question: What instruments do governments have to control health care developments? The following chapter is an attempt to answer this question.

5.3 Health (Care) in Constitutions

Regarding health care, governments cannot stay on the sidelines for the simple reason that provisions in national constitutions and international agreements oblige them to act. In countries with a system of social health insurance, this constitutional norm is elaborated by statutory law, which regulates the provision, finance, organization, and quality of health care services.[70] Consequently, even if governments choose that health care should move as far as possible to the right side of the continuum, i.e., leaving things increasingly to the market, the obligation to satisfy national constitutions and international agreements forces them to control that market. Both national constitutions and international agreements are clear about this matter.[71]

As for international agreements, two Articles of the Universal Declaration of Human Rights, accepted in December 1948, are important in the context of this chapter.

First of all, it is stipulated in Article 3 that "everyone has the right to life, liberty and security of person." Furthermore, it states in Article 25, part 1, that "everyone has the right to a standard of living adequate for the health and well-being of himself and of his family, including food, clothing, housing and medical care and necessary social services, and the right to social security in the event of unemployment, sickness, disability, widowhood, old age or other lack of livelihood in circumstances beyond his control."[72] Simply put, the signatories of this declaration, coming from all over the world, including Russia and China, sincerely promised each other to look after their fellow citizens in need, thus intending to make the world a better place.[73] Consequently, we find statements about governments' responsibilities regarding health in almost each and every single constitution; that is, if a country has one. As for the European Union, this includes the former communist countries.[74]

Because of this, it seems rather safe to assume that formulations regarding governments' responsibility for their citizens' health are typical of the way Europeans want to relate to one another. As I wrote in the first chapter, European political culture is deeply imbued with a sense of general duty to aid the needy. Constitutional or comparable legal formulations regarding health (care) are a consequence of that sense of duty, which may be considered an expression of a European interpretation of the concept of solidarity, resulting in collective arrangements for social security and health care. No wonder, therefore, that the draft Treaty for a Constitution for the European Union also includes the spirit of solidarity with the poor and vulnerable members of society.[75] Respect for human dignity, solidarity, combating social exclusion and poverty, and a social market economy that recognizes and promotes the role of social partners in society are elements of the draft, which refers to a European history of taking one's fellow citizens into account. Consequently, health and health care are also included in the draft. In this respect, it is formulated in Article II-35 that every citizen is entitled to medical care under the conditions of national arrangements and practices. Here, the European Union has a supporting, coordinating, and complementary role regarding the protection and improvement of public health (Article I-16). In a way, the draft European Constitution reiterates what was included in the "Charter of Fundamental Rights of the European Union," as agreed during the Nice summit of 2000. Then, it was stipulated that "everyone has the right of access to preventive health care and the right to benefit from medical treatment under conditions established by national laws and practices."

This historic and cultural background of solidarity in the formulations of the constitutions of the countries of the European Union is not necessarily a feature of other political cultures. For example, the Arabian and Asian cultures, have differing views. I will not deal with all these views but, instead, I will limit myself to the United States, a country which is of particular importance in the context of this book. I found that, in the Constitution of the United States, not a single word is written about the federal government's responsibility regarding the health of American citizens. One might assume, however, that, as in the European Union, health (care) in the United States is the responsibility of each separate state. This suggests an

American subsidiarity principle. To find out whether this was correct, I examined the constitutions of 42 American states, thus covering 84% of the American federation.[76] This showed that, whereas all 42 states emphasize the importance of education for their citizens in their constitutions, 27 states (64%) have not written a single word on health (care). Of the remaining 15 states, 8 limit their attention to provisions for insane, blind, and deaf and dumb people. Mostly, this attention is closely related to the state's responsibility for penal institutions. In fact, Florida and Hawaii are the only states that may be considered to have formulations regarding their government's responsibility in health matters comparable to the countries of the European Union. Apparently, American culture has no room for collective health care arrangements. Such arrangements are perceived to be an unacceptable limitation of personal freedom.

An important point is whether constitutional formulations regarding health care actually make a difference for governments taking action in this area. This is not necessarily the case. After all, although former communist countries also had such formulations, they were of very limited meaning for those who did not belong to the powerful elite. After the fall of communism in Russia, its population's health worsened drastically, despite the transition to democracy. On the other hand, the communist state of Cuba is known to have had a high-quality, universally accessible health care system. Moreover, the United States, having hardly any constitutional formulations on health (care), has extensive health care organizations such as Medicare and Medicaid.

Constitutional formulations as such, therefore, are rather meaningless. The only consequence of constitutional formulations with regard to health and health care is that governments have to do something about them. They are "instruction norms," demanding that governments promote these ideals of basic social law and create conditions favourable to their pursuit.[77] To a greater or lesser extent, therefore, health care is always governments' business. What this implies for daily practice in democracies results from the interpretations of the constitutional formulations through processes of democratic decision-making. If, however, the constitutional norm has been elaborated in statutory law, for example the Sickness Fund Act of the Netherlands, this can make a difference, because it makes it possible for patients to claim health care through legal actions.[78]

It is important for democracies of the Western world that research has shown that good health, and with it good health care, is by far the highest priority for people. In this respect, a 1983 poll within the European Community showed that 81% of interviewed people ranked good health very high among the different interview categories.[79] The electorate, which is prepared to pay for solidarity in their health care systems, also believes that combating illnesses should be a prominent objective of society.[80] To put it even more strongly, having paid for it through taxation or premiums, the electorate believes that it has a legal right to health care. Limitations, in this respect, other than those for strictly medical reasons, are not acceptable. For social-pluralistic democracies this is, by and large, the point of departure for interactions between the government and the electorate, with the latter playing a zero-plus game. Either directly through a national health system or indirectly through a system of social insurance, however, health care expenditure at the macro level of society has to compete with other items of public spending, like education, defense, and cultural matters. Therefore, although it is an item of the constitution, the electorate cannot force governments to fulfil all its health care demands, even though, by law, governments are obliged to do at least something.[81] Consequently, constitutional formulations are not as absolute as the electorate wants them to be. Also, those who hold the view that "the patient expects, and has a right to expect, the best medical care at an acceptable cost" suffer from wishful thinking.[82] Constitutional formulations only refer to a limited obligation to try.[83] They leave room, therefore, to expand or to limit the right to health care in accordance with available financial means. And this is exactly what happens in daily practice. During the prosperous times when the welfare state was created, health care, together with items of social security, received a considerable share of a growing wealth pie (see chapter eight). When the recession made this no longer possible, governments found themselves in a delicate position. This was not only because scrapping an already existing provision was very difficult to contemplate, but, even more so, because the electorate's attachment to good health care remained unchanged and, thanks to scientific and technological developments, opportunities to combat disease continued to increase. It is meaningful that a recent Eurobarometer survey showed that only 5% of the population of the European Community were prepared to accept lower public spending on health care, whereas 50% wanted even higher spending.[84] In other words, where, due to times of economic recession, governments are forced to play a zero-minus game, they see themselves confronted with an electorate that wants to continue a zero-plus game. In the words of Friedman, therefore, at the beginning of an economic recession, governments enter a time of "catching rattlesnakes barehanded."[85] The only instrument available for that job is finance. I will return to this topic in the next chapter.

5.4 An Aging Population

Particularly over the past ten years, all governments of the countries of the European Union have made the aging of the population a central item of health care policy. The problem will accelerate at the end of this decade, when the baby-boomers from just after the Second World War will retire. In this respect, the European Commission predicts that the number of people over 65 years of age will increase from 16.1% of the total European population in the year 2000, to 22% in 2025, and to 27.5% in 2050, whereas the proportion of people 80 years and older, being 3.6% in 2000, will grow to 6% in 2025, and to 10% in 2050.[86] According to some, this may lead to a "distribution battle between generations" (author's translation).[87] It has been calculated for the Netherlands that the money spent in 1995 on general old age state pensions, other pensions, and health care, which was 20% of each Dutch guilder around the beginning of the 1990s, would, if policy stays as it is, increase to 35% in the year 2010.[88] The financing of this growing consumption load will increase pressure on younger people to cough up a bigger share of the increasing premiums. It remains to be seen if they are willing to do so. In the United States, an organization called Lead or Leave, a pressure group of some 1,000,000 members that was established to promote the interests of younger people and to demand a decrease in the public debt, is opposing the American Association of Retired People (AARP).[89] The elderly, so these youngsters argue, are responsible for the increasing public debt because of the benefits they receive.[90] Another pressure group, called Americans for Generational Equity (AGE) is demanding a fairer distribution of benefits and burdens between generations, pleading for "intergenerational equity."[91]

There seems to be no reason to leave aside comparable developments in the countries of the European Union. It may be true that, for the time being, governments of the European Union will have fewer problems, given the results of the Eurobarometer surveys of 1993 and 1996. They show a high level of agreement among citizens on the point of view that those who work should pay taxes in order to make it possible for elderly people to live a decent life. Of the Danes, 60.1% thought so; of the British, 45.9%; and the Spaniards, the Dutch, the Portuguese, and the Irish scored 45.7%, 42.4%, 41.2% and 40.7%, respectively. In Greece, Italy, Luxembourg, Belgium, and Germany the percentage was a little lower, whereas France had the lowest score with 25.9%.[92] Altogether, the "social contract" among the citizens of the European Union still seems to be in good shape, particularly when it comes to long-term care, and a private health care sector is widely opposed.[93] So far, therefore, European citizens appear to demonstrate a reasonable level of solidarity with elderly people. However, due to ongoing demographical changes, this is no guarantee for the future. This future may well lead to a "civil war between the green and the grey."[94] After all, from a certain point in time, that solidarity will be at the expense of younger people's own material wealth. In this respect, it is worth mentioning that 30,000 young French people took to the streets in Paris in 2003 to protest the—in their view—overly generous pensions that old people enjoy.[95] In conclusion, it cannot be ignored that the governments of the European Union will also be forced to cope with conflicting interests between generations.[96]

To some extent, one might say that conflicting interests are arising already. As an example, I refer to parliamentary discussions in the Netherlands around the end of the 20th century. Here, the "problem" was a surplus in the annual public budget, a fact unheard of for many years. There were several alternatives for spending this surplus. Reducing public debt, so that the Dutch could afford new debts if unemployment were to increase and an aging population was to cause real problems, was one of them. Shifting responsibility for the future to the individual citizen by deciding to reduce taxes was another. Or, finally, the Dutch could decide to invest in education and health care, because they were the depressed areas of society. Of course, the solution was found in the incremental middle course.

Meanwhile, although compromise and incrementalism are still characteristics for decision-making, policy measures directed at dealing with the problems of an aging population are being carried out all over Europe. They include disincentives for pre-pension retirement, postponing the age of retirement, and the termination of index-linked pension benefits.[97] Germany passed legislation in 2004 to cut present state pensions from 53% of average salaries to 46% by 2020. Also, in 2004, the Italian government proposed to increase the retirement age from 57 to 60. Moreover, in 2003 the Austrian government decided to phase out the right to early retirement with full pension by 2013, and in the same year the French government increased the number of working years necessary for civil servants to qualify for a full pension from 37.5 to 40 by 2008.[98] In addition to this, one can think of policies directed at increasing labor participation by women, or jobs that are adapted to incapacitated people.[99]

The question is, however, whether we can afford a policy of incrementalism in this respect. Regarding this, Judt suggests the possibility that, around the year 2010, the moment when the baby-boomers will retire, "the presence of an enormous group of frustrated, bored, unproductive and, in the end, sick old people, can cause a big social crisis"[100] (author's translation). One can argue about statements like these, since frustration and unproductiveness of elderly people will probably not be that serious, because many of them will enjoy ample pension benefits. Moreover, many elderly people contribute, for example, to social services in society. However, these ample pension benefits, when combined with a small labor pool of elderly people, could create an overheated economy, with stressed young families with children, wage explosions, and conflicts between generations. It should be taken into account that time and money are scarce assets for young families with children. Families like these in the Netherlands, for example, have 30% less to spend than families without children, compared to 15% less as the European average.[101]

Meanwhile, worries about illness and growing health care consumption by elderly people remain pertinent.[102] In the Netherlands, one in eight citizens was over 65 years of age in 1995. This 12.5% of the population absorbed almost half of all health care consumption. In addition to this, elderly people use a great deal of medication, and they consume 75% of home care in the Netherlands.[103] There is no reason to assume that, apart from the southern European countries, where, for cultural reasons, care for the elderly is organised considerably differently, comparable figures from other members of the European Union will differ very much in this respect.

There is no general agreement as to the health care consequences of an aging population in financial terms. American research, on the one hand, led to the conclusion that it is not the very old (over 80 years) but the "younger old" (between 65 and 80 years) who consume relatively more expensive high-technology care. Furthermore, British research concluded that "pressures arising from demography and morbidity are likely to have a modest impact in the future." And, indeed, rather generally expected rising health care costs as a consequence of an aging population may turn out to be lower than anticipated because of life long better nutrition and social conditions for elderly people. Next to this, an on-average improved education may positively affect the life styles of elderly people. American research has shown that the proportion of elderly people requiring assistance with their daily activities halved between 1976 and 1991. Finally, British research has led to the prediction that the total burden of disease would fall by two-thirds by 2051, due to increasing levels of fitness in successive generations.[104] On the other hand, Dutch research (which, in contrast to the American research, included long-term care for the elderly) found that health care costs increase exponentially from age 50 onward.[105]

Looking ahead to the next chapter on scientific and technological developments in health care, societies may be forced to determine which medical interventions are thought to be important and to whom. It is not unreasonable to assume that the answer to this question will be based on a comparison between health gains and their associated prices. Empirical research has shown that it is deemed acceptable for younger people to get preference; even elderly people think so. As an example, American research showed that saving the lives of eleven 60-year-old people was deemed to equal saving the life of one 30-year-old person. Similar research carried out in Sweden came up with the result of one QALY (Quality Adjusted Life Year) for a 30-year-old person per six QALYs for a 50-year-old person and 19 QALYs for a 70-year-old person. Consequently, politics will have to consider whether it is acceptable for society to prioritize access to health care for different groups of people.[106] This naturally leads to a discussion of ethical aspects of health care.

5.5 Ethics

About ten years ago, I had to explain the functioning of the Dutch health care system during a congress of Austrian hospital managers in the city of Innsbrück. There were quite a number of nuns among the audience. As usual, there was time for questions after I had finished speaking. It was my bad luck that, during the evening before, Austrian television had broadcast a Dutch program on euthanasia, and, coincidentally, the chairman of the congress had been the TV presenter for that program. Apparently, the Dutch program had shocked the Austrians. There was not a single question on my presentation. Instead, I was treated as if I were the Dutch hangman himself, purposely bringing helpless people to death, and, therefore, a murderer. I do not recall exactly how I answered the many questions on euthanasia, but I am sure I must have defended my country, knowing that, although the Dutch have rather liberal ideas on matters like euthanasia, abortion, and drug abuse, they are not an inconsiderate people. The difference between Austria and the Netherlands in those days was mainly that, in the latter country, topics like euthanasia could be discussed openly. There was no way this could be done in Austria at that time.

With the same openness, in the 1970s abortion had already become a matter of public debate in my country. In contrast, the Irish still rejected abortion in the late 1990s. Even then, a part of the Irish population wanted to amend their constitution so that it would contain a phrase that abortion should be prohibited, no matter what the circumstances. So, even if an expectant mother knew that her unborn baby would be mentally or otherwise handicapped, abortion was not to be allowed. The life-time health care costs this would bring to the Irish society would have to be accepted. Furthermore, IVF appeared to have become a matter of party politics in Italy, resulting in a referendum in 2005.[107]

Meanwhile, the liberal Dutch are very reluctant to donate their organs in the case of death. In this respect, they are very low in the European ranking. Dutch policy forbids using the organs of dead humans unless there is a written approval. It is a policy of "no—unless." In contrast, the Belgian regulation is a "yes—unless." These examples implicitly refer to ethics in health care, which has increasingly become a topic of government regulation over the past two decades, also at the European level.

As for euthanasia, for example, the Netherlands considers this to be a crime, but, since 1994, there has been no prosecution of euthanasia if certain conditions of carefulness were met: i.e., (1) the euthanasia must have been performed with the full and free consent of the patient, whose suffering was unbearable without any prospect of recovery; (2) it must have been performed in a medically correct way in consultation with a second doctor; (3) the local coroner had to be informed, and he, in turn, had to inform the public prosecutor; and (4) one of the five regional evaluation committees, composed of a doctor, a lawyer and an ethicist, had to check the conditions of carefulness. In November 1998, a new regulation on euthanasia reporting came into force, involving the public prosecutor only after the evaluation committee has made its report.[108] In November 2000, this practice of non-prosecution was legally regulated. As of April 2002, an amended law came into force, which further outlines the role of the evaluation committee. In Belgium, euthanasia was legally regulated by law in May 2002. Here, the criteria of carefulness are extensively described.

As for organ transplantation, as a second example, Greece and Spain were among the first countries to provide legal regulations (1978 and 1979, respectively). Belgium did so in a law of June 1986, whereas Germany introduced legal provisions in November 1997.[109]

Reading all these legal arrangements makes it very clear that ethical issues are at the center of these types of medical interventions. Governments have a special conditioning and correcting role here, which underlines that the production and consumption of health care goods and services cannot simply be compared to the production and consumption of other goods and services, because here, aspects of human dignity, self-determination, and personal integrity are involved. This being so, it may even be decided to consult the citizens in ethical matters explicitly by holding a referendum, as did the Italian government on IVF in 2005.

A positive side-effect of these legal arrangements is that, for example, the shroud of secrecy which surrounded euthanasia has been broken. Legalization has facilitated a widespread acceptance of life termination. Consequently, the number of reported cases of euthanasia in the Netherlands increased by almost 25% during the final decade of the 20th century.[110] In the words of Ansieau, legal regulations have facilitated a "decriminalization of euthanasia."[111] It is a topic that can be discussed these days. But it is by no means a topic of general policy agreement. On the contrary, because discussions on euthanasia combine ethical, moral, religious, human, and cultural aspects,[112] there will probably never be general agreement on how to act. As recently as March 2002, the Standing Committee of European Doctors adopted a resolution taking a clear position against any form of assisted suicide.[113] At the European level it is meaningful that a September 2003 resolution legalizing active assistance dying was accepted by a small majority of 15 against 12 in the Social, Health, and Family Affairs Committee of the Council of Europe.[114] Further proof of the delicacy of ethical questions in health care is the fact that the European commission has set up several groups of advisors regarding the relation between technology and ethics. In 1991, the commission had already established a group of advisors on the ethical implications of biotechnology. In 1993, this advisory group adopted an opinion on products derived from blood or human plasma, which was followed in 1994 by a report on the ethical implications of gene therapy.[115] More recently, the commission set up an independent, pluralist, and multidisciplinary European Group on Ethics, which is a consultative body to the European Commission on ethical questions regarding new technologies. Genetic screening and the use by employers of genetic information about their (potential) staff members are items of concern to this group. Happily, the group since has expressed as its opinion that the use of genetic testing in the context of employment is, in principle, ethically unacceptable.[116] That does not mean to say, however, that it will never happen. Finally, in 2000, the WHO also recognized the importance of ethical issues in health care by adding "health and ethics" as a special European Health for All target to its program.[117]

Given all these ethical aspects of health care, it is no wonder that health care providers are also trying to find ways to deal with them. The creation of medical or clinical ethics committees has been one response. In the 1960s, these committees had already emerged in the United States, where they have become part of the hospital establishment. The setting up of comparable structures in European hospitals happened considerably later.[118] They now exist, offering a forum for "discussing a variety of different moral judgments and allow opinions on difficult situations to be expressed."[119] Such a forum may be composed of medical experts, focusing on questions such as whether to provide certain treatments and developing ethical guidelines, or they may represent a bottom-up approach, involving all hospital staff.[120] The general impression one gets from the literature is that dealing with ethical questions in hospitals is still in a development phase. It will probably be so for a long time to come.

All in all, ethical questions regarding health care constitute an important peculiarity for the economic order, at national as well as supranational levels. Governments, as the keepers of the common good and of norms and values, cannot remain on the sideline in this area. Given the predicted developments to come in medical science and technology, it may even be expected that ethical matters will become increasingly significant. If it becomes possible, for example, to implant electrodes in a person's brain through which that person's personality can be influenced, this will certainly raise enormous ethical disputes.[121] And what about having people walking around with a gene-pass?[122] What about people's privacy? What about solidarity and equity if neuro-electronic interfaces make it possible to neutralize paralysis?[123] Will it be only the better-off who can afford this, or will we include it in the basic coverage package? And how will we guarantee that human cloning is only to the benefit of free citizens? The delicacy of topics like these is evident from the results of several research projects. A Spanish poll of some years ago, for example, revealed that 73% of respondents wanted their government to do everything to prevent investigations and experiments in cloning, with 81% in favor of legal measures to forbid it.[124] Although there is now a realistic prospect of improving human nature by cloning, making humans less vulnerable to certain diseases,[125] this implicitly augments the ethical issues surrounding health care. To give a final example, how do we prevent biotechnology from reaching a state of development which makes it inherently "non-masterable and unpredictable"?[126]

Ethics is a relatively new area of health care, but it may be expected to become a major factor in political decision-making.

5.6 Summary

This chapter dealt with the dilemmas for governments that, regarding health care, want to move to the right side of the continuum. It showed that maintaining solidarity among citizens is difficult to combine with the introduction of market principles. Only second-best markets are feasible. Furthermore, restrictive policies are hampered by the many different parties involved in the health care process. These two factors together lead governments to pursue policies of incremental change, taking small steps one at a time. Further obstacles are caused by constitutional obligations, the aging of the population, and ethical issues. They force governments to interfere extensively in the production and consumption of health care goods and services.

6
Health Care Dynamics

Developments in health care are to a considerable extent determined by the immanent dynamics of the health care process. These dynamics make health care a very difficult item to control in any democratic economic order. In order to explain these dynamics, I define health care as *a complex and dynamic process of continuous innovation, i.e., of constantly changing new combinations of science, technology, organization, politics, economics, and (medical) culture.*

Based on the generally accepted distinctions between *cure* and *care*, on the one hand, and *extramural* and *intramural*, on the other,[1] the workings of this definition can be illustrated with help of the following diagram.[2]

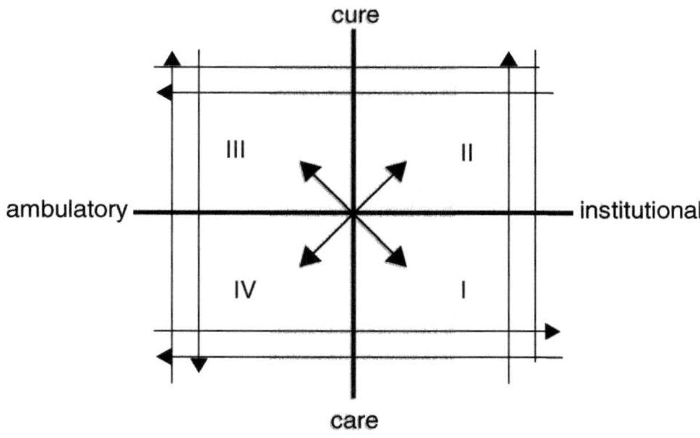

Cure refers to short-term medical interventions directed at correcting a health problem. *Care* deals with long-term medical attention, often for chronic conditions.[23] *Institutional* cure or care involves in-patient facilities, like wards and hospital premises. *Ambulatory* care or cure occurs without these facilities.

The diagram shows four quadrants of health care. The first, institutional care, refers to institutions for the mentally retarded, psychiatric hospitals, and nursing homes. The second quadrant includes acute hospitals, university clinics, specialized hospitals, and the like. In both quadrants, supply is institutionalized. The differences between these quadrants are largely determined by their level of complexity. The third quadrant includes the wide range of health care services that are delivered in outpatient clinics. Short-term psychotherapeutic interventions also belong in this quadrant, as do visits to the dentist, the physiotherapist, and the general practitioner. The fourth quadrant refers to the large variety of clinical and social (support) services needed to help (former) patients stay self-reliant. Preventive medicine also belongs in this quadrant, as do domiciliary or home-care services.

Among these four quadrants, three types of dynamics can be distinguished. Firstly, there are *horizontal dynamics*, i.e., movements from II to III and vice versa, as well as those from IV to I and vice versa. A few examples may illustrate these dynamics. The introduction of a mobile version of the lithotripter made ambulatory treatment possible for patients with a specific kind of kidney stone, instead of hospitalization (II to III). Developments in pharmaceuticals helped certain schizophrenic patients to carry on in society with ambulatory support instead of remaining dependent on institutional care (I to IV). The vice-versa movement in the horizontal dynamics is obvious: if ambulatory cure or care no longer helps, then institutional cure or care is the only alternative.

Secondly, there are *vertical dynamics*, i.e., movements from III to IV as well as from II to I, and vice versa. For example, the patient who is admitted to hospital after being badly injured in a traffic accident will be transferred to an institution for the physically handicapped if a spinal cord lesion is one of the consequences of the accident (II to I). People who were formerly admitted to a nursing home if they could no longer walk may nowadays have a hip replacement (I to II). People with mental disorders who can no longer be helped by a general practitioner may have to rely permanently on ambulatory mental health care (III to IV).

Thirdly, there are *diagonal dynamics*, i.e., movements from II to IV and from III to I, and vice versa, which include various types of aftercare; for example, follow-up care after the treatment of breast cancer or carcinoma of the colon, or a kidney transplant after a period of haemodialysis. And if, in the coming years, research on Alzheimer's disease leads to the invention of an effective drug, institutional care in nursing homes may start a diagonal dynamic from I to III.

Transitions between the quadrants of health care are becoming increasingly common, leading to an ever more holistic view of integration. Transition may even have already become a matter of national policy. There is a deliberate search for so-called "seamless care." Moreover, health care professionals may work in more than one quadrant. Furthermore, we see the emergence of hospital-based home care. It should be mentioned, finally, that most of the dynamics in the diagram are initiated by health care providers, facilitated by scientific and technological developments. Sometimes, however, they simply emerge when the health care provider (or patient) decides to "another way," with the government in a conditioning and/or correcting role.

To see if and how governments can influence this dynamic process, I will analyze the foregoing definition of health care in more detail. To make things more manageable, I will deal with the six elements of science, technology, organization, politics, economics, and (medical) culture separately. I start with the last element.

6.1 Medical Culture

Many have said that medicine is not yet a very exact science.[4] Of course, medicine can benefit from scientific input, but "culture intervenes at every step of the way."[5] Because of this, it is understandable that there are many differing views and opinions on the treatment of patients among medical doctors, resulting in differing medical cultures. In documenting these differences, Payer distinguishes between Cartesian thinking in France, Romanticism in Germany, Empiricism in England, and aggressiveness in the United States. Valuing thought, French diagnosis is based on logic and theory, taking into account the whole patient and his environment (the French speak of the *terrain*). In contrast, German Romanticism values feeling. Its proponents, unlike the Cartesians, do not see the world as a machine, but as an organism with an interplay of opposing forces. This attitude is in the German character and, thus, influences the German way of approaching medicine. For the British Empiricists, all knowledge comes from experience instead of thought and theory. This view has influenced the whole of British society. Whereas, for example, the European continent has drawn up legal regulations in anticipation of disputes, British law is based on interpretations of disputes that have already come up.[6] This attitude has also influenced medicine in Britain. You do not intervene unless experience has proven that intervening is the right thing to do. The aggressiveness of American medical treatment is characterized by doing everything you can to combat disease. Medicine means, in fact, a war on disease.

These cultural prejudices influence the daily practice of medicine, as well as patients' attitudes toward and appreciation of their doctors. Let me give a number of examples.

Research in France has shown that patient appreciation for the French doctor is positively correlated with the number of prescriptions the doctor writes. British doctors prescribe fewer drugs per capita than their French, German, and American colleagues. The British patient is less likely to have heart surgery (a chance of 1:2), and even less likely to have coronary bypass surgery (a chance of 1:6), compared to an American patient. Because of this attitude, it is said that economy is the most striking characteristic of

British medical care.[7] A Spanish doctor treating a wound may use two sutures, because he is paid for treating the wound, whereas his Belgian and Austrian colleagues may use six or even more sutures because they are paid for the number of sutures.[8] Some ten years ago, figures showed that Portuguese women had by far the highest number of Caesarean operations in Europe, a fact which cannot be explained by physical differences between Portuguese and other women. The rumored explanation is that Portuguese gynecologists are paid extremely well for this intervention. In France, women may have plastic surgery because they want to be happy. In contrast, in Sweden women are supposed to accept their body as it is. Most American women who undergo breast surgery want their breasts to be enlarged. Their French colleagues want them to be reduced.[9] The Germans see their doctor twelve times a year on average, compared to the French, British, and American average of five times a year.[10] In Germany, there are some 120,000 drugs on the market, ten times as many as in Iceland.[11] For American doctors, death is regarded as an ultimate failure in medical skills. Their British colleagues regard death as something physiological, which may even be hoped for.[12] Finally, American doctors perform more diagnostic tests than their colleagues in France and Germany. They prefer surgery to the use of drugs, and when they prescribe drugs, they use the more aggressive ones.[13] In this respect, Mechanic reveals that, in the 1970s, the rate of American surgical operations per capita was twice as high as that in England and Wales.[14] Altogether, the examples given demonstrate that, indeed, health care is not a very exact science. Medical culture plays an important role. Changing these cultural aspects of health care will take considerable time, if it is feasible at all.

The same applies to other cultural differences which also have an influence on health care. One example would be people who for religious reasons refuse to have vaccinations. As a second example, care for the elderly in the Southern countries of Europe is, to a considerable degree, the responsibility of relatives. In Spain, for example, 72% of home care was provided by family members in the mid-1990s.[15] In the Netherlands, people are used to thinking that care for the elderly should be part of the health care system. A change in citizens' attitudes in this respect, which the Dutch government seems to be pursuing, will take considerable time.

Finally, though not directly labeled as culture but nevertheless related to it, philosophy and opinions have their influence on the health care process. It is hard to deny their influence on health care activities that are not so much based on scientific evidence but on personal assessment. Let me give a few examples.

Research in New York has shown that doctors diagnose the need for a tonsillectomy quite arbitrarily.[16] Psychotherapy sessions used to be a very time-consuming process. They could easily last for more than one year. Due to the increasing workload of the therapists, something else had to be tried. In the mid-1980s, the alternative became short-term interventions, sometimes as few as eight sessions, which, depending on the nature of the problem, delivered comparable results.[17] During the 1960s, health was defined as an optimal combination of physical, mental, social, and environmental factors; in short, the WHO approach. Nowadays we accept that the ideal differs from reality. Consequently, health care professionals try to teach people to cope with the ailments of life. During the second half of the 1970s, the Dutch government started to reconfigure Dutch psychiatric hospitals, transforming them into small-scale facilities with more privacy for patients. About the same time, the Italians closed down psychiatric hospitals completely. The same Dutch government, shortly after having completed the reconfiguration, changed its mind and started to develop sheltered homes. Now, for the Dutch, the initial signs of too much optimism are becoming evident, whereas Italian families are experiencing difficulties in dealing with the psychiatric problems of their relatives.

In conclusion, the prevailing societal philosophy and opinions often cause changes in health care without any scientific evidence that these changes add value to the health care delivery process.[18] Therefore, influencing "common wisdom" might be an effective way for governments to reform their health care systems. As an example, in January 2004, the Dutch Minister of Health simply declared that the basic coverage package would no longer include psychotherapy after 30 sessions. To support this decision, he could have cited Lasch, who accused psychotherapeutic professionals of making "extravagant claims for their expertise," setting themselves up as doctors "not only to sick patients but to a sick society."[19]

However, because it has been forecasted that the effectiveness of psychotherapy may increase due to developments regarding brain research,[20] governments' attitude towards psychotherapy may change in the future.

6.2 Science and Technology

In order to bring some structure to these two elements of the definition, I will distinguish between two separate aspects of the influence of science and technology on developments in health care: (1) the recent past and the future of science and technology itself followed by (2) the marketing of medical technologies and the means governments have to control scientific and technological developments.

6.2.1 The Past and the Future

In 1967 Kahn and Wiener published a famous list of 100 technological innovations predicted to occur with great probability before 2000. Fourteen items on that list had to do with improving, restoring, or controlling the human condition. They all have, in fact, become reality. Moreover, even some of their other 35 less probable or even far-fetched predictions (presented in two other lists) have occurred or are currently being tested with promising results.[21] In the last half-century, developments in health care science and technology have been amazing, particularly those that occurred during the first three decades after the Second World War. As a consequence, and using a broad definition of the term *technology*, i.e., "drugs, devices, and medical and surgical procedures used in health care, *and the organizational and supportive systems within which such care is provided*" (italics mine),[22] technological developments are estimated to have contributed to a 50% increase in health care expenditure over the past decades.[23]

It would be wrong, however, to assume that the present state of medical knowledge and capabilities is the consequence of a deliberate search for methods to combat disease alone. Many important discoveries were the result of willpower, determination, chance observation, and the good luck of interested individuals.[24] For example, the discovery of penicillin (1941) was an accident, rather than a consequence of scientific research. The creation of cortisone (1949), which together with penicillin caused a therapeutic revolution, was unanticipated. As for psychiatric illnesses, the 1950s saw six new types of drugs for the treatment of schizophrenia, which, in large part, were discovered by chance. Meanwhile, despite the unexpected discovery of important drugs, the real causes of many diseases are still unknown.

In particular, the year 1950 caused a "paradigm shift" which separated medicine's past from its future. Streptomycin was discovered and, combined with PAS (para-amino salicylic acid), appeared to be very effective for the treatment of tuberculosis. For over 100 years before 1950, the dominant paradigm in medicine had been "the germ theory," and research was directed at finding effective treatment for infectious diseases with tuberculosis as the biggest challenge. Thanks to streptomycin and PAS, treatment efforts could shift to non-infectious diseases like cancer, strokes, and heart attacks. But, again, willpower and determination were decisive. For example, during the 30 years after the Second World War, hundreds of thousands of chemicals were investigated as potential cancer treatments to find no more than 30 that proved to be of any value.[25] Heart transplantation became possible, thanks to the fortuitous discovery of azathioprine. Furthermore, statistics, instrumental to epidemiologists, started to provide the means for mass-scale prevention measures. Finally, randomized controlled trials, although intensely debated, came into use for the evaluation of the effectiveness of the many drugs that came on the market in the period 1950–1960.[26]

All in all, "it is [. . .] a distinctive feature of post-war medicine that many doctors and scientists attempted, against all odds, to take on 'the insoluble.' "[27] Their attempts even included self-experimentation.[28] Their achievements, however, "did not arise from a profound understanding of the nature of medical problems but, more often than not, from chance or luck or some technological development."[29] Medicine is so influenced by exogenous factors that one can rightfully argue that it is only partly an exact science. It is first of all an occupation and only on occasion a profession.[30]

Particularly in the United States, state funding during and after the war contributed enormously to health research.[31] The then-established institutions, like the National Institute of Health and the National Cancer Institute, were funded with billions of dollars.[32] All this medical research would help, it was believed, to make the world a better place. Scientific innovations during and shortly after the war contributed to the "big bang" in medicine. The many research activities being pursued had important spill-over effects for further developments. In other words, medicine was on the rise, and it developed its own internal dynamic. This dynamic has six themes.[33] The first two themes concern the coincidental discovery of antibiotics and steroids, as well as the "interconnectedness" of medical research. The rise of "clinical science," the third theme, became the dominant ideology in the 1940s. Training specialists and promoting research to advance medical knowledge created an atmosphere of optimism. Zeal and the desire for knowledge stimulated the belief that, eventually, most medical problems could be solved. Furthermore, patients became "interesting clinical material" on whom ambitious doctors could perform experiments, hoping for publication in well-known medical journals.[34] The fourth theme is the enormous development of pharmaceuticals. The discovery of sulphonamides, antibiotics, and cortisone produced huge potential markets with very attractive profits. Because of this, the pharmaceutical industry started to invest heavily and attracted many chemists. Le Fanu characterizes the period 1940–1975 as "the golden age of drug discovery."[35] Technology, the fifth theme, also played a role. Contrary to drug discovery, however, technology is highly intentional. It tries to find specific answers to defined problems.[36] Le Fanu distinguishes between three main categories: (1) life-sustaining technologies (intensive care, ventilators, dialysis, and pacemakers); (2) diagnostic technologies (CT scanners, MRI scanners, ultrasound, PET scanners, angiography, and cardiac catheterization); and (3) surgical technologies (joint replacement, intraocular lens implants, chochlear implants, the pump, operating microscope, and endoscopy).[37] Although all these themes contributed to the rise of modern medicine, the sixth theme, concerning "gifts from nature" or "the mysteries of biology," is equally important. While there are some who give doctors and scientists the credit for the ascendancy of modern medicine and devalue the mysteries of nature, it is undeniable that nature has played an enormous role in the development of medicine. Doctors and scientist who fail to acknowledge this role, overestimating their intellectual capacities, claiming knowledge they do not possess, and believing that medicine can solve any problem, will experience frustration if therapeutic innovation declines.[38]

Since most of the achievements in health care were realized in the 20th century, particularly in the second half, this era has been labeled "the health century,"[39] during which health care developed into a "health industry."[40] In retrospect, it is amazing how quickly the image of health has changed completely. If one had predicted human organ transplantation halfway through the 20th century, one would have had a fair chance of being thought mad. But in 1956, the first kidney transplant (between twins) was done, followed by the first liver transplant in 1963; and in 1967 the world was awed by the first heart transplant. Nowadays, these interventions have waiting lists in many countries. Indeed, the aforementioned six themes have, together, definitively changed the focus of health care from caring to curing. And the end is not in sight yet. Here, the most fundamental contributor has been, still is, and will continue to be the computer. Computers, together with laser techniques, biomedical research, developments in pharmacology, and so on, will continue to contribute to further developments. Already, digital imaging, drug-coated stents, oral cancer treatments, minimally invasive surgery, sepsis treatment, implantable devices, and microscopic cameras are a reality.[41] They may be expected to diffuse rapidly.

The American Food and Drug Administration points to advancing computer-realted technology, molecular medicine, home- and self-care, minimally invasive procedures, combined device/drug products, and organ replacements and assists as exciting new developments in health care. The Dutch Council for Public Health and Welfare adds to this list technologies that may contribute to improving efficiency and labor conditions.[42]

As for *computer-related technology*, one may point to many developments serving the consumer. Here, the internet plays a determining role. Consumers will increasingly surf the internet in order to find information regarding their health and, if necessary, how their health problems can be solved. Around 2000, the number of websites with health (care) information already numbered more than 100,000. It is likely that this number will continue to increase. Surveys suggest that 75% of all web users have accessed health information.[43] The positive side of this development is that it contributes to patient empowerment. On the negative side, these patients may be exposed to unreliable information or unreliable medical products. Another negative aspect is the fact that access to the internet is still limited to the relatively young and more educated members of society.[44] This may create a "digital divide."[45] On the other hand, the internet has also taken a leading role in the development of E-health, which has been defined by the Dutch Council of Public Health and Welfare as the use of information and communication technologies, and particularly internet-based technology, to support or to improve health and health care. E-health offers opportunities for health care professionals to receive profession-related information at the right moment and in the right place, thus contributing to improved quality, efficiency, effectiveness, and accessibility of health care. Furthermore, E-health has the potential to improve the relations between provider and consumer. Like the internet, E-health also offers a mixture of opportunities and threats. Regarding the latter, the possibility of infringement of privacy is a serious problem. Apart from the internet and E-health, computer-related technologies will continue to deliver new diagnostic and therapeutic opportunities. CT, MRI, and PET scans will be perfected. Telemedicine is spreading rapidly,[46] and "virtual medicine," which creates three-dimensional images of organs, is on the move. In order to restrain extreme optimism, however, it should be mentioned that making these opportunities a common part of the health care process depends to a large extent on the willingness of medical professionals to do so. In this respect, expectations prevalent during the 1960s that electronic patient dossiers might deliver enhanced opportunities for diagnosis and therapy have not become reality in a way that might have been possible had medical professionals reached agreement among themselves on the desirable use and content of such dossiers.

Regarding developments in *molecular medicine and biotechnology*, knowledge about the genetic components of diseases is rapidly increasing. Research about different aspects of biotechnology (diagnostics, drugs, vaccines, tissue engineering, gene therapy, xenotransplantation) may in the shorter or longer term offer new opportunities to improve the human condition.

As for *combined device/drug products*, many new applications like the insulin pump and time-release tablets have been developed during the past decades. By combining different technologies, new devices like biosensors and micro-electronic pumps, which can be implanted, may be developed. Coating new hips with antibiotics in order to prevent infections is a further example of new technology.

Minimally invasive technologies (which started with the heart catheter in 1929) will increasingly replace traumatic operations. Since the beginning of the 1980s, laparoscopic intervention has been used regularly for the treatment of appendicitis, as well as for gall-bladder operations. Minimally invasive technologies are also being used increasely for heart surgery as well as for neurosurgery. In Canada, computer-supported laparoscopic bypass surgery, with a beating heart, was done for the first time in 1999. Since 2000, dozens of patients have been treated this way worldwide.

Predicting the future for *organ replacements and assists* is very difficult. For the time being, the availability of donor organs will be the critical point for further development. Although the artificial kidney of 1944 and the heart-lung machine of 1951 have been very important developments in health care, to a large extent the production of artificial organs appears to be limited to special components, like heart valves. Organ assists, however, like the pacemaker, first implanted in 1960, increasingly support the functioning of organs (intra-aortal balloon pumps) or serve to bridge the time before a donor organ is available (ventricle device). As medical technology advances, more organ assists, based on a combination of (micro)-mechanical, micro-electronics, and material technology, are expected to become available.

Computer technology will also affect *home- and self-care*. In this respect, tele-monitoring patients in their own living environment may contribute to diagnostics and treatment from a distance. Biosensors will allow doctors to monitor patients' condition remotely and to take correcting measures if necessary. Trans-mural home-care technology will increasingly replace hospital admission.

Finally, there is the vast area of brain research, where psychopharmacology and micro-electronics are important factors. Magnetic stimulation of muscles and limbs, neurohelmets that improve the storing and processing of information in the brain, as well as enhancers that improve mental functioning are no longer fiction.[47]

The impression one gets from these (possible) future developments is that it is particularly (information) technology that rules. But what about medical science? If we follow Le Fanu, it seems as if "the age of optimism"[48] regarding the future of medicine began to end, for several reasons, at the beginning of the 1980s.[49]

First of all, he observes a "marginalisation of clinical science" in the United States. In this country, the number of young doctors wishing to undertake postdoctoral medical research halved between 1968 and 1978. Apparently, young doctors cannot resist the seductive lure of high incomes which they can generate in procedure-based medical specialties like cardiac catheterization. These young doctors appear to suffer from the "young physician–Porsche syndrome."[50] Consequently, the clinical scientist may become "an endangered species."

Secondly, the pharmaceutical industry has not, in general, come up with many important new drugs recently.[51] The 1960s saw some 70 new drugs coming to the market each year. In the 1970s, this number was halved. In addition to this, many of the new drugs introduced in the early 1970s were, in fact, more expensive varieties of older and cheaper drugs. Moreover, shocking failures were exposed. The sleeping pill thalidomide, for example, caused babies to be born with missing limbs. Governments rightfully reacted by imposing very strict regulations on the introduction of new drugs. Consequently, the development time for each new drug had increased by ten years by 1980, with the development costs for each new drug escalating to £150 million by the 1990s, from £5 million in 1960. Though understandable, the new and very strict regulations acted as a disincentive to innovation. According to Le Fanu, the pharmaceutical industry, out of frustration (not being able to find effective drugs for the treatment of cancer or dementia, for example), turned to so-called life-style drugs (for impotence, for baldness, for obesity, or what have you).

Thirdly, medical technology seems to be out of control, with doctors doing far more tests than necessary. Testing has become an end in itself. It would appear that doctors suffer from "medical vampirism."[52] Here, finance also plays a role, since each and every test has to be paid for, thus generating income for the doctor in health care systems that are based on insurance. However, the other side of the coin is that, particularly in the United States, but now also on the European continent, lawsuits against doctors who did not do everything possible are on the increase. Doctors may easily be charged with negligence. Out-of-control technology is also an aspect of health care given to patients in their final days, with people "hopelessly entrapped by machinery more sophisticated than the ethics governing its use."[53] Here, however, technology itself is not the problem. The problem is doctors' lack of self-control, according to Le Fanu. And often the patient's relatives want a doctor to do everything he or she can to prolong life.

Altogether, the developments in clinical science (decreasing interest in medical research), pharmaceuticals (retarding innovation), and technology (overuse) have, according to Le Fanu, caused the end of "the age of optimism." In his view, there is no longer any reason to be optimistic about the future of health care. It may be an over-reaction, however, to be pessimistic. After all, no one knows what the future will bring. It is worth mentioning that, in the 1980s, a new paradigm emerged based on two very different specialties: epidemiology and genetics.[54] The first is a social theory, arguing that diseases like cancer, heart disease, and strokes are caused by unhealthy life-styles. Changing those life-styles could contribute to health. As for genetics, a few amazing developments during the 1970s opened up the possibilities of identifying abnormal genes in several diseases. This new paradigm, according to Le Fanu, "is striking testimony to the declining power of empirical therapeutic innovation."[55] As yet, however, the new paradigm has not fulfilled its promise. There is still a considerable gap between anticipated benefits and reality. And Le Fanu is right: the causes of many diseases are still unknown (multiple sclerosis, rheumatoid arthritis, psoriasis, Crohn's disease, et cetera).

6.2.2 Marketing Medical Technologies

The heart of enterprise is innovation: innovation in products, in methods, and in markets. Innovation seems to be a condition for survival. Innovation is so important that, for example, a failure rate of around 90% for new consumer goods is apparently not enough to slow down the creation and marketing of new products.[56]

In the framework of this book, it is not necessary to consider the way innovations are dealt with in general terms, because starting in 1960s and 1970s, a wealth of literature has been published on the subject.[57] It is important, however, to pay attention to the question of how *medical* innovations, be they diagnostic techniques, surgical procedures, or drugs, become part of medical practice. In particular, this is important from the perspective of governments' capabilities to control health care developments. In fact, if we take it as a given that if industry perceives the promotion of innovations to be a useful way of bringing new products to the health care market, the diffusion of such an innovative product, i.e., "the process by which the use of an innovation spreads and grows,"[58] is relevant in the framework of this book, because, unlike innovations outside the health care sector, innovations in health care need multiple acceptance from different stakeholders with differing interests in order to realize a successful launch. McKinlay distinguishes a general pattern of seven stages of innovation[59]:

1. *Promising Reports*
   The career of an innovation quite often begins with the publication of enthusiastic reports regarding remarkable results which have been achieved through its use or application. This happens increasingly through the mass media, like magazines and newspapers.[60]
2. *Professional Adoption*
   This stage is directed at mobilizing as much influential support as possible from interested parties. The aim is to get organized commitment from potential users, like medical specialists and hospitals.[61]
3. *Public Acceptance*
   Following its adoption by professionals and hospitals, the innovation is accepted by the general public, which has started to believe that the innovation means an improvement in health care and, therefore, should be available. In other words, there is public demand for the innovation.[62]
4. *Standard Procedure*
   In this stage, the new technology or procedure loses its status as an innovation and becomes a standard procedure, which is generally accepted as the most appropriate way of dealing with a particular health care problem. Its effectiveness or desirability is judged to be so important that it takes courage to question its added value. The innovation is now halfway through its life cycle. Nevertheless, it has still not been subjected to any formal evaluation. Instead, its position is secured by comparative observational studies.[63]
5. *Randomized Controlled Trials*
   Observational studies never really test the effectiveness of an innovation. For this, randomized clinical trials (RCT) are appropriate. In order to do this, however, several objections have to be overcome because use of the innovation has become the norm in the medical field with different interest groups and reputations invested in its continuing success.[64]
6. *Professional Denunciation*
   If RCTs lead to criticism of what has become a standard procedure, this almost always leads to defensive reactions from the medical establishment. There are, of course, many ways of discrediting the results of an RCT that

challenge some standard procedure. McKinlay refers to widely employed techniques like restricting the application of the results and depicting RCTs as impractical, ivory-tower activities which are of no use to the real medical world.[65]

7. *Discrediting*

At a certain point in time, the erosion of support for the innovation sets in. The once-enthusiastic claims for its efficacy begin to be modified. Its claim of universal application is adjusted and it is claimed that only certain types of patients or stages in diseases can be served by it.

Sometimes, an innovation's career is ended by a scandal. However, "more often it is simply eclipsed by some other rising star, and just drops out of public view. The innovation no longer enjoys public attention, little prestige is derived from association with it, cheaper alternatives become available, and so forth [. . .]. Discrediting or discard usually occurs only when a *replacement* becomes available."[66]

Some remarks have to be made regarding these phases. First of all, it should be taken into account that the introduction of an innovation may be preceded by years of research that was not directly related to the innovation. The concept of a cardiac pacemaker, for example, was formulated in 1928. It took another 30 years, however, before this device was implanted for the first time. Furthermore, the CT scanner, introduced in the beginning of the 1970s, is based on a mathematical theorem dating to 1917.[67] Secondly, it should be noted that it is not necessary for each and every innovation to pass through all of the separate seven stages. Depending on the possibilities the innovation opens up, it may be accepted more readily.

6.2.3 Government Control?

All in all, science and technology can be regarded as boosters of opportunities in health care, whereas medical professionals and patients will exert pressure on governments and third parties to ensure that the developments benefit them. In the framework of this book, therefore, it is important to ask whether governments of democracies are able to *control* scientific and technological developments regarding health care.

Unlike governments of communist countries, democratic governments' instruments in this respect are rather limited, since one of the fundamental characteristics of Western democracies is that the production of goods and services is, to a large extent, a matter of private enterprise. Governments have to tolerate this, in principle. What governments can do, however, is condition and correct private enterprise. In fact, governments do this so intensely that private enterprise in Western democracies does not mean free enterprise[68] (see 1.1.3). Consequently, when it comes to health care, governments can condition the research potential of universities by limiting their budgets, but they cannot prevent industry from putting the results of its research activities on the health care market. The only thing governments can do is to condition and to correct the supply side through competition, price, and quality regulations.

The demand side is another story. Here, almost all governments of the European Union have (legal) instruments that condition the use of high technology, i.e., medical devices which are technologically complex and so expensive that governments want their availability to be restricted.[69] These instruments boil down to the need for hospitals to have special governmental permission for the purchase of expensive devices (MRI scanners, PET scanners, et cetera), as well as for the performance of complicated medical interventions (cardiac surgery, transplants, neurosurgery, et cetera). Because there is a lot of money involved here, governments try to control the diffusion speed through policies of restricted availability.

However, one can argue about the effectiveness of such policies. First of all, these policies do not affect, other than through conditioning and correcting, the private health care market, which is not dependent on collective financing. Secondly, as time goes by, expensive devices may become cheaper, and medical interventions may become less complicated, thus reducing the need for special permission. As an example: the CT scanner, once an item of special permission, has become cheaper and has been perfected. Therefore, since the 1990s, the governments of many countries of the European Union have no longer thought it necessary to control its use by restriction policies. Comparable developments can be observed in the United States. Here, between 1964 and 1972, a total of 23 states and the District of Columbia tried to control the acquisition of expensive equipment by adopting "certificate-of-need" laws. Furthermore, through federal legislation in 1974, newly established health systems agencies were expected to regulate the purchase of new equipment by hospitals in 205 health-service areas. Both initiatives failed because political skills enabled some to bypass the regulations, and the regulations did not apply to doctors in private practice.[70]

Regarding the effectiveness of restriction policies for the use of high technology, it is useful to deal briefly with the outcomes of research into the diffusion speed of four items/procedures of high technology (CT scanners, linear accelerators, lithotripters, and cardiac surgery), a task I undertook at the end of the 1980s.[71] My research showed that governmental attempts to control diffusion were not very effective. Take the CT scanner, for example: by the end of 1984, 44% of the scanners installed in Italy were owned by private health care institutions.[72] In Greece in 1985, 50% of all CT scanners were in the hands of self-employed specialists outside hospitals[73]; and this increased to 82% in 1991.[74] In Germany, private practitioners owned 37% of all CT scanners in 1985.[75] Despite the fact that the government introduced purchasing regulations in December 1985, this figure had increased to 44% out of 594 CT scanners installed in 1988.[76] Also in Germany, out of a total of 78 NMRs in 1988, 47% were in the hands of self-employed specialists.[77] More recently, there were only three PET scanners in Germany in 1995, by 2002 there were more than 90, most of them installed in the offices of ambulatory specialists.[78] German hospitals even refer patients to these self-employed specialists for diagnosis. The health care systems of these three countries have important market elements. And where a market functions, governments cannot forbid practitioners from making use of new opportunities. However, in a country like Portugal that has a National Health Service, the location of heavy medical equipment is also rather independent from hospitals, leading to a situation where hospitals reimburse private clinics for the use of this equipment. It has been reported that 69% of CT scanners, 75% of lithotriptors, and 86% of MRI scanners are installed in private Portuguese clinics.[79]

Now, one might assume that governments of countries with nationalized health care systems would be in a better position to control the technological developments. This is not necessarily true. The development of heart transplants in the United Kingdom is illustrative. Here, the first two transplants at Papworth were paid for by the local health authority. The next six transplants, however, were funded by the private National Heart Research Fund. A further seven were covered by a special grant from the Ministry of Health, whereas a donation of £150,000 per annum from a philanthropist covered the costs of transplants from September 1980 to September 1982.[80] Governmental control of the diffusion of heart transplants was rather inadequate, therefore. Moreover, even if the British government had held firm intentions regarding this, there still was the British population, which, excited by media interest, was very much in favor of their doctors' performing heart transplants. A 1968 poll, in this respect, revealed that the 67% of British citizens supported heart transplantation.[81] Furthermore, Irish hospitals, functioning in a health care system which is 75% financed through general taxation, have also started to organize fund-raising activities to assist with purchasing expensive medical equipment, asking the department of health for financial support to cover operating and maintenance costs.[82]

Apart from the influence of the private health care market and philanthropic organizations as boosters of new health care opportunities, the research also showed remarkable differences between countries which cannot logically be explained. Figures for cardiac surgery in 1985 (per million population), for example, were 850, 300, 440, and 385 for the Netherlands, the United Kingdom, Germany, and Greece, respectively.[83] It is difficult to assume that, for medical reasons, the Dutch would have to be operated on almost twice as often as the Germans. Furthermore, it is difficult to give a rational argument, based on health care considerations, that explains why in 1985 the German ratio of scanners to population was three times higher than that of the United Kingdom. Apparently, differences in medical culture between countries play a role as well. As a further example: in the mid-1980s, the price of drugs in the Netherlands was about 25% higher than in other countries of the European Union. The consumption of drugs per inhabitant in the Netherlands, however, was the lowest in the (then) European Community.

Now, if we define planning as *information processing of decisions about future actions in a coordinated and controlled way*, the facts outlined above make it hard to maintain that the introduction and diffusion of high technology takes place in a coordinated and controlled way. Whether a country has a national health care system, or one that is based on social security, or a system with important market elements, medical technologies develop in their own way. They justify their application by their very existence. All economic theories that claim that the market is likely to take precedence over planning initiatives are proven right where medical technology is concerned. The best thing a health care system can aim for is to slow down the diffusion speed. Manufacturers, professional organizations, sponsoring, donations, and public pressure, mostly mobilized by patient unions, constitute barriers to coordination and control that can hardly be overcome. No matter what system, this means that, as McKinlay rightfully observes, the state and third parties eventually do not act on the basis of reliable evidence, but on the basis of some combination of professional, organizational, and public pressure, and to the extent that they do act, the financial position of a country, its social-cultural values, and the degree of pluralism in its democracy are the determining factors. Moreover, these actions are undoubtedly influenced by the fact that politicians have to take into account that most of the electorate say health is their first priority in life. Because of all this, it is hard to apply rational principles to the spread of medical technology or to explain the imbalances that prevail. As an example: research revealed that the United Kingdom had such cardiac surgery over-capacity that it could even treat patients from other countries, while at the same time the United Kingdom had far fewer lithotripters than many comparable other countries.

Finally, I also count among science and technology the educational and training capacities of universities. Since, to a large extent, the financing of universities is a matter of public spending in many countries, governments can control health care developments by limiting university budgets or by imposing enrollment restrictions on certain types of training. Here, the Netherlands produces some unfortunate examples. Dental care is one of them. In 1982, the number of newly enrolled dental students was 465. A enrollment restriction imposed in 1987 reduced this number to 120, and two faculties that trained new dentists were closed.[84] The government subsequently realized that, due to a shortage of professionals, dental care had become a problem, so the enrollment restriction was slowly lifted beginning in 1998. At the moment, it is 300. It has been predicated that if this number is not increased further, the Dutch will have a shortage of dentists of 14% by the year 2012. Similar control measures affected the training of general practitioners. The Netherlands, however, was not the only European Union country that imposed enrollment restrictions. For example, France did so in the early 1970s,[85] as did Belgium in 1995.[86]

6.3 Organization

The next element is organization, by which I mean the way economic orders arrange and control the health care delivery process. Here, too, one can observe large differences between countries. An important point, in this respect, is a country's geography. Vast but thinly populated countries, with people living in clusters in remote areas, mostly have their health care system organized along *geographical lines*, in regions that are responsible for the provision and administration of health services. With an average density of 16.5 inhabitants per square kilometer, Finland's regional administration, for example, is divided into five provinces, each with its own department of social affairs and health, which are part of the general state administration. Finnish local administration is in the hands of 444 communes, which enjoy a large measure of autonomy regarding the provision of primary health care for their population. These communes are also responsible for specialist treatment. For this purpose, the country is divided into 21 inter-communal districts, each with a central hospital, a psychiatric hospital, and other special provisions.[87] A comparable structure exists in Sweden, a country with a density of around 20 inhabitants per square kilometer. Here, responsibility for health care services is entrusted to 21 county councils and one large municipality. Their work is regulated by legislation. The other 288 municipalities, with populations ranging from 5,000 to 700,000, are responsible for social services, childcare, schools, and care for the elderly, as well as care for disabled people and psychiatric patients. At its basic level Swedish health care is organized in primary care districts, each of which may have one or more of the 950 local health care centers. Hospital care is provided through about 90 acute hospitals, ranging from regional hospitals to central county and district county levels, with the latter ones having at least internal medicine, surgery, radiology, and anaesthesiology as specialties. Highly specialized care is provided in six medical regions through cooperation between county councils. Geographical conditions also determine the way a country organizes its emergency care. In this respect, for example, the university clinic of Tromsö, Norway, a country with 13.9 inhabitants per square kilometer, has a helicopter trauma team available around the clock, covering an area with a diameter of 1,000 kilometers. Furthermore, this country uses telemedicine when assisting in medical interventions that are carried out at far-away outposts.

Another geographic reason to organize a health care system into regions may be the fact that the country is mountainous. Here, although distances measured in straight lines may not be that great, the time to get from one place to another may be a reason for regionalization. Austria is one example. As a second example, the Azores islands, an autonomous Portuguese region in the middle of the Atlantic Ocean, spend around 25% of GDP on health care. The distance to the Portuguese mainland is so far, however, that the establishment of a relatively extensive infrastructure became inevitable. In 2000, the country of Suriname spent 9.4% of GDP on health care, which, compared to the spending level of the countries of the European Union, is a very large amount of money. Nevertheless, 32% of the country's population is not insured against medical costs.[88] Suriname, however, is a large and thinly populated country, not surrounded by wealthy countries with well-established health care systems, as is, for example, Luxembourg. The necessity of a relatively extensive health care infrastructure is comparable to that of the Azores islands. Finally, big cities that have many people living in a relatively small area may be regarded as a special geographical case. This may lead countries to decide to arrange their health care system in such a way that it allows them to pay specific attention to the health care needs of city dwellers.

Next, the arrangement and control of the health care delivery process may be organized along *functional lines*. In this respect, in the Netherlands, for example, there has been a countrywide historical distinction made between hospital care, psychiatric care, care for the mentally retarded, and long-term care (e.g., nursing homes). They all have their own provisions, their own budgets, and their own associations. As for psychiatry, institutional and ambulatory care have been separate sectors for many years. Referring back to the quadrant approach discussed in the beginning of this chapter, however, we see an increasing integration, particularly between the different long-term care sectors, between ambulatory and institutional psychiatric care, and between acute hospitals and nursing homes. The merging of these different types of institutions is no longer an exception.

Arranging and controlling health care delivery may also be organized along *political lines*. An example is Spain, which recently decentralized its health care system so that its regions can to a considerable extent decide autonomously on health care matters. A comparable structure was introduced in Italy some years ago. Political lines are also involved in a country like Germany. Here, the federal political structure is important as regards investments in health care facilities. France has a large public health sector, in addition to a private one that works not-for-profit as well as a private one that works for profit. The CEOs of the first sector are appointed by the Minister of Health. Politics also plays a role in those countries that have delegated the arranging and controlling of health care delivery to municipalities, which for that reason can also be the owners of facilities.

One can furthermore distinguish *administrative lines*. For example, England has 28 Strategic Health Authorities which are responsible for the oversight of health care planning and delivery in their geographical area, which means that they, in fact, operate as the local headquarters of the NHS. Scotland has one central senior executive health department, with NHS boards being the administrative subdivision of the country. Ireland, where the current organization has been in place for more than 30 years, is considering new administrative arrangements which involve the appointment of a National Health Services Executive, who would be directly responsible to the Minister of Health, as well as a three "pillar" system of health care delivery: (1) primary, community, and continuing care; (2) a national hospitals office; and (3) a shared services department. Existing delivery systems will be subsumed into the new structures, and many of the other bodies will be merged or subsumed into new structures.[89]

Finally, *religion* may be a distinctive organizational characteristic, as is the case, for example, in Belgium and Austria.

In line with my definition of health care, one may conclude that the element of organization is already a dynamic phenomenon by itself. People in industry, in governments, and in general, always tinker with the organizations they create. The organization of health care is no exception to that. To give two recent examples: (1) the Danes have just decided to rearrange their regional structure, clustering the arrangement and control of health care delivery around a number of university centers; and (2) the Dutch have set up 85 so-called regional indication agencies countrywide in order to come to independent, integral, and objective conclusions about people who need long-term care. These continuous organizational changes have already determined the health care world for decades. They do not make that world a stable one. On the contrary, together with the other dynamics, they create a very turbulent external environment for those who work in health care. Whether this is favorable for the quality and reliability of health care delivery remains to be seen. The same applies when it comes to effectiveness and efficiency.

6.4 Economics and Politics

Finally, we have two elements left: economics and politics. I have purposely positioned them at the center of my definition, because they are the heart of the matter. Together, they are the most important determinants of any collectively financed health care system. The reasoning in this respect is very simple. If there is no money, there is nothing one can do. In this regard, McKee et al. rightfully observe that "health and wealth are inextricably linked."[90] And if there is no political will, promoters of a sound health care system, accessible to each citizen, will expend their energy to no avail. As was pointed out in the introduction to the first chapter, the United States is a good example of this. Although around 14% of the United States GDP is spent on health care, there are nevertheless some 44 million people who are not insured or are underinsured. At the start of his administration, President Clinton tried to change this situation. We all know that he did not succeed. Apparently, there is no political will in the United States to support change in this respect. Cuba is an opposite example. The country, being poor, nonetheless had, compared to other countries in the region and even to the whole of the South American continent, an excellent universally accessible health care system, free of charge. Apparently, within its limited available financial means, Castro's government had made health care a high priority for the citizens of Cuba (together with education, for that matter). Admittedly, in contrast to the perceived inequitable capitalistic world, the assumed benefits of a communist society, financially supported by the Soviet Union, have been a strong motive for this Cuban policy. When Russian financial support stopped, however, the system started to deteriorate. Then there is South Africa, where around the turn of the millennium it was decided to carry through a financial redistribution between the nine provinces, implying that the richer ones had to make financial sacrifices to benefit the poorer ones. One unintended effect of this was that the Western Cape province, the richest in the country, in order to reduce its public spending, closed down hundreds of beds in psychiatric hospitals around Cape Town. Patients had to return to their communities. Psychiatric community care to support them, however, failed for the simple reason that the provincial government could not afford to pay for it. Finally, we have Suriname. Before it became an independent republic in 1975, its health care system was unparalleled in the Caribbean region, except for Cuba. Due to political squabbles which have lasted for decades, however, health care is now in a deplorable state with a lack of facilities and many people uninsured.[91]

For the countries of the European Union, it was true for a long time that, on average, there was the money *and* the political will to maintain a sound health care system, based on the principle of solidarity between the rich and the poor, the healthy and the sick, the young and the old. This was a reflection of the will of the people, who, according to a substantial body of research, see good health and health care as their first priority in life. And they want their fellow citizens to enjoy the same. Wanless's 2001 report for the United Kingdom, for example, reveals that 80% of the population believe that the NHS is critical to the British society and should therefore be maintained, while 75% of the people want to retain universal access.[92] Similar research for Finland delivered a result of 95%.[93] Apparently, the citizens of the countries of the European Union have certain moral and cultural motives, albeit to differing degrees, to strive for equity and justice, based on the notion that this is essential for a prosperous and civilized society. This is the foundation for the establishment of the European welfare states. Health care has received its share in this respect.

All the same, it should be kept in mind that a strong economy has been the mainstay for the development of the welfare state and, with it, for the expansion of health care systems within the European Union. After all, what arguments would one have to adopt in order to assume that people living in developing countries do not see good health and health care as a first priority in life? The only reason I can think of is that people living in those countries have accepted the fact that the money to fulfill their wishes is simply not there for most of them.

For the countries of the European Union, the money was there, thanks to strong economic growth. The cultural climate of those countries was imbued with a sense of general duty to aid the needy, and in the framework of democratic decision-making, political coalitions within the member states, therefore, could rather easily decide to meet the electorate's wishes for health care provided through a collectively financed system. In the words of Cyert and March, these coalitions were viable to make the payments that were needed to keep the members of the coalition together. Worded differently, there was sufficient *organizational slack*; i.e., there was room to do things which would not have been done under a tight budget.[94] That this coincided with an acceleration in health care opportunities was also no problem, thanks to that same economic growth. Consequently, health care financing became an open-ended affair in most countries of the European Union. This relaxed approach became a problem when, in the mid-1970s, economic growth slowed. Because of this, organizational slack quickly evaporated. Then, finance appeared to be, in fact, the only effective instrument for governments to cope with the new situation.[95] From that moment on, the governments of the countries of the European Union, some firm, some frenetic, have tried to maintain the collective aspects of their health care system, while at the same time trying to include new health care opportunities. One can wonder if this approach will hold in the end. In the words of Wanless: "in a world where patient expectations are rising rapidly and people are increasingly looking for health services which offer greater personal choice in non-clinical services, it may not be acceptable or equitable to meet all of these additional demands through public financing."[96]

6.5 Summary

Based on the definition of health care as a complex and dynamic process of constantly changing new combinations of science, technology, organization, politics, economics, and (medical) culture, this chapter analyzed those six elements against the background question of how this process can be controlled. It showed that influencing the cultural aspects, if it is feasible at all, takes a very long time. Furthermore, governments in democracies that are based on the principle of private enterprise must, in principle, tolerate scientific and technological developments in health care, although they can take conditioning and correcting measures. The effectiveness of these measures has to be questioned, however. The same applies for organizational measures. Consequently, the determining factors are economics and politics, with finance as the overall instrument to widen or to constrain health care developments, against the background of equal access in a society whose health care system is based on the principle of solidarity.

7
The Influence of the European Union

According to the Maastricht Treaty of 1992, health care in the countries of the European Union is, together with social security, subject to the principle of subsidiarity, which implies that each member state is free to choose its own organizational and financial arrangements regarding the production and consumption of health care goods and services. Nevertheless, the internal market requires that EU citizens be provided a level of health services of a certain quality in accordance with professional norms. Articles 152 and 153 of the Maastricht Treaty, as well as EU agreements regarding the protection of human rights, are (also) meant to enforce this requirement.[1] My argument in this chapter is that, as a result of ongoing European economic integration, the subsidiarity principle will be slowly eroded with respect to health care, because continued collective financing of health care will encounter problems similar to those resulting from the attempts to combine economic objectives with objectives of social policy regarding social security. In other words, though individual member states may want to administer their health care systems without restriction, this will become increasingly difficult as a consequence of ongoing economic integration; and thus the principle of solidarity in health care will be effected. Looking at the developments since 1975, we may conclude that, despite the subsidiarity principle, the European Commission is slowly taking the lead in getting control of the financial aspects of health care. Though the Commission's role, in this respect, still seems mainly to be assisting the member states, a more directive role should not be excluded, if it were only because the member states' governments, taking into account their constitutional obligations, are very much interested in an optimal balance between the costs and benefits of their health care systems. I will deal with this influence of the European Union in the second section of this chapter, whereas the third section will go into some adjustment problems following from the EU's enlargement of 2004. Before doing so I will address in the first section the difficulties one encounters when attempting to compare health care systems.

7.1 Comparing Health Care Systems

In chapter five, I defined a health care system as the infrastructure which governments have established for people to have their health problems solved. More precisely, it is the legal and organizational framework directed at producing, distributing, managing, regulating, supervising, coordinating, and controlling health care activities in order to realize defined health care values. This framework is very much determined by historical, cultural, and political traditions. Therefore, health care systems are sometimes labeled socio-historic constructions[2] which can differ considerably from one country to another. Because of this, comparing health care systems is a difficult and rather arbitrary matter. I consider three approaches useful in dealing with this complex subject.

The first (and, in fact, a very simple one) is Field's distinction between five basic types, or analytical constructions, varying from, on the one hand, a system in which all the decisions regarding health care production and consumption are the governments' prerogative, and, on the other hand, a system in which governments are not involved at all.[3] Although this approach is in line with Eucken, it is far too simple to be of use when comparing health care systems of democracies which claim that their health care systems are based on the solidarity principle. After all, a government which has committed itself to the production and consumption of health care goods and services for its citizens must at a minimum monitor whether reality is in accordance with this commitment. Otherwise, in situations where a market system for health care prevails, governments have to ensure its accessibility for all their citizens.

Combining different sources of funds with different methods for paying providers, the Organisation for Economic Co-operation and Development (OECD) comes up with seven models that vary from, at one end, the voluntary out-of-pocket model to, at the other end, the public integrated model. In the first model, service flows, as well as financial flows, are the result of interaction between a health care consumer and a health care provider. In this model, the government has no role. In the public integrated model, the government is both the principal insurer and the principal provider. Here, all health care staff is on the government's payroll, consumers are compulsory insured, receive services in kind, and pay their share through premiums or general taxation, with facilities being state-owned. Reasoning in rough outline, one could say that the first model is ruled by the market and the seventh model by the government. The OECD's approach is exactly what it says: a model. The reality of health care systems, however, always shows a mixture of one or more of the seven models.[4]

As a third way of comparing health care systems, it is rather common for the countries of the European Union to distinguish between two types of systems: *social security systems*, which take a Bismarckian approach, on the one hand, and *national health systems or services*, which take the Beveridge approach, on the other. Social security systems can be differentiated into those which have social insurance and third-party payers providing reimbursement insurance (Luxembourg, France, and Belgium) or benefits-in-kind (Germany and the Netherlands). National health systems are predominantly financed through taxation, i.e., through either national, county, or municipal or a mixture of the these forms of taxation (United Kingdom, Denmark, Sweden, Finland, Portugal, Spain, Greece, and Italy). Though at first sight this distinction between social security and national health systems seems rather simple, if one looks at the differences in more detail, as has been done in the following table,[5] it becomes evident that the situation is actually quite complex.

National Health Systems	Social Security Systems
Financed through general taxation	Mainly financed through (income-related) premiums
Universal coverage	Coverage through funds or mutualities per profession,region, or otherwise
Public infrastructure	Public/private infrastructure
Physicians on payroll	Self-employed physicians, paid by "fee for service"
High degree of state interference	Private ownership
Government controlled	Complex structure with many interested parties

Source: Vos, P. de: *Hoe gezond is de Europese Gezondheidspolitiek?*

So, although this distinction is very common, its usefulness is rather limited because in reality health care systems are quite often a very detailed mixture of both models, since both national health systems and health care systems based on social security may have important *market elements*, e.g., a public/private mix. In fact, classifying health care systems along the lines of public/private (and, within the latter, for-profit/not-for-profit) is as easily defensible as classifying them as shown in the table above. But, here again, reality is more differentiated than the latter distinction suggests. Health care provision in the Netherlands, for example, almost completely organized in private foundations, is for the most part financed by a system of premium levying, complemented by limited governmental subsidies. In a true private sector, i.e., professionals and institutions working for profit, one is free to invest in health care, taking into account only the conditioning and correcting role governments have in the economic order in general terms. Some argue, therefore, that we can distinguish between three types of health care systems.[6] France, Italy, Greece, Spain, Portugal, and Ireland, for example, have considerable private health care markets.

The distinctions outlined here are, for different reasons, not very helpful in comparing health care systems. Firstly, this is because they represent a rather static approach. Like the economic order in general, health care systems are a dynamic phenomenon, as I argued in chapter six. Consequently, comparing health care systems in detail produces a plethora of facts which may be outdated soon after they have been collected. Secondly, even if two countries' health care systems are, for example, both labeled a national health service, the differences between the two can be very significant. The same applies for health care systems based on social security. These differences can be further demonstrated, with the following short inventory.

The Dutch health care system is considered a social security system. In fact, it is a mixture of a social security system, legalized with the Sick Fund Law of 1964, compulsorily insuring all Dutch citizens under a certain income level against sickness, and a national health service, legally arranged in 1968 by the Exceptional Medical Expenses Act, covering all citizens for long-term care.

Both the Netherlands and France are considered to have a social-security based health care system. In the Netherlands, the general practitioner serves as a gatekeeper for referrals to medical specialists. The French, however, could until very recently visit a medical specialist directly without restrictions and as often as they wanted, a phenomenon called "medical nomadism."[7]

Some countries count the cost of nursing-home care as part of their health care expenditure. The Danes, however, do not. To them, these costs are an item of social security expenditure.

In 1997, Denmark had 465 hospital beds per 100,000 inhabitants, but for France the figure was 877. In 1999, Ireland had 226 general practitioners per 100,000 inhabitants, but the Belgians had 405. In 1997, France had 46.4 self-employed pharmacists per 100,000 inhabitants, compared to 17.5 for the Netherlands.[8]

Within national health services, countries like the United Kingdom organize the financing of services through general taxation. Over the course of time, however, general taxation contributions decreased from 100% in 1948, the year the NHS was established, to 82.6% in 1988, the difference coming from NHS contributions, local authority rates, and patients' own payments.[9] In Sweden, taxation at the county level is important, while in Finland, the municipalities play a large role.[10]

Some countries of the European Union have an independent department of health services, whereas others combine health care with social affairs, employment, the environment, women's affairs, or even sports.

Countries with health care systems based on social security may have, in fact, a national health service when it comes to investment in facilities. In this respect, investment decisions may be decentralized to county level. Here, the example is Germany.

Furthermore, health care systems may have differing dynamics. The Italian national health service, for example, a system based on compulsory social insurance, is the result of a transition process that was completed around the end of 1984.[11] Before that, the system was characterized by important market elements. While the system has been decentralized, resulting in rather autonomous decision-making by the regions, market elements still have a considerable role. The United Kingdom, which has opened its NHS to internal competition to diversify supply and to increase purchasing power,[12] provides another example of the dynamics of health care systems.

All in all, comparing European health care systems in detail reveals an enormous diversity.[13] This diversity would also be present even if we limited the comparison to, for example, the way different countries have organized their systems of social health insurance.[14]

Detailed comparison between EU countries would reveal that it is impossible to discover a common line of rationality, consistency, planning, and control as regards the organization of their health care system. These systems cannot be explained by normal logic. Instead, they are ruled by this creed: so many people, so many opinions. Two examples may illustrate that concepts like rationality, consistency, planning, and control are of limited meaning in health care.

Years ago, the famous British television series *Yes, Minister* presented a much-appreciated episode featuring a newly built hospital which stayed empty because there were no patients. You may think that this is fiction, but it is reality. In the city of Leuven, Belgium, a public hospital was enlarged by 250 beds. Due to planning regulations in the 1980s, most of these new beds have not been used as hospital beds, but rather have been used by students. The same thing happened in Brussels. There, a newly built hospital was never opened and is used now as an office for a trade union. Events like these, however, should not be interpreted primarily as the consequence of health care policy missteps. They seem to be more the result of inadequate policy coordination between different governmental departments.

In April 2001, the Dutch television news revealed that 30% of acute hospital beds were not in use, due to a shortage of staff. The Dutch government believed that pumping hundreds of millions of guilders into its health care system could solve the problem, which was the consequence of almost 20 years of economizing, including reductions in education and training capacities (see 6.2.3). It will take the Dutch years to get things going smoothly again. Staff shortages are a problem more countries of the European Union will have to face in the near future, particularly when it comes to physicians.[15]

In conclusion, with regard to the health care systems of the countries of the European Union, the reality is that each country acts as it likes. Cultural and administrative traditions largely determine the ways in which separate countries set up their health care infrastructure. Such an infrastructure reflects a country's "interlinked belief system," which, through democratic processes, has crystallized into a concrete set of (legal, administrative, and physical) organizational forms governing the allocation of resources and the distribution of authority and power.[16] Comparing health care systems other than in rough outline, therefore, is rather useless. What all systems do have in common, however, is the objective of making good quality health care accessible to all citizens, be it through private insurance or a mechanism of collective financing. If, therefore, there is to be a convergence of the health care systems of the individual countries of the European Union, finance and quality will be the instruments of change. Reading "between the lines" of reports from Brussels supports this conclusion.

7.2 Policy Lines From Brussels

As stated in chapter five, this book is about health care and not about health. Therefore, as far as the European Union is concerned, I will not deal with its involvement in health matters other than noting that its commitment, in this respect, is enormous and very much differentiated, and this commitment dates back to long before it became an official activity under the terms of the Maastricht Treaty.[17] Topics like food control, pollution, agriculture, product safety, employment, the environment, energy, fishery, and so on all appear, in one way or another, to be health-related. A 1995 report of the European Commission is a good illustration of this health-relatedness.[18] Furthermore, instruments of European market-making, like the Single European Act (SEA), appear to have spillover effects for health care; i.e., directives from Brussels regarding, for example, safety and health at the workplace,[19] the mutual recognition of diplomas, and working time directives, do not leave health care untouched.[20] This led the European Health Management Association to conclude "that the relationship between health services as a major sector of Member States' economies and the SEA are intertwined in such a complex manner that it is virtually impossible to separate them."[21] These spillover effects, however, are also not the focus of this book. For decades, there has already been an increasing cooperation at the level of the European Union, with the support of the European WHO office, on public health matters like health promotion, health education, health information, cancer, cardiovascular diseases, accidents, suicides, AIDS and other communicable diseases, drug abuse, and so on. By 1984, the countries of the European Union had already adopted 38 Health for All Targets for the European region, which were adjusted in 1998 into 21 targets for the 21st century. Establishing targets, however, is one thing; implementing strategies to achieve them is quite another.[22] These public health matters will also not be dealt with.

What is important in these health-related/public health topics, however, is that they demonstrate increasing cooperation at the European level. Admittedly, each of the reports covering these topics points to the fact that health care is ruled by the subsidiarity principle, but reading them carefully in a chronological sequence gives one reason to suspect that this principle may have been at least partly eroded, and will at any rate not prevent a certain convergence regarding several health care matters. After all, one may expect that closer cooperation and mutual consultation between governments will lead to mutual learning. Mutual learning may, in turn, lead to acting collectively, which, again in turn, may lead to the creation of a Union-wide health policy. Consequently, increasing cooperation in health and health care at the level of the European Union may affect the self-reliance of health care systems of national economic orders. Components of those systems, like finance and quality, which are very important for governments, could in the not-too-distant future be relatively easily lifted to the European Union level. This section examines this point of view based on the developments to date, which I have classified in three categories: (a) *political considerations*, (b) *practical regulations*, and (c) *rulings of the European Court of Justice*. It should be noted that, first of all, the different categories may interact: i.e., political considerations may result in practical regulations, and vice versa; rulings of the European Court of Justice may lead to political considerations, et cetera. Secondly, the different categories are not mutually exclusive: i.e., political considerations may at the same time be practical regulations.

7.2.1 Political Considerations

This subsection gives an overview of *political considerations* at the level of the European Union over the past 25 years. On the one hand, these considerations demonstrate a growing need for cooperation between national governments. On the other hand, they are also an expression of the need for governments to lean on each other in the attempt to control developments in health care throughout Europe. The need for cooperation and mutual support will to a certain extent eventually lead to supra-territorial decision-making at the level of the European Union regarding those aspects of health care systems, particularly finance and quality, which do not directly touch upon the principle of subsidiarity. After all, there are no substantial differences in interests here between member states: They all want efficiency, effectiveness, and high quality care to be characteristic of their health care systems. The points that are relevant, in this respect, are presented in italics.

In 1978, the ministers of health of the then European Economic Community agreed that *something had to be done about the costs of health care.* That "something" implied the desirability of *exchanging information and developing plans for communitarian cooperation.*

At the end of 1982, the European Commission informed the Council that it had investigated the costs of health care as part of the costs of social security, which had led the Commission to conclude that the costs of health care formed the major part of social security budgets. In this report, and to my knowledge for the first time, *health care providers were criticized for inefficient and ineffective treatment procedures. Introduction of "competition" within the system, it was thought, would contribute to improvement.* Furthermore, the Commission proposed concerted action at the community level to control further developments. Proposed items for such action were *(a) planning of staff, (b) evaluation of medical technologies, (c) comparison of drug prescriptions, (d) comparison of treatment costs, (e) health indicators and information systems,* and *(f) health education and "self-help."*[23]

Next, during a debate in the European Parliament in 1983, one member argued that *the time had come to establish and launch a European health policy.*[24] From that moment on, Brussels increased its involvement in health and health care. And very soon this involvement included, in addition to health and health policy issues, the costs of health care. But this involvement was not very effective. Each country still had to sort out these problems on its own. Nevertheless, the costs of health care became a shared problem between governments. This was illustrated, for example, during the 1984 informal meeting of health ministers during which the *increase in health spending* was discussed.

The 1992 Maastricht Treaty gave the European Union new competencies for international cooperation. As in 1982, joint action of member states was recommended for health promotion and health protection, as well as for subsidizing medical and health policy research, and "*the establishment of international information systems.*"[25]

In the 1992 recommendation of the Council (92/442/EEC) on the *convergence of social protection objectives and policies*, member states are expected to ensure *access to necessary health care*, as well as to develop a *high-quality health care system.* In 1993, the European Commission set out a framework for action in the field of public health based on the fact that, among other things, "*cost containment remains a topic of major concern in the 1990s especially in the context of the present recession and the budget constraints on public expenditure growth.*" One of the other challenges in this report appears to be "*better structuring and financing of health systems to minimize costs, cutting out ineffective treatments and evaluating medical equipment and medicines in cost/benefit terms.*"[26] Furthermore, a 1993 report of the Committee on Environment, Public Health and Consumer Protection of the European Parliament provides a comprehensive overview of public health issues, including "*comparable/compatible health data and indicators [and] health care costs,*" whereas the Economic and Social Committee of that parliament argued for "*transparency of medicinal product prices.*"[27]

Next, a 1995 Council report dealt with an analysis of the *impact of containment measures on the quality of the health care systems*, including the item of equal access.[28] Furthermore, this report revealed that the European Commission financed several projects in both Central and Eastern European Countries (CEEC) and the New Independent States (NIS), regarding the "*reform of the financing system including budget programming and allocation, cost containment measures, payment of care-providers, health insurances issues, etc.*," as well as the "*reorganisation of health services, in particular to make care increasingly less hospital- and community-based, including privatisation issues.*"[29] Also in 1995, the European Commission launched a proposal on a community health monitoring system. One of the domains such a system would have to cover was *the costs of inpatient as well as outpatient care and the costs of pharmaceutical products*.[30] Finally, in its 1995 report on the future of social protection, the European Commission called upon the Council of Ministers to "*acknowledge the importance of developing a framework for debate on the future of social protection in which Member States and the Union could pool their efforts towards improving the workings of their social protection system* [health care included] *and make them more employment-friendly and more efficient.*"[31]

Then, we have the 1997 report of the European Commission on the modernization and improvement of social protection. This report deals with the European health service's *needs to improve efficiency, cost-effectiveness and quality of health care systems in order to be able to meet the demands that will arise from an aging population and other factors.* If we add to this then Commissioner Flynn's statement that "*a Community policy on public health which ignored the development and effectiveness of health systems would be wholly inadequate*," it is difficult to see how national health care systems can remain beyond the reach of the ongoing process of European integration. All the more so, since, also in 1997, the European Commission proposed that it could "*combine the efforts of member states regarding the improvement of efficiency and effectiveness of health care systems, while assessing at the community level the initiatives of individual member states directed at minimizing costs*" (author's translation).[32]

In May 2000, the European Commission proposed, while "*fully respecting the responsibilities of the Member States for the organisation and delivery of health services and medical care*," a new public health framework one of the three priorities of which was to put in place a *comprehensive health information system* in order to "*provide policy makers, health professionals and the general public the key health data and information that they need.*" And, once again, the reader was informed that "*the costs of health care are a major charge on national budgets and one that is continuing to grow as resources chase rising demand.*" In view of this, "*Member States are trying to improve the cost-effectiveness of their health systems in order to accommodate new priorities while also respecting budgetary constraints. To meet this challenge, they require better and comparable data and information, e.g., on health status and the effectiveness of particular health interventions. The Community has the potential to provide much of this.*" Here, for the first time to my knowledge, the Commission openly argued that it could make a difference in a way that individual member states could not. The European Commission maintained that, with the proposed public health framework, with its "limited" budget of €300 million, it would be able to "*make a positive impact on the health of the Community citizens and on making health systems in Member States more effective,*" thus providing real community added value. Finally, the European Commission assumed that promising outcomes would result from implementing its proposals, including making information available to national, regional, and local health authorities which "*will assist them in developing policy and in decision-making by providing up to date and comparative data on health trends and developments, and by establishing benchmarks to measure progress and effectiveness of health interventions and strategies.*"[33] Meanwhile, in November 2000, the European Parliament adopted a resolution calling on the European Commission to anticipate that "*the collection of statistics and comparable data* [which] *would lead to best practice being applied.*"[34] Just before the end of 2000, the European Commission published a report on the health care consequences of an aging population in which it said that "*comparing health care systems and treatment methods in order to trace 'good practices' is of utmost importance for health care systems and an optimal use of social security finances*" (author's translation).[35] Helpful, in this respect, was the establishment in 2000 of an "Open Method of Coordination" for the European Council, which was meeting in Lisbon. Based on mutual learning, this method was meant to facilitate the delivery of indicators and benchmarks of "good practice," the establishment of monitoring systems, the development of policy guidelines, and so on.[36]

A further report of the European Commission appeared in 2001, in which an *"open coordination" for health* was promoted. Among the topics for such open coordination were "*defining targets and objectives on the European level, defining, quantifying and qualifying indicators and benchmarks, and monitoring, analysing and evaluating the achievements in the Member States.*" Furthermore, the European Commission advised that it would "*develop a framework for definition of common quality standards and best practice at Community level [. . .] which could cover quality standards, criteria for good medical practice, rules on equivalence of competence and medical practice, hospital accreditation, medical prescription, etc.*"[37]

Furthermore, it is meaningful that the health ministers of the European Union, during their meeting in Malaga in February 2002, agreed to focus on four health care themes: *(a) European cooperation to enable better use of resources; (b) information requirements for patients, professionals, and policy-makers; (c) access to and quality of care; and (d) reconciling national health policy with European obligations.*[38] It is also meaningful that Brussels plans to introduce, again,[39] *a common EU health insurance card by 2005.*[40] This would be supported by those who see the integration of all health insurance systems as a medium-term prospect.[41]

Finally, in 2003, participants in a "high-level reflection process," including 13 ministers of health, all on a voluntary and personal basis, invited "*the Commission to facilitate information sharing at European level on possible available health care, existing supply of care, entitlements and procedures, costs, prices, adverse incidents, patient records, nomenclature of conditions, treatments and products and continuity and quality of care across the Union. [. . .] Action could include support to networking and developing databases.*" All of these can be found in the framework of the EU public health program for 2003–2008.[42]

Where do these developments leave the subsidiarity principle regarding health care? In this respect, my argument is as follows.

In the first chapter of the book, I referred to the fact that coming to agreement on a common European competition policy took some 25 years of debate, negotiating, and compromising. The introduction of the Euro has a similar history. Agreement on these items of European integration implied that national economic orders had to transfer power of decision-making from the national to the supranational level of the European Union. I also assumed that, over a comparable time span, some sort of European social policy would emerge. Meanwhile, social policy is becoming increasingly harmonized at the European level, which will undoubtedly affect the subsidiarity principle.

Now, let us look at the history of European political interference in health care matters. Some 25 years ago, this involvement began, somewhat hesitatingly, with health ministers exchanging their worries about the rapidly increasing costs of health care. The reason for this was simply that each of them had become convinced that something had to be done within his or her member state to get control of health care developments. But also, each of them had to find solutions individually within their member state. At the European level, for a long time, practical interference remained focused mainly on health-related and public health matters, resulting in increasing cooperation in these areas. But governments could no longer deny the fact that, as had already been argued by the European Commission in 1982, health care costs formed the major part of a country's social security budget. No wonder, therefore, that this exchange of worries by the ministers of health was accompanied by proposals to cooperate in controlling the costs. Since then, we have read about increasing efficiency and effectiveness, about establishing a common database, about transparency of medical product prices, about containment measures, about comparable health data, about benchmarking, about good practices, and so on.

It seems to me that this ultimately will lead to a harmonization of health care activities at the European level. Four arguments, in combination, support of this point of view.

First of all, for decades, health care was thought not to be important enough to receive specific attention within the European political framework. Far behind the Common Agricultural Policy, it was a minor part of social policy. Since 1999, however, we have had a European Directorate for Health and Consumer Protection (DGXXIV). We may assume that this directorate will increase its focus on health care matters throughout the European Union.

Secondly, the European Commission has expressed that it sees itself as qualified to add European value to health care systems, starting with the setting-up of a database with comparative information.

Thirdly, there is increasing interest in a European health insurance card, combined with a European health insurance system. If this becomes reality, we may safely assume that pursuing efficiency and effectiveness on providing health care will be high on the insurers' agenda.

Finally, and most importantly, the information technology is now available.

Now, assume yourself to be the European Commissioner responsible for health, meeting regularly with the ministers of health from the member states, knowing that, in health care, each country acts as it pleases and also knowing that the relational picture of all the parties involved in health care resembles a wheelbarrow full of frogs, accepting that the developments in health care (finance excepted) are difficult to control, and, in particular, realizing yourself that all those member-state ministers have to do their utmost to live up to their constitutional obligations regarding their citizens' health, what would you do?

You would persuade those ministers to work closely together on all those aspects of health care which do not directly touch upon the principle of subsidiarity, and which could benefit each of them individually. Finance is such an aspect. In line with the ongoing harmonization of social policy, therefore, financial harmonization in health care provision matters is a logical next step. It may take another ten years, but it will come. And this can even be done while maintaining the idea of subsidiarity. After all, health ministers working together to get control of health care in financial terms implicitly admit that they are not capable of doing that individually. This, in turn, legitimizes action at the European Community level in accordance with the principle of subsidiarity as formulated in the preamble of the Maastricht Treaty.[43] Consequently, there will come a time when health care provision will have to be delivered in line with European Union cost and price regulations. In addition to this, it is not unreasonable to assume that the use of new technologies, except for the strictly private health care market, will also be subject to EU policies. Even now, initiatives to harmonize technology assessment at the EU level are underway. In this respect, the EU-funded ECHTA project (European Collaboration on Health Technology Assessment) has proposed gathering and distributing health technology assessment findings to decision-making bodies of the respective member states through the establishment of an EU clearing house.[44] Following this line of argument, the European Union may realize that Union-wide planning, based on centers of excellence, could deliver a more cost-effective way of ensuring high-technology care in some specialized areas.[45]

In the longer term, developments like these may have serious consequences for the managerial freedom of health care providers. I will return to this topic later.

7.2.2 Practical Regulations

National governments, applying the territoriality principle, mostly limit their activities regarding health care to legal arrangements for their own citizens through nationally recognized insurers. However, regardless of whether the European Union further integrates economically, the citizens of Europe will always go abroad. They may do so because they want to spend their holiday in the sunny parts of the European continent, their job may require them to work temporarily elsewhere, or they may want to spend wintertime in a more agreeable climate. No matter what the reasons are, however, during their stay in another member state, they may meet with an accident or they may become sick and need medical care. And since it is not unlikely that the seriousness of their illness will make it impossible for them to return immediately to their country of residence for medical treatment, it is appropriate that member states set up arrangements to deal with the unexpected health care needs of foreigners. The governments of the European Union have done so extensively by establishing *practical regulations* regarding health care for their citizens in other member states. In 1958 the territoriality principle was mitigated for the purposes of providing health care for immigrant workers. From that moment on, they and their families were entitled to health care in their country of residence. This entitlement was limited, however, to immigrant workers from member states. Thirteen years later, in 1971, the European Council introduced regulation No. 1408/71 regarding the application of social security schemes to employed persons, self-employed people, and their families, in the case of moving within the European Union.[46] From this regulation followed a number of so-called E-forms. The forms most frequently used to obtain health care abroad are—

1. E-111, which secures emergency services for the insured and their relatives in a situation of displacement. Since 1996, this form has also granted permission to obtain dialysis and oxigenotherapy services, and since 2001, it has granted health services to pregnant women before the 38th week of gestation.
2. E-112, which grants health coverage for the insured and their relatives. This form is used for treatment in another state which is not available in the country of residence. In addition, it applies to continued assistance for the insured and his relatives.

3. E-113 authorizes hospitalization in a different member state.
4. E-114 makes it possible to receive significant treatment in another member state. In 1982, the list of the treatments was specified (orthopaedic prosthesis, orthopaedic shoe gear, hearing aids, wheel chairs, et cetera).
5. E-119 guarantees the right of the unemployed, and their relatives, to health care when they are looking for a job in another member state.
6. E-120 certifies the right to benefits for pension applicants.
7. E-126 grants reimbursement for benefits in kind.
8. E-128 is a health care arrangement for workers and students who are engaged in official study courses.

For most of these forms, the urgency criterion applies.

As discussed previously, these kinds of arrangements have been established independently from further European integration. They are practical arrangements from the insurance side "*in case something happens.*" In financial terms, the significance of this type of cross-border care is very limited, on average amounting to less than €2.00 per capita in 1998, with Luxembourg as an exception.[47] Natural obstacles like language, distance, lack of information regarding the foreign health care system, administrative procedures, and traveling time, play an important impeding role.

Patients are not the only ones whose movement is very limited. Free movement of health care staff is also rather insignificant. Research on the first ten years of implementation of the free movement of persons made it clear that, for example, the number of physicians moving abroad was limited to 0.21% of the overall workforce.[48] Despite the way free movement was discussed shortly before the latest enlargement of the European Union, which suggested that European health care professionals would be constantly traveling around within the European Union, this appears not to have happened to any significant extent thus far. Generally speaking, we know very little about the effects of free movement on professionals, with the exception of doctors.[49] Overall, so far the right of people to move freely has not led to doctors' exoduses to and from countries within the European Union. Not only language, but also cultural and social barriers, as well as restrictive policies of national governments, play an important role here. As for the latter, the lack of mutual recognition of formal qualifications and, even more so, national regulations regarding continuing education, appear to impede free movement. National restriction policies, however, may lead to intervention from the Court of Justice in Luxembourg.

Another type of practical arrangement is cross-border activity regarding health care provision. We see an increasing number of cross-border cooperation projects on a structural basis among health care providers throughout Europe. Research by the European Hospital and Health Care Federation (HOPE) in 2003 identified no less than 169 projects, with 28 along 37 common borders, involving a few hundred health care institutions.[50] The research shows a wide range of cooperation objectives, varying from emergency care to telemedicine, sharing of expensive equipment, human resources, research projects, funding issues, et cetera. Cross-border projects seem to be to the benefit of all parties involved. Patients are no longer confronted with traveling long distances; hospitals benefit from the sharing of facilities; insurers can contribute to the reduction of waiting lists while, for health care systems, the principle of economies of scale applies.[51]

Regarding these cross-border projects, two additional remarks should be made. First of all, they appear to be bottom-up processes. Authorities, though interested, are not particularly involved. Secondly, apart from the lack of a legal framework,[52] funding issues, for example, patient reimbursement, as well as administrative differences, are key problems. Insurers, however, appear to be cooperative. As an example, the Dutch CZ group insurer, together with the German AOK Rheinland, developed a simple International Health Card for their clients, which gives them free access to all basic medical specialist care anywhere in the EU region Meuse–Rhine.[53]

It is not very likely that, in the near future, cross-border projects will lead to the creation of a single health care system for the European Union. Nevertheless, health ministers of the European Union have expressly declared their intention to increase their involvement and actively participate in these types of arrangements.[54] Politicians may, therefore, like the partners in the projects, see their involvement as an opportunity to learn. That learning process may contribute to a (further) erosion of the subsidiarity principle regarding health care systems.

7.2.3 Rulings of the European Court of Justice

In 1978 and 1979, the European Court of Justice (ECJ) had already ruled that insurers always have to give authorization for treatment in another country of the European Union if that treatment was indicated for the person involved and the necessary care could be provided within a reasonable timeframe in that person's country of residence. Although these rulings were important for the formulation of regulations regarding the free movement of persons, they did not fundamentally touch upon the principle of subsidiarity regarding health care. As long as governments saw to it that the necessary care could be provided within a reasonable timeframe within their countries, authorization to go abroad could be refused. And this is exactly what happened. Things changed with ECJ rulings some 20 years later. Below, I present some important illustrative examples.

To begin with, the Decker and Kohll rulings of 1998 regarding ambulatory treatment in a neighboring country without prior permission subordinated the subsidiarity principle to the free movement of persons, goods, and services. The initial reaction of governments was that the Decker and Kohll rulings explicitly and exclusively had consequences for ambulatory care. Institutional care, they assumed, would stay out of reach.

This assumption was proved wrong by the ECJ's rulings in the Smits–Peerbooms cases of July 2001. Without prior authorization, a Dutch citizen, Mrs. Smit, received multidisciplinary Parkinson's treatment in a German clinic. She paid for the treatment in Germany and proceeded to present the bill to her Dutch insurer. That insurer refused reimbursement, arguing that the German treatment was unusual among professionals, that adequate treatment by a contracted Dutch provider would have been possible, and that the German treatment did not add medical value.

A 36-year-old Dutch citizen, Mr. Peerbooms lapsed into a coma as a consequence of a car accident. The attending neurologist advised his relatives to take him to an Austrian clinic, where he came back to consciousness through intensive neurostimulation treatment. At that time, the Netherlands employed this kind of treatment only on an experimental basis for patients under the age of 25 years. In Austria, the relevant treatment was already fully covered by the insurer. The Dutch insurer refused reimbursement, arguing that adequate treatment would also have been available in the Netherlands.

Both Smits and Peerbooms went to the ECJ. At stake was, primarily, the question of whether hospital care should be considered an economic activity which, therefore, was subject to the free movement of goods and services, and, secondarily, whether prior authorization for such an activity was necessary.

The national governments involved set up their defense, arguing that (a) there is no question of payment if the patient receives treatment free of charge, or, in the event that the patient has paid, this payment is fully or partly reimbursed; (b) labeling the health care items in question as an economic activity would only apply if the provider had a profit motive; and (c) social insurance systems could not be considered as free economic activities governed by the terms of the treaty because patients concerned would neither be capable of deciding for themselves on the nature, the content, and the scope of the necessary care, nor on the price of it.

The ECJ did not go along with these arguments and ruled that while European Community law does not detract from the power of member states to organize their social security systems, member states must, nevertheless, comply with the principle of freedom to provide services when exercising that power. It held that it was not necessary for patients to pay for the service rendered as a condition for labeling the treatment a service. Furthermore, the ECJ ruled that prior authorization would obstruct patients from having their treatment abroad. Such a barrier would only be legitimate for reasons of general interest. This would be the case if treatment abroad would (a) result in a serious threat for a balanced system of social security, (b) threaten the objective of a balanced service delivery for all citizens, and (c) endanger the maintenance of treatment capacities and medical competences.

In conclusion, according to ECJ rulings, treatment in hospitals is not exempted from EU regulations regarding the free movement of goods and services. This also applies for systems with service delivery in kind. The problem behind all this is that, while the ECJ acknowledged the right of member states to define the coverage package, it also appears to have called for a European-wide consensus on what should be covered and what should be deemed evidence-based. Indirectly, the consequence is that European jurisprudence marginalized the territoriality principle as it applies to health care systems, while, as a side effect, national insurance regulations have been extended to health care providers all over Europe.

In principle, the foregoing also applies to voluntary health insurance. That too, is an economic activity which is subject to EU regulations. In this respect, in most member states voluntary health insurance exists as part of a legal systems of social security. Here, the EU regulation is that health insurance that is part of a statutory system of social security is excluded from the EU competition directives. It depends, however, on how one defines social security. In dual systems, like the Netherlands, it is not certain beforehand that the competition directives do not apply. If we add to this the fact that private insurers are complaining about the tax advantages of mutual health funds and voluntary not-for-profit insurers, while accusing them of misusing their dominant position, one can safely predict that the ECJ still has much work to do in order to clarify this issue. For example, currently (in 2005) being heard is a case of a private insurer who is accusing a Belgian mutual health fund of misusing its dominant position by offering voluntary additional insurance at a price that no private competitor can beat. It is not difficult to imagine other developments which could decrease member states' capabilities to uphold their voluntary health insurance based on solidarity.

Finally, there is the question of whether health care institutions can be considered an "undertaking." According to EU competition policy, each entity engaged in economic activities is an undertaking, regardless of its legal status or the way it is financed. In this respect, the ECJ has ruled furthermore that, for an undertaking, the profit motive is not necessarily a decisive criterion. Consequently, non-profit organizations and charitable institutions may also be labeled undertakings. Moreover, the ECJ holds that it is irrelevant who the owner of an undertaking is or whether it is governed by private or public law. Consequently, government agencies are also undertakings. All in all, the only way for an organization *not* to be defined as an undertaking is if its activities can be considered non-economic. Here, the ECJ is to be very strict, arguing that if such an activity can also be taken up by a private organization, one cannot label it as being non-economic. Altogether, this means that health care organizations pursuing social objectives do not by definition remain free from competition regulations at the level of the European Union. The distinctive argument is "whether a given health care institution acts so differently from private undertakings so that a private company, working in the same way, could not, in principle, hope to make a profit. Whether the health care institution actually seeks to make a profit is irrelevant. An economic activity can therefore be defined as one that can be carried out to realise a profit, even if this does not actually happen. An activity that is only possible on a non-profit making basis is different from an economic one because it is not guided by economic motives but, instead, by the principles of solidarity and of social protection." In this respect, a recent ruling from the European Tribunal of First Instance is meaningful, because it labeled the purchasing activities of a buyers' co-operative, not having a profit motive, as a non-economic activity because of the purely social character of those activities, based on the principle of national solidarity.[55]

Altogether, the discussion on the definition of an undertaking shows that health care institutions are potentially subject to the rules of European competition policy. They are considered to be undertakings. Ownership or profit motive are not important in this respect. What counts is that they are engaged in economic activities. Even if the majority of their activities are non-economic, this does not automatically apply to all their activities.

There are several ways, however, to label activities as being non-economic. One way is to think of activities as a sovereign state affair. Then, however, the state has to prove that it is necessary for it to execute those activities itself. Delegating their execution to other organizations, and still claiming them to be non-economic, may not hold in court.

All in all, it is highly possible that reforming health care by introducing market elements may subject these systems to the rules of European competition. In other words, stipulating the free movement of persons, goods, and services among health care systems may infringe the principle of solidarity.

7.3 Enlargement

Adding to the health (care) policy issues of European integration is the latest enlargement of May 2004.[56] Of the ten new members, eight have a communist history. But this does not mean that their health care systems are alike, i.e., centrally controlled and directed. Consequently, comparing these health care systems is just as difficult and arbitrary as is the case with the 15 countries that were already members of the European Union before May 2004. The problems of integrating these eight new members, however, are manifold. Particularly problematic is the fact that there is an enormous economic gap, with their GDP in 2001 being less than half the average GDP of the 15 members. Even adjusted for purchasing power, the difference is considerable.[57] The relative poverty of these new members is reflected in their citizens' health. Life expectancy at birth is considerably lower than in the 15 pre-existing member states; death rates compare unfavorably; and the number of people reporting long-standing illness is substantial. Much of this is caused by the lack of an adequate health care infrastructure, i.e., health care facilities which can be quickly and easily accessed. It is estimated that 25% of the mortality gap (between birth and the age of 75 years) can be explained by failures in medical care. Furthermore, new pharmaceuticals and new surgical techniques which came into use in Western Europe from the 1970s on were only rarely introduced in the East.[58] While a lot remains to be done to improve the health status of the people who just joined the European Union, much was already done during the transition process. A well-known example is the Phare program of 1989, an important source of assistance, contributing no less than 36% of total development finances for Central and Eastern Europe in 1999, directed at systems development (sustainable financing, hospital management, primary care development, information systems, human resources, et cetera). Furthermore, the European Bank for Reconstruction and Development and the World Bank contributed their share. The WHO appointed "liaison officers" to support health policy-making in transition countries. Individual countries of the West took initiatives for bilateral support, whereas individual hospitals started twinning projects.[59]

It took some time before health and enlargement became a substantial item on the political agenda of the European Union. From about the turn of the century, however, EU presidents started to organize specific health and enlargement conferences.[60] From those days on, health care and enlargement became a topic of political interest at the European level.

First of all, this interest focused on public health, and in particular such items as health and safety, communicable diseases, and alcohol and tobacco.

As for health and safety, is should be realized that for the 15 preexisting member states the costs of inadequate safety measures were already estimated to be between 2.6% and 3.8% of GDP, or 1% to 5% of operating profits in most sectors. Reducing risks to health and safety may in the longer term increase productivity and profitability.[61] Health and safety measures should take account of the need for a level playing field in an (integrated) EU business community.

Regarding communicable diseases, the reality is that in the 15 preexisting member states mechanisms for surveillance and control differ widely and are undersourced. Here, political action by the European Union should deliver greater benefits than would be realizable if each member state acted on its own, if only because communicable diseases know no national frontiers.[62]

Finally, concerning alcohol and tobacco, EU politics will have to deal with existing differences regarding anti-smoking policies between member states. Some countries are relaxed in this respect; others have imposed severe measures. Here, the ambiguity is that the European Union is, first of all, an economic entity "where trade appears to trump health at all turns."[63]

Comparable ambiguity exists about pharmaceutical policy within an enlarged European Union, i.e., a desire for free trade on the one hand, and the wish to regulate pricing in the framework of cost containment on the other. Intellectual property rights, regulations about the provision of new drugs, reimbursement policies, parallel imports, reference prices, positive lists, et cetera, are all items that must be considered in the design of a pharmaceutical policy for the European Union.[64] Such a policy deserves to be high on the EU's agenda because pharmaceutical spending has reached a level of 10% to 15% of total health care spending, a growth which has outpaced that of inpatient and outpatient care in most countries of the European Union.[65]

Furthermore, there is the freedom of movement of persons, which may have consequences for the labor market in health care. Also, patients are free to travel abroad for their treatment. If patients do so in considerable numbers, this may affect the health care infrastructure in their country of residence. As for the labor market, there is the problem of mutual recognition of medical training, in addition to the fact that there are remuneration differences. Medical specialists from the new entrants with accepted qualifications may, for income reasons, prefer to apply for positions in the 15 preexisting member states. At the same time, these member states may try to recruit physicians from the new member states due to the shortages in medical staff they are experiencing. As it is, there is not much known in quantitative terms regarding these aspects of enlargement. Nevertheless, there is concern about the impact of free movement. The European Commission, however, expects this impact to be limited.[66]

Next, there are considerable price differences. Charges for hip replacements, for example, may differ sevenfold between EU countries.[67]

All in all, the enlarged European Union will face a tremendous challenge in attempting to adjust and streamline the many different aspects of health care. In analyzing this process, Dubois and McKee distinguish between two hypotheses.[68] The first one emphasizes the convergence of health care systems based on the transition to a market economy. Under the second hypothesis, institutional diversity between the member states is the starting point. The first hypothesis suggests that the health care systems of the former communist countries are likely to pursue the standards of the West, expecting them to become more economically viable, responsive, and compatible with the market economy. Consequently, these health care systems will become similarly exposed to the exogenous challenges faced by the health care systems of the West. The second hypothesis takes into account the diversity of national circumstances, suggesting that different histories and different contexts lead to different transformation paths. The authors do not express a preference regarding the two hypotheses. However, since the new former communist members allocated on average 6.2% of GDP on health care, compared to 8.5% in the 15 preexisting member states,[69] and given the fact that the people of those former communist countries enjoy a relatively poor health status, with their GDP being considerably lower than that of the West, it seems logical to assume that investing in the health care infrastructure is inevitable if one wants to approach Western health care standards in a not-too-distant future. But upgrading that infrastructure "is pretty much a linear function of economic growth."[70] Given what their GDP growth rates have been up till now, however, it will take the former communist countries some decades to reach the Western standards. The question is whether it is wise to follow such a policy. In line with what I said in section 1.3.3, the West should realize that, for the sake of a continuously (politically) stable European Union, the differences in health care standards should not be too large. Investing in the health care infrastructure of these new member states seems appropriate, therefore. Specific structural funds of the European Union could be the instrument to do this.

7.4 Summary

In line with the Maastricht Treaty, health care in the countries of the European Union is subject to the subsidiarity principle, which implies that each member state is free to choose the organizational structure and financial arrangements. Thanks to the ongoing European economic integration, however, this subsidiarity principle is slowly being eroded. This does not mean, though, that the health care systems of the countries of the European Union will converge into a universal one, because the organizational and financial arrangements differ too greatly. Convergence will concentrate on two aspects, finance and quality, which can be relatively easily brought onto a common footing. Given political considerations at the EU level over the past decades, the European Commission will probably take the lead in designing this type of convergence policy. It also seems wise for the European Commission to supervise upgrading the health care infrastructures of the new entrants with a communist history.

8
Investing in Health Care

This chapter and the next one deal with developments in health care since the end of the Second World War. It should be noted that, for the first 10 to 15 years after the Second World War, there is hardly any useful aggregated information available, either quantitative or qualitative. An analysis in financial terms, therefore, must start in 1960. From that time on, the countries of the European Union started to collect data systematically. These data have been collated by the OECD.

In retrospect, the 40 years from 1960 to 2000 can be divided into a period of growth in health care expenditure, lasting from 1960 to 1980, followed by a period of reform, which started around the beginning of the 1980s and is still continuing. This chapter is limited to the first period. During this period, the combined influence of organizational, medical, political, and economic change led to the creation of the "health industry."[1] I will deal with these four types of change in separate sections, and I will conclude the chapter by going into the rising criticism regarding this industry, which started around the mid-1970s.

8.1 From a Closed System to an Open One

For the first 10 to 15 years after the Second World War, hospitals in general, as well as other health care institutions, functioned more or less in isolation from society. These institutions, many of which were established by religious congregations, formed a world of their own, characterized by devotion and decent poverty. This was reflected in the composition of the administration in which mother or father superior, minister, priest, or rector, were amply represented. This explains why hospitals' annual reports of those days reported extensively on spiritual matters. These reports sometimes even started with a real sermon or the results of examinations of the nursing-staff-in-training on theological subjects.

Medical staff and medical performance were extensively reviewed. Individual medical staff members were listed as well as the diagnoses per specialty. Otherwise, information was limited to the training of nurses, disciplinary regulations, compensation of the costs of further education and training, promotions, jubilees, and, once in a while, mention of a representative council for those employed by the hospital.

The hospitals' daily practical operation was under the leadership of the medical superintendent, who could be assisted by a deputy, usually female, who had specialized in nursing matters. It was very exceptional to have a business administrator as a member of the board. Doctors were held in high esteem, were very well looked after, and received all types of fringe benefits. In the case of psychiatric hospitals and institutions for the mentally retarded, doctors could live on the organization's premises, paying modest rents, and having their houses and gardens maintained by the organization's technical staff.

In contrast to this closed world, the business community of those days was already paying extensive attention to the international economic situation, reviewing companies' positions in the market. Government interference in the economic process, particularly regarding fiscal policy and trade relations, was a regular theme in their annual reports. Economic trends were assessed, and there were complaints about an overstrained labor market, which was assumed to lead to wage increases that were not in line with increases in productivity. The importance of research and development was underlined regularly, and the term *customer service* came into use.

In short, unlike the health care world, the business community paid attention to the external environment as a matter of course. Insofar as health care institutions did this at all, their focus was mostly limited to the immediate external environment.

To understand these differences, it is important to realize that, after the war, much of the industrial capacity of the countries of Europe was destroyed. Rebuilding that capacity was, therefore, the first priority of European governments. In line with this, the costs of labor had to be kept as low as possible. This could be done by a centrally controlled wage policy, or, for countries with a health care system based on social security, by keeping the premiums as moderate as possible. In short, governments' health care policy, while making use of financial instruments, was directed at decelerating the speed of extension, thus creating room for industrial investment.

For hospitals, the financial instruments were price control and limitations on the creation of new capacities. Where social insurance companies performed an intermediary role, they had to use up their financial reserves. General practitioners saw their fees frozen, and home-nursing services had to cope with a limitation in subsidies. Of course, this had financial consequences for health care institutions.

Meanwhile, health care providers had to handle a strongly increasing demand. Therefore, it was no exception in those days for hospital patients to be accommodated in the corridors for the simple reason that the wards were overcrowded.

The financial problems of health care providers became even more severe because of the increasing exodus of religious congregations. Instead of drawing a labor force from their own ranks, whose members had never heard of a collective labor agreement, an eight-hour working day, or democracy in labour relations, and who had a holiday of no more than a few days per year for a religious retreat, these congregations had to enter the labor market with its accompanying terms. Working in health care thus became a job or a profession, instead of a calling. In this respect, it should be realized that replacement of one congregation member of the "old style," i.e., working 12 hours per day, 7 days per week, took more than two employees from the labor market. Consequently, the costs of labor more than doubled. The resulting price increase could only partly be compensated for by an increase in the price of medical services. With governments persisting in their policies of scarcity, and not directing developments, the only thing that hospitals, i.e., mostly congregations, could do to bridge the gap between their revenues and the costs of increasing medical consumption was to draw on their own financial reserves. These financial reserves, for that matter, could be considerable because of substantial legacies and benefactions.

From the 1960s on, the world of health care was transformed very rapidly from a closed system into an open one. More and more, health care came to be seen as a business characterized by fast growth and increasing complexity. It was no longer a world in itself, and those in charge became convinced that the hospital organization should not be considered in isolation but in the context of the environment at large. Mother and father superior, as well as the minister, the rector, and the priest, disappeared from the administration and were replaced by professionals.[2] The business administrator entered the hospital boardroom, and religious convictions became less dominant. Medical and technological developments accelerated, resulting in a boom in diagnostic and therapeutic opportunities. As a consequence of these developments, staff increased, particularly paramedics and medical auxiliary staff like physiotherapists, laboratory assistants, analysts, technicians, and social workers. General hospitals in the Netherlands, for example, saw a growth in staff members of 25% during the period 1968–1972, and overall employment in health care in OECD countries almost doubled during the period 1970–1990.[3] In short, hospitals entered the third phase of medical science and technology, i.e., "the modern era of the biological revolution, the development of machine-based technology, and the appearance of extended longevity, with a corresponding increase in rates of chronic diseases."[4]

With regard to mental health care, a change in treatment philosophy came about. Categorization, small-scale accommodation, smaller groups, and deconcentration characterized this change. As for the "technology" of psychiatric treatment, an extreme differentiation was carried through. In no time at all, this aspect of health care developed several distinctive "technologies" or models. Based on two main streams, behavioral psychology and psychoanalysis, psychotherapy was differentiated into a large number of side therapies (family therapy, group therapy, therapy on analytic lines, the Rogerian approach, et cetera).[5]

There was an increasing interest in treatment outside institutional walls. Treatment in outpatient clinics developed rapidly, and day treatment became popular. Cooperation between different types of institutional care got off the ground, whereas in the hospitals, patients became clients, and public relations became policy items: the flower and fruit stall, the hairdresser and the beauty parlour, the television room and the restaurant became enduring elements of hospital accommodation.

In the beginning of the 1970s, with the nuns, deaconesses, and lay brothers almost all gone, personnel departments got off the ground, and it soon became clear that their job was not only to provide adequate staffing, reduce absenteeism, and set salary conditions, but also to take care of matters like career policies, assessment systems, and social counseling.

Meanwhile, the increasing complexity of health care organizations, resulting from medical-technological developments and a strong increase in staff, caused these personnel departments to create solutions for an increasingly complex communications network. At the same time, changing opinions in society regarding labor relations resulted in a strongly growing culture of consultation. Although that culture labelled its instruments differently, e.g., employee participation, work-progress discussion, or grievance committees, each of these instruments was an expression of the democratization of labor relations.

Starting in the beginning of the 1970s, health care organizations began to engage in continuously developing or adjusting organizational structures with the help of external management consultants, who were quite often professionals in areas of social work. The old-fashioned tripartite structure of the medical staff, the nursing staff, and the support staff of the 1960s was replaced by the matrix structure of the 1970s, implicitly acknowledging that health care can also be considered as a range of production processes, each of which needs specific inputs. Policy preparation and consulting platforms were set up. Memoranda were written in which new organizational structures were explained, policy plans unfolded, missions were presented, and ideas on the future were expressed.

Contrary to the situation in the business world, the democratization of labor relations in health care organizations was viewed as an objective, worth to pursue in its own right. Moreover, an important difference with health care organizations was that creating democratic labor relations in the business world was not sought so much in complex structures and platforms of consultation, but in creating opportunities for co-decision-making by employees. Business leaders pursued management flexibility by delegating responsibilities and authority to lower organizational layers, thus offering employees the opportunities to develop their talents. There was an extension of duties, job rotation, process design, education, and training.

Although to the bigger companies, economies of scale were thought to be very important, pursuing that objective was carried through while maintaining controllability and flexibility through a policy of decentralization, taking into account central guidelines. Management teams were small, directed at improving decisiveness, because this was believed to increase the flexibility the market demanded.

In short, the democratization of labor relations in business life was expressly connected to promoting personal responsibility in the workplace. When the economy stagnated around the beginning of the 1980s, this philosophy was also applied to the carrying out of cost reduction programs.

8.2 The Authority of Medicine

During and after the Second World War, the United States took the lead in the further development of health care. The countries of Western Europe followed some time later, due to the fact that their immediate priorities lay with recovering from the devastation of the war.[6]

During the war and the two decades thereafter, great strides in health care knowledge were made in the United States, with American medical faculties teaching students many new ways to combat disease. At that time, medical academicians considered themselves to be doing good work for society.[7] Medical faculty members had a certain disdain for commercial activities, did not patent their discoveries, were satisfied with relatively low salaries and adhered to high standards of intellectual honesty. Those who entered medicine were advised to do so out of a desire to serve the public, accepting that they would not become wealthy from medical practice.[8] Nonmonetary rewards, like recognition from peers and society, were thought to be more important than financial gains. In the words of Ludmerer, "the currency of academic medicine was not dollars but publications, appointments, titles, memberships, and awards."[9]

Furthermore, medicine was highly appreciated by the public at large, not least as a consequence of some striking medical achievements during the war. During that time, an antidote to chemical weapons was discovered and research was stimulated which culminated in the synthesis of cortisone. Surgery on the battlefield influenced the development of heart surgery, and, of course, there was the discovery of penicillin.[10] These war-related innovations created a "critical mass," which, together with developments in the pharmaceutical industry, contributed to a chain reaction of further progress.[11] Moreover, the euphoria after the war victory "released a surge of pent-up utopian energies."[12] Medicine could help to make the world a better place, it was believed. Consequently, medical research funding in the United States during the first two decades after the war increased to staggering heights, from $87 million in 1947 to over $2 billion in 1966, of which the major part was federal government financing.[13]

The easy availability of federal funds for research, together with achievements in bio-medical research and the adulation of the public, created a "golden age" for medical schools, particularly in the 1950s and 1960s,[14] during which medical education became a "national enterprise."[15] Many students entered American medical schools, causing the number of MD graduates to increase by almost 230% over the period 1960–1980. But medical schools, their number having increased by around 45% over the same period,[16] were not only established to train doctors. They were also places to practice "clinical science," which caused medicine to evolve from "a single broad area of practice into a federation of diverse disciplines."[17] In contrast to a primary objective of medical education being "training for uncertainty," and making students "alert to the exception,"[18] specialization and sub-specialization apparently were thought to deliver more certainty in combating disease. Moreover, specialized training was intended to develop the specific skills necessary for the use of new technological equipment and the application of new and complicated procedures. Consequently, new categories of medical specialties (gastro-enterology, endocrinology, medical oncology, clinical pharmacology, et cetera), together with the necessary auxiliary staff and infrastructural capacities (for example, intensive care units) became part of the medical world.[19]

The countries of Western Europe soon followed the United States. In the 1970s, the number of kidney specialists in the United Kingdom, for example, increased around fourfold as a consequence of an increasing demand for dialysis and transplantation. The greater opportunities to treat coronary heart disease led the number of cardiologists to almost double; that of haematologists quadrupled once certain types of leukaemia and lymphomas could be treated; and the number of psychiatrists doubled once mental illness came to be seen as a treatable disorder.

In short, medicine developed into a highly sophisticated enterprise, able to deal with a large range of human illnesses. And the public, becoming increasingly health conscious, loved it. After all, except for suiciders, nobody wants to die unnecessarily. Consequently, particularly in the United States, health policy became based on the assumption that a nation's health depended on the quality and quantity of doctors.[20] Furthermore, a nation's health was believed to contribute to its competitiveness.[21] Investing in medical education and research, therefore, was perceived as an economic benefit to the country.[22]

No wonder, then, that doctors and what they did were much appreciated. Society itself granted supreme authority to the medical profession, making it preeminent, and the assumption that "doctor knows best" was not questioned. Particularly during the early and middle decades of the 20th century, when doctors were primarily dealing with acute diseases, the medicine's authority was clear and unchallenged.[23] As a consequence, particularly in the United States, for almost a quarter of a century after the Second World War, the medical establishment was hardly questioned, either by the public or by governments. There were no questions about the necessity and scope of specialization, and there were no worries about the optimal mix of specialists and general practitioners, or the increasing level of medical testing.[24] Through the conjunction of professional associations and with state support, the medical establishment had gained a monopoly over its work. This monopoly position was political in character, "involving the aid of the state in establishing and maintaining the profession's preeminence."[25]

Interestingly, it was the academic medical world itself which, in the 1960s, expressed criticism about these developments, believing that the proper balance between specialists and general practitioners had been disturbed. From over 80% in the 1930s, by the mid-1960s the numbers of American medical students who planned to enter general practice had dropped to only 15%; the rest wished to specialize.[26] Furthermore, medical testing evolved into overinvestigation. Throughout the 1970s, the number of medical testing in the United States doubled, leading some to speak of the syndrome of "medical vampirism," because patients in hospitals could become anemic as a result of blood loss caused by too much blood testing. Sometimes they even needed blood transfusions.[27] All in all, technology and testing became ends in themselves, with doctors failing to exert self-control over their newfound powers.[28] It can be argued that health care in the 1970s came under the influence of the "technologic imperative," which commanded that all possibilities available be used for the treatment of patients.[29]

Though all this may be true for "the glory days of medicine" of the 1970s,[30] it is an oversimplification to blame the medical establishment for the fact that, during the period 1960–1980, medicine went "out of control,"[31] an observation which is in itself debatable. After all, the positive aspects of the developments in medical care are many. More illnesses became curable, the average length of stay in acute hospitals decreased, turnover in the use of hospital beds increased, treatment in outpatient clinics expanded enormously, et cetera.[32] In short, despite the negative aspects like overinvestigation, overall medicine became more effective and efficient.

We also should mention the health-conscious public, which started to regard health care as a basic right, which led to an increased demand for doctors and medical services.[33] This health-conscious public also expected doctors to do everything possible to combat disease. Negligence, increasingly led to legal proceedings. As an example, the number of legal cases against obstetricians in the United Kingdom tripled between 1983 and 1990.[34] Lawyers in the United States, and increasingly in the countries of the European Union, are making a lot of money litigating medical malpractice cases.

Also, the idea that health care is a basic right has been reinforced through legislation. In this respect, the introduction of Medicare and Medicaid in the United States in 1965 is exemplary. Its introduction should be appreciated in a historical context. It was the time of President Johnson's "War on Poverty," the Civil Rights Act of 1964, and the Voting Rights Act of 1965. In short, those were the days of the belief in the manageability of a fair and just democratic society. The introduction of Medicare and Medicaid was in conformity with this belief, as it was meant to bring elderly and poor people into the same health care system that already served the more affluent citizens, of whom 75% were privately insured in 1965. In short, the objective was to create a classless health care system.[35] But this creation had its price, since spending on Medicare and Medicaid programs, increased fourfold from 1971 to 1976, from $14 billion to $56 billion, and overall health care costs experienced annual double-digit growth for more than a decade.[36]

The consequences for health care provision in the United States were enormous. Almost overnight, it considerably broadened health care's potential to generate income. Uninsured patients, who before the passage of Medicare and Medicaid would be treated free of charge because they were "interesting clinical material"[37] for (teaching) hospitals, now became financially interesting. Based on a fee-for-service system, under the terms of the new legislation, each treatment and investigation became reimbursable with public and private third-party payers. This caused clinical services to grow rapidly, thus generating income for hospitals; it caused a change in the attitudes of doctors, who now stood to benefit financially; it caused an erosion of the charitable mission of hospitals,[38] and it caused interest in clinical scientific research to decrease, because graduates preferred making money in private practice.[39] Focusing on academic medical centers, Ludmerer therefore rightfully observes that the introduction of Medicare and Medicaid transformed them from charitable institutions into "vendors of services."[40] Consequently, health care became big business for hospitals and medical training institutions, conducted by CEOs who, in turn, consulted external experts for advice on investing, accounting, reporting, cost-cutting, administrative procedures, and information systems,[41] paying them fees of up to 2% or 3% of the institution's revenues.[42] By the 1980s, "academic physicians were being compared with corporate executives, stockbrokers, and financial scoundrels in their greed and self-serving behaviour."[43] They turned from service-maximizers into profit-maximizers.[44] Finally, in accordance with the changing ethical landscape, medical schools established formal relations with pharmaceutical companies, exchanging research grants for patents. They even started their own companies in order to be able to exploit their scientific discoveries.[45]

This also caused the medical establishment to overrate its position in society, abusing the public's and the government's appreciation. In other words, the *esprit de corps* that prevailed shortly after the Second World War had changed by the 1970s into arrogance, with doctors claiming that all their demands should be fulfilled as a matter of course. Medical schools in the United States had grown fat and affluent, their revenues increasing from $882 million in 1965 to nearly $21 billion in 1990.[46] During the 1980s, they bought every new piece of equipment available without wondering whether it would add value to the health care process.[47] Acquiring the newest technologies became part of the "medical arms race" between competing hospitals. Research from the 1970s showed that hospitals with more competitors had higher costs of care, higher staffing levels, and more high-technology equipment.[48] But despite the constantly increasing costs of health care, physicians' interest in health care policy, according to an American economist, started and ended with only two directives: (1) "give us money" and (2) "leave us alone."[49] Medical faculties started to gaze inward, focusing on their rights and entitlements, and no longer acted as guardians of the nation's health.[50] This detached, arrogant behavior was fostered by the lack of a sensible governmental health care policy, not only in the United States but in almost all countries of the developed world. In the era of belief in the manageability of a fair and just society, flushed with revenues derived from a long period of economic growth in the 1960s, governments allowed health care to develop without control, vision, leadership, and the political will to forge a sensible health care policy.[51]

8.3 Health Care Expenditure in the Countries of the European Union

The picture that results from the previous section, though mainly based on the developments in the United States, applies unrestrictedly to the countries of the European Union. Here too, the medical establishment was entrusted with authority. Furthermore, it should not be forgotten that, in the countries of the European Union, the period 1960–1980 was also a time of belief in the manageability of society through planning, in the idea that the trees of prosperity would grow up to heaven, and that governments were capable of looking after their citizens from the cradle to the grave. In this social climate, solidarity between the rich and the poor, the healthy and the sick, the young and the old was taken for granted. Health care policy was no exception in this respect. On the contrary, during this period, the need for universally accessible and equitable health care became self-evident. Consequently, in the 1960s, the countries of the European Union introduced or extended legalization meant to improve universal access to health care for all citizens. As a result, the percentage of the population covered by compulsory health insurance increased during the period 1960–1996 to (almost) 100% in the majority of EU countries.[52] National constitutions were also brought into line with the then-existing ideas on solidarity (see section 5.3). In terms of first chapter, also in health care matters, we also started to move to the left side of the continuum. The floodgates of health care were opened. In health care systems that were based on social security, open-ended financing became the norm, which implied that each and every new health care item, and there were many, was automatically included in the benefit package. As an example: the costs of health care in the Netherlands increased by almost 13% annually over the full decade of the 1970s.[53] Illustrative of the Dutch government's reluctance to interfere, in this respect, is the fact that even though in its 1965 annual report, the Dutch National Health Tariffs Authority was already warning the government that things would get out of hand financially, it took another 18 years before the government reacted substantially with the introduction of budgeting in 1983. In addition, EU citizens also became more health conscious and demanding, making good health an ever higher priority in their lives.[54]

The differences, however, between the United States and the countries of the European Union are threefold:

First of all, there is a difference in financial regulations. The United States seeks to finance health care mainly through the market for private health insurance. Medicare and Medicaid are instruments created to guarantee access to health care for the elderly and the poor. The market for private health insurance, together with Medicare and Medicaid, would then, indeed, create universal access for the American population, were it not for the fact that millions of Americans under the age of 65 are too well off to benefit from Medicare and Medicaid but, at the same time, too poor to buy their health insurance on the market.[55] The countries of the European Union mainly have chosen to finance health care for all citizens through either (general) taxation, or through a system of (compulsory) collective social security, with citizens, employers, and employees paying a premium and with governments' direct contributions quite limited. Within this model, variations between EU countries can be observed. Additionally, the market for private health insurance in the countries of the European Union is, in comparison with the United States, (still) rather limited. Moreover, the concept of a private health insurance market in the countries of the European Union is questionable. In the Netherlands, for example, technically about one-third of the population is privately insured. Their inclusion in groupings (civil servants, health care personnel, and so on) is so prevalent, however, that in practice, many privately insured persons participate in a specific collective.

Secondly, during the period 1960–1980, it was typical for some countries of the European Union to deal with health care through a corporatist model of providers and insurers with representatives of the government in the role of observers. In this model it was not the market, but the outcome of negotiations between health care providers and insurers (the social middle field), which was decisive for the developments in health care.

Thirdly, due to the devastations of the Second World War, Europe has lagged a bit behind the United States when it comes to health care developments.

None of these differences, however, detracts from the fact that, in the countries of the European Union, the authority of medicine also became firmly established. Consequently, in those countries, developments in health care also accelerated, which resulted in growing health care expenditure.

The acceleration of health care developments in the EU, which started around the beginning of the 1960s, was reinforced by two factors of political economy. First of all, the countries of Europe, once they had reasonably recovered from the devastation caused by the Second World War, started to benefit from a long period of economic growth, which made it possible for governments to stop their policies of scarcity. Secondly, some of these countries had government coalitions, mostly liberal-Christian-Democrats, which adhered to the principle of laissez-faire, thus leaving developments in health care to the parties concerned in a corporatist model.[56] Often, governments stood on the sidelines, letting things take their own course. Health care was even thought not to be important enough to merit a separate ministerial department but, instead, was often combined with social affairs. Austria was probably the first EU country to recognize the societal importance of health care with the establishment of its federal ministry of health in 1972.[57] These two factors combined, strong economic growth and governments standing on the sidelines, were very favorable for health care providers to make up for time lost just after the end of the war. In health care systems based on social security, policy change in this respect was often initiated by those involved in the daily health care delivery process, i.e., providers and insurers. Due to the change in government policy, they could afford to play a zero-plus game, winning a prize with every draw, and being able in every case to present a bill to another party: the providers to the insurers, the insurers to the insured, the insured to the employers, and, in the end, by raising prices, the employers to the consumers. It is no wonder that, particularly since the mid-1960s, the costs of health care have increased tremendously as a consequence of a powerful expansion of hospitals, a rapid growth of medical and technological opportunities, and a strong increase in staff numbers and wage levels. At the beginning of the 1980s, general hospital beds in the European Region of the WHO had increased by 25%, medical staff by 50%, and nursing staff by 66%.[58] Furthermore, based on the idea that a civilized society should look after its vulnerable citizens, several countries started to invest heavily in long-term health care facilities, bringing an end to campus accommodations. Consequently, as illustrated in the next table, total health care expenditure as a percentage of GDP increased dramatically.

Percentage of total expenditure on health of GDP[59]

	1960	1965	1970	1975	1980		1960	1965	1970	1975	1980
Germany	4.8	5.1	5.6	8.1	8.1	Ireland	4.0	4.4	5.6	7.7	8.7
Austria	4.4	4.7	5.3	6.4	7.0	Italy	3.9	4.6	5.5	6.7	6.8
Belgium	3.4	3.9	4.1	5.5	6.3	Luxembourg	n.a.	n.a.	4.9	5.9	6.6
Denmark	3.6	4.8	6.1	6.5	6.8	Netherlands	3.9	4.4	6.0	7.7	8.3
Spain	n.a.	2.7	4.1	5.1	5.9	United Kingdom	3.9	4.2	4.5	5.5	5.8
Finland	4.2	4.9	5.6	5.8	6.3						
France	4.3	5.3	6.1	7.6	8.5	Sweden	4.7	5.6	7.2	8.0	9.5
Greece	2.9	3.1	3.9	4.0	4.2						

Taking into account only those countries that have figures for the whole period of 1960–1980, we can see from the table that the average increase in health expenditure as a percentage of GDP was almost 80%. For Ireland, the Netherlands, and Sweden, the figure more than doubled. We should consider, however, that relating health expenditure to GDP has limited meaning.[60] After all, if GDP growth stagnates, as was the case in the 1970s, and if health expenditure is kept constant, its relative share will increase. Nevertheless, for the purposes of getting an idea of the developments, it seems appropriate to relate growth in GDP per capita to health expenditure per capita.[61] In order to do so, while acknowledging that, because of classification problems and difficulties regarding value comparisons,[62] comparing health care expenditure data between countries is "a hazardous business,"[63] I used macro-economic figures from different OECD data sources. Comparison across countries of these macro-economic figures "yields reliable results."[64] The following graph relates the weighted average of growth in health expenditure per capita for the countries of the European Union to the weighted average of growth in GDP per capita over the period 1960–1980.[65] In interpretating these developments, it should be taken into account that, particularly for the first ten years of this period, several countries had no figures available. The Netherlands, for example, did not produce a first overall insight into the costs of health expenditure until 1977. Consequently, over the first ten years of this period, the graph covers roughly 62% of the European Union's population. For the next ten years the coverage percentage is about two-thirds of that population.

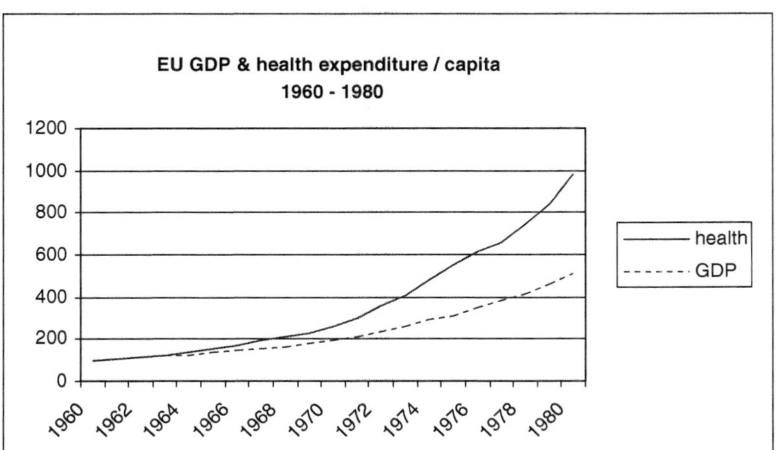

Based on different OECD health data sources.[66]

The graph shows that health expenditure per capita increased considerably more than GDP per capita, in indices from 100 in 1960 to, respectively, 985 and 512 in 1980.[67] As stated earlier, the graph presents a weighted average of the countries of the European Union. A more detailed analysis of the OECD Health Data makes it clear that: (a) In 1960, one can distinguish between "big spenders" (Germany, Sweden, the United Kingdom) and "low spenders" (Ireland), with Austria, Finland and Italy having an intermediate position. The ratio between "low spenders" and "big spenders" per capita was approximately 1:5 in 1960. (b) "Low spenders" show a considerably steeper increase in health expenditure than "big spenders" (Ireland from 100 in 1960 to 1,254 in 1980), thus changing the ratio between "low spenders" and "big spenders" to 1:2.5. (c) Countries having an intermediate position in 1960 came near to or surpassed the spending level of the "big spenders" in 1980. (d) Small countries and big countries demonstrate a comparable development pattern. (e) The United Kingdom, having the purest nationalized health system, shows a relatively moderate increase (from 100 in 1960 to 520 in 1980).

The increase in expenditure per capita, however, does not necessarily mean that EU societies became healthier during this period. Distributional aspects have to be taken into account. After all, figures on economic growth may tell us how the economy is doing overall, but not necessarily how people within that economy are doing.[68] I will come back to this subject in chapter ten. Although the increase in expenditure per capita is partly the result of making up for the arrears incurred since the end of the Second World War, other factors also came into play:

First of all, as stated earlier, the strong economic growth which started at the beginning of the 1960s made spending on health care more affordable.

Secondly, the exodus of religious congregations from the labor pool caused an upward pressure on wages, bringing them more into conformity with wider labor market salaries.

Thirdly, increasing health care opportunities made it necessary to attract additional staff.

Fourthly, health care had and still has to deal with the so-called Baumol effect.[69] The starting point for this effect is the linking of wage increases to productivity increases when negotiating new labor terms in the framework of collective bargaining agreements. In general, wage increases will be more easily agreed by employers when they do not surpass increases in productivity. In the framework of market conformity, however, agreements in important branches of industry will have a spillover effect on other branches which, by their nature, are incapable of realizing comparable productivity increases. Because it is very labor intensive, particularly in the care sectors, health care is such a relatively less productive branch. Consequently, increasing wages in health care will lead to higher prices with every new round of wage negotiations. It seems to me that differences in productivity between industrial sectors and health care are the most important reason for the

Part One
A Changing Social Context

above-average increase in the costs of health care. Furthermore, apart from measures of control and organization, it is unlikely that the health care branch can realize considerable increases in productivity because of the nature of medical service delivery. Diagnostics and therapy can only partly be standardized. Mechanization and automation can be employed far less than in other industries. This leads to the conclusion that, with ongoing productivity increases in the industrial sector and wage increases linked to those productivity increases, the discrepancy between the price level in health care and the general price level will increase. It may be concluded, therefore, that health care is caught in a "productivity trap." Market conformity in remuneration will lead to increasingly disproportionate price levels, while paying less than labor-market terms will make health care an unattractive sphere of employment, particularly in times of economic growth.

Finally, an increasing appreciation for good health may be caused by the availability of more health care opportunities.[70] If this is correct, Say's law of supply creating demand would apply, with citizens expecting that everything medically possible should be included in the coverage package. For governments in democracies, it is very difficult to ignore these expectations. In this respect, Poland is a good example of citizens wanting their government to catch up in health care after the country became democratic. Research in 1993 showed that more than 90% of the population wanted their government to improve Polish health care.[71] A corrolary is also true: Health care opportunities, once included in the coverage package, are very difficult for governments to remove. It may create uneasiness among citizens. Looking ahead to a subsequent chapter, we take note of research among the Dutch which shows that the percentage of people who are worried about their own health increased from 20% in 1958 to 46% in 1995.[72]

The period 1960–1980 was the time when countries of the European Union started to establish or extend their welfare states. In the terms of the first chapter, a period of strong economic growth, which lasted around seven years, apparently created sufficient "organizational slack" to start a trend which probably would not have developed had the economic climate been less prosperous. This trend was also inspired by the belief in the manageability of society, propagated by governments in which Social Democrats and Christian Democrats took part.

In retrospect, it is easy to argue that the creation of the welfare state was based on too optimistic a view about the possibility of planning societal developments. The medical breakthroughs of the 1960s (chapter six) could just as easily have caused political reservations about the advisability of including all the new health care opportunities in a universal coverage package. This did not happen because it was widely believed that a fair and just society could be created and managed in a way that would last.

The previous graph suggested that health care received more than its fair share of the increase in GDP during this period. Such a suggestion is considerably mitigated, however, by the next graph.

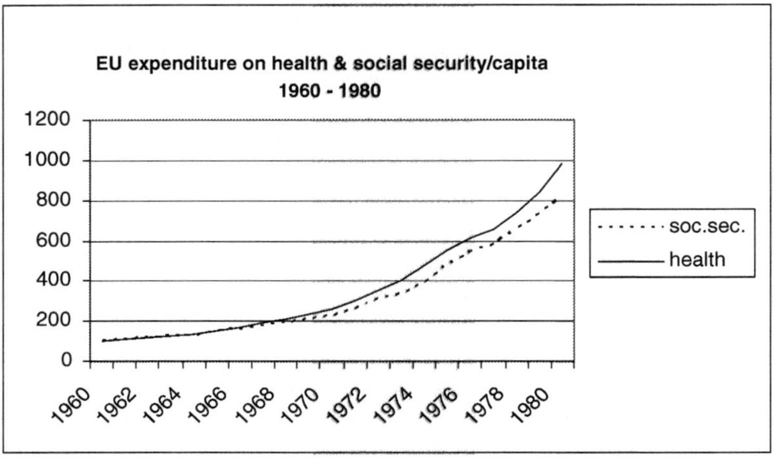

Based on different OECD health data sources.

In this graph, the growth in health care expenditure at the EU level on a per capita basis is compared with that of social security. It shows that, during the period 1960–1980, the growth in health care expenditure is not particularly unique. Social security received a comparable share of society's "organizational slack." It was only during the second half of the 1970s that health care expenditure started to expand, and then only relatively.

8.4 A Changing Tide

By the final years of the period 1960–1980, the "age of optimism" ended. Pessimism about the claims of future advances in medicine had gained a foothold within the medical establishment. The number of doctors wishing to undertake postdoctoral research decreased, because clinical science, it was believed, had been exhausted. The number of genuinely new drugs fell sharply,[73] and lawyers, on behalf of their clients, interfered increasingly with medical practice. Moreover, medical innovation in the 1980s was mainly characterized by fine-tuning, while the causes of many diseases remained unknown (multiple sclerosis, rheumatoid arthritis et cetera).[74] Finally, the new paradigms of the 1980s, i.e., the "the social theory" (epidemiology) and "the new genetics," proved "to be blind alleys, quite unable to deliver on their promises."[75]

As for social theory, McKeown's ideas, launched in the 1970s, proposed that instead of emphasizing expensive hospital-oriented medical services, money would be spent far more effectively, and health care would be considerably cheaper, if people were stimulated to change their life-styles and if pollution and poverty were reduced. The adoption of a "healthy life-style" would lower the incidence of many diseases, it was assumed. In fact, promoting a healthy life-style, very much to the pleasure of governments, became a new religion, which linked the use of "alcohol with breast cancer, coffee with cancer of the pancreas, yoghurt with cancer of the ovary, vaginal douching with cancer of the cervix, regular use of alcohol mouthwash with cancer of the mouth and red meat with cancer of the colon."[76] According to this hype of "healthism," even electricity pylons and sewing machines, and more recently mobile phones, were assumed to be a health threat. As it turns out, many of these claims were unfounded. For example, it was assumed that a healthy life-style would lower the incidence of heart disease. Research conducted in 1997 among 125,000 participants, however, showed that adopting a healthy life-style (stop smoking, start exercising, lower your cholesterol level) "had no effect on stopping them from dying from heart disease."[77]

Cholesterol-lowering drugs became very profitable for the pharmaceutical industry. By the mid-1990s, people spent over £3 billion a year because of their cholesterol obsession.[78] In short, by the mid-1990s many human pleasures (sex, tobacco, alcohol, smoking, various foods, et cetera) had come to be perceived as a threat to health. Le Fanu's verdict on this development is that the McKeown's social theory (see p. 376) "is in error in its entirety," not fulfilling its promise of preventing thousands of deaths each year, because it ignores "the inescapable laws of biology."[79]

Regarding genetics, Le Fanu observes a hiatus between anticipated benefits and reality. Nevertheless, the value of shares in companies engaged in genetic engineering initially shot up on the stock exchange market. So far, however, genetic engineering appears to be an expensive method for producing drugs that either existed already or are of only marginal therapeutic benefit. Since 1995, only a few biotechnology drugs represent significant therapeutic advances, for example, a vaccine against hepatitis B and erythropoietin (EPO), which stimulates the production of red blood cells. The working of genes is not yet sufficiently understood to expect biogenetics to create a breakthrough in medicine.[80]

Because of this, according to Le Fanu, modern medicine, though very successful in the 1960s and 1970s, is approaching its high-water mark. First of all, this is because most things that are medically possible were done during the period 1960–1980. Secondly, research on several age-determined diseases has not produced impressive further medical progress. Thirdly, the rate of medical innovations is declining, with chemists finding that "they are scraping the bottom of the barrel of chemical compounds that can be synthesised and screened for their therapeutic potential."[81] Finally, though medical research is defined as "the art of the soluble," it is not clear at all whether diseases like multiple sclerosis or leukaemia are curable.[82]

Altogether, modern medicine, despite its successes in the recent past, is trapped in a fourfold paradox,[83] according to Le Fanu. To underline his point, Le Fanu, first of all, points to the fact that the number of doctors regretting their decision to enter medicine has increased from 15% in 1966 to 50% in 1988. Secondly, despite the progress made in medicine, the percentage of people who are worrying about their health has increased considerably. Thirdly, there is the imbalance between, on the one hand, an enormous cost explosion over the past decades, and, on the other hand, a relatively small gain in the health of the population. Finally, an increasing number of people are turning away from modern medicine, seeking alternative treatment instead. Worldwide, alternative medicine accounts for over $60 billion a year in health care expenditures. About half of the American population are investigating alternative treatment opportunities. In Italy, the number of people using alternative medicine doubled between 1991 and 1999[84]; in a Swedish study among primary care patients in 1998, 15% of respondents regularly sought alternative medicine[85]; in Great Britain, there are more alternative medical practitioners than regular general physicians[86]; and a German survey of 1997 showed that 84% of respondents would like to see an extension of natural methods in medicine.[87] Meanwhile, we see that conventional American medical schools, (such as Harvard and Columbia) stimulated by a worldwide WHO campaign, are integrating alternative medicine into their curriculum.[88] In 1992 the United States established a National Center for Complementary Alternative Medicine with a budget of $2 million. Around the turn of the century, this center's budget had increased to $90 million.[89]

In summary, Le Fanu's view on the future of medicine is not too optimistic, to say the least. It may be reassuring, however, to remember that nobody knows the future. There may very well come a time when we do know the working of genes and are able to use this knowledge to our benefit.

Another point of criticism is the accusation that modern medicine has been overdoing things. In 1974, the American scholar Illich had already accused the medical world of not allowing people to arrange their lives independently.[90] He introduced the term *iatrogeneses*,[91] referring to the medicalization of society, and differentiated this concept into (a) clinical iatrogeneses, (b) social iatrogeneses, and (c) structural iatrogeneses. As for clinical iatrogeneses, he claims, for example, that health care expenditures for many diagnoses and treatments do not deliver results, or only do so insufficiently. Social iatrogeneses refers to a number of phenomena which result from social over-medicalization and reduce people's capabilities to cope with the ailments of life. Structural iatrogeneses, finally, has to do with the medical establishment's using a technical model which inevitably results in manipulated maintenance of life, rather than providing healthy answers to human suffering. According to the author, the only reasonable answer to this threefold iatrogeneses is a political program directed at limiting the influence of the medical establishment and at the same time supporting people in regaining their ability to looking after their own health as much as possible.[92]

Illich schocked the medical establishment with his ideas and traveled the world for a while. In retrospect, we have to note that his views hardly changed anything. That does not mean, however, that Illich was talking nonsense, since we now know that the damage to people's health caused by iatrogeneses has become a major health care problem. In the United States, almost 100,000 patients die annually as a consequence of this "disease." Estimations for the Netherlands, in this respect, vary from 4,700 to 9,700 per year.[93]

Specifically focusing on psychiatry, in 1971 the Dutch psychiatrist Foudraine launched his attack on the psychiatric medical establishment, arguing that psychiatry was trapped in the classification of mental deviations, labeling them wrongly as diagnoses.[94] Within five years, Foudraine's explosive analysis had been reprinted in 28 editions in the Dutch language and had been translated into several foreign languages. The psychiatric establishment, however, felt offended, and in no time labeled Foudraine as a revolutionary, a psychopath, and a charlatan.[95] Disappointed with these reactions, Foudraine sought refuge with Bhagwan Shree Rajneesh, and in psychiatry things went back to "normal" again.

Then there are Malleson and Taylor. Malleson introduced the term *sickness industry* in 1973, exposing the weaknesses of the medical profession and the ineffectiveness of many medicines created by the pharmaceutical industry,[96] while Taylor criticized the "medical-technological complex."[97] The American sociologist Fox warned against the medicalization of social problems,[98] a tendency that was supported by the WHO definition of health as an optimal combination of physical, mental, social, and environmental factors.

Finally, the WHO joined the ranks of critics in 1983, arguing that health policies since the Second World War had set a dangerous course. Instead of promoting healthy life-styles, preventing disease, and investing in community care, the bulk of health budgets has been used for the establishment of "disease palaces," a policy which was strongly supported by the public, encouraged by doctors, and led by politicians. This occurred without an effective structure for health planning or an adequate system for the assessment of the real value of new developments.[99]

So there is a body of literature in which authors have tried to critique the influence of the medical establishment on society. The effects have been limited, however. This is understandable, because the period 1960–1980 was a time for celebrating health care and those who could deliver it. The public became ever more impressed by medical opportunities, thus making itself "a prisoner of the medical profession."[100] During these developments, governments in many countries stood on the sidelines for a long time.

Slowly, however, the idea that medical care is only one of the factors which contribute to people's health began to spread more widely during the 1970s. As a consequence, the "Great Equation: Medical Care = Health" came under attack, and it became clear that the economic law of diminishing returns also applies for health care.[101] People became increasingly critical of their doctors' capacities, which resulted in an increasing demand for a "second opinion," and governments expressed their criticism by demanding transparency, accountability, and "value for money." Slowly, the profession's privileged position started to lapse and people started to realize that it could even be taken away.[102] The era of celebrating the medical profession faded away, and the image of doctors was adjusted to reflect reality.

That image was even further compromised in the 1990s, when it was revealed that a considerable part of the (American) medical establishment (doctors, hospitals, laboratories, medical schools) was guilty of fraud (billing for services not rendered, falsifying diagnoses, generating fictitious billings, fabricating medical episodes, reclassifying patients into more profitable DRG categories,[103] et cetera). These criminal practices are estimated to amount to between $100 billion and $500 billion a year.[104] Fraud, however, is not exclusive to health care[105]; nor is it an exclusively American phenomenon. In Italy, for example, a group of general practitioners were suspended in 1998 for bribery, which involved referring patients to a private center for radiological examinations.[106] In the United Kingdom, estimates of £115 million yearly are given for prescription fraud.[107] And, of course, health care experiences "normal" fraud, like pilfering, medical consultants using payroll time for their private practice, bribery by construction companies, et cetera.[108]

It is no wonder, then, that governments and insurers have implemented policies to counter health-care-related fraud. At the end of the 20th century, the British established the NHS Counter Fraud Service. In the United Kingdom patients, pharmacists, dentists, opticians, doctors, and hospital consultants, as well as health care staff, all engage in fraudulent practices, together stealing £150 million from the health services each year. The newly established fraud service aims to reduce this fraud to an absolute minimum in ten years. As in the United States, professional counter-fraud officers have been appointed to achieve this objective.[109] Since 1999, in the Netherlands, countering fraud has become a cooperative effort between health insurers, which established a fraud protocol in 1998.[110] Still, research conducted in 2003 delivered proof of fraud totalling over €5,000,000.[111] Luxembourg has set up a Surveillance Committee to counter "unjustified deviation" from the fee schedule for medical interventions. Two administrative bodies can even suspend providers from the health insurance system for a certain period of time or fine those who break the rules.[112] Meanwhile, initiatives have been taken to reach a European policy on fraud control. This has already resulted in the drawing up of "The European Healthcare Fraud and Corruption Declaration" in 2004, which, among other things, calls for the creation of a European Healthcare Fraud and Corruption Office, a not-for-profit center for counter-fraud and corruption work.[113]

8.5 Summary

Shortly after the Second World War, the medical scene started to change fundamentally. Due to some important medical breakthroughs in pharmacology and technology, health care opportunities increased enormously. A relatively long period of prosperity which started around the beginning of the 1960s, made it possible to provide the financial means necessary to include the new treatment methods in legally defined benefit packages. All the more so because the 1960s and part of the 1970s was a time when society was believed to be manageable. Health care received its reasonable share of public finances during these prosperous times, and the medical establishment was invested with considerable authority. As a consequence of these favorable times, health care expenditures in the countries of the European Union as a percentage of GDP increased, on average, by almost 80% during the period 1960–1980. The tide started to change at the end of the 1970s. Critics warned that medicine had been overdoing things, that it was out of control, and that the economic law of diminishing returns also applied to health care. Later on, medicine's image was further damaged when the fraudulent behavior of doctors, hospitals, and laboratories, in the United States as well as in countries of the European Union, was exposed.

9
Health Care Reforms

The changes that have occurred, and still are occurring, in EU health care systems since the beginning of the 1980s may lead one to conclude without exaggeration that health care—whether examined from the delivery, the financial, or the organizational perspective—finds itself in turbulent times. If one analyzed developments since 1980 in detail, one could easily come up with several hundred reforms. And if one were to include the different ways EU governments are pursuing current reform objectives, the list would be extended considerably. Analyzing health care reforms this way, however, would lead to an unreadably dense and very topical inventory of facts, an inventory which, for that matter, would be outdated immediately after completion.

However, the objectives of all health care reforms[1] can be summarized under two main headings: (1) improving the quality of care and (2) cost containment. Nevertheless, the daily reality of health care reforms is more complicated than this simple summary suggests, since interested parties in the health care process may look at these two categories from different or even opposing perspectives. Quality of care, for example, can be observed from the patients' perspective (what do we want?) or from the providers' perspective (how can we perform better?). In addition, quality of care and cost containment may easily be conflicting objectives. A government which, as a means of containing costs, allows waiting lists to develop, may have to accept the resulting negative effects on quality of care which, in turn, will raise opposition from consumers. The medical professional who is tied to prescription guidelines (which governments believe to contribute to cost containment) may believe that this hinders his intention to offer the highest quality of care possible. Furthermore, a government which introduces prescription charges for pharmaceuticals may believe this will contribute to cost containment; the patient may see it as a financial transfer which negatively influences quality of care as well as equal access (which is also a government objective). Finally, a government which chooses to decentralize its health care system, making it possible for local governments and citizens to influence health care policy development, in the belief that this will improve quality, may find that such decentralization has a negative impact on the objective of cost containment.

Furthermore, analysis of health care reform measures indicates that they often overlap. Prescription guidelines, for example, may be directed at cost containment and, at the same time, may also be directed at improving prescription practices. Similarly, regulations directed at empowering patients may at the same time influence quality of care.

Consequently, any classification of reform measures will always have a degree of arbitrariness introduced by the classifier. My arbitrary classification of the health care reforms introduced since the beginning of the 1980s is constructed around four themes.[2] The objective of this classification is to describe the developments in health care against the background of the basic values of solidarity and equal access.

I start with health care reforms that can be perceived as a continuation of the developments which started in the previous period (1960–1980). In chapter eight, I described the changes in the health care world during this time as a transformation from a closed system to an open one. With this openness have come external demands for improved performance. Health care professionals and health care institutions, as well as health care insurers, have had to learn to accept that the external environment is increasingly minding their business. The generic term for this development is *accountability*.

The second theme is organizational reform. Such reforms may relate to the system, the structure, or the process of health care delivery. Some of the changes in this area are induced by the immanent dynamics of health care (chapter six); others are a consequence of changing health policy.

The third theme comprises rationing and priority-setting. Both terms refer to cost-containment concepts. How priorities are set and how health care is rationed will be clarified by examining some of the ways governments try to convey to their citizens that the provision of health care goods and services is (also) subject to the problem of scarcity.

The final theme is cost containment, which can be approached in several ways. Cost-containment measures can be directed at a reduction of services and the introduction of cost-sharing. Such measures can also be aimed at reducing the income of providers and the profits of the pharmaceutical industry or increasing the efficiency and effectiveness of health care delivery. Furthermore, the implementation of prevention programs, as well as cost-shifting from public budgets and taxes to health insurance programs, can also be seen as cost-containment measures.[3] Describing all these types of cost containment would go beyond the scope of this book. Therefore, I will limit the discussion to a description of some cost-containment activities which are directed at influencing the costs of health care in directly financial terms.

Going into the four themes in extensive detail would make this book unreadable. However, given the objective of this chapter, it is not necessary to deal with each and every single health care reform item of each and every single EU country. It is sufficient to sketch what is going on in the countries of the European Union by examining a cross section of items which together may give an impression whether, regarding health care, EU countries are moving to the right side of the continuum, i.e., the toward market.

9.1 Accountability

Accountability means that one can be called to account by others, from which it follows that one has to accept responsibility for one's decisions and actions towards others.[4] Accountability may apply to all aspects of performance. Submitting oneself to appropriate external scrutiny has long been the norm in the business world; this is now also true in the world of health care providers, at both the individual and institutional level. Where accountability in business life is mainly an issue in the relation to the shareholders, in health care, those responsible for the daily operations have to deal with a range of stakeholders, notably the government, patients, and insurers. These stakeholders have an obvious interest in what is going on in health care. They want to be informed, they want to receive value for their money, they want to be able to influence policy, and they want health care delivery to be of high quality, evidence based, and cost effective. In short, the term *accountability* refers to a transparent process of health care provision, with everybody knowing where he or she stands, and with a clear description of rights and duties. In business, the architecture for this interpretation of the term accountability is called corporate governance,[5] which refers to the organizational framework which has been set up to ensure that companies are managed in the interests of their owners.[6] Comparably, in health care, we speak of health care governance, which is an umbrella term for a whole range of activities undertaken in the interests of stakeholders. It presupposes some form of external scrutiny, for example, through reporting, auditing, inspection, performance monitoring, or external inquiry.[7]

In summary, through health care governance, the health care world has become the focus of society at large, with different stakeholders involved in its daily operations. This new trend in the external environment can be found in many governments' reports in the countries of the European Union. A well-known example, in this respect, is Tony Blair's first White Paper of December 1997.[8] It stipulated that NHS Trusts would be required to embrace health care governance fully, including responsibility for quality of care, rigorous scrutiny of costs and performance, human resources development, staff involvement in management matters, board meetings in public, et cetera. And to emphasize that the British government of 1997 was serious about this change of policy, the White Paper also stated that, "when performance is not up to scratch in NHS Trusts there will be rapid investigation and, where necessary, intervention," with the ultimate threat of the removal of the NHS Trust Board.[9]

That health care has entered the era of accountability can be illustrated with several examples. Changing responsibilities of hospital boards, performance measurement, benchmarking, community involvement, methods of cost-effectiveness improvement, et cetera, can all be seen as aspects of accountability. I have chosen to elaborate two aspects: quality improvement and empowerment of patients. The first because it has changed the established health care world into one of continuous learning; the second, because it has enabled consumers to play a groundbreaking role in the health care process.

9.1.1 Improving Quality

The peculiar thing about quality in health care is that it was hardly an issue until around the beginning of the 1980s. Apparently, quality was taken for granted during the first three-quarters of the 20th century. But if we consider what has happened since the 1980s, it seems as if there is an assumed negative correlation between the focus on quality of care and the financial constraints imposed on health care providers. Suspicious people may conclude, therefore, that governments fear that financial constraints may endanger the quality of care that people have gotten used to. Perhaps that is why, since the 1980s, that quality has become an item of regulation and management in all countries of the European Union.

The problem with quality, however, is that it is a "container" concept. That is to say, it is like a container which is loaded with a huge range of instruments which, separately or in combination, are directed at improving the quality of health care. The use of these instruments may focus on the structure or the organization of the health care system; it may be directed at input aspects like the training of professionals or the way they organize their work; it may be aimed at improving aspects of health care management; or it may be concentrated on patients' satisfaction. The container concept, therefore, includes items like practice guidelines, evidence-based medicine, peer reviews, cooperation between professionals, certification and recertification of physicians, outcome measurement, patients' safety, medical malpractice, public disclosure of performance data, purchasing policy, workers participation, accreditation of hospitals, benchmarks, best practice, and so on.

Improvements regarding all these separate aspects may certainly contribute to improving the quality of health care delivery, provided that one takes an integrative view, i.e., the aim should be total quality control, which "makes quality a responsibility to be shared by all the people in an organization." Thus, hospitals which, for example, have set up a quality-control department, may miss the boat if they forget to communicate quality improvement objectives to all the different disciplines working in the organization.[10] Governments imposing quality legislation may expect a higher "return on investment" if that legislation has been drawn up in close consultation with those who have to implement the new rules.

In the framework of this book, it is not necessary to deal separately with each and every single quality item one can think of for each EU country. An overview which gives a random but representative cross section of the developments is sufficient to illustrate that improving the quality of care has become part of the turbulent times which started in the 1980s.

Around the start of the 1990s, many EU countries introduced legislation, established specific institutions, or decided on regulations focusing on the quality aspects of health care.

Sweden introduced such regulations in 1994 through its National Board of Health and Welfare, followed by legal arrangements in 1997 which demanded that quality in health care "systematically and continuously be developed and assured."[11] In the framework of this legislation, health care workers became obliged to integrate quality assurance activities continuously and methodologically into their daily routines. Since then, health care quality monitoring has been broadened in its scope to include not only the technicalities of the health care process, but also the totality of health services provided to patients, their relatives, and the public at large. Furthermore, national quality registers were developed through cooperation among the Federation of County Councils, the National Board of Health and Welfare, and the Swedish Society of Medicine, which were meant to support local initiatives regarding quality improvement in clinical departments. In 2001, forty such registers were operational across the country, each of which is national in scope. Furthermore, several county councils have set up quality committees to support hospitals and health centers in the development of quality assurance systems.

Austria established a legal framework for the implementation of a nationwide quality assurance program for hospitals in 1993. It forced hospital owners and managers to implement quality assurance through the setting-up of quality commissions charged with initiating, coordinating, and supporting measures of internal quality assurance.[12] The Austrians, therefore, considered quality assurance to be primarily a task of the hospitals themselves, whereas the federal government, together with the Structural Commission and the Länder, were necessary to create the requisite external conditions. After this legislation was enacted, eleven Austrian hospitals started a pilot project in 1997 directed at intensifying the focus on patients and staff and improving health status and the use of resources by identifying and comparing both processes and outcomes. The project involved the commitment of 230 employees and the participation of 62 departments, plus around 3,000 people through indirect channels.[13]

Through ANAES (Agence Nationale d'Accreditation et d' Evaluation en Santé), France set up procedures for quality control in 1996, including the (compulsory) accreditation of public or private hospitals and the (voluntary) audit of self-employed professionals. ANAES also prepares practice guidelines for the entire medical profession.[14] In 1996, thirty recommendations were published regarding clinical practice, relating to diagnoses, treatment, and supervision of certain conditions. Furthermore, ANAES published 200 recommendations for general practitioners in 1998, together with 250 for medical specialists. Another mechanism for quality improvement is continuous education, which has been compulsory since 1996 and is paid for by the health insurance funds. The relationship between professionals and health insurance funds was renewed under a 2002 law directed at agreement regarding different types of good practice. Meanwhile, the 1996 Ordinances made it compulsory for health care institutions to be accredited in order to be able to continue to provide treatment. As part of this process, hospitals are evaluated on dimensions like quality of care, information given to the patient, medical records, general management, risk prevention, et cetera.

In 1979, the Dutch Association of Medical Specialists and the Dutch Association of Medical Directors of Hospitals established the Institute for Health Care Improvement. This independent institute is very active in the field of quality assurance for medical specialists, nurses, allied health professionals, and health care institutions.[15] The Netherlands passed a law on quality for health care institutions in 1996. Apparently, this law was unsatisfactory, because in 2002, the Minister of Health wrote a letter to the Dutch parliament proclaiming that health care institutions should take rigorous action to implement a structured, programmed quality system in order systematically to measure, improve, redesign, and control quality of patient care. In 2003, the Minister of Health published a catalogue of kick-off measures to be introduced in 2004: (1) benchmarking in primary care for all general practitioners and ten pilot hospitals; (2) the introduction of indicators for safer and better care; and (3) a program on quality, innovation, and efficiency with priority on patient safety and patient-centered delivery of care. All of these measures were to be under the supervision of the Inspectorate of Health Care.[16]

Finally, as part of the Health System Modernization Act of 2003, the government of Germany submitted a draft bill calling for the establishment of an independent institution in order to improve patient information, develop standard treatment for major diseases, and perform cost-efficiency analyses for prescription drugs. Moreover, the proposed institution would (1) produce scientific papers and recommendations related to the quality of reimbursable services; (2) issue recommendations regarding reference prices for prescription drugs; (3) issue recommendations for certification of providers; and (4) issue recommendations for the development of disease management programs for chronic diseases.[17]

As a result of all these quality initiatives, health care providers have to meet an increasing number of quality standards which are sometimes rather narrowly defined. In reaction to that, many health care institutions have set up quality departments which are staffed with salaried quality specialists. Although this has mostly happened without additional funding, these institutions have to live up to the new quality demands if they want to qualify for two of the health care requirements of the 1990s: accreditation and certification. In order to meet the required criteria, they may, as is the case in the Netherlands (based on the Individual Health Care Professions Act of 1993), even have to record the qualifications of each individual professional in a register, which has to be kept up to date.

These examples serve to illustrate developments in accountability in health care since the 1980s, as far as quality of care is concerned. They do not represent the complete picture, since in each of the countries mentioned more activities directed at improving quality of care have been undertaken. The reader can be assured that comparable initiatives have been taken in the other countries of the European Union.

9.1.2 Empowering Patients

The most important health care buzzword since the 1980s has been "patients." Their position in the health care delivery process has been reinforced considerably. This is a consequence not only of their increasing awareness, aided by access to the internet, but even more so the result of the legalization of their rights. Most EU governments have enacted laws which have transformed the patients' position in the health care process from one of object into subject. Patients have become "clients." Because of this, phenomena like second opinions and informed consent have become more widely recognized. Furthermore, patients have strengthened their position in society. The power of patients as pressure groups, enjoying political support, is an important phenomenon in EU democracies. Regularly measuring patients' satisfaction with their health care system is one of the consequences of this development.[18] As in the previous subsection, the changing role of patients in health care will be illustrated with a number of examples from different EU countries.

In an attempt to be more specific on this topic, the British government listed a range of patients' rights and health care standards the NHS was expected to meet in its Patients' Charter of 1991. As for rights, among other things, the Charter provided that patients have the right to (1) receive health care on the basis of clinical need, regardless of ability to pay; (2) be given a clear explanation of any treatment proposed, including possible risks and alternatives, before a decision regarding treatment is taken; (3) access their health records and be guaranteed that health care staff will deal with these records confidentially; and (4) choose whether to take part in the medical research and training programs of medical students. Among the standards which the NHS is expected to meet, first of all, is respect for the privacy of patients, their dignity, and their religious and cultural beliefs. In addition to this, we find a number of instructions related to the organization of the health care process (the ambulance has to arrive within 14 minutes in urban areas; a specific appointment time in an outpatient clinic should be met within 30 minutes; before discharge from the hospital, arrangements, if necessary, have to be made for follow-up care; et cetera). A review of the Charter, emphasizing the importance of local instead of national charters, was published in 1998.[19]

Ten years later, in 2001, Austria also considered the idea of a Patients' Charter, to be drawn up under Article 15a of the Austrian Constitution. Its content would be very similar to the British Charter, except for two additional aspects: (1) representation of patients' interests and (2) enforcement of claims for loss or damage. In addition to this, the Austrians introduced the idea of a patients' ombudsman to investigate complaints.[20]

In 1992, Denmark passed a law obliging doctors to inform patients of their condition and treatment options. Since that date, doctors must have a patient's permission before they can start or continue treatment. In 1998, further legal rights were introduced, focusing on issues like access to information, sharing a patient's medical information by doctors with third parties, and the patient's right to decide on treatment options.[21]

Finland introduced legislation on patients' rights in 1993 which provided for their rights to information, informed consent to treatment, access to any relevant documents, and protection of their autonomy. Furthermore, as in Austria, a patients' ombudsman was introduced by this law. A review regarding the functioning of the law in 1996 revealed that patients' active participation and access to information needed to be improved, and the idea of an ombudsman was amended so that a patients' ombudsman had to be introduced in each health care organization.[22]

After years of parliamentary discussions, Belgium accepted a law on patients' rights in 2002. Here, too, an ombudsman was introduced.

A variant of the patients' ombudsman can be found in Portugal, where every public medical institution has a so-called Users' Office where patients can complain about any aspect of the national health service. Alternately, patients can be referred to the Medical Association or they may choose to go to court directly. The majority of complaints appears to be related to organizational issues such as waiting times or service amenities. Meanwhile, under the coordination of the Ministry of Health, a National Observatory of Users' Offices was established in 2000 to support the Health Administration.[23]

Apart from several legal arrangements which are comparable to those in other EU countries (the Health Care Complaints Act 1994, the Medical Treatment Agreement Act 1995), the Netherlands has a special position regarding patients' rights. First of all, patients' organizations are represented in national platforms and institutions which deliver recommendations to the government regarding the development of health care policy. Secondly, and in particular, patients or clients have a say in the management of individual health care institutions. The latter is based on a 1996 law on client participation in health care institutions, which gives clients' representative platforms a say in decision-making at the institutional level. Based on this law, the institutions' management must consult clients' representatives in matters like the appointment of management staff, investment intentions, determining the yearly budget, et cetera.

All in all, the change of health care from a closed system into an open one has created a situation where health care providers are increasingly accountable to patients. This has been manifested in a changing involvement of patients in the health care delivery process. Patients have become subjects to which medical professionals and institutions must respond in terms of both behavior and quality. They increasingly hold the medical world responsible for their comings and goings, and they may successfully sue health care providers in cases of malpractice. American physicians paid $9 billion for malpractice insurance premiums in 1991; fees for lawyers alone accounted for 40% of total malpractice costs in that year.[24] In short, patients want to be taken seriously and they want to be dealt with on equal terms. They may also take legal action if timely treatment is denied or if the quality of delivered care is below reasonable standards, the Dutch sickness funds being a recent case in point.[25] Undoubtedly, the fact that, on average, patients are more educated and informed these days plays an important role. However, it also seems that the spirit of the current time contributes to the changing climate. This climate has taken down the medical establishment from its pedestal. Phenomena like second opinions and the increasing number of lawsuits regarding medical malpractice also suggest that people are getting used to seeing medicine as just another field of professional activity in which making mistakes is just as normal as in any other occupational activity.

Furthermore, the end of this growing influence of patients on the health care process is not yet in sight. The future will increasingly be determined by patients in two ways: Firstly, European governments increasingly want their health care system to be demand-driven. The Dutch government, for example, has formulated this health care policy explicitly. As a consequence, individualized budgets for long-term care, which make it possible for patients to select their own providers, is an increasingly popular phenomenon in the Netherlands. Secondly, with the help of the internet, patients will be ever better informed. They may even go to see their doctor with a computer printout which, in their view, could be relevant to diagnosing what could be wrong.[26] Furthermore, since 1990, in the United States there has been a National Practitioner Data Bank where patients can find individualized performance information of medical specialists.[27] The state of Massachusetts even passed a law in 1996 to make it possible for the public at large to ask for the number of mistakes that individual doctors have made. In addition to this, through the internet, the outcomes of accreditation procedures may be placed in the public domain.[28] Consequently, the internet may function as an electronic pillory, so to speak.[29] At any rate, health care providers will be forced to adapt to the development of the internet; and governments, like most Swedish county councils, will support them.[30] The International Data Corporation predicted a few years ago that the internet market would grow 60% annually, increasing to $78 billion in 2003. For health care, this growth was estimated to be 58% worldwide. Illustrating the speed of the developments in this respect is a German online survey of 2000, which showed that 38% of respondents used health information on the internet at least once a month.[31] One may safely assume that health care consumers will increasingly surf the internet, searching for information on the more than 20,000 medical and health-related websites that existed at the turn of the millennium.[32]

Finally, patients find growing mutual support through the phenomenon of self-help groups. Germany has over 70,000 such groups already, a large number of which are active in health matters. In accordance with the German social security law, health insurance agencies have to support these groups financially.[33] Austria has some 600 self-help groups which offer assistance for specific health problems.[34] Recently, Spain has also experienced the emergence of self-help groups.[35]

9.2 Organizational Reforms

Organizational reforms in health care systems in EU countries are many. They may be a natural consequence of the health care dynamics (chapter six), or they may follow from deliberate changes in (political) views on how health policy and health care delivery should be designed. They may be initiated by health care professionals or institutions, or they may be demanded by insurers or patients. They may, furthermore, be motivated by arguments like cost-containment, effectiveness, efficiency, quality improvement, workload, task performance, et cetera.

A government, as in the United Kingdom, may choose to reform a centrally controlled health care system into one that involves regional or local-level layers directing the system's operating and health policy development, or, as in the Netherlands, a government, may reform its health care system by transforming health care insurers into the directors of the health care delivery process, believing that this is a suitable method of deregulation. Scientific and technological developments may make it possible to increase treatment in outpatient clinics, thus making health care delivery less dependent on the availability of hospital wards. If we believe that continuity of care contributes to quality, different health care providers and institutions may seek closer cooperation through merging, thus aiming at some form of integrated or seamless care. If developments in pharmacology make it possible to discharge psychiatric patients from large mental hospitals, the reform alternative can be accommodation in sheltered homes. If waiting lists for hospital admission become too long, patients who can afford to do so may choose to opt out, turning to the private health care circuit and taking out supplementary insurance. Furthermore, governments may pursue policies of privatization, in the belief that this contributes to efficiency and effectiveness, as well as to a reduction of bureaucracy. Finally, governments, as well as health care providers, may believe that the market principle is an alternative for collective financing, and thus introduce co-payments, cost-sharing, or reductions in the coverage package.

One way or another, all these reforms may have organizational consequences for a health care system's design, as well as for its management. In the present discussion, I limit myself to elaborating three examples of organizational reforms: decentralization, the phenomenon of internal markets, and several forms of private initiatives.

9.2.1 Decentralization

Governments of the European Union regard decentralization to be "an effective means to improve service delivery, to better allocate resources according to need, to involve the community in health decision-making and to reduce inequalities in health."[36] As argued in section 6.3, geographical circumstances may provide an argument for a decentralized health care system, as is the case in the Scandinavian countries of the European Union.

Denmark, for example, has had such a system since the beginning of the 18th century, with municipalities and counties playing an important role in the financing and delivery of health services. However, with the 1970 reforms of the country's administrative structure, which reduced the number of counties from 24 to 12 and the number of municipalities from over 1,300 to 275, both centralization and decentralization were achieved, with state tasks delegated to counties and responsibility for hospitals reassigned from municipalities to counties. On the other hand, and more recently, Danish municipalities have had to pay counties for each day any patient stays longer than is necessary in a hospital while waiting for a place in an old people's home. This has forced municipalities to do something about the problem.[37] In order to achieve better coordination between somatic and psychiatric facilities through the establishment of smaller units in the community, psychiatric care and care for disabled people was decentralized from local boards to the counties in 1976. According to the European Observatory on Health Care Systems, a serious consequence of decentralization in Denmark is unequal access to health care in different counties. Apparently, Danish politicians consider self-governance to be more important than geographical equity.[38]

In Sweden, responsibility for health care has also been decentralized to local governments for a long time, except for national policy development, legislation, and supervision. Responsibility for care of the elderly and the disabled, as well as long-term psychiatric care, however, are affairs for the municipalities. Here too, municipalities have to pay for "bed-blockers," i.e., patients whose medical treatment has been completed but for whom no municipal or institutional care is available.[39] Since the 1970s, financial responsibility has been further decentralized within each county. The degree to which this has been done, as well as how it is organized and managed within counties, varies considerably. However, since the end of the 1970s, cost containment has become an important issue for all counties.[40]

In Finland, municipalities are responsible for health care arrangements, although the relevant regulations are scanty. There appear to be significant variations between municipalities in both clinical practice and in the delivery of services. According to a 2000 review, this was also the case for per-capita expenditure on health.[41]

As discussed, the Scandinavian EU members have a long history of decentralization. Other EU countries started this process more recently.

Portugal, for example, coming from a national approach, established a decentralized system of five regions in 1993. Delegating responsibility to the regions was limited, however, to autonomy over budget setting and primary care. Hospitals are still a national affair, as is planning. An attempt to decentralize further within the regions was initiated in 1997 with the establishment of regional contracting agencies, making these agencies responsible for resource allocation through the implementation of contracting with hospitals and health centers. As for hospitals, decentralization was directed at allowing lower-level managers to exert greater power to deploy resources through the creation of Responsibility Centers in 1999.[42]

In Spain, the decentralization process started with the creation of 17 autonomous regions. This process, through which these regions received considerable public management power, including authority over health care, was completed in 2003. The autonomous regions bear responsibility for health care financing, organization, provision, and management.[43] Responsibility for planning and regulation, however, is a matter of co-responsibility between the center and local governments. Furthermore, since the Spanish health care system is financed out of general taxation—most taxes are centrally raised and regions have limited fiscal autonomy—the power of the center over developments in health care remains very strong.[44] In contrast, through this decentralization process, the role of Spanish local governments in the health care process has, as in Denmark, decreased.[45]

The reforms made in the United Kingdom in 1991 were, firstly, directed at increasing efficiency, quality, and patients' choice through the establishment of market-type mechanisms, which represented a shift away from hierarchical, or vertically integrated, forms of organization toward models which are based on a separation between providers and purchasers of health care through contractual relationships. Secondly, the reforms were meant to change the highly centralized health care system, which dictated an identical structure and function for all the organizations that make up the NHS, into a more organic one which enables the adaptation of structure and processes to local and individual needs.[46] Related to this was an intended devolution of decision-making as a response to the prevailing "regulatory and administrative bulimia."[47] Nevertheless, providers and purchasers remained accountable to the regional offices of the NHS Executive. In addition, the NHS Executive exerted strong control over the district health authorities and hospital trusts in matters of planning and service priorities.[48] Overall, British deregulation, which involved removing whole layers of regulation to make it possible for organizations to innovate and compete, has, so far, been more rhetoric than reality, according to Walshe.[49] Nevertheless, the British intend to decentralize further in the coming five years by converting NHS Trusts into Foundation Trusts, thus giving them more freedom. Performance monitoring remains a national task conducted through the Healthcare Commission, however.[50]

Drawing partly on the British experience, Italy started a process of devolving formal power and authority to regions in 1992. This gave regional health departments more autonomy in policy-making, health care administration and management, resource allocation, and control. Based on legislation enacted during the period 1997–2000, devolution of power to the regions was extended, including fiscal federalism which transferred the funding of the Italian national health service from the central to the regional level, thus strengthening the fiscal autonomy of the regional health departments. Furthermore, during the 1990s, a process of delegation was carried through, transforming local health units and tertiary hospitals into autonomous bodies with greater financial and decision-making autonomy, thus creating a UK-like internal market.

A peculiar feature of decentralization in Germany is the delegation of power to corporatist actors. Here, there is no devolution of power from the federal government to the so-called Länder, since the latter already existed before the federal republic was established. An opposite devolution is taking place, requiring the Länder to pass certain rights and responsibilities to the federal government.[51]

9.2.2 Internal Markets

As was argued in chapter five, combining solidarity with market principles is difficult to accomplish. Some EU governments, therefore, have settled for second-best options, labeling them internal markets or quasi-markets.

A well-known example, in this respect, is the United Kingdom where, based on the NHS and Community Care Act of 1990, an internal market was introduced. Realizing that the existing central tax-based system was, compared to other countries, quite effective in containing growth in health care expenditure, and taking into account that "the NHS is the closest thing the English have to a religion,"[52] the focus for the internal British market was on the way services were organized, managed, and delivered. Reforms in these areas were expected "to increase the flexibility and efficiency of the system and to enhance the quality of health care,"[53] while maintaining tax-based financing and preserving (almost) free access. Behind the ideas on the internal market was a strong belief in the superior efficiency of the private competitive sector. Private-sector-like changes would increase efficiency in the NHS, it was assumed. To achieve this objective, a competitive environment also had to be established for the NHS. The instrument employed to effect this expected change was competition. Competition between providers of both hospital and clinical services, it was believed, would increase efficiency and improve the quality of services, thereby increasing consumers' satisfaction. In short: the British government wanted "to squeeze more out of the system"[54] without fundamentally changing it.

The basic idea for implementing competition was a distinction between purchasers and providers of health care. Providers would deliver health care services on the basis of contracts with purchasers. Purchasers could be distinguished into two types. Firstly, there would be the district health authorities, who in the new system would have to identify and select the services needed, and contract these services out to various providers. The second type of purchaser would be those general practitioners who would act as fund-holders, managing a budget to secure a certain range of hospital and primary care services for their patients. Purchasing responsibly, it was assumed, would not only increase the quality of care for the fund-holders' patients, but could also result in budget surpluses which could be diverted to expanding the range of services. Furthermore, fund-holders were expected to cash in the personal incentives the new approach was assumed to offer. By purchasing responsibly, they would be able to increase their number of patients, which would raise their per-capita income.

On the provider side, hospitals were transformed into "trusts," which were obliged to compete with each other for contracts with district health authorities, fund-holding practitioners, and private insurers. Although the trusts remained public sector organizations, they became considerably more autonomous to enable them to play the internal market game. Nevertheless, the NHS management executive retained power through monitoring the trusts' financial performance and business plans. In 1994, around one-third of British general practitioners had obtained the status of fund-holder, while 90% of hospitals had become trusts.[55]

It is important to mention that the British ideas on the internal market were first implemented during Thatcher's Conservative administration. Because of that, they were criticized from the beginning by Labour, which was then in opposition. Tony Blair was said to be against this type of reforms for three reasons: first of all, because they had caused the NHS to experience exhausting organizational changes and an escalating bureaucracy; secondly, because the Conservative ideas were said to be based on a blind ideological faith that the market is a more efficient instrument to get value for money; and thirdly, because in Labour's view, the real Conservative agenda was to commercialize and privatize the NHS.[56] In contrast, Blair presented himself during his election campaign as the guardian angel of the NHS with statements like: "We created the NHS. We will save it. And we will save it for the better."[57] Once he was in office, however, apart from changing the vocabulary, it took years for changes to materialize. For that matter, the changes that did materialize can be labeled as "warmed-up neo-liberalism,"[58] i.e., "clothing right-wing ideas in progressive language."[59]

An important point is whether the new approach did, indeed, improve the flexibility and efficiency of the system, since that is what is was all about. Research carried out after some years of experience was rather inconclusive. It did, on the one hand, show that fund-holders were more able to challenge hospital practices and to demand improvements. In addition to this, fund-holders appeared to be more careful in prescribing new and costly drugs, choosing generics more often. On the other hand, the British National Audit Office concluded in its first evaluation report in 1994 that, although fund-holders realized savings as purchasers, these savings were not used for quality improvement or a reduction of waiting lists.[60] Furthermore, referral patterns hardly changed and consumers' free choice did not expand significantly. Apparently, changes like these are expected to take effect only gradually.[61] Meanwhile, since 2003, the idea of a hospital trust seems to be out of favor with Scottish politicians because of the assumed unnecessary bureaucracy it has created.

The United Kingdom was not the only EU country which saw the creation of an internal market as a way to improve cost containment. Italy did so with its second phase of health care reform in the early 1990s. Here too, reforms led to increased managerial autonomy for hospitals and local health units, whereas a partial purchaser-provider split was introduced to promote competition. And here too, the new arrangements were expected to increase responsiveness to patients' needs and demands. Contrary to the situation in the United Kingdom, however, (1) patients retained their free choice of provider; (2) contracts were not identified as the way to negotiate price, volume, and cost; (3) a per-case system was introduced in the hospital sector; and (4) cost containment from the demand side ranked high on the political agenda. Each of these arrangements was based on a more general set of structural changes directed at introducing managed competition among public and private providers. The 1999 reforms deepened the delegation process while simultaneously reinforcing the regulatory and monitoring role of state authorities.[62] Central power was reinforced by explicitly stating that the regions would be held financially accountable for their deficits. These deficits would have to be covered by heavier regional taxation or by increasing co-payments. Room to maneuver in this way was, in fact, rather limited, given the strongly centralized general and payroll taxes, with co-payments already at a relatively high level.[63]

Although not directly labelled as countries creating an internal market, Portugal, Denmark, Sweden, Spain, and the Netherlands have introduced internal market-like changes in the financing and provision of health care.

Portugal decided in 1996 that new hospitals would have to adopt a more entrepreneurial management style. In 1998, regional health authorities began to establish regional contracting agencies, whose mission was to develop expertise in analyzing, negotiating, and decision-making regarding public financing of health services. The power of these agencies was rather limited, however, since they had very small budgets. Moreover, their influence over providers was limited. As for the new management style, in 2003 new legislation was enacted which converted 30% of public hospitals into "hospital companies."[64]

In Denmark, several counties have experimented with negotiated contracts and goal-setting for hospitals. Such contracts include activity levels and provide activity-based financing and even bonus arrangements for treatment in specific areas. Although such contracts are not legally binding and do not include sanctions, they do have an effect, since persistent failure could lead to salary cuts or changed employment conditions for the responsible managers. Finally, several counties have applied internal market-like practices by introducing competitive bidding among private and public suppliers, particularly for auxiliary services (laundry, catering, cleaning, et cetera), and in some cases even for clinical activities.[65]

As for Sweden, 14 out of 26 county councils established separate purchasing organizations in 1994 which were operating at county, district, or municipal levels. These purchasing organizations are assumed to have increased competition among providers,[66] albeit with serious concerns that market-based mechanisms would negatively influence social equity. In the mid-1990s, therefore, the term *cooperation* started to be used instead of competition.[67]

In the early 1990s, some regional health services in Spain introduced a contract program, characterized by negotiating between third-party payers and hospitals regarding the hospitals' activity levels. During the 1990s, information systems measuring hospital performance improved significantly, quality indicators were established, and aggregate measures of activity were defined. Developments like these made it easier to compare the performance of individual hospitals.[68]

A final example of the introduction of internal market-like changes in health care can be found in the Netherlands, where, as a consequence of the health insurance system's First Phase Amendments Act of 1989, sickness funds started to bear real financial risk. This act introduced budget payments from the central fund to the sickness funds to cover the costs of benefits. An additional source of financing to cover these costs was provided by flat-rate contributions which sickness funds received from their members. The amount of flat-rate contributions could differ between sickness funds, depending on how cost-efficient they were in the use of their budgets. It was hoped, therefore, that the flat-rate contributions would be an incentive for sickness funds to increase efficiency and cost-effectiveness in their operations.[69]

To conclude this section, it should be noted that the EU also includes countries which deliberately did not consider the introduction of an internal market for health care. France is an example. Here, French culture and the historically strong role of the state are the explanation. Moreover, French patients already enjoyed free choice of doctors, the fee-for-service system raised provider activities, and waiting lists are rare.[70]

Undoubtedly, implementing internal market ideas has brought about positive changes in health care management.[71] During the first period (chapter eight), health care management, especially in hospitals, basically involved "minding the shop," with an open-ended financing system abundantly delivering the necessary financial means. In those days, management in health care was a relatively easy job. From the 1980s on, with the introduction of the idea of a health care market, health care managers, providers, and insurers alike had to start to think in market terms, taking notice of their competitive position in that market. To those who did so, it became clear that on the market, quality and price are the determining factors. This explains their increasing attention to quality measurement, quality improvement, and management accounting systems. The last item might deliver useful signals for the measurement of efficiency and effectiveness of the organization's daily operations, as well as of the profitability of their products.[72] Management accounting systems could deliver an insight into the cost structure of their products, help to determine a satisfactory price for the products produced and distinguish between profitable products and unprofitable ones, and make it possible to detect losses and wastes and separate the costs of idleness from the costs of production, et cetera.[73] In short, the introduction of market ideas contributed fundamentally to developments in health care management. The times of "minding the shop" were over; instead, managers had to be capable of bearing responsibilities very similar to those of their colleagues in business life. With that, health care management became a challenging and demanding job.

Two points should be made in this respect. Firstly, compared to many other businesses, health care management is still a relatively young profession. In this respect, the OECD rightfully observes that, in most OECD countries, "hospital management systems are in their infancy."[74] Further professionalization, therefore, is needed and may be expected.

Secondly, health care management occurs in organizations that have relatively independently functioning professionals. This demands particular types of leadership and control which, to a certain extent, differ from those in organizations which are not characterized as professional.

Thirdly, despite the fact that health care management, particularly in hospitals, will increasingly resemble management in other businesses, it will continue to be considerably more restricted by governments' regulatory demands. I will come back to these points later.

9.2.3 Private Initiatives

To begin with, it should be kept in mind that private initiatives in health care are not as unique as the title of this section might suggest. Apart from the fact that, in many countries, general practitioners and medical specialists, as well other health care professionals, are self-employed, many hospitals (both for-profit and nonprofit) also exist as a result of private initiative. In Germany, the share of doctor-owned hospitals is growing, particularly for specialized hospitals.[75] For-profit hospitals in France, furthermore, account for no less than 40% of all French hospitals and 20% of all inpatient beds. These private for-profit hospitals are small, with an average of around 70 beds. They tend to specialize in certain areas and are hardly involved in emergency admissions. Their involvement with patients needing long-term care or psychiatric treatment is even more marginal.[76] Austria has around 50 small private hospitals, which are run by private individuals or companies and account for 5% of all Austrian hospital beds. They are mainly sanatoriums. Admission depends on a patient's ability to pay and the extent of the patient's insurance.[77] Furthermore, Greece is exceptional because its government prohibited the establishment of new private hospitals during the period 1983–1992, while at the same time trying to absorb part of the existing private hospitals into the public system. In 1992, the restriction on the establishment of private hospitals was lifted. People were so dissatisfied with the public system that they increasingly turned to the private circuit.[78] Also, a country like Spain has traditionally contracted-out between 15% and 20% of its hospital needs to private not-for-profit providers.[79] Finally, it is possible for a patient to have a private bed in a public hospital. The United Kingdom's NHS, for example, has 3,000 authorized amenity beds, of which the majority are on ordinary wards.[80]

However, these already existing private initiatives in EU health care systems are not the focus of this section. What is interesting in the framework of this book are those private initiatives which can be seen to be a consequence of the reform process that started around the beginning of the 1980s. Since then, those who are daily involved in health care delivery have started to explore new ways of providing services. Many private initiatives directed at improving efficiency and quality of care were initiated in almost all spheres of collectively financed health care systems. Cooperation between different health care providers, the merging of different institutions, pursuing integrated care and seamless care, and pioneering new methods have become the order of the day. Most governments of EU member states, while keeping an eye on the basic values of solidarity and equal access to their health care systems, have welcomed these private initiatives. Some of them have even stimulated these developments through specific legal measures, and in some cases governments themselves took the lead in trying to involve private business in health care projects. All in all, the reform phase stirred up many innovations in health care delivery. For many of these innovations, to some extent and to differing degrees, a (quasi-) market for health care came to the fore.

For practical reasons, private initiatives in this section are classified along three lines: (1) those initiated by health care providers, often with support of insurers; (2) legal measures intended to create room for private initiatives; and (3) governmental initiatives to involve private business in health care.

As for private initiatives initiated by health care providers, I follow the inventory which was devised by the Dutch Health Management Forum in 1999.[81] Many items on this inventory have also been applied in other countries of the EU. The forum distinguishes between private initiatives by public providers, which are directly related to patient care, on the one hand, and additional services, on the other. Private initiatives in the first category are, for example, special arrangements directed at rapid treatment of particular categories of patients (based on a contractual relation between an employer and a provider, with the employer paying for the extra services), nursing homes, establishing nursing capacity for people fleeing countries with cold winters, hospitals with wards for different classes or special hotel facilities outside the hospital, or separate specialized treatment centers that also perform interventions which are not covered by the health insurance scheme (cosmetic surgery). As for the second category, additional services, one can think of hospitals providing fitness facilities or sports clinics, home-care organizations installing alarm systems in private homes of elderly people, rehabilitation centers starting private companies for the development of orthopedic instruments, physiotherapists providing supplementary services like fitness and prevention programs, and hospitals creating independent laboratories which provide blood tests for the market.

Regarding private initiatives by private providers, one can also distinguish between those initiatives which are directly related to patient care, on the one hand, and extra services, on the other. Examples of the first category are private home-care organizations, private nursing homes, and special institutions for terminal patients. The second category comprises services like television or telephony provided by private firms in hospitals, hotel facilities for relatives of admitted patients, and health resorts.

Regarding legal measures intended to create room for private initiatives, Sweden provides a good example. During the 1990s, a lot happened in this country. Some county councils, like Stockholm, took the strategy of privatizing the ancillary services as much as possible. The operations of one hospital were even sold to a private investment firm, with the building remaining state property. This novelty raised the debate in Sweden as to whether private profit-seeking organizations would be as capable of providing health care of equal quality and accessibility as the existing not-for-profit organizations. Meanwhile, due to waiting list problems, several specialized inpatient clinics had started to provide treatment on a contract basis for publicly funded patients. In 1998, it was estimated that, of total health expenditures, 3% was attributable to private health care. The majority of private hospitals tend to concentrate on care which requires minor investments in equipment. Recently, two private emergency hospitals were established in Sweden. Due to long waiting times for certain medical interventions during the 1980s (hip replacements, cataract surgery), patients who could afford it financially turned to private clinics, which caused a growth in private providers, particularly in the larger cities.[82] As for care for the elderly in Sweden, 240 entrepreneurs were active in 1999, employing 2,500 people. Some of these entrepreneurs are from a religious congregational background. Also, in Dutch health care policy, we see increasing governmental support for private initiatives. This can be illustrated by a policy evaluation regarding the so-called independent treatment centers for the provision of outpatient treatment and day surgery. From 1998 on, the bureaucratic/political establishment's appreciation of this phenomenon slowly evolved from "a necessary evil" (combating waiting lists) into "a useful provision" (contributing to market dynamics).[83] This has been expressed by a liberalization of corresponding legal regulations directed at removing or relaxing the conditions for the establishment of independent treatment centers. As a result of changes made in 2003, establishing an independent treatment center no longer depends on the existence of waiting lists; formal cooperation between hospitals and these centers is no longer necessary; and the insurer's view is no longer important. To date, it is not yet clear if, in the future, independent treatment centers may work for profit. The 2003 Minister of Health left this point open to discussion in the framework of a fundamental change of the health care system.[84] In 2005 the minister, however, did not explicitly exclude the profit motive from health care provision.

Finally, let us consider governmental initiatives to involve private business in health care:

"Let me say at the outset that partnerships between the public and the private sector are a cornerstone of the Government's modernisation programme for Britain. They are central to our drive to modernise our key public services. Such partnerships are here and they are here to stay."[85] Thus said the British Secretary of State for Health, Alan Milburn, in 2000, expressing a decisive Labour government policy to modernize the NHS. At the macro-level, this would be achieved by introducing the private finances that the government could not afford. At the micro-level, this would be achieved by pursuing value for money through the transfer of risks and associated costs to the private sector, which otherwise would have to be borne by the public sector. A further advantage would be the expected benefits of greater expertise, efficiency, and innovation that the private sector was assumed to possess. Therefore, private management of hospitals could be part of the deal.[86]

In fact, this policy option was nothing new. In the early 1990s, the then Conservative government had similar ideas, confusingly labeling them as Private Finance Initiatives.[87] Limiting the interest in PPP/PFI to hospitals, the British government started enthusiastically with a first contract signed in 1997. By the spring of 2003, a total of 117 contracts with hospital trusts had been signed, with an approved investment of £3,2 billion.[88] Now, how profitable are these constructions to the public sector?

To begin with, it is important to note that the British hospital infrastructure was neglected for a prolonged period. There was little hospital building until the 1960s, since the government's focus at that time was on housing and education. Of the 1962 hospital plan for over 200 (re)construction schemes, only one-third had been realized by 1976 when public investment was curtailed, and between 1980 and 1997 only seven public schemes were completed. Consequently, in the 1990s, the NHS was burdened with "an outmoded and worn-out estate, a significant part of which predated the First World War, and a backlog of maintenance."[89] It is no wonder, then, that the decision to finally modernize the hospital infrastructure would cost British taxpayers enormous amounts of money as a consequence of political shortsightedness in the past. Thus, the decision was made to modernize with private funding. And private investors appeared to be very willing, assuming health care to be a profitable market. After all, the only interest of the private parties in PPP/PFI is making money. And here, private partners appear to be very successful. In this respect, a 2004 evaluation report by the British Association of Chartered Certified Accountants (ACCA) is revealing. It shows that the annual capital costs for 13 hospitals built under PPP/PFI are at least £45 million higher than if they had been built under the government's capital charging regime, even though these newly built hospitals are considerably smaller than the old ones they replaced. As for the latter point, it has been calculated that, in order to compensate for the additional charges and interest costs, the number of beds for the first 11 hospitals built under PPP/PFI was reduced by more than 30% than was deemed necessary according to the existing governmental planning figures.[90] Extra capital costs, furthermore, caused an increase of 26% in the trusts' budget in 2003 compared to 2000.[91] Thanks to these extra costs, 6 out of these 13 hospital trusts face financial problems. These capital costs leak out of the health care system. Had the hospitals been built under the government's capital charging regime, the capital costs could have been recycled within the health care system. Because of this "leaking out," £125 million has to be injected into the NHS on an annual basis to keep it in steady state in relation to the government's capital charging regime.[92] Furthermore, the report shows that the hospital trusts are paying a risk premium of about 30% of the total construction costs to ensure that the new hospitals are built on time and in line with the available budget. All in all, the ACCA researchers concluded that the private partners in these projects, contrary to the government's assumption, do not experience any risk at all, because all payments are guaranteed by the government. Banking consortia, construction companies, and service providers, the latter two regularly connected, are the ones who benefit from PPP/PFI constructions, not the taxpayers. Consequently, in the end, these taxpayers are the ones who have to cough up the money. In addition, the Netherlands Board for Hospital Facilities correctly observes that the very long time-span of PPP/PFI contracting may easily be at odds with the unpredictable and rapid changes taking place in health care.[93] These changes require flexibility; long-term fixed contracts are an impediment in this regard.

As for private management of public hospitals, the assumed advantages of greater expertise, efficiency, and innovation are very difficult to prove. Previous Australian experience, in this respect, produced such negative results that after the first two PPP/PFI projects, the state of Victoria abandoned its attempt to seek a private operator for the third one. Indeed, the privatization of Australian public hospitals has caused so many problems that a special committee of the Australian parliament recommended in 2000 that "no further privatisation of public hospitals should occur until a thorough national investigation is conducted and that some advantage for patients can be demonstrated for this mode of delivery of services."[94]

Meanwhile, the PPP/PFI train thunders on. In Portugal, the present government has chosen private investment in state-owned health care facilities as one of its priorities for its health agenda. It is assumed that this will improve the Portuguese health care system by providing capacity while at the same time guaranteeing value for money spent, through cooperating with private business in the building, maintenance, and operation of health care facilities. Furthermore, it is thought that cooperation with business will transfer the risks to private investors and, through this, alleviate the government's public investment burden. In 1995, the management of a new 600-bed hospital near Lisbon was contracted-out to a private consortium. Meanwhile, legal provisions have been enacted to create the necessary framework for the further implementation of actual partnerships. The Portuguese government intended to launch ten public–private-partnership hospitals before 2006 with private investment, public financing, private management, clinical services, and public ownership.[95] In Spain, some regions experimented in the early 1990s with contracting-out to private companies the integrated management of services in several health areas. The Valencia region contracted-out hospital services in two health areas to private for-profit organizations, based on a long-term agreement.[96] Due to persistent underfunding of capital investment in the health care infrastructure, some local health authorities and hospital trusts in Italy have developed pilot programs over the past few years involving a public–private mix in project financing. To date, legal issues concerning the role that private business can play in managing public health organizations limit the scope of these experiments.[97]

9.3 Rationing and Priority Setting

Around the beginning of the 1980s, governments started to realize that developments in health care were getting out of hand. The situation of an ever-growing share of public funds absorbed by health care objectives, regularly in double digits during the 1970s, had to be addressed. For the implementation of restructuring policies to proceed, however, the public at large, and in particular consumers and providers, would have to start to realize that the process of production and consumption of health care goods and services is not as self-evident as people had come to believe. To put it another way, people had to get the message that health care goods and services are also subject to scarcity. This was not an easy task for governments to accomplish. For example, in 1998, a representative population survey in Germany showed that the majority of respondents favored unlimited funding for health services, arguing that the extra money required should be gained through savings in other areas.[98] Similarly, the British King's Fund argued that "there can be no doubt that any strategy which could be interpreted as limiting the comprehensive nature of the NHS [. . .] will cause a public furore of considerable proportions."[99] Governments pursuing rationing policies will always face opposition from (part of) their electorates. Realizing this, and acknowledging the delicacy of the matter, governments therefore phrase their rationing policies in rather vague terms. The next subsection attempts to illustrate this point. After that, some more substantial ways of rationing, e.g., priority setting, will be dealt with.

9.3.1 On Rationing

Scarcity raises distribution problems, and, with that, forces governments inevitably to pursue a balanced approach between demand and supply. Against this background, several EU governments have organized campaigns to communicate the scarcity message to their citizens.[100] Scarcity, so it has been argued, forces rationing and priority setting in health care. After all, not everything that is possible medically is feasible financially. Although the message was clear, implementing it was quite another story.

First of all, implementation encountered difficulties because several EU countries have no defined list of health care items that are provided through collective financing. The United Kingdom, for example, grants a large degree of discretion about the range of services actually provided, with the Secretary of Health in a position to decide "to such an extent as he considers necessary to meet all reasonable requirements."[101] Also, countries like Sweden, Portugal, and Italy do not have explicit lists of services to be provided, although some of these countries have attempted to define the content of a homogeneous benefit package.[102] Even countries like Germany and the Netherlands, for example, which do have a defined coverage package, face similar problems, however. In other words, having decided on the content of a coverage package does not make decision-making regarding the exclusion of specific items from that package any easier. As a consequence, discussions and proposals on rationing mostly resulted in rather general principles and guidelines.

A Finnish report of 1994, for example, written by a special task force, contains no specific recommendations. The report was a plea for transparency in decision-making, taking into account principles of human rights, self-determination, equality, and justice, while distinguishing between the political and the clinical level as regards the application of these principles. Ongoing discussions on this topic in Finland by the end of the 1990s culminated in a so-called high-level consensus meeting in 2000. But, again, the appropriateness of its outcomes remained vague. Health care, it was argued, should be provided on fair and equal grounds. The effectiveness of services should have a central position, and the Finnish health care system should be built on a sound financial foundation.[103]

Sweden also formulated rationing principles. First of all, human rights are central: regarding health care, individuals have equal value and equal rights irrespective of their personal position in society. Secondly, rationing measures should take into account the principles of need and solidarity, with resources focused on the individual or sector in greatest need. Thirdly, the principle of cost-effectiveness should be followed, e.g., health care delivery should be in accordance with a reasonable relation between costs and effects, measured as improved health and a higher quality of life. The third principle was subordinated to the other two principles. When they were raised to the Swedish political/administrative level, the discussions resulted in four levels of priorities: (1) care for life-threatening acute diseases and diseases that, without treatment, would cause prolonged disability and/or premature death, as well as care for serious chronic diseases, palliative care in the final phase of life, and care for people with reduced autonomy; (2) prevention measures that had documented benefits, rehabilitation, et cetera; (3) care for less serious acute and chronic diseases; and (4) care for reasons other than disease or injury.[104]

The Netherlands, which received a report on the limits of health care in 1986,[105] expected a special committee to solve the problem of determining the content of the benefit package. In its 1992 report, this committee developed a ranked ordering of four criteria: necessity, effectiveness, efficiency, and individual responsibility. Health care items which satisfied these four criteria would have to be included in the benefit package.[106] But here too, theory differed from practical implementation, if only because most of the four criteria can be debated.

So, altogether, rationing is a rather theoretical exercise in "muddling through elegantly."[107] It is also a highly sensitive topic politically, and it does not deliver many options for dealing with the scarcity problem in practice. What we see in practice, therefore, is that health professionals, working in the daily process of health care delivery, "ration" simply by adjusting needs to means. In the words of the British Medical Association, this involves "the denial of treatment on grounds other than simple clinical judgement."[108] More generally, if the means to fund a health care system on the basis of a collective scheme are inadequate, one has to bring the needs for health care in line with what is financially feasible.

Meanwhile, one of the problems with rationing policies is rationality itself. There are those who have attempted to judge the contents of a benefit package on the basis of criteria like uncertainty, information asymmetry, and fundamental importance.[109] Others have even developed econometric models for the establishment and financing of a basic insurance package.[110] These attempts, however, leave unaddressed the fact that there is a considerable difference between formulating rationing ideas at the macro-level and their implementation in practice. One can, for example, easily decide at the macro-level to limit the finances of hospitals, but the consequences of such a decision have to be dealt with at the micro-level of hospital care. And if, in this respect, measures to improve effectiveness and efficiency of health care delivery have been exhausted, further rationing has to be left to the ingenuity of those who are directly involved in the health care delivery process, particularly the medical specialists and the nursing staff. At the micro-level, therefore, rationing "continues to be implicit and controlled by the medical profession."[111] It is "ultimately individual clinicians, and clinicians acting together with colleagues in clinical directorates and similar groupings at institutional level, who actually manage the process."[112] They are the ones to decide on the treatment program, the use of resources, how to deal with waiting lists, et cetera. This has always been so, and always will be.

Although the concept of rationing as such is rather vague, in daily practice it has become a substantial consideration through the use of strategies for priority setting regarding the demand side as well as the supply side of health care.[113] Since the 1980s, both sides have been the focus of policymakers. As for the demand side, one can think of items like cost-sharing and co–payments. On the supply side are items like capacity planning, technology assessment, appropriate care, financial constraints on hospitals, and waiting lists. Some of these items have a direct financial impact, either for consumers or for providers. They will be dealt with as part of the fourth theme of this chapter. For the completion of the present theme, I will deal with three selected items of priority setting on the supply side. I start with technology assessment in a separate subsection, the reason for this being that, over the course of time, it has become an established field of research on its own throughout the European Union.

9.3.2 Health Technology Assessment

In the sixth chapter I concluded that it is very debatable whether the introduction and diffusion of expensive health care technologies can be viewed as a rational process. In contrast with other technologies, marketing research before the production and launching of something new, including calculations about when a potential market will be fully served, is quite unknown in the medical technology field. The starting point for the introduction is far more that a new technology, be it a drug or a medical device, promises to fulfill needs that could not be fulfilled before, or has the potential to deal with them in a cheaper and more efficient way. The question of effectiveness, i.e., does the new technology fulfill its promise, and does it really add a new dimension or value to the health care process? mostly comes *after* the new technology has become a standard procedure.

This last point illustrates a more general problem besetting most health care systems in the European Union, namely, the repeated adoption of unevaluated innovations. What is worrisome is the way in which just about all innovations slip into the health care systems of many countries without proper evaluation, either before or during an innovation's career. The legal assumption that a suspect is presumed innocent until proven to be guilty appears to apply to medical innovations as well. They are assumed to be effective until they are shown to be ineffective. This has consequences for the first part of my definition of planning—the processing of information regarding decisions on future actions (section 6.2.3). It is obvious that, before information can be processed, two factors must be evaluated, namely, the completeness of the information and its reliability. There is quite a lot of research proving (always after the fact) that new technologies were introduced without adequate evaluation. In order to cope with this problem, governments have taken an interest in technology assessment for some decades now.[114] During the period at issue, almost all EU countries have one way or another engaged in using this technology assessment to control the costs of health care. They do this by listing expensive technologies that need explicit government permission to be purchased, or by putting specific committees in charge of decision-making. The following cross section is an illustration of the general picture in this respect.

Luxembourg uses a list of pieces of costly, specialized medical equipment which cannot be purchased without special authorization by the Ministry of Health. The list is revised every three years. The authorization process includes consultation with the Permanent Hospital Committee, an advisory board composed of representatives from the government, the Union of Sickness Funds, hospitals, and health professionals. In order to prevent hospitals from purchasing expensive equipment without authorization, a 1998 law provided that the state would pay 80% of the respective costs, with the rest to be supplied by the insurance funds.[115]

Belgium has special accreditation criteria for the use of expensive technology. If a hospital fails to meet these criteria, not only can reimbursement be refused, but it is also possible that the hospital budget will be cut by 20%. Technology assessment is done by technical councils composed of representatives from the health insurance funds, health care providers, and university experts. Input from economists, statisticians, epidemiologists, or engineers is minimal. Consequently, attention to cost-effectiveness is often lacking. In 2000, Belgium did not yet have a formal national program or institute for health care technology assessment. Due to the increasing costs, proposals have meanwhile been formulated to try to control the use of expensive technologies.[116]

In 2001, Italy had no national agency responsible for the promotion and financing of technology assessment activities. The regional Centre for the Assessment of Biomedical Equipment, established in Trieste in 1989, can be considered to be Italy's first experiment in technology assessment. In 1997, the Ministry of Health funded this center to monitor the dissemination of major health technologies. In Veneto, a regional Centre for Technology Assessment and Quality Improvement in Health Care was established in 1993 with the objective of carrying out integrated assessment of individual technologies, i.e., technology assessment from an epidemiological, clinical, and economic perspective.[117]

In Spain, the introduction of health technology assessment took place in two phases: a first wave of institutional design in the mid-1980s, and a second wave in the mid-1990s. During this second wave, in 1994, the Spanish National Office of Technology Assessment was established. Its functions and organization were enlarged and reformed in 1999, in the sense that several regional agencies were created. Since then, the regional approach has become important in Spain, since it contributed to the improvement of available data on evidence-based medicine and cost-effectiveness.[118] Furthermore, some Spanish regions are involved in "horizon scanning," i.e., proactively identifying new technologies that could be included in the benefit package.[119]

Although the United Kingdom has had a health technology assessment program since 1993, which was funded as part of the NHS Research and Development Programme and which aimed "to ensure that high quality research information on the costs, effectiveness and broader impact of health technologies is produced in the most effective way for those who use, manage and work in the NHS,"[120] assessment activities remained rather scattered[121] until, in 1999, the National Institute for Clinical Excellence (NICE) was established in order "to create greater national harmony in the use of health technology."[122] NICE is an independent organization which has to assess new health technologies based on substantive criteria, such as (1) does the new technology promote clinical excellence? and (2) does it contribute to an effective use of available health care resources?[123] Additionally, like the Spanish, the British are engaged in "horizon scanning" at a unit of Birmingham University, i.e., identifying new technologies that are likely to affect the NHS with a view to encouraging their evaluation and assessing their clinical potential and cost-effectiveness.[124] Horizon scanning may contribute to prospective policy-making.[125]

With its Drug Reimbursement Scheme (GVS) of 1991, the Netherlands created an explicit assessment process regarding the coverage of outpatient drugs. Under this scheme, these drugs are appraised for their therapeutic value compared to other drugs.[126] The GVS, therefore, can be labeled a reference price system for pharmaceutical reimbursement, directed at limiting public reimbursement without restricting choice.[127] The initial effect of the introduction of GVS was price convergence to the reimbursement level, resulting in an overall price reduction of around 5%. The pharmaceutical industry reacted by introducing high-priced new drugs into the market. This led the Dutch government to decide to halt reimbursement for innovative drugs for a number of years. Due to a growing list of new drugs waiting for approval, this policy could not be maintained. Therefore, since 1999, after assessment of their therapeutic value and costs, new drugs can be reimbursed in line with their premium price. In the same year, the ministry also introduced guidelines for pharmaco-economic research which producers have to follow when submitting new drugs for market approval. As of 2005, the assessment criteria included the results of pharmaco-economic research.[128]

Finally, Denmark established its Institute for Health Technology Assessment (DIHTA) in 1997. Providing information, counseling, education, and training regarding health technology assessment, as well as contributing to quality development, are among DIHTA's objectives. The organization works in close cooperation with the counties. Health technology assessment is done in cooperation with clinical departments, general practitioners, health administrators, clinical scientists, researchers, and representatives from the medical technology industry. DIHTA's advisory board is made up of 22 members, representing the main stakeholders in the Danish health care system at the political, administrative, and industry level. It also receives multidisciplinary advice from its scientific board. With its annual budget of 25 million Danish crowns, DIHTA employs a multidisciplinary staff of ten full-time members, complemented with an external expert staff of seven members on a part-time basis.[129]

Thus, altogether, there is a lot going on regarding health technology assessment in the countries of the European Union. At national, regional, and institutional levels, governments are trying to control the use of technology through assessment. But does it work? In this respect, a recent study on eight countries which are involved in health technology assessment delivers some interesting results.[130] It shows, firstly, that there are considerable differences between countries with regard to aspects like the transparency of the assessment process, appeal procedures, and composition of assessment teams. Secondly, different countries assessing the same new technology may come to different conclusions regarding its effectiveness. Thirdly, negative assessment outcomes may be overruled by political intervention or court rulings with a possible consequence that, fourthly, assessment organizations reverse their initial conclusions. Finally, most health technology assessment focuses on matters of effectiveness. For health technology assessment ever to have a chance of being an effective rationing tool, however, more attention should be paid to cost-effectiveness. In this respect, the Dutch decision to include pharmaco-economic criteria when determining whether a new drug should be included in the benefit package is a step in the right direction. Finland and Portugal have decided to follow the same road.

Nevertheless, three problems regarding health technology assessment remain. Firstly, health technology assessment is very costly and time-consuming, so that, given the speed of technological development, it is highly likely that, by the time the assessment is completed, the technology concerned has been replaced by newer technology.

Secondly, it is impracticable to control all new technologies that come onto the health care market each year. Understandably, therefore, most assessment is limited to the expensive devices and procedures. For example, in the Netherlands, health technology assessment deals with around 3% of total health care costs and around 9% of all hospital costs.[131]

Thirdly, how can governments forbid the introduction of a unevaluated technology, especially in a health care system with important market elements, if there are no compelling reasons for governments to condition or to correct? Furthermore, the very existence of a private market for health care can create obstacles for governments that want to control the use of expensive technologies in their public hospitals. In Portugal, for example, with 67% of the expensive medical equipment in use installed in private clinics, even public hospitals make contracts with private clinics for the use of their equipment. Would a government dare to forbid that?[132] In this respect, it should be realized that if a new technology is paid for by private insurance, or by private individuals, this will exert pressure for public insurers to follow.[133]

Finally, there is the aspect of financing the assessment. Correct reasoning requires one to add the assessment costs in order to establish the real costs of expensive technology. I agree that doing so would not deliver much benefit for each individual EU country. But if health technology assessment would be raised to the level of the European Union, making it a combined affair, assessment effectiveness could increase considerably. Such an EU-level approach would have to start with reaching agreements on matters like the interpretation of the assessment task, the procedures to follow, as well as the methodology to be used. It is difficult to see why such an idea would not be feasible. After all, at the EU-level, we already have the European Agency for the Evaluation of Medical Products, the European Medicines Agency, and the Committee for Proprietary Medicinal Products.[134] Moreover, technology assessment has nothing to do with a country's medical culture. Technology is neutral. One can either use it or not.

9.3.3 Two Other Examples of Priority Setting

As stated in the introduction to this chapter, each of the four themes can be illustrated with many examples. With regard to priority setting, two other examples are presented below: waiting lists and clinical guidelines.

The phenomenon of waiting lists is well known in quite a number of EU countries. They are the consequence of a too-limited capacity, either in facilities, in equipment, or in staff numbers in relation to demand. Such a situation may lead to what the Dutch in the 1990s started to call a "care gap," i.e., the difference in financial terms between what the then government coalition was prepared to supply and what those involved in health care delivery thought was necessary. In one of its yearly "Health Care on Account" reports, the Federation of Dutch Health Care Organizations calculated this difference for all institutional health care provisions to be 0.8% yearly during the period 1996–2000.[135] The government, however, which was strongly focussing on reducing public debt (its main priority in those days), was not prepared to offer any consolation for many years. Health care institutions, so it was argued, had to economize on their budgets and had to work more effectively and efficiently, thus increasing productivity. Subsequent reports of the Federation in the following years in which claims for more financial means were well substantiated did not change the government's position.[136] Consequently, waiting lists grew in acute hospitals, in long-term care, and in ambulatory mental health care, as well as in home care. When, at the beginning of the 21st century, things had really got out of hand, with citizens even going to court to force insurers to live up to their legal obligations, the government had to give in. Comparable developments can be observed in other EU countries.

Denmark, for example, where waiting times were also too long, had to reach an agreement on goals for maximum allowable waiting times for specific treatments, to be achieved by the end of 1995. This agreement forced the government to come up with extra financial incentives. However, because general legislative guarantees appeared not to work, a more differentiated approach based on assessments of the impact of waiting times for different patient groups was followed beginning in 1999. Since 2000, targets have been set for a number of life-threatening diseases (some serious heart conditions, and some types of cancer). Due to these measures, the overall percentage of patients waiting for treatment for more than three months has fallen from 32% in 1995 to 21% in 1998. In the latter year, 71% of patients were treated immediately, 14% within a month, and 8% had to wait more than three months.[137]

The government of Portugal took the phenomenon of waiting lists seriously in 1994 when it launched a special program to cope with this problem by contracting with private health care institutions. After that, the policy to reduce waiting lists was extended several times by granting extra funding for hospitals and surgical staff. After a change of government in 2002, this policy was revised and exchanged for a policy of involving more private hospitals (for-profit as well as not-for-profit) to cope with the problem. Nevertheless, by mid-2002, of more than 120,000 patients waiting for surgery, almost 70% had endured an unacceptable delay.[138]

In Sweden, there was much political discussion in the 1990s regarding accessibility, e.g., waiting times and treatment. In 1992, a National Guarantee of Treatment was introduced with the objective of reducing waiting times. A patient who had to wait more than three months could demand treatment elsewhere, even outside the county of residence.[139]

Finally, in the United Kingdom, the administration which came to power in 1997 faced a serious waiting list problem. For years already, this had been a major source of concern within the NHS. Illustrative of the seriousness of the situation are the commitments the new Labour government made: (1) a wait of no more than 18 (!) months for a hospital inpatient admission; and (2) a reduction of the number of people on waiting lists by 100,000 by the time of the next election (that is, after six years). Despite these commitments, however, in the beginning of 1999, the number of patients who had been on waiting lists for between 12 and 18 months had increased by around 65% compared to the time when the new government took office.[140]

These examples show that sometimes waiting lists may be a consequence of deliberate restraint policies, with governments setting other priorities. Consequently, priority setting in health care is of an "inherently political nature."[141] At other times, governments may not have sufficient financial means. It is not always clear which argument applies. But no matter what causes waiting lists, three things can be concluded.

Firstly, those who work in daily practice have to do the resulting priority setting. They are the ones who have to decide on who comes first. Decision-making, in this respect, is not necessarily always based on health conditions.

Secondly, those who can afford it will bypass waiting lists by taking private health insurance or by seeking health care abroad. Particularly in the United Kingdom, waiting lists increased the proportion of the population who had taken private medical insurance in the beginning of the 1990s to 13%. This number was expected to grow to over 50% by the turn of the century.[142] This development did not materialize, however.

Thirdly, in the longer term, governments in democracies appear not to be able to ignore the problem of waiting lists forever. Sooner or later, public protests force them to do something about it.

The second example of priority setting concerns the performance of medical professionals and institutions. Here, over the past decades, several methods of standardization have been explored based on best practice, evidence-based medicine, accreditation, or clinical guidelines and protocols. They are all meant to increase the cost-effectiveness of medical performance. Health care institutions and medical professionals of all EU countries are involved somehow in all these types of standardization, sometimes through private initiatives, sometimes through apparent coercion by insurers or governments.

In this respect, the Dutch Association of Medical Specialists, together with the Dutch Association of Medical Directors of Hospitals, established the Dutch Institute for Health Care Improvement (CBO) in 1979. The institute's programs include the development of medical guidelines and indicators, as well as dissemination of best practices. However, it is up to the individual doctor whether to follow the CBO's programs. In only a very few situations is funding of treatment related to acting upon issued guidelines. For the rest, guidelines are simply an advice which medical professionals can follow or not.[143]

In Denmark, the Copenhagen Hospital Corporation introduced an accreditation system for all hospitals in the area in order to be able to compare hospital performance and to encourage self-regulation. In 1998, an independent Centre for the Evaluation of Hospital Activity was established in order to strengthen the quality of care and promote the efficient use of resources. In 2002, it was decided to develop indicators for clinical quality that could be used for comparison between (departments of) hospitals. The intention was to make this information publicly available.[144] Practice guidelines are, to a large extent, produced by the different medical colleges.

In France, quality of care and the evaluation of medical performance became issues in the mid-1990s. The French addressed these issues in two ways. Firstly, through the aforementioned organization ANEAS, they designed and disseminated a system of practice guidelines. Secondly, they emphasized the need for continuous education. ANEAS's practice guidelines are recommendations which doctors are required to follow. In 1998, ANEAS issued 200 recommendations for general practitioners and 250 for medical specialists, mainly concerning drug prescriptions or the provision of medical examinations. Failure to follow the recommendations could lead to financial penalties for the doctor concerned. Meanwhile, research on the effects of the recommendations has shown that doctors have modified their prescription behavior. The percentage of prescriptions that did not comply with recommendations decreased from 19% in 1994 to 8% in 1996. The system of penalties, which was hardly used, was abolished by the end of 1999.[145] A new legal arrangement in March 2002 made it possible for professionals and insurers to conclude targeted agreements on good practice.[146]

Belgium introduced a Minimal Clinical Summary in 1998 which was intended, among other things, to follow hospital compliance with accreditation criteria. Belgian social insurers and physicians concluded an agreement on standards of quality of care in 1993. In 1997, evaluation committees were established in hospitals, not only to assist in the improvement of the quality of care, but also to install quality indicators into the financing system.[147]

Finland introduced national guidelines on quality assurance in 1995 and 1999. Here, the guidelines included the promotion of patient-oriented services, as well as the incorporation of quality assurance as part of the daily activities of health care providers.[148]

With its National Health Plan for 1998–2000, Italy established a procedure for institutional accreditation of public and private health care providers based on an assessment of the quality of their infrastructure as well as human resources, and including methods to address the effectiveness and appropriateness of health care interventions. Furthermore, the plan envisaged a national program for designing and applying clinical guidelines with the involvement of relevant parties at macro-, meso-, and micro-levels. The underlying idea was to steer the behavior of medical professionals toward effective and appropriate service delivery. In accordance with the plan, a National Program for the Elaboration, Dissemination, and Evaluation of Clinical Guidelines was established, directed at designing and disseminating guidelines on treatment of the most prevalent health conditions, especially back pain, hypertension, cervical cancer, breast cancer, and angina pectoris.[149]

As a final example, in the United Kingdom, the issuing of clinical guidelines, as well as medical auditing, is the responsibility of the respective Royal Colleges.[150] The central government is the authority engaged in the development of a national framework for performance assessment in the NHS. This framework will cover six dimensions, among which is "effective delivery of appropriate care." The framework is meant to underpin accountability agreements between regional NHS offices and health authorities on the one hand, and these authorities and primary care groups, on the other, with the development of standards expected of clinical professionals as one of the most important areas of regulation.[151] NHS hospitals are not subject to formal regulation through accreditation systems. Instead, nongovernmental organizations like the King's Fund offer accreditation services which have been taken up by NHS hospitals as well as by private clinics.[152] One of the first results of the government's proposals to regulate professional performance assessment was the publication of clinical indicators and high-level performance indicators in 1999.[153]

So, altogether, there is a lot going on in the countries of the European Union regarding attempts to regulate medical performance. Best-practice examples, clinical guidelines, accreditation and evidence-based medicine, as well as protocols can all be seen as attempts to "rationalize" medical performance and as "proof" of cost-effectiveness. Priority setting by medical professionals along these lines would require them to follow these attempts, because they assume to provide "a secure knowledge base that can provide rational foundations for clinical decisions."[154] They have the "smell" of science, and through that limit the freedom of professional autonomy. This is, by and large, the implicit assumption of governments and insurers. The problem with this assumption, however, is, firstly, that clinical guidelines, evidence-based medicine, and protocols are based on the treatment of an "average patient," not a specific patient.[155] Secondly, the first encounter between a medical professional and the client is not about "what works?" but about "what's wrong?"[156] This judgment dilemma, of "meaning-making,"[157] is an intrinsic and inescapable imperative for clinicians,[158] and with it uncertainty in professional practice is inevitable.[159] Thirdly, studies on the effectiveness of medical performance take so much time that, by the time an agreement has been reached on guidelines, there is a fair chance that new innovations have meanwhile rendered them obsolete.[160] In summary, guidelines, evidence-based medicine, protocols, et cetera, may be seen as an attempt to create some scientific-bureaucratic rationality (you follow the rules, and you perform responsibly and cost-effectively), but the problem of uncertainty (chapter eight) remains. This may explain why following clinical guidelines is almost never enforced and at best strongly advised.

9.4 Cost Containment

As argued in the introduction to this chapter, cost containment is one of the two main objectives of health care reforms. It is an objective which does not necessarily have to be achieved through financial measures. Clinical guidelines and medical protocols, for example, can at the same time be instruments of quality improvement and methods of cost containment. Similarly, organizational reforms may simultaneously lead to greater involvement of health care personnel in health policy development and financial savings. In these examples, cost containment is an indirect and pleasant byproduct of reform policies. This type of cost containment is not the focus of this fourth theme, however. On the contrary, its focus is on direct financial reforms.[161] First, the theme deals with developments regarding pharmaceuticals, because pharmaceuticals represent an ever-growing share of health care expenditures. A number of financial measures have been applied to examine the issue. In the framework of this book, copayments and coverage limitations are of particular importance. The same applies for the second item, cost-sharing. The final subsection will go into the financing of hospitals, for two reasons: Firstly, hospitals consume more than half of a country's health care budget; secondly, reforms in hospital financing give an indication of the current developments in hospital management.

9.4.1 Pharmaceuticals

As for reforms in the pharmaceutical field, a complicating factor is that pharmaceutical companies contribute not only to a population's health. They are also an important source of employment. The German pharmaceutical industry, for example, provides employment for 115,500 workers in 1,100 companies. France is also an important producer, with 300 firms employing 90,000 people. In addition to this, French wholesalers employ 15,000 people, and Belgium has a dynamic pharmaceutical industry which saw an increase in employment of 23% during the period 1987–1997, compared to 12% overall for private business.

There are considerable differences between countries regarding drugs consumption. In the United Kingdom, for example, the level of prescribing is between 30% and 80% lower than in Italy, Germany, and France. Denmark is also not a big consumer in this respect, with a spending level of only 0.7% of GDP compared to 1.3% on average for the other EU countries, the United States, and Japan.

Meanwhile, overall expenditure on pharmaceuticals in EU countries has reached a level of between 10% and 15% of the total health care budget.[162] Understandably, therefore, all EU countries have taken measures to get control of spending on drug consumption. The following is a summing-up of these attempts. Here, apart from some incidental comments, copayments are left out, since they are the topic of a separate section.

As for the pharmaceutical industry, the United Kingdom had already started to regulate profits in 1957 through a voluntary, non-statutory Pharmaceutical Price Regulation Scheme. Under the 1999 Health Act, the government acquired the power to impose statutory price and profit controls on those companies that chose not to sign up for the voluntary scheme. In France in the 1980s, the profit margins of manufacturers, wholesalers, and pharmacists were regularly reviewed and adjusted downwardly. Since 1994, there has been more cooperation between the government and the National Union for the Pharmaceutical Industry through "framework agreements," of which over 140 had been signed by 2004, covering 97% of turnover. Germany presents a dichotomy in this respect. On the one hand, it has regulated the distribution of drugs through wholesalers and pharmacies in detail. On the other hand, its regulations regarding pricing by the industry and proof of efficacy are very liberal.

Governments try to control the price of pharmaceuticals through a variety of measures. Italy revised the distribution margins downward in 1994. Moreover, the country's government imposed a nationwide drug expenditure budget. Spain reduced the profit margin for wholesalers from 12% in 1997 to 9.6% in 1999. Finland introduced a regressive formula for determining pharmacy profit margins in 1997. Belgium and Denmark introduced price freezes in 2000, and the latter country also imposed (temporary) price ceilings and price cuts. Since 1993, when Germany introduced "spending gap" regulations, physicians' associations and the pharmaceutical industry have had to pay for overspending.[163] Similar developments can be observed in Italy, where private companies, wholesalers, and pharmacists are responsible for paying 60% of the costs of exceeding the nationwide drug expenditure budget.[164] Also popular is the idea of reference-pricing, allowing the price of a drug not to exceed that of a certain average of comparable drugs in a number of other countries.[165] Reference-priced drugs, which accounted for 15% of the German drug market in 1997, have since grown to more than 60%.[166] The pharmaceutical industry countered reference-pricing partly through above-average increases in the prices of non-referenced-priced drugs.[167] People who prefer these non-reference-priced drugs have to pay copayments. Finally, there is cost-effectiveness pricing with pharmaceutical companies seeking eligibility for reimbursement having to submit economic studies to prove the effectiveness of their products. Canada in 1995, and Finland in 1999, introduced such a requirement.[168]

Additional measures of control include the substitution of generics for trademarked counterparts, as well as the shift to parallel imports. The peculiar thing with generics is that they are very popular in some countries and almost non-existent in others. Generics in Denmark, for example, accounted for 49% of total pharmaceutical expenditures in 1999, which is far more than in France, 2% (of reimbursable drugs); 1% in Belgium; or Spain, only 0.2% of total public pharmaceutical expenditure in 1999. It is likely that the copayment level, as well as the price difference between generics and trademarked drugs, played a role here. In Austria, for example, prices for trademarked drugs are generally only 10% above those of generics. Besides, generics are not always available.[169]

A very important control measure is the screening of the need for and the effectiveness of drugs. In this respect, in 1982 the Irish had already deleted about 900 over-the-counter medicines from the list of reimbursable drugs and medicines.[170] The Netherlands started need and effectiveness evaluations in 1996. This resulted in the removal of a large number of reimbursable drugs from the coverage package.[171] Here, the distinction between positive and negative lists is important. Negative lists, as opposed to positive lists, represent drugs which are no longer reimbursable. Most EU countries have these types of lists. Once they exist, they are updated regularly. Spain, for example, introduced a negative list in 1993 which excluded almost 900 drugs from public funding. After updating this list in 1998, a further 830 were excluded. France set up its Commission on Transparency in 1999. It reevaluated drugs in accordance with defined criteria, declaring 835 ineffective between 1999 and 2001, and removing 84 from the French positive list in 2003.

Finally, there are several measures directed at drug prescription practices. The Danish Institute for Rational Pharmacotherapy, established in 1999, for example, develops guidelines and provides information for the rational use of pharmaceuticals. A similar organization, Pharmacet, was established in 1996 in Belgium. The British introduced a system of indicative prescribing budgets for general practitioners in the beginning of the 1990s. Denmark and Sweden have special pharmaceutical committees to promote effective prescription behavior. Additionally, most counties in Denmark have units that undertake medical audits, although, in contrast to the situation in Austria, doctors who persistently fail to adhere to prescription guidelines are not likely to be financially penalized.

Do all these measures of control significantly influence drug expenditures? The answer is uncertain. In most EU countries, pharmaceuticals expenditure as a percentage of total health care expenditure increased considerably. Taking as a starting point the year 1980 (=100), increases varied between EU countries from a relatively low figure of 106 for Belgium in 1997 to a relatively high figure of 197 for Sweden in the same year.[172] Only Germany experienced a decrease to 95 in 1996, probably as an initial result of the introduction of the spending gap during that period.

We will never know what the increase would have been if EU governments had not taken all these control measures, including the screening of pharmaceuticals for their effectiveness. To begin with, the effects of increasing copayments are not clear from the available material. Modified copayment rules in Italy, dating to 1994, for example, only marginally influenced the share of public expenditure on pharmaceuticals (from 59% in 1996 to 57% in 1999). Spain, on the other hand, saw an increase in public expenditure on pharmaceuticals from 100 to 245 over the period 1990–1998, with copayments as a percentage of total public expenditure decreasing from 100 to 70.

As for governments dealing with pharmaceutical companies regarding the prices of drugs, it is likely that expenditures would have been considerably higher had governments left price-making completely to the market. In this respect, developments in the United States, where drug prices are not regulated,[173] are rather disturbing. Here, prices for prescription drugs increased by around 18% per year during the 1990s. Today the figure is still 15%,[174] with Americans currently spending some $200 billion a year on drugs.[175] Contributing to this development have been the effective lobbying, marketing, and legal activities of American drug companies. In 2002, the pharmaceutical industry employed 675 lobbyists, more than one for each member of Congress, at a yearly cost of over $90 million.[176] In addition to this, the industry gives copiously to political campaigns[177] and tries to buy "fiscal influence" at the federal and state level.[178] Furthermore, acknowledging that doctors are a big target, American drug companies paid for 60% of their continuing medical education in 2001, under the guise of marketing.[179] The objective is, of course, to influence doctors' prescription behavior. Apparently, the American pharmaceutical industry has been very successful in pursuing this objective, since prescription drugs' share of the overall pharmaceutical market tripled during the period 1980–2000.[180] And, of course, pharmaceutical companies try to influence consumers directly. Ordering medication through the internet, the so-called "pill channels,"[181] is on the increase, while a good deal of health information in doctors' waiting rooms is supplied by the pharmaceutical industry.[182] Furthermore, as for legal activities, the industry employs small armies of lawyers who have been successful in extending the patents of brand-name drugs from about eight years in 1980 to about fourteen years in 2000.[183] Finally, the pharmaceutical industry did not hesitate to exploit the fear among Americans surrounding the anthrax attacks after September 2001, 11, claiming to be "part of the nation's defence system."[184]

Drug companies are very aggressive in defending their market position. This is understandable, since the stakes are very high. In 2001, the net return of ten American drug companies on the Fortune 500 list, whether measured as a percentage of sales (18.5%), of assets (16.3%), or of shareholders' equity (33.2%), was astonishingly high compared to the other companies on that list, which had to settle for a net return on sales of only 3.3%.[185]

Profit margins of the five European pharmaceutical giants[186] (GlaxoSmithKline, AstraZeneca, Novartis, Roche, and Aventis) are similar to those of their American counterparts.[187]

Although one could argue about the morality of such high net returns, the problem is more the way the pharmaceutical industry defends its relatively high pricing policies.[188] Here, the first and foremost argument is that the industry needs an enormous amount of money to cover the costs of its research and development activities.[189] In 2001, the industry claimed that these costs were about $800 million for each new drug.[190] The reality is, however, not only that this amount has been estimated to be eight times too high, but also that the bulk of the research work is done in government and university laboratories, i.e., with public finances. This research is the real basis for the development of innovative drugs. For example, the American Institutes of Health found in 1995 that 16 out of 17 scientific papers which led to the discovery and development of five top-selling drugs (Zantac, Zovirax, Capoten, Vasotec, and Prozac) came from outside the pharmaceutical industry.[191] This may explain why American drug companies have close connections these days with universities, which may even lead to "the merging of commercial and academic interests,"[192] with drug companies hiring faculty members as consultants, paying them nicely, but claiming monopoly rights on their discoveries in return, or at least establishing business relations of mutual interest.

Apart from this, drug innovations are not as numerically impressive as the pharmaceutical industry wants us to believe. Regarding this, Angell comes up with a figure of only 12 innovative drugs introduced per year during the period 1998–2002, out of a total of 415 new approved drugs.[193] The majority of the rest are so-called "me too" drugs. They are the industry's main business. They are imitations of preexisting drugs, with very small alterations that are just enough for them to be classified as new by the American Food and Drug Administration. This practice is called the "evergreening" of drugs.[194] These drugs are not more effective in treating diseases than the preexisting ones. Therefore, they have to be marketed to gain a place among the other drugs. And this is where most of the industry's money, around 35%, goes: marketing. Marketing has diverted the pharmaceutical industry from its original purpose of discovering and producing useful new drugs. Instead, the industry has become a "marketing machine" to sell drugs of sometimes dubious benefit. And for this it "uses its wealth and power to co-opt every institution that might stand in its way, including the U.S. Congress, the Food and Drug Administration, academic medical centres, and the medical profession itself," according to Angell.[195] There are even cases of bribery and fraud in the generic drug approval process.[196] As for the medical profession, drug companies appear to offer medical doctors large bounties, up to $12,000, for each patient they enroll in clinical trials testing the effectiveness of new drugs.[197] If the history of the pharmaceutical industry was one of promoting drugs to treat diseases, it often seems to be the opposite these days, with drug companies promoting diseases to fit their drugs.[198]

All in all, there is a huge gap between the pharmaceutical industry's rhetoric of working for the benefit of humanity and its practices. The reality is that the pharmaceutical industry, like any other corporate entity, is just big business with all the usual trappings, including the phenomenon of CEOs overpaid with huge salaries and generous stock options.[199] The consequences of this "corporatization" are often negative. One example would be the underproduction of necessary childhood vaccines, because the profits they deliver are assumed to be too small.[200]

Meanwhile, for several reasons, the tide seems to be turning against the pharmaceutical industry. Firstly, people no longer believe that the high prices of drugs are a necessary condition for research and development, because they realize that this is not the industry's core business. Secondly, insurers have started to negotiate considerable discounts, while at the same time using lists of preferred drugs (formularies). Thirdly, American pharmaceutical companies may soon find themselves caught in the crosshairs of federal investigators (the Justice Department, the Food and Drug Administration, the Federal Trade Commission, and the Department of Health and Human Resources) regarding their pricing, sales, and marketing policies. Already, one pharmaceutical company has had to pay a fine of $875 million.[201] Finally, the flow of really new and innovative drugs is decreasing. These are all signs that the prosperous times for the pharmaceutical industry may be over. Some drug companies that have started to realize this have meanwhile introduced discount cards for low-income American senior citizens in an attempt to improve their present image as "the most resented industry."[202]

As a further consequence, the industry has started a process of downsizing. Pfizer announced in 2003 that it planned to save $2.5 billion by closing five research centers worldwide, and Merck announced a layoff of 4,400 employees in the same year.[203]

Compared to the United States, the countries of the European Union are way ahead when it comes to regulating prices and availability of pharmaceutical products. This has greatly benefited members of the European Union. For example, a recent estimate shows that Italians pay 53% of what Americans pay in cash for the same brand-name drugs. For the French, the Swedes, the Germans, and the British, these figures are 55%, 64%, 65%, and 69%, respectively.[204] Nevertheless, there still are considerable differences between member states regarding drugs prices and policy. These member states should realize, however, that due to the aging of the population, more drugs at affordable prices may be necessary. Therefore, it would be wise to create a unified European market for drugs by regulating market entrance and price-making at EU level. It is hard to imagine what the objections would be to the recent idea of the Belgian Minister of Health regarding raising the regulation of certain drugs to the EU level.[205] It would not subvert the subsidiarity principle, as all member states could jointly benefit from this kind of common approach. To be sure, I am absolutely not against private business making a reasonable profit, but a net return on sales of 18.5%, or on shareholders' equity of 33.2%,[206] as was the case in the United States in 2001, seems more like taking advantage of sick people.

Despite all the criticisms made regarding the pharmaceutical industry, however, its positive contribution to the developments in health care should not be forgotten. The pharmaceutical industry has played an important role in increasing effectiveness and efficiency in health care provision. Preventing hospital admission, decreasing the average length of stay in hospitals, as well as substituting treatment in outpatient clinics and day care facilities for in-patient treatment, for example, would certainly not have been so successful had it not been for the availability of effective drugs.[207] Moreover, research indicates that the availability of new drugs has a potentially positive influence on employees' productivity.[208]

Still one more point has to be made. It may be true that the rate of medical innovations is declining, with chemists finding that "they are scrapping the bottom of the barrel of chemical compounds that can be synthesized and screened for their therapeutic potential" (see 8.4); and it may be true that over the period 1998–2002 only 12 innovative drugs were introduced out of a total of 415. Nevertheless one of those 12 might have meant a breakthrough in combating a thus far untreatable disease. Because of this possibility, few would really like to see the pharmaceutical industry slowing down its research activities.

9.4.2 Cost-Sharing

In their attempts to contain the costs of health care, all governments of the European Union resort to measures which reduce the collectively financed part of their health care systems. In the terms of this book, this means that governments are moving to the right side of the continuum, leaving things increasingly to the market and stressing people's personal responsibility for their health. The instruments governments use, in this respect, are out-of-pocket payments, user charges, copayments, co-insurance, deductibles, limiting the coverage package, and conversion methods. Although these notions refer to different ways of shifting the balance from collective to private financing, they are all instruments of cost-sharing, meant to influence the demand side of health care. The latter term combines all the attempts to move heath care to the market by (partly) shifting payment for services to the consumers.

If one reviews what is going on in the countries of the European Union in this respect, the first thing that catches the eye are the huge differences between countries in the share copayments make up of total health care expenditure, varying in 2003 from 2.7% in the United Kingdom to 44.6% in Portugal.[209] Furthermore, cost-sharing measures are enormously diverse despite their common increasing importance as a source of financing health care.[210]

Belgians, to begin with, saw copayments (e.g., patients paying a certain fixed amount of the cost of a service with a third party paying the rest[211]) increase from 12% to 17% during the period 1987–1994. From 1998 to 2002, this increase was 27%. Another Belgian method of cost-sharing was the conversion of acute and chronic hospital beds into beds for rest and nursing homes, as well as into beds for psychiatric care homes. This conversion resulted in savings for the insurance companies because patients in the latter types of institutions have to pay a much higher share of the costs.[212] In Italy, user charges for outpatient care were increased from 15% in 1982 to 50% in 1991.[213] Germany, with a long tradition of cost-sharing, introduced copayments in the 1980s for in-patient hospital days, rehabilitative care, and ambulance transportation. The country markedly increased cost-sharing measures in 1997.[214] Austria saw a rise in out-of-pocket expenses from 16.3% in 1980 to 25.1% in 1996.[215] Finally, although the United Kingdom's NHS funding is limited to only 2% from user charges, prescription charges for drugs, which had already been introduced in 1952 and increased 18 times since then,[216] rose by 300% over the period 1971–1993, adjusted for inflation.[217] Other EU countries show similar developments, with pharmaceuticals as the main item for policy action.

Related to increased cost-sharing is the phenomenon of different types of voluntary supplementary insurance in addition to statutory systems, for coverage of services not included in the compulsory scheme. In Belgium, for example, additional insurance for hospitalization, is growing steadily (by almost 30% during the period 1993–1996) and covered around 30% of the population in 1999. Although its turnover is still small, this country also has a growing for-profit insurance market.[218] In the United Kingdom, voluntary private health insurance expanded dramatically during the 1980s, particularly as a result of employment-based schemes. Coverage through the private insurance market peaked in 1990, applying to 11.5% of the population.[219]

The reason people take out voluntary supplementary insurance appears to relate to decreasing benefits under statutory schemes or dissatisfaction with the functioning of the health care system. In France, for example, voluntary health insurance is developing rapidly due to the demand for better coverage and the slow but significant erosion of the statutory coverage package. In 1960, voluntary supplementary insurance covered 33% of the population; in 2000 this figure was 86%. However, the quality of supplementary insurance coverage in France varies with social status and level of income, with over 50% of the low-income population having no supplementary coverage.[220]

Since the beginning of the 1980s, Sweden has also seen a growing interest in private health insurance, with many citizens wishing to avoid waiting lists for certain medical treatments.[221] The voluntary health insurance market in Denmark, though small, is becoming increasingly popular.

Although voluntary health insurance traditionally mainly covered dentists, drugs, and eyeglasses, nowadays people also seek insurance for treatment in private hospitals, largely as a consequence of long waiting times and assumed "poor service" in public hospitals.[222] Among the reasons Portugal is experiencing a growth in the private insurance market are difficulties in accessing the country's national health service and dissatisfaction with its services.[223] In Austria, supplementary insurance is offered by private for-profit insurance companies. Reducing waiting times for tests and therapeutic services are among the reasons why around one-third of all Austrians have taken out this supplementary insurance.[224]

There are considerable differences between EU governments regarding the tax aspects of cost-sharing and voluntary supplementary insurance. Some governments appear to encourage voluntary supplementary insurance. In Portugal, for example, tax incentives dating to 1998 have stimulated high-income earners and companies to take out private insurance.[225] Tax-expenditure subsidies in this country are estimated at 4.8% of direct tax revenue, or between 0.2% and 0.3% of GDP.[226] In Belgium, tax exemptions apply to all households, which means that Belgians can deduct their copayments and supplementary insurance, beyond a certain amount, on their income tax forms.[227] In Britain, where private insurance appears to be heavily skewed toward higher socioeconomic groups, the government introduced tax relief in 1991,[228] while Italy established tax benefits for supplementary health insurance in the late 1990s.[229] On the other hand, the 28% of the Danish population who took out private voluntary insurance in 1998 could not deduct the related premiums from their taxable income.[230] Finally, a 1998 Swedish law prohibited the deducting of private insurance premiums from one's personal income tax.[231]

All in all, as regards cost-sharing as an instrument for cost containment, policies of EU governments reveal a patchwork of different attempts to introduce the market into health care provision, albeit with detailed regulations to protect those who cannot participate in that market. I will come back to this matter in the next chapter.

9.4.3 Financing Hospitals

During the period 1960–1980, reimbursement for hospital activities was, in the majority of EU countries, hardly more than letting third parties or the government pay the bills that hospitals sent out. The parameters were simple (bed-days, medical interventions, laboratory test, fee-for-services, et cetera), and financing was open-ended. The more you did, the more you could bill, and the more money you got paid. This mechanism was an incentive to push up treatment prices and to increase the number of beds and keep them occupied by patients for as long as possible. This increased a hospital's income as well as the income of the self-employed medical specialists working in it. Things like controlling efficiency of hospital operations or evaluating the quality of services were hardly heard of. When, finally, around the beginning of the 1980s, governments started to realize that health care costs would get of hand completely, they also discovered their lack of means to control costs. The introduction of budgeting, therefore, was almost the only logical start, since other instruments were hardly available.

Budgeting as an instrument of cost containment has several advantages. First of all, it is a simple instrument. By declaring period t-1 to be the basis, one can easily decide that the corresponding finances will be the (prospective) budget for period t. Secondly, a budgeting system can be introduced very quickly. And exactly this road has been taken by many EU governments since the beginning of the 1980s, some a little bit earlier, others considerably later. Italy had already introduced budgeting by the second half of the 1970s;[232] Finland in 1993;[233] but Luxembourg not before 1995.[234] And, of course, there were differences between countries as regards the cost items to be included in the budget. But the simple principle was the same everywhere. A third advantage of budgeting is that this instrument can be used repeatedly if one wants to economize quickly, simply by imposing budget cuts. This path has also been followed by several EU governments. The Netherlands, for example, introduced a budgeting system in 1983 and 1984 for hospitals and long-term care institutions, respectively, followed by generic budget cuts of 2% in the following three years. The Danes acted likewise, but with a higher overall percentage cut.

Initially, budgeting proved to be very successful. It forced hospital managers to economize and to improve effectiveness and efficiency. Despite an increasing demand for health care, most hospitals and other health care institutions initially appeared to be able to cope with the imposed financial constraints, which is, for that matter, also an indication that their "organizational slack" was considerable. In the Netherlands, for example, the annual growth rate in hospital expenditure was 8.7% in the pre-budget period of 1978–1982. Budgeting reduced this growth rate to 1.3% during the period 1983–1988. However, budgeting, as it was introduced for hospitals, and subsequent budget cuts have only had a temporary effect. Governments cannot continuously use this approach without endangering quality of care, which is an equally important concern of government policy, or causing serious financial difficulties for hospitals. For example, 34% of Dutch hospitals had operating cost overruns in 1992.[235] A further criticism of imposing budgeting on hospitals is that is does not accurately reflect the relationship between hospital activities and funding.[236] However, two American views appear to be of help here.

The first is the idea of "managed care," which refers to a variety of hospital payment plans through which third-party payers try to contain the costs of hospital care by strictly controlling medical interventions and the use of resources with an eye toward increased efficiency and effectiveness.[237] Particularly in the United States, managed care has expanded enormously through health maintenance organizations (HMOs). In 1995, over

50 million Americans were enrolled in managed care plans, compared to less than 9 million in 1980.[238] In recent years, the number has further increased.[239] While the initial HMOs were non-profit organizations, in the course of the 1980s they became dominated by investor-owned for-profit corporations,[240] with, as in normal business life, CEOs being paid an average salary of $255,000 per year plus stock options ranging from $2.8 million to $15.5 million.[241] The benefits of HMOs are not uncontested, however. HMOs are criticized for denying patients' needs, limiting access, and placing profits before patients. These criticisms were one reason why state governments enacted around 120 regulations addressing these issues in the late 1990s.[242] A 1999 American survey revealed that only 37% of respondents felt that managed care organizations "do the right thing."[243] Furthermore, in the same year, 42 American states established rules governing "drive-through deliveries," meant to counter irresponsibly rapid dismissals from hospitals.[244]

It is important to note that HMOs have contributed considerably to changing the power relations between health care providers (doctors and hospitals) and payers. Providers were in control of the financial developments until around the beginning of the 1980s. The introduction of prospective budgeting systems can be pointed to as the dawning of a new era, to be sure, but with the introduction of managed care in the American health care system, power shifted essentially from providers to payers.[245]

American ideas on managed care are slowly gaining a foothold in EU countries. The Irish branch of BUPA (a British voluntary health insurer), for example, generated opposition from physicians when it insisted on detailed information before admitting psychiatric patients, including the diagnosis, prognosis, and expected date of discharge. Apart from the fact that this policy stigmatized patients, it also caused serious delays in admission. Similarly, an Austrian report from the beginning of the 1990s mentioned that Austrian hospital managers increasingly inform physicians that no beds are available for resource-intensive patients.[246] In general, however, to date, EU countries while seeing the advantages of managed care, seem unprepared to take the risk of endangering the quality of care which may be a consequence of uncritically imitating the American approach. Nevertheless, the technicalities of managed care, particularly the information systems needed to control medical performance, are considered positively.

However, the other American idea of setting a fee per case, determined by the patient's diagnosis, has meanwhile been embraced by many EU countries. Most countries started to explore this new approach carefully by limiting DRG payment to some specified medical interventions on an experimental basis, and slowly extending the new practice to other health conditions. Portugal, for example, introduced a DRG system in 1997, covering around 10% of medical interventions. By 2002, this coverage had increased to 50%.[247] Others initially restricted the use of DRGs to only part of the country, to a few medical specialities, or to a particular item of health care costs. In Spain, the testing of DRG pilots started in the second half of the 1990s in a few autonomous regions.[248] Finland started to use DRGs in only three hospitals districts in 2000, followed by three more in 2001,[249] whereas Belgium introduced a restricted DRG-based reimbursement system for pharmaceutical expenditure in hospitals in 1997.[250] Ireland has had an operational DRG system, covering 492 acute-care cases, since the late 1990s.[251]

It took the Netherlands some six years of deliberations before a DRG experiment, limited to a number of hospitals, could start. The country devised its own version, labeling its system "DBCs" (Diagnosis Treatment Combinations). The differences from DRGs are fourfold: (1) coding under DBCs is done after treatment and not before, as is the case with DRGs; (2) patients can be coded in more than one DBC; (3) coding is the responsibility of medical specialists instead of special personnel; and (4) DBCs include payment of physicians. The use of DBCs started in 2005 and is expected to be fully implemented within three years.[252] This Dutch variant of DRGs, and the way the system works, can lead health care providers to classify patients after treatment in the most remunerative DRG, thus resulting in "up-coding" or "DRG creep."[253] As regards the latter, the American Health Care Finance Administration has already charged several hospitals of up-coding by using inconsistent coding methods.[254]

Finally, the United Kingdom, which implemented a contracting system in the 1990s, is working on a refinement of hospital contracting practices in order to ensure that the costs of particular treatments are more accurately reflected in contract prices. In this respect, the NHS Case Mix Office has been developing "health-related groups," a British version of DRGs.[255]

The use of DRGs, with countries mostly excluding sophisticated medical interventions, has important consequences for hospital management because it forces negotiations over the price of DRGs with insurers.[256] In order to do this successfully, hospitals must have a complete understanding of their cost structure (see section 9.2.2). Consequently, management information systems are of the utmost importance. All EU countries working with DRGs are active in this area. French hospitals, for example, are involved in the Programme to Medicalise Information Systems (PMSI), which was introduced in 1983 in direct response to Medicare in the United States. PMSI developed significantly during the 1990s. Furthermore, since 1991, French hospitals have been required to evaluate their operations by producing a Standard Discharge Summary (RSS), which contains information on the nature of treatment, the examinations carried out, the diagnosis that led to hospital admission and associated diagnoses, as well as possible complications. The next step is to integrate the RSS into one of the 512 patient groupings for the classification of hospital stays, which are adapted from the American DRG system.[257] In the same vein, the Spaniards developed a new information system (Minimum Basic Dataset) which covered almost all hospitals in 1999. This information system is supposed to contribute to linking hospital contracting with levels of activity and quality issues.[258]

9.5 Summary

The objective of this chapter was to describe the trends in the development of health care systems against the background of the basic EU values of solidarity and equal access. Doing so in detail would have required presenting an enormous amount of facts, which would have made the book unreadable. Because of that, I selected of a number of items which together give a general indication of whether, with regard to health care, the countries of the European Union are moving to the right side of the continuum, as introduced in the first part of the book, i.e., choosing for the market. The selected items are classified according to four reform themes. The first theme is accountability, illustrating that the health care world is increasingly being called to account by several other stakeholders in the health care process. This theme was elaborated by means of two examples: improving quality of care and empowering patients. The second theme is organizational reform, which may be a natural consequence of health care's immanent dynamics, or the intended consequence of decisions taken by stakeholders. The theme was elaborated in three directions. Firstly, processes of decentralization as initiated by EU governments were dealt with. Secondly, attention was paid to private initiatives initiated by providers and/or facilitated by adjusting governmental regulations. Also, governments' role was sketched. The third theme, rationing and priority setting, was explained in the context of the rationing concept, followed by more explicit examples like health technology assessment and the phenomenon of waiting lists in health care, as well as clinical guidelines and protocols regarding medical performance. The fourth theme, finally, was cost containment, one of the two main objectives of health care reforms. As an illustration of the developments in this respect, government policies regarding drugs, cost-sharing, and financing hospitals were elaborated in three subsections.

10
The Effects

The reforms in health care which have been carried out during the past decades were meant to contribute to quality improvement and cost containment, while maintaining the equity principle. And, indeed, medical practice based on guidelines, protocols, or evidence-based medicine can increase the streamlining and predictability of professionals' performance. Decentralization of a health care system can lead to more involvement of local stakeholders in the development of health policy. Prospective budgeting has forced hospital managers to analyze the health care delivery process from the perspectives of efficiency and effectiveness. So has the rise of the internal market. Empowering patients has contributed to the maturation of the relation between health care providers and consumers, whereas health technology assessment has mitigated the "easy market" image of health care. Finally, cost containment measures regarding pharmaceuticals and the introduction of cost-sharing methods may have made consumers more aware that health care has its price.

Nevertheless, in relation to the basic values of the EU health care systems, i.e., solidarity and equity, one wonders if health care reforms have been carried through without harming these values. In this respect, many EU countries report developments which support the impression that health care reforms have had a negative impact. Belgium has experienced large increases in copayments that have made health care increasingly unaffordable for low-income groups.[1] Estimated cost-sharing in Denmark increased, in relative terms, by 26% between 1986 and 1995,[2] and Irish citizens saw user charges for private accommodation in public hospitals increase by no less than 1,100% in 20 years.[3] Finally, in the Netherlands, the number of unpaid bills (both specialists' and general practitioner's), as well as unpaid insurance premiums, doubled in 2005.[4] Now, there is nothing wrong with reforms like cost-sharing measures or reducing the coverage package, i.e., introducing the market into the health care system, provided that everyone can afford to participate in that market. Acknowledging that such participation is not possible for all their citizens, EU governments, therefore, have taken actions to prevent people from being excluded by making exemptions to the (new) rules in order to uphold the basic values of their health care systems. This is what the first section of this chapter is about: equity.

In the second section, attention will be paid to the managerial consequences of all the regulations that have flooded the health care world since it entered the era of accountability. Increasingly, individual health care providers are complaining about the administrative burden they have to endure. Compliance with these new administrative requirements, they claim, has come at the expense of the time they can spend on what they are there for: helping patients effectively and efficiently. This may be one of the reasons why "burn-out" and disinterest among medical professionals are on the increase. A study by the London-based Policy Studies Institute found that the proportion of doctors working "with regrets" about their chosen career increased from 14% in 1966 to 58% in 1986.[5] One may safely assume that a repetition of this study today would result in a considerably higher "with regrets" percentage. Since then, after all, most of the administrative burden has been put on the medical professionals' shoulders. Health care managers have also had to cope with an increasing administrative burden. Part of this is reasonable, some of the administrative tasks seem to exist only to satisfy bureaucratic needs, and some can be labeled the consequence of institutionalized mistrust. The latter phenomenon has led to a management paradox; i.e., on the one hand, health care managers are expected to behave as business-like entrepreneurs and, on the other hand, that behavior is constrained by very strict control mechanisms which are, in turn, a particular interpretation of the accountability principle in health care.

In the third and final section of this chapter I will assess the balance of all the reform measures EU governments have carried out since the beginning of the 1980s. Here, I will deal with the question of whether cost containment has been successful, and I will speculate about the future in this respect. More specific, I will deal with the question of what may be expected regarding further developments of EU health care systems, including the consequences for their defining principles of solidarity and equity.

10.1 On Equity

One of the factors which causes an upward pressure on public health expenditure is "moral hazard" caused by consumers who believe that they are entitled to all that is medically possible because they have paid for it through premiums or taxes, or by providers who think similarly. Moral hazard, therefore, refers to excessive and unnecessary utilization of health care resources. In order to counter this behavior, one can let consumers pay for (part of) health care consumption by introducing cost-sharing measures, assuming this will make them more aware that health care also has its price.[6] Here is where the market for health care starts. The advantages are threefold. Firstly, it may decrease the demand for unnecessary health care, with consumers no longer visiting their physician for trivial reasons. Secondly, it will reduce upward pressure on public expenditure. Thirdly, it can raise revenues to supplement the public health care expenditure budget.[7]

The problem with introducing a market to health care this way, however, is that it may be at odds with the fundamental values of EU health care systems: solidarity and equity. After all, introducing a market is one thing; the ability to participate in that market is another. And since cost-sharing measures for acute care, as well as the exclusion of services from reimbursement, put a greater strain on the budgets of lower-income households compared to higher-income ones, these measures may negatively influence the equity principle. In this respect, it should be noted that there is evidence that health care consumption by lower-income groups is more responsive to cost-sharing measures than that of more wealthy groups.[8] Consequently, lower-income groups' demand for health care may decrease for financial reasons. However, these negative influences may be mitigated if health care consumers can take supplementary insurance to offset cost-sharing measures. But apart from the fact that it is not always possible to take supplementary insurance, consumers may not be able to pay the extra premium. All in all, due to the delicate relationship between the market and the solidarity principle, the introduction of cost-sharing measures in health care is not as simple as it may seem. Because of this, these measures are often a topic of intense political debate in EU countries. In practice, therefore, cost-sharing measures tend to be rather incremental deviations from the status quo, coupled with specific regulations to exempt vulnerable groups of citizens designed to uphold the equity principle.

The delicacy of cost-sharing measures can be illustrated by several side effects which accompany their introduction. First of all, cost-sharing measures may easily provoke popular protest. In France, for example, an overall increase in copayment rates in 1967 had to be withdrawn one year later because of demonstrations of public discontent. After that, it took 25 years before the French government dared to introduce a cost-sharing measure again.[9] Likewise, attempts by the Italian government to introduce copayments for hospitals stays in 1989 and for hospital emergency services in 1994 had to be withdrawn because the Italian people refused to accept them.[10] Similarly, the Spanish government was confronted with a sudden outburst of public opposition when it tried to introduce some moderate cost-containment measures in 1991, because the Spaniards believed this to be an attempt to privatize the health care service.[11] In general, cost-sharing does not seem to be acceptable at all in Spain, and therefore politicians currently "refuse to legislate for it."[12] Finally, the Danish government did not introduce user charges for visits to general practitioners and hospitals because it feared a reduction in the use of the services concerned by the poor.[13]

Secondly, health care providers may disregard or bypass cost-sharing measures. Hospital patient charges in Greece, for example, have had a minimal effect, because hospitals simply did not levy the charges for administrative reasons, whereas Portuguese providers disregarded levying charges because of the bureaucracy involved.[14] In Ireland, the exclusion of certain drugs from the list of reimbursable products in 1982 resulted in the prescription of newer and more expensive alternatives because they were free. Consequently, the 1989 Irish Department of Health restored two of the delisted categories, pain-killers and anti-acids, to the list of reimbursable products.[15]

Thirdly, there is a lack of consistency regarding cost-sharing measures, making them a matter of trial and error. Cost-sharing measures may ebb and flow with changes in a country's political constellation.[16] Portugal, for example, introduced substantial cost-sharing measures in 1982 which were abolished after the 1986 elections. In 1987, such measures were even thought to contravene the Portuguese constitution, but after the constitution was amended in 1989, cost-sharing measures were re-introduced in 1992.[17] The Dutch government introduced co-insurance in 1997 for those insured under the Sickness Fund Act of 20% of medical costs up to a yearly maximum of €90 (excluding GP visits, basic dental care, and hospital costs of pregnancy), as well as a daily copayment for hospitalization services of €3.62, but it abolished these measures in 1999.[18] The Germans reduced cost-sharing in some areas during the 1970s but increased them again some time later;[19] while France introduced rationalization plans for health care as frequently as every 18 months on average during the final two decades of the 20th century.[20]

The latter point may also be regarded as an indication that governments do realize that the use of cost-sharing measures may easily be, or may be assumed to be, at odds with the basic values of solidarity and equity in health care. While attempting to introduce cost-sharing methods, therefore, governments enact corresponding regulations to preserve solidarity and equal access by exempting specific (groups of) citizens from cost-sharing measures. Without such regulations, cost-sharing would cause inequity in the financing and receipt of health services.[21] Exemption regulations can be very detailed. France, for example, has three types of exemptions. Firstly, some exemptions are linked to a person's health status, and exemptions are granted in particular for people who are suffering from one of 30 (!) specified long-term illnesses (diabetes, AIDS, cancer, psychiatric illnesses, incapacitating diseases, et cetera). The second type of exemption is linked to the nature of the treatment provided (treatment in hospitals, infertility treatment), and the third group of exemptions applies to special cases (people involved in accidents, pregnant women, disabled children, et cetera).[22] Germany, as a second example, also has detailed exemption regulations. First of all, Germans on very low incomes and those on unemployment benefits or social welfare are exempted from cost-sharing regulations, except for hospital treatment. Secondly, children up to the age of 18 years are exempted, except for co-insurance payment for crowns, dentures, and copayments for transportation. Thirdly, all cost-sharing for other sickness funds' members regarding pharmaceuticals, non-physician care and transport (except for hospitals and rehabilitation centers) is limited to 2% of a single person's yearly gross income. This threshold is lower if two or more people are dependent on one income. For the latter group, co-insurance payments for crowns/dentures are also lower. The fourth category of exemptions concerns chronically ill people who have spent at least 1% of their gross income on pharmaceuticals, non-physician care, and transportation. Above this level, they are exempted for the further duration of that chronic illness. In contrast to the third category, however, this exemption applies only to the individual person concerned.[23] Finally, Greece has a copayment rate for pharmaceuticals of 25%. However, the country has special regulations for the treatment of certain diseases, including Parkinson's disease, diabetes, heart diseases, rheumatoid arthritis, tuberculosis, chronic obstructive pulmonary disease, ulcerative colitis, Crohn's disease, and liver diseases. Again, we see a very detailed regulation of exemptions.[24] Similar exemption regulations can be found in the other countries of the EU.

Introducing cost-sharing measures, as well as exempting people from these measures, requires the setting up of administrative systems to ensure, among other things, that the revenue side has to be higher than the cost of collection. In this respect, the Portuguese discovered in 1995 that the financial impact of copayments accounted for only a little over 1% of the running costs of hospitals and health centers.[25] Similarly, in 2001 the Austrians were considering the abolishment of a simple cost-sharing measure introduced in 1997 regarding visits to a general practitioner because of the corresponding costs of administration involved.[26]

Where exemption regulations apply, the costs of administration to protect equal access must not be underestimated.[27] The more people are exempted, the more extensive the administrative system has to be. The Italian government, for example, having introduced copayments for prescription drugs in 1991 but exempting the 25% of the population who were responsible for 75% of the total public pharmaceutical expenditure, raised the question, whether the costs of administration did not exceed the intended savings.[28] Furthermore, the British government in 1989 restricted free vision testing and the supply of eyeglasses, to 40% of the UK population (children, full-time students, low-income individuals, registered blind citizens, and people suffering from specific eye diseases), which raises similar questions.[29] The same question applies to pharmaceuticals since, during the mid-1990s, 84% of pharmaceutical prescriptions in the United Kingdom were dispensed to people who claimed exemptions.[30] Obviously, exemption regulations are time-consuming and costly to administer.

One can wonder, therefore, whether cost-sharing measures contribute significantly to cost-containment. This is very doubtful. Firstly, the share of cost-sharing versus overall health care expenditure needs to be taken into account. In countries with a relatively low level of cost-sharing in total health care expenditure as, for example, the Netherlands and the United Kingdom, the measure has a negligible effect on overall expenditure. In countries with a relatively high level—for example, Portugal—the effects of cost-sharing may be neutralized through voluntary supplementary insurance or through exemption regulations for specific (groups of) citizens. Furthermore, if cost-sharing amounts are set too low, they will not sufficiently discourage consumption. If, however, they are set too high, people may take supplementary insurance, with governments applying exemption regulations for those who cannot afford such insurance.[31] In both cases, again, consumption will hardly be affected.[32]

Besides this, there is the problem of exempting elderly people, which many EU countries do. Leaving aside the fact that many elderly people have sufficient financial means to be excluded from exemptions, it is questionable whether this measure is sustainable with the number of elderly people growing as a percentage of the population.

On the other hand, one can wonder what would become of people who cannot participate in the health care insurance market if governments had not made exemption regulations. Here, the experience of Finland is interesting. According to the European Observatory Report of 2002, Finland has no exemptions from user charges for low-income groups. These people have increasingly sought subvention through the social welfare system. A survey from 1996 showed, however, that the share of households in the lowest income group that had to resort to assistance from relatives and friends or to municipal support to cover their medical expenses increased from 2.1% in 1987 to 8.4% in 1996 (relatives and friends) and from 3.2% to 7.3% (municipalities).[33]

Finally, I wish to raise the matter of vouchers. The United Kingdom uses vouchers to help certain priority groups in the area of ophthalmic services for children and those in low-income groups. In 1996/1997, almost 4 million vouchers were issued.[34] Comparable measures were taken in Sweden in relation to pharmaceuticals. In 1999, approximately 975,000 people, representing more than 10% of the population, had special cards which entitled them to free pharmaceuticals.[35] Finally, Italy introduced a voucher system for lower-income groups in 1993 so that the destitute were effectively exempted from personal contributions for medicines.[36]

Surveying the different cost-sharing measures as practiced in the countries of the European Union, it is difficult to escape the conclusion that their cost-containment effects are very limited. Although these measures are the main instrument for influencing the demand for health care,[37] in general they do not restrict health care spending because of the impact of exemption regulations and the option to take supplementary insurance. Furthermore, one can question whether it is correct to require consumers to share costs. After all, a patient who enters the health care world has only limited influence on what he is advised to consume. Consequently, one can argue that cost-sharing is a punishment for the patient who listens to his doctor.[38]

When applied to first-contact services, cost-sharing may limit demand.[39] But this type of cost-sharing would be at odds with the equity principle. The same would be true if cost containment were pursued through a reduction in the coverage package. In this respect, Saltman and Figueras correctly observe that the effect of cost-containment measures depends on the services to which they are applied, as well as on the broader context of the provider–payment system, i.e., the supply side of health care. This suggests that the individual medical practitioner's performance and the organization of institutional health care delivery, as well as the market for pharmaceuticals and medical technologies, are promising areas for implementing cost-containment measures successfully. In this scenario, excessive utilization would be countered more effectively through supply-side incentives, including the management of clinical activities.[40]

Anyway, the room for further increasing cost-sharing measures in order to contain the costs of health care, leaving aside their assumed effectiveness, seems very limited for EU countries,[41] particularly because we do know that introducing cost-sharing in health care systems with universal coverage negatively affects equal access for low-income people.[42]

Among the fundamental values of EU health care systems is the idea that people should have equal access to health care according to need. The financial circumstances of the patient concerned, therefore, are assumed to have no significance in the decision as to who is treated first or who will be treated and who will not. Combining cost-sharing with exemption regulations as previously described can considered to be an attempt to live up to this promise. But does it really work that way? This remains to be seen.

How acceptable is it that Finnish people have to turn to their friends, relatives, or municipality to meet their health care costs, as has been alleged? A 1997 Belgian survey concluded that one-third of the population had difficulties in paying for medical care, with 8% of the families questioned occasionally postponing medical care (particularly dental care) for financial reasons.[43] Similarly, surveys conducted in Stockholm County in 1993, 1995, and 1996 indicated that between 20% and 25% of the population did not seek medical care at least one time per year for financial reasons, with people on low incomes being more strongly affected than other groups.[44] Furthermore, a study in 2001 found that 3% of the Swedish population refrained partly or wholly from medical consultations for financial reasons, with 4% saying they did so to try to avoid buying prescription drugs.[45] Research in the United Kingdom, to give another example, gave strong evidence of systematic inequalities in access to diagnosis and treatment for cardiac services, as well as for after-cancer treatment for low-income groups, whereas Finnish research revealed "inappropriate socioeconomic differences," i.e., under-utilization of services by low-income groups, regarding coronary bypass operations, hip replacement, and cataract surgery.[46] Finally, the idea of a "no-claim bonus" for those insured under a collective insurance scheme also has to be mentioned. The Germans have considered this idea but have not gone ahead with it so far[47]; the Dutch, however, have introduced it. This will probably influence equity in a negative way, because people may postpone a necessary visit to their doctor for financial reasons. After all, receiving a bonus of €200 at the end of the year is a welcome extra for many Dutch families.

Equity problems also occur at the micro-level of health care delivery. Providers must, in addition to their professional responsibilities, increasingly take account of financial considerations regarding the use of scarce resources. This is rationing at the level of the individual professionals. They ration, however, without having any publicly endorsed criteria to guide them in doing so. This leads to "an impossible 'double bind' for the health care professional, and to inequality in decisions made—an inequality which remains invisible since all these decisions remain implicit."[48] Despite all the attempts to assist the professional by making rationing criteria more explicit (for example, the Oregon experiment and the priority list of the Swedish county of Dalarna), in the end it is the individual professional who makes the final decisions. These decisions are not always based on medical criteria alone. On the contrary, there are indications that maintaining equal access is not always the determining factor in medical decision-making. Socioeconomic status or age, for example, may well influence decision-making regarding the elimination of waiting lists.[49] In this respect, research in Seattle revealed that medical criteria and social-medical aspects, as well as a patient's personal characteristics, sense of responsibility, compliance, age, and social factors led to "people-like-us"-decisions at the level of the medical professional.[50] Decisions like these are difficult to subject to accountability procedures.

Problems of equal access are also manifest as regards voluntary (supplementary) insurance. In France, for example, 20% of the population, in particular those belonging to lower-income groups, could not afford to take out supplementary insurance for the coverage of cost-sharing measures in the beginning of the 1990s.[51] However, through the Universal Health Coverage Act of 1999 (CMU), the French government provided supplementary insurance coverage for these people. In fact, the CMU is an exemption regulation on economic grounds.[52] In Ireland, half of the population has voluntary private health insurance. Of the other half, according to research in 2003, 42% said they did not take voluntary insurance because they could not afford to pay the premium.[53] With regard to premiums for supplementary health insurance, which have to be paid privately in Spain, a price elasticity of 0.44 has been calculated for the period 1972–1989, i.e., a 10% increase in the premium results in a reduction in demand by around 5%.[54] In the Netherlands, in 1995, when dental care for people of 18 years and older was removed from the coverage package for those insured under the terms of the Sickness Fund Act, around three-quarters of the population took (limited) supplementary insurance. Among those not included were more than half of all elderly Dutch citizens and people with low incomes.[55] As for the latter, the number of contacts with a dentist decreased. In contrast, visits to the dentist were more frequent in Spain for people with supplementary insurance.[56] Furthermore, there are indications in the Netherlands that, after introducing, in the late 1990s, a cost-sharing measure for people insured under the terms of the Sickness Fund Act, low-income people reduced their drugs consumption.[57] In the United Kingdom, private insurance appears to be heavily skewed toward higher socioeconomic groups, and private coverage drops sharply after the age of 65 when employment-based coverage ceases.[58] Because of long waiting lists, high co-payments, and the often unsatisfactory quality of services (particularly in the central and southern regions), Italians who can afford to pay the extra insurance premium seek care outside Italy's national health system.[59] In Spain, it is suggested that the existence of voluntary health insurance may increase inequity with negative consequences for the health of poorer people,[60] whereas in Ireland providers face incentives to offer private patients preferential treatment in public hospitals.[61]

Finally, there is the problem of the increasing cost of voluntary health insurance. Research in the United Kingdom in 2000 found that 58% of subscribers considered voluntary health insurance to be too expensive. Yearly price increases of premiums above inflation were 5% between 1991 and 1996. In particular, individual premiums, compared to group premiums, increased substantially. This was enough reason for the UK Office of Fair Trading to recommend that subscribers should be warned about the probable increase in voluntary health insurance premiums. The same increase in premiums for voluntary health insurers has occurred in other EU countries, showing that the yearly growth rate in premiums for individual subscribers is considerably higher than the yearly growth rate of per-capita total expenditure on health.[62]

Apparently, EU governments understand that equity is somewhat difficult to achieve. Some of these governments, therefore, have taken specific policy measures directed at reducing health inequalities by improving the health of the worst off in society. The United Kingdom, for example, after having concluded that health inequalities were widening,[63] developed a national framework for assessing the performance of the NHS based on six dimensions, among which fair access to services for black people and ethnic minority groups is included.[64] The establishment of 26 Health Action Zones, particularly located in areas of social and economic deprivation, was one of the actions taken.[65] In Denmark, inequalities in health care have also received increasing attention in recent years. Significant, in this respect, were the results of a comprehensive national study on mortality and life expectancy conducted between 1987 and 1998, which showed that the mortality rate for Danes with no vocational training was almost 80% higher than that of more educated people. Unfavorable living conditions, more unhealthy work environments, and a much higher mortality rate for chronically unemployed/underemployed people were said to be the cause of this difference.[66] Reducing existing large inequalities in health status and health care between geographical areas in Italy is the mandate of national and regional planners in the framework of the National Health Plan 1998–2000.[67] With its 1982 Health Care Act, Sweden stipulated the importance of equal access to health services for the entire population, with special attention to vulnerable groups (elderly, immigrants, and early retirees).[68] Furthermore, three out of four Swedish citizens believe that they will have to pay extra insurance or save money in order to be able to receive health care when they are old, whereas participants in a focus group expressed their fear that people who are already socially excluded would be particularly disadvantaged in the future because of the "Americanization" of the Swedish health care system.[69] In a 1995 survey in Spain regarding the question of whether the Spanish health care system delivered the same services to everyone, 31% of respondents thought that treatment was influenced by social status.[70] Finally, France demonstrated that the objective of equity was believed to be more important than cost containment when it passed its CMU legislation in 1999.[71]

When assessing these effects on equity, the cumulative effect should be taken into account.[72] This involves not only supplementary premiums and reductions in the coverage package (pharmaceutical products, physiotherapy), but also increases in rents, the prices of energy, increasing municipal levies, and so forth.[73] In the Netherlands, the number of tenants spending over 25% of their income on rent increased from 5% in 1981 to 25% in 1993, whereas increases in the levying of local taxes meant that people on lower incomes lost an additional 1.9% of their disposable income in the beginning of the 1980s, and this increased to 3.7% twelve years later.[74] The groups eligible for the previously mentioned exemption regulations are particularly affected by this, which is an EU-wide phenomenon. The Belgian General Report on Poverty of 1995 is a revealing illustration of poverty's impact where access to health care is involved.[75] Looking back to chapter four, there is the potential danger, if it does not already exist, that EU countries are creating a split in their societies where access to health care is concerned. As long ago as 1995, a French author spoke of "*des soins à deux vitesses*," meaning that "either we find the means to assist patients to exercise their rights by easing their access to public health care, or parallel health care structures of 'special precariousness' will increasingly develop, which will confirm a two-speed health care system" (author's translation).[76] Similarly, the Germans speak of a "*Zwei-Klassen Medizin*," i.e., one type of health care for those who can pay for it and another for those who cannot.[77] As long ago as 1996, the latter group was the focus of congresses with eye-catching themes such as "Health Care for the Poorest in Europe,"[78] "Competition and Solidarity,"[79] "Solidarity and

Inequality,"[80] and "Social Exclusion and Regeneration."[81] Themes such as these would have caused us to frown when governments started to reform their health care systems in the beginning of the 1980s. They are also themes which reveal much about the well-intentioned attempts to tackle the problems. On a positive note, we should point out that during the 1990s, a "*medical card*" or "*carte santé*" was introduced in several places within the European Union which guaranteed a certain minimum of health care for those who could not pay (Charleroi, Barcelona, Ireland, and the Lower Rhine area near Strasbourg).

In addition, there is another split in society: the distinction between "the deserving" and "the undeserving,"[82] which leads, among other things to preferential treatment for people with a job. In the beginning, political circles in the Netherlands were opposed to this possible type of split regarding access to health care. Nevertheless, the Dutch government slowly gave in. By the mid-1980s, a Dutch minister of social affairs still argued that "we in the Netherlands implicitly assume that, whatever inequalities we will accept, we will not accept inequalities in health and length of life" (author's translation).[83] In 1995, while the then Minister of Health, Welfare and Sport still said that she was not afraid of a split in health care,[84] less than one year later she allowed those who were employed to have priority for operations, albeit on a temporary basis.[85] And whereas she did not reject priority treatment outside normal surgery hours,[86] she reversed her opinion during subsequent debates in the lower house of the Dutch parliament.[87]

All in all, although equity of access according to need is still a defining principle of EU health care systems that commands popular support, there is every reason to worry about whether this principle will hold. At best, the overall picture which emerges is that "there are no grounds for complacency. The risk continues in many health care systems that the most disadvantaged do not receive the services they require in relation to their needs."[88] Pessimism about its sustainability is widespread. People fear further limitations in the coverage package; they expect that they will have to pay extra charges to cover their health care needs when they are old; they observe that some groups are treated as more deserving regarding their health care needs; and they foresee an American-like two-tier health care system with good-quality health care for those who can afford to pay for it and basic, second-rate services for those who cannot. In this respect, it is important to note that there is no difference between countries with national health care systems and those which are based on a social security system. Class-based access problems, for example, also appear to exist in social health insurance countries like Austria, Belgium, and Germany.[89] Nevertheless, the belief in equal access for all citizens, i.e., the moral basis of collective health care provision, is still the defining principle for EU citizens.[90] In the context of the present international political economy, it will be very difficult for EU governments not to let some of those citizens down further.

10.2 Regulation

Emphasizing accountability has caused an increasing administrative workload for health care providers, be they individual professionals or health care institutions. In order to acquire some control over health care providers and the quality they deliver against costs, other stakeholders, particularly governments and insurers, have burdened health care providers with an increasing mass of paperwork during the past decades. When this new approach to health care provision started at the beginning of the reform process in the 1980s, this was understandable. After all, during the period 1960–1980, the medical establishment had developed an arrogant, self-willed attitude, believing that it was not answerable to other stakeholders, simply demanding more money (and getting it) and otherwise wanting to be left alone (and getting that, too). Imposing accountability regulations, therefore, apart from the financial necessity, can be considered to have started a kind of punishment drill in reaction to decades of non-compliance by the medical establishment. But if one defines regulation as "sustained and focused control exercised by a public agency over activities which are valued by a community,"[91] and looks at how far regulating health care has proceeded to date in EU countries, one can wonder if the present accountability "regime" has not evolved into "overkill." This section examines this issue.

In its 2001 report, the American Hospitals Association stated that American hospitals have to deal with over 30 regulatory agencies at the federal government level alone. In addition to this, these hospitals have to comply with regulations issued by agencies at the state level or by non-governmental organizations. Medicare and Medicaid have regulation rules and instructions totaling 130,000 pages, which is three times the length of the federal tax code. Furthermore, in order for centers for Medicare and Medicaid services to qualify for participation in a survey process regarding certification, they have to go through a state operations manual several thousand pages long. Many of these regulations are pointless, overdone, causing much unnecessary paperwork. As an example: an American case study concerning an elderly patient who was admitted to a hospital with a fractured hip, found that filling out forms, submitting records, seeking authorization, and collecting data for several regulators, required the staff of the emergency department to spend 50% of its time on administrative tasks. For inpatient surgery, staying in a nursing home, and home health care, the figures were 37%, 33%, and 44%, respectively.[92]

Regulating health care in the United States, meanwhile, has grown to such proportions that it is no exaggeration to speak of a regulatory industry, catalyzed in particular by accreditation processes for hospitals. The total costs to the American health care system of accreditation activities by the Joint Commission on the Accreditation of Healthcare Organizations (JCAHO) alone lie between $425 and $850 million annually.[93] To receive JCAHO accreditation, American hospitals have to satisfy the prescriptions of a manual of 725 pages, containing 500 standards.[94] Walshe calculates that the costs of regulation by a selected number of seven regulatory agencies are almost $950 million annually. And this is only the tip of the iceberg, because most of the costs of accreditation fall on the organization that has to be regulated.[95] Meanwhile, the accreditation process for American hospitals starts to resemble a form of policing, since many regulatory agencies appear to employ more lawyers than doctors, giving the accreditation process a more or less judicial structure.[96]

In addition to this there are many regulations regarding cost containment. American hospitals have had to establish committees to review utilization of resources and to assure quality. They have to admit external committees to review the records of hospitalized patients from the perspective of the necessity of certain treatments. They have to comply with "certificate of need" regulations in order to be able to prove that the purchase of equipment was necessary. In short, the host of regulations that has flooded American hospitals over the past decades have made them among "the most regulation-burdened industries in the country,"[97] with doctors and nurses spending up to 50% of their time on paperwork for the collection of data demanded by external agencies.[98]

The consequence of all these regulatory measures has been that the number of administrative employees in hospitals and other provider organizations in the United States increased sixfold from 1972 to the beginning of the 1990s.[99] Similar developments in regulating health care systems (though maybe a little less rigid) have occurred in EU countries.

In the United Kingdom, the growth of health care regulation has grown sharply since 1997, when the new Labour government announced the establishment of NICE (see section 9.3.2) and the Commission for Health Improvement. After that, three new agencies (the National Clinical Assessment Authority, the National Patient Safety Agency, and the Modernization Agency) were added to the "increasingly crowded regulatory landscape."[100] All these agencies have established administrative and procedural prescriptions that health care providers have to live up to. They have issued more or less extensive manuals that providers have to follow. For care homes, regulation prescriptions are laid down in an 81-page manual; for independent health care providers (acute hospitals, maternity services, psychiatric clinics, day surgery units, et cetera), 221 pages were needed.[101] Meanwhile, NHS organizations complain about the "regulatory or inspectorial overload and fragmentation—too many regulatory agencies or oversight mechanisms, each making considerable demands for information, and sometimes conflicting with each other over the data they seek or the requirements they impose." Taking into account the fact that NHS organizations have to interact with at least 16 different agencies which regulate and oversee them, in addition to being performance-managed by the department of health and other supervisory authorities, these complaints are understandable.[102]

In Portugal, responsibility for regulation lies with the General Directorate of Health. Here, regulatory mechanisms are highly normative with extensive legal provisions. The country has numerous and sometimes very restrictive controls over pharmaceuticals, the purchase of high technology, the training of staff, et cetera; and it has established a Court of Accounts which regularly conducts external audits of Portuguese national health service performance.[103]

In Denmark, regulation at state, at county, and at municipal levels is managed through a number of formal and informal mechanisms (laws, circulars, economic restrictions, incentives, education, authorization, negotiation, information).[104]

The introduction of DBCs in the Netherlands has forced hospital managers to spend between €200,000 and €300,000 per hospital on software to be able to comply with the demands for information from the inspectorate for health care, from several insurers, and from research institutes. These stakeholders appear to think up their own diverging information needs. Fulfilling these needs costs hospitals a lot of money. According to a Dutch hospital manager, "the new system is made up of an endless number of new incentives, new rules and new control mechanisms" (author's translation).[105]

The Belgium health care system, finally, is extensively regulated by federal, regional, and municipal authorities. Federal authorities exert control over financial and economic aspects of health care. They fix accreditation standards for both hospitals and doctors. They determine the levels of insurance premiums and the amount of public subsidies, and they play an important role in capital investments. As of 1990, specific legislation reinforced the possibility of state intervention in the processes of forming contracts and agreements, including the introduction of correction mechanisms if budgetary limits are exceeded.[106]

Increasing regulation results in an increasing number of administrative support positions. The consequential expenses are estimated to amount to 15% of total national health spending. Medical professionals believe this to be excessive and argue for a reduction in overhead spending as a source of cost savings. Compared to other service industries, however, there is nothing special about health care overhead spending. American law firms, investment banks, and accounting firms, for example, saw employment in professional support staff increase by 77% during the period 1980–1992. Furthermore, in most American industries, overhead expenses fall between 20% and 35% of gross expenses, whereas technologically complex sectors (pharmaceuticals, electronics) show a figure of almost 75% of gross expenses. The same applies, for example, in European consumer-related businesses, which have to operate under "legislative, legal, product safety, sales, marketing, employer, occupational safety, environmental, financial, tax, construction and other regulatory responsibilities."[107] Compared to this, an increase of 52% in the costs of health care administration during the period 1980–1992 is relatively modest. Health care, therefore, is just going along with the general developments in society.[108] There is one important difference, however. In general, commercial services industries and industrial production firms will pass on increasing overhead expenses to their prices, taking account of their competitive position on the market. They may also compensate for these increasing expenses through measures which increase their productivity. In this respect, however, health care finds itself in a difficult position for two reasons. First of all, increasing overhead expenses have occurred during a period of price constraints, with governments and insurers pre-fixing (lower) health care budgets. Many regulatory demands have to be carried through without financial compensation. Increasing overhead expenses, therefore, have to be recovered through productivity gains. Here, and secondly, the Baumol effect mentioned in section 8.3 applies, particularly for the long-term care sectors.[109]

Although the rise in overhead expenses in health care compared to other sectors in society has been relatively modest, governments have nevertheless proclaimed their intentions to reduce bureaucracy. The Blair government of 1997, for example, promised to free the NHS from bureaucracy (to the tone of £1 billion in savings) during his first term by stripping away the bureaucracy of the internal market.[110]

Similarly, the Dutch government installed a committee to advise it on how the administrative burden of Dutch health care could be decreased. The committee, reporting in 2002, pointed to three causes of the rise and existence of this burden. The first cause was the fact that health care has to operate in a hybrid external environment characterized by multi-conduction with conflicting signals and movements which contribute to mutual distrust, thus creating the image of an unreliable government, hesitating health insurers, demanding consumers, and stubborn health care providers. Secondly, all actors in health care demonstrate opportunistic behavior, concentrating on the margins in regulations or trying to find loopholes. Thirdly, the fact that health care provision is, by definition, directed at individuals, means that extensive systems of control, procedures, and accountability have been created in such a way that, in principle, every single health care delivery item can be related to an individual case. Together, these causes have created a fertile environment for the growth of administrative obligations. The committee, distinguishing between the costs of compliance with and enforcement of the regulations, concludes that these costs, totalling €1 billion, could be reduced by around 30%.[111]

Some years later, however, neither the British nor the Dutch can say that they have reduced bureaucracy in health care.

Three other effects of regulating health care since the reform processes started in the beginning of the 1980s have to be mentioned. First of all, the health care world has turned into a patchwork of organs, institutions, committees, laws, regulations, agencies, services, advisory committees, and counseling bodies. Consequently, those involved in health care spend much of their time on coordinating, negotiating, consulting, and adjusting in order to maintain some oversight of the developments.

Secondly, health care has become the domain of technocrats. The regulations and calculation methods that have flooded health care over the past decades are produced by policy staff of governmental or insurers' offices, most of them without any experience regarding daily health care delivery.

Finally, the power relations between the actors in health care have changed. Insurers have turned into policy initiators instead of followers, and governments have increasingly taken the lead as regards the direction of health policy.

Finally, and most importantly, it has to be mentioned that, despite the enormous investments made, "it is remarkably difficult to tell what impact hospital regulation has had on the performance of hospitals or on the quality of care."[112] The same applies for other health care sectors.

10.3 The Emerging Picture

As stated in the introduction to the ninth chapter, since the start of reforms in the beginning of the 1980s, the health care community in the countries of the European Union has experienced turbulent times. In this respect, probably the most fundamental change is that the external environment is increasingly minding health care's business. Openness has been transformed into a multi-layered structure of accountability. Health care providers have to respond to the (combined) demands of different stakeholders, and these demands are many. Since they have already been extensively described in chapter nine, they will simply be summarized as follows.

The quest to improve quality caused the development of a range of instruments focusing on the structure, the process, and the outcomes of health care delivery. Several quality assurance systems have been implemented; hospitals have hired special quality-assurance staff; external agencies with expertise in quality matters have been hired for support; and annual quality reporting has been added to the task of health care managers.

Patients saw their position in health care reinforced. Governments developed patients' charters, took legal actions to give patients a say in the health care delivery process, appointed patients' ombudsmen, and established national platforms to involve patients in the development of health policy.

Health care providers have carried through organizational reforms, motivated by factors like cost containment, effectiveness, efficiency, quality improvement, workload, task performance, et cetera. Organizational reforms also have followed from changing political views on how health policy as well as health care delivery and control systems should be designed. Decentralizing the health care system was one of the options here, on the assumption that this would contribute to improvement of service delivery and greater involvement of the community in health care decision-making.

A much applauded idea has been the creation of an internal or quasi-market for health care. This second-best option, since a real health care market was not feasible, was expected to increase the flexibility, effectiveness, and efficiency of health care systems, as well as to improve medical performance. To achieve this, competition between providers and insurers has been introduced. Special agencies have been set up to assist providers in the processes of contracting, negotiating, and decision-making on the quasi-market. So far, however, there is a difference between theory and practice, since there is remarkably little evidence that competition between health care organizations does improve performance.[113] Nevertheless, competitive bidding between private and public suppliers, particularly regarding auxiliary services and sometimes even for clinical activities, has become a normal affair.

Health care providers took the opportunity to develop private initiatives, extending their range of products that could be put on the market and exploring new ways of providing services. Governments facilitated this development by relaxing legal conditions in order to create room for private initiatives. Governments even have chosen to be involved directly through partnerships with private business.

Meanwhile, governments have started to convey the message to their citizens that health care also has its price, and that, due to increasing demand, public financing of new developments in medicine can no longer be taken for granted. As a consequence, rationing in health care has become a topic of interest in almost all EU countries. Discussions and proposals on rationing, however, have mostly resulted in rather general principles and guidelines phrased in terms of human rights, self-determination, equality, and justice. Nevertheless, in daily practice, rationing has been implemented on a large scale through the use of strategies for priority setting on both the demand side of health care as well as the supply side. Since the 1980s, both sides have been the focus of health policy-makers. On the demand side, cost-sharing measures have been introduced throughout the EU, while on the supply side items like capacity planning, technology assessment, evaluating appropriateness of health care, financial constraints, and waiting lists have received increasing attention.

Through technology assessment, governments at national or regional levels have started to try to control the use of new (and expensive) health technologies, particularly focusing on their cost-effectiveness. However, the existence of a private health care market appears to have produced obstacles to control. Furthermore, a lot still has to be done regarding the differences between EU countries in areas like the assessment process, appeal procedures, and the composition of assessment teams. Finally, technology assessment is a costly and time-consuming affair, while the speed of technological developments makes it impossible to assess every new technology.

As for waiting lists in hospitals, most EU governments have argued for a long time that, by economizing on budgets, while at the same time working more effectively and efficiently, productivity in health care provision could be increased to such an extent that the problem of waiting lists would disappear automatically. Public dissatisfaction with the length of waiting times, however, has forced most EU governments to increase available capacity.

Also, the development of guidelines and protocols, as well as evidence-based and best-practice medicine, can be considered instrumental in times when balancing supply and demand is necessary, because they may increase the cost-effectiveness of medical performance. In line with this, medical performance has to be standardized. Health care institutions and medical professionals of all EU countries have become involved in this type of standardization, sometimes through private initiatives and sometimes as a result of apparent coercion by insurers or governments.

Next, cost containment through direct financial measures became a crucial item of health care reform, if not the most important one. Controlling the price of pharmaceuticals, changing the distribution margins, cost-sharing by consumers, establishing a national budget for pharmaceuticals, influencing prescription behavior, substituting generics for branded drugs, assessing drugs' effectiveness, reference-pricing, et cetera, have all been governmental initiatives to get control of ever-increasing expenditures on pharmaceuticals.

Furthermore, cost-sharing measures have been introduced and have become the most frequently used instrument of cost containment over the past decades. Since measures like these may directly influence the equity principle, governments all over the EU have enacted exemption provisions to protect vulnerable groups of citizens from cost-sharing.

Finally, reimbursement for hospital activities has changed fundamentally. Open-ended financing has been terminated and prospective budgeting has been introduced, followed by subsequent budget cuts in many countries. The next step was the introduction of new methods of calculation and pricing, and the development of ideas on managed care and diagnostic-related groups, through which governments and insurers have tried to get a grip on hospital performance by strictly controlling medical interventions and the use of resources. Consequently, management information systems have become essential for the collection of a range of data regarding the measurement of costs and the quality of care. These relatively new demands have made health care an interesting and profitable field for producers of health information technologies. In 1997, they had already sold $15 billion-worth of products to health care organizations, an amount estimated to have increased to $25 billion in 2000.[114]

All in all, these reforms have fundamentally changed the world of health care provision. Its casualness has disappeared, providers are held accountable for their performance, and patients have started to realize that health care also has its price. However, the most important question of all is whether EU governments have succeeded in achieving the main objectives of health care reforms—improving quality and containing costs—while at the same time maintaining the equity principle.

Regarding the attempts to improve the quality of care, it is useful to follow the distinctions made by Donabedian in the 1980s. He distinguished between three aspects of health care quality: (1) structural quality, (2) process quality, and (3) outcome quality. The first aspect refers to the input of resources necessary for health care provision, including credentials of personnel, staffing ratios, availability of medical equipment, et cetera. Process quality regards the follow-up of instructions and guidelines by those involved in the health care delivery process, whereas (3) outcome quality refers to the changes in a patient's health condition after treatment. Of course, outcome quality is what matters most.[115]

Taking these distinctions as a starting point, it has to be observed that, despite all the time and money spent on structural and process quality, hardly anything is (yet) known about improvements in outcome quality. Legal regulations regarding quality, the setting-up of special quality committees, accreditation systems, the hiring of staff specialized in quality matters, the implementation of quality assurance methods, surveys on patients' satisfaction, auditing, monitoring, clinical guidelines, ideas on disease management, et cetera, have all led to an increasing workload, higher costs, more insight, and more transparency as regards structural and process quality, but we simply do not know if all this has also contributed to outcome quality. What is more, we hardly know how structural quality is linked to outcome quality, and there is only limited research available on the relation between process quality and outcome quality.[116] Perhaps this explains why, through excessive and oversimplified use, the quality theme has gradually become somewhat worn out.[117]

Meanwhile, consulting firms are making a lot of money by selling their quality assurance systems, their accreditation methods, their utilization review systems, and their disease management practices to health care providers. But, again, we do not know the effect of these activities on outcome quality. American research on the effectiveness of utilization review systems in hospitals, for example, has not provided to date a systematic answer regarding their effects on costs and quality of care.[118] Furthermore, there is only limited systematic evidence that clinical guidelines and disease management have reduced costs or improved quality.[119] Indeed, though regulations that have flooded health care providers during past decades, it is very difficult to ascertain their impact on quality of care.[120] Comparable conclusions can be drawn for nursing homes in the United Kingdom and the United States, for which it is has been said that "a decade of quite aggressive and forceful [...] regulation appears to have yielded only modest improvements in performance and quality."[121] And, most importantly, despite all the quality initiatives regarding structures and processes of health care provision "the variation in quality of care by physician or by hospital is immense."[122] Quality, therefore, is still "a matter of trust."[123] And since quality starts with the physician, working on outcome quality demands more than structural and procedural regulations, no matter how useful they may be. It demands partnership between managers and professionals who come to mutual agreement on the expectations and objectives of health care delivery in an organizational climate that motivates people.[124] This is different from the image of policing, which seems to have become increasingly characteristic these days of the application of clinical guidelines, accreditation procedures, utilization reviews, et cetera.

As for cost containment, we have already seen that cost-sharing as it is currently practiced hardly contributes to this objective. Furthermore, the many regulations enacted regarding pharmaceuticals has not prevented spending on drugs from becoming an ever-growing part of total health care expenditure, and changes in the financing of hospitals have not resulted in decreasing expenditures on in-patient care. In addition, a few more items assumed to contribute to cost containment have to be reviewed. First of all, ideas on managed care, coming from the United States and increasingly favored by EU governments and insurers, have to be dealt with.

Despite their poor image (section 9.4.3), there is no definite proof that managed care organizations (MCOs) in the United States have a negative influence on quality of care. In contrast, research has shown that the quality delivered by managed care organizations is comparable to that delivered under traditional indemnity insurance.[125] Whether they contribute to cost containment is another story. In this respect, it is argued that MCOs realized cost savings in the 1980s by enforcing substitution of treatment in outpatient clinics for hospitalization, as well as by reducing the average length of stay in hospitals. However, comparable developments can be observed in the countries of the European Union, which in those days did not follow managed care ideas. It is true for both the United States and the countries of the EU that scientific and technological developments have mainly caused these changes, with MCOs pushing health care providers to such an extent that the average length of stay in American hospitals fell substantially more than it did in hospitals in EU countries. But substitution and reduction of the average length of stay in the United States failed to hold down the increase in total costs, as overall Medicare spending rose at an annual rate of no less than 9.5% between 1985 and 1997. It is no wonder, then, that American corporate executives deemed the costs of health care to be a "major" (60%) or "top" (35%) concern at the beginning of the 1990s.[126] Although Medicare spending slowed down somewhat from 1997 on, this was caused by a combination of other factors, like an increase in the number of enrolees and a reduction in provider payments (hospitals and physicians).[127] Reducing provider payments was not a particularly American phenomenon. EU countries enacted similar measures.[128]

Another strategy of cost containment is competition between MCOs, since employers have several MCOs to choose from and employees may easily change their MCO. Consequently, MCOs that performed relatively poorly financially went bankrupt, and the whole sector experienced financial troubles. A pre-tax profit margin of 2% in 1997 is an indication of the worrisome experience of MCOs.[129]

An response to these developments for both providers and MCOs has been mergers. While, in 1975, most American physicians worked in solo practice, today less than 25% do. Then, three-quarters of all community hospitals were independent; today most American hospitals belong to a network. The economies of scale that were assumed to materialize from merging appear to be very modest, however, except for mergers that have led to hospital closures.[130] The real reason for the merging of providers seems to have been to increase their market power so that it would be easier for them to resist MCOs' pressures to cut prices. For MCOs, the reason for merging has been mostly to increase the number of enrolees, which made it possible to negotiate bigger discounts.[131] And did all this contribute to cost containment? Given the fact that MCOs' premiums increased by 6% to 8% on an annual basis in the late 1990s, this is highly questionable.[132]

Until around the turn of the millennium, EU countries had, in general, tried to contain the costs of health care directly through the use of relatively simple instruments, such as those dealt with in the previous chapter. They also tried indirect ways of controlling their health care systems, like setting yearly maximum spending levels, decentralizing (management) responsibilities, screening the effectiveness of drugs, restrainting capacities, et cetera. And, like their American counterparts, EU providers and insurers have also tried to strengthen their position in the health care market by merging, trying to realize vertical as well as horizontal integration. MCO-like behavior, however, with health care providers becoming the "vassals of the marketplace,"[133] is relatively new for EU countries. In this respect, it would be wise for EU countries to take account of the American developments when introducing American-like methods of cost containment. The same applies for (variants of) DRG-like calculation methods, which are embraced at present by most EU governments. An important advantage of these methods is that they are a step in the direction of real health care pricing. An important disadvantage is that they demand an increase in regulation and control measures.[134] Both can make health care even more expensive than it is already.

There is another reason to be very critical of American "success stories" regarding managed care and competition. The fact that the United States already spent 7% of GDP on health care in 1975, a figure which doubled in the following 25 years, should make us suspicious. The American method of controlling health care costs has been to hire commercial enterprises for accreditation, utilization review, informatics, the development of guidelines, and what have you. The object lesson of this policy is that privately based controls regarding the costs of medical care do not work. In contrast, the simple methods used so far by EU governments appear to work better.[135] Nevertheless, for both methods, the question remains whether it is possible to contain the cost of health care while at the same time maintaining equity. I will come back to this.

What have been the effects of all these simple measures on containing health care costs in EU countries since 1980? For an answer to this question, the next graph, which is comparable to the one in chapter eight, relates the weighted EU average expenditure per capita on health care to the weighted growth of GDP per capita. Again, the figures are from OECD sources in US$ (PPP). However, in contrast to the graphs in chapter eight, covering around two-thirds of the population of the 15 EU countries from before May 2004, coverage in the following graph is around 95%.

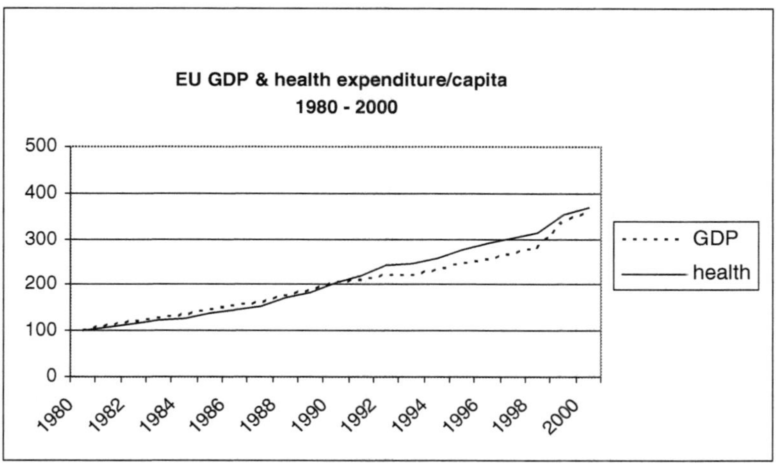

Based on different OECD health data sources.

The divergence in the lines shown in the first graph in chapter eight, with an increase in health care spending per capita over 20 years almost twice as high as the increase in GDP per capita, has disappeared. The development during the period 1980–2000 is reasonably in line with growth of GDP, although, apparently, spending on health care tends to exceed growth of GDP. In interpretating the graph, it should be kept in mind that around the beginning of the 1980s the whole idea of the welfare state became subject to reassessment. Spending on social security, for example, was restrained by the introduction of stricter regulations regarding eligibility, reach, and extension of social security provisions. As in chapter eight, in the next graph the growth in health care spending per capita is related to that of social security spending per capita.

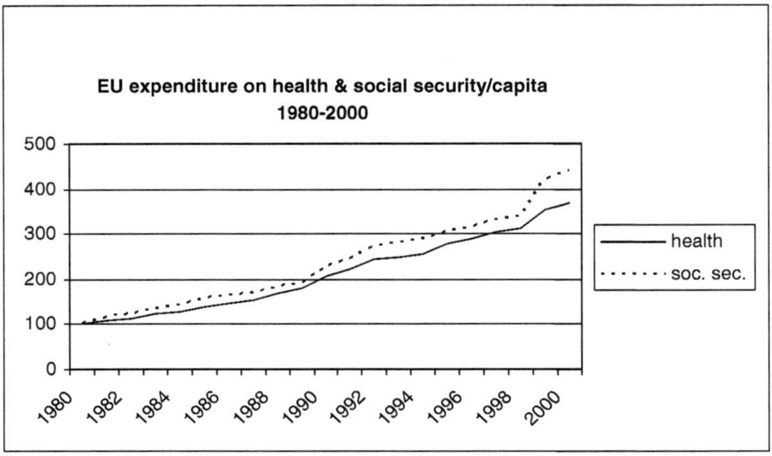

Based on different OECD health data resources.

If we compare this graph to the second graph in chapter eight, it is interesting to see that, while during the period 1960–1980 health care spending per capita grew considerably more than social security spending per capita, the roles were reversed during the period 1980–2000. The final graph suggests that EU governments have succeeded in getting control over the growth in health care spending, even better than social security spending. Both suggestions are too optimistic, however.

As for the developments in spending on social security, research has shown that, despite the general atmosphere of the welfare state's being in crisis in recent decades, reality is too complicated to enable one to draw such far-reaching conclusions. I will come back to this in the next chapter of the book.[136]

The developments in health care spending during the period 1980–2000, however, are not so much the result of governments' starting to control their health care systems and, after years of neglect, attempting to put their affairs in order financially by putting a ceiling on yearly health expenditure growth or by introducing cost-containment measures (as reviewed in chapter nine). After all, it is not too difficult to impose a system of budgeting, followed by subsequent budget cuts, after one realizes that finances have for long been provided too thoughtlessly. Furthermore, it is not too difficult to cut salaries of health care personnel and lower reimbursements for medical specialists. Both are relatively easy steps to take, but they result in "onetime savings."[137] After a certain point, budgeting will loose its effectiveness. Moreover, one cannot cut salaries and tariffs endlessly, and there is a limit to capacity reduction.

Altogether, the period from 1980 to 2000 can, for many EU governments, be considered as a time of catching-up after a long absence in terms of financial authority. Cost containment during this period, however, has hardly been more than skimming off the "organizational slack" (chapter one) which health care providers had acquired during earlier years. The big advantage has been that the period 1980–2000 has forced health care providers to think about efficiency and effectiveness. But once all the organizational slack has been skimmed off, and nothing more can be squeezed out of health care providers, it will be interesting to see how governments will show that they are capable of real cost containment without harming the equity principle. Real cost containment assumes the capability to control (future) developments in costs. In a society where the production and consumption of goods and services is largely a matter of private enterprise, governments have only limited power to do so.

Speaking bluntly, the period 1980–2000 can be labeled as the period of "cleaning up the mess." No party in particular can be blamed for this mess. Instead, it is the consequence of a kind of "collective misconduct"—misconduct by providers and consumers who thought health care was "priceless"; misconduct by insurers who for too long have operated as a serving hatch for money, only functioning as an intermediary between patients and providers,[138] and misconduct by governments who failed, or did not have the courage, to interfere. We are now nearing the end of cleaning up the mess from the past. The question, however, is, if not the methods we have used for cleaning up this mess have laid the foundations for the creation of another mess in the near future. I will deal with this in the final part of the book.

As regards the effects of cost containment on equity, we saw already (section 10.1) that governments have taken a range of (very detailed) measures aimed at the demand side of health care in order to protect certain (groups of) citizens and preserve the principles of solidarity and equal access. The effectiveness of this policy can be questioned. More important, however, is the question of whether cost containment has affected equity negatively. On the demand side, despite exemption regulations, it is still true that vulnerable people experience difficulties accessing health care services. We saw that in Finland an increasing share of lower-income households had to turn to relatives and friends to have their medical bills paid; a 1997 Belgian survey concluded that one-third of the population had problems paying for medical care, sometimes leading these people to postpone that care; 3% of Swedish people refrained wholly or partly from medical consumption for financial reasons in 2001; in the Netherlands, low-income people reduced their drug consumption as a consequence of the introduction of cost-sharing measures; and in Spain, equity may be harmed because poorer people cannot afford to pay the premiums for voluntary health insurance.

As for cost-containment measures on the supply side, limited capacities in the United Kingdom led to systematic inequalities in access to diagnosis and treatment for cardiac services, as well as for after-cancer treatment. Finland experienced underutilization of services by low-income groups when it came to coronary bypass operations, hip replacements, and cataract surgery. In the Netherlands, preferential treatment for people with a job came to be accepted, whereas privately insured patients in Germany appear to be treated faster and better than those with social health insurance.[139] In general, limited capacities have led to rationing in favor of higher socioeconomic groups in society.

The problem is, however, that assertions regarding decreasing equity cannot be substantiated with longitudinal quantitative information. We may know something about equity problems at a certain point in time, but we do not know if they have become worse over the course of time. In itself, this is remarkable. After all, governments mostly have a fair estimate in advance of the financial effects of the implementation of cost-containment measures on total health care spending. Furthermore, they have set up specific administrations to oversee exemption regulations. But there is hardly any information about what I call the drop-out effects. The Dutch government, for example, excluded the first IVF treatment (€2,000) from the coverage package as of January 2005. One may safely assume that not every candidate for such a treatment could privately afford to pay this amount of money. However, there is no insight into this effect in quantitative terms. Regarding the effects of cost-containment measures on equity, governments apparently opt for an ostrich policy, a "ready-fire-aim" approach, waiting for their citizens' reactions, and, if necessary, adjusting. That the Dutch re-included the first IVF treatment in the basic package again, albeit with a certain method of co-payment for this type of treatment, is an example of the "ready-fire-aim" approach.

The fact that there is hardly any quantitative longitudinal information available regarding the equity consequences of cost-containment measures is no reason not to be worried. After all, health care reform measures are characterized by incrementalism, with each step by itself not having a clearly noticeable effect on the equity principle, if only because, so far, "reform proposals that would threaten solidarity never achieved a political majority."[140] But the accumulation of a number of incremental reform measures may, over the course of time, reduce the equity principle; i.e., the aggregation of cost-containment measures may lead to a strategic change with the economic priority of achieving sustainable funding considered to be more important than maintaining the equity principle.[141]

Apparently, governments and citizens are not optimistic about the future in this respect. We saw already that 75% of Swedish citizens believe that they will have to pay extra premiums or save money in order to be able to afford health care when they are old. A survey of German health care institutions and organizations found that over 60% of respondents believe that further rationing in health care is unavoidable.[142]

Research in the Netherlands in 1995 showed that 82% of the population believed that, by 2020, those who can afford to pay more will receive better care.[143] Subsequent Dutch research in 2005 made it clear that a large majority of respondents are worried about future costs and capacities of Dutch health care.[144] Furthermore, the Dutch fear that, due to the new health insurance system introduced in 2006, a considerable number of citizens will be without insurance. As a last example, pointing to the pressures from demographic change, developments in medicine, consumerism, information technology, and a general rethinking of the welfare state concept, the British wonder if it will be possible "to maintain equity and comprehensive care." Furthermore, they ask themselves if the pressures of demand will "force a reassessment of what health services are provided free at the point of use."[145]

It is not unlikely that these fears, which arise as a result of moving to the right side of the continuum, will materialize in the near future. Even now, governments are showing reluctance regarding reimbursement of new, expensive drugs for certain treatments, and they are hesitating to recognize specific phenomena of physical distress as diseases. As a consequence of ongoing scientific and technological developments regarding health care, questions like these will increasingly be part of governments' agendas. They will augment the tension between setting the overall level of health care spending that is financed collectively and paying for innovations that find their way onto the health care market. In this respect, it is important to point to research which found a positive correlation between growing wealth and health care spending. It shows that, "after a certain level of income, an increase in earnings is accompanied by a disproportionately sharp rise in health care expenditure."[146] American figures show that personal consumption of privately bought medical services as a percentage of total personal consumption increased from 5.3% in 1960 to 10.3% in 1980, and then to 15.3% in 2000.[147] In a society where the government sets the overall level of spending and is not prepared to include medical innovations in the coverage scheme, people who can afford to do so will choose to opt out, turning to the private health care market within their country or outside, thus creating in a natural way a two-tier health care system.

Moreover, governments that are not willing to include new health care opportunities in the coverage package may expect popular protests. The United Kingdom, for example, has for a long time chosen to restrict the funding of the NHS. For years, its spending on health, measured as a percentage of GDP, has been among the lowest of the countries of the EU. This has led to an obsolete physical health care infrastructure, long waiting lists and waiting times, and an increasing number of British citizens choosing treatment abroad. This was the British way of controlling the costs of health care. Realizing that the effects of this policy were no longer acceptable, the British government has decided to let health care expenditure grow in five years to the EU average level. The consequence of this change in policy will be that the United Kingdom will experience the same problems of cost-containment that other EU countries are facing already.

The problems with a sector like health care are at least threefold.

First of all, innovations will increase pressure on public financing since, in general, the public expects new health care opportunities to be automatically included in the coverage package.

Secondly, the speed of innovation will set limits to collective financing. In this respect, it is no exaggeration to say that each week new devices and drugs are poured into the health care systems. Neither is it an exaggeration to say that, in health care, once a need is met, another is discovered. Progressive pressure is characteristic of health care.[148]

These two aspects together cause a meaningful upward pressure on health care spending and thus on demands for collective financing. This is nothing new. It became obvious once we started to invest in health care. Since governments have implemented reform measures, however, the financial effects resulting from progressive pressure caused by the sector's innovativeness could, so far, be reasonably absorbed by policies of "cleaning up the mess." Consequently, health care spending as a percentage of GDP did not rise dramatically after governments started to reform. But, as stated before, we are nearing the end of the period of "cleaning up the mess". However, innovation is probably here to stay. Moreover, health care will remain a labor-intensive affair. Then, continued collective financing of innovation will cause the share of health care spending as a percentage of GDP to rise. All the more so because an extra upward pressure on spending as a consequence of an aging population cannot be excluded. Such an upward pressure will further be reinforced by rising and more complex demands for health care. In this respect, demographic projections for the Netherlands for the period 2000–2020 show an increase in the prevalence of, for example, diabetes mellitus, cardiovascular diseases, heart failures, and dementia of 36%, 44%, 42%, and 41%, respectively.[149] In a recent German study, upward pressures like these have led researchers to anticipate an annual growth in expenditure on health care of around 6% to 2020.[150]

A third problem with health care is that its innovation is unpredictable. We do not know, for example, if and when the pharmaceutical industry will come up with an effective drug to treat Alzheimer's disease. If it does, it could save society enormous amounts of money, although the drug will surely be very expensive in the beginning. We also do not know if it will ever be possible to treat multiple sclerosis effectively. But if it becomes possible, that too could save society much money. However, while innovation does not necessarily mean that it will make health care more expensive, the problem is that governments cannot count on the contrary.

The ultimate consequence of this development is that, in the context of the present-day international political economy, the upward pressure resulting from innovations in health care will force governments to limit the extent of collective financing, i.e., limiting the basic package, and leave the rest to the market. This, surely, will not make governments popular with many of their citizens (which, by the way, explains government policies of incrementalism and of postponing decision-making). In this political climate, health care providers and insurers may take it for granted that governments will do their utmost to postpone choosing a "rational and clear-cut package of services"[151] as long as possible. And while postponing they will "tighten the screws" on providers and insurers, sparing consumers as long as possible because of constitutional promises. Despite the subsidiarity principle, it may be expected that "Brussels" will offer a helping hand. After all, subsidiarity becomes an option if member states cannot cope on their own. The cynical point in all this is that, as soon as the economy becomes strong (again), governments may resume embellishing their health care "cathedrals,"[152] without being sensitive to the argument that doing so will make the task of (further) economizing more difficult when the next recession forces them to do so.

Behind all this is the fundamental question of whether health care must be considered a public good at all costs. During the time when the welfare state was established, when it was widely believed that society was manageable, the answer to this question was generally in the affirmative. This remained so during the first years of the reform process, but gradually, reform measures have resulted in developments which have given us reason to modify the meaning of "public." Phenomena like opting out, preferential treatment, exemption regulations, excluding specific items from the coverage package, et cetera, have implicitly made it clear that health care is not an *inherently* public good.[153] It is a public good in so far as we are willing to define it as such. Reviewing the developments in health care during the past decades, it seems that we are becoming, apparently, less willing. However, defining the "public-good aspects" of health care, which is what you do when you define a package of services, offers only a very temporary solution because of health care's immanent dynamics. In fact, these dynamics make the task of defining the public-good aspects of health care a continuous affair, which is impracticable. It is conceivable, however, to make the question as to how far health care should be considered a public good a regular topic (say every five years) of a solidarity debate in (the European) parliament. Such a debate could result in decisions to either increase taxation in order to fund increased public spending on health care, to find a trade-off with other items of public spending, or to leave increasing provision to the market.[154] Of course, cost-saving innovations should be included in such a debate.

The present state of the international political economy is not favorable to these ideas. The focus remains dogmatically on the market as the only alternative, with reducing the costs of labor as the paramount objective for reasons of global competitiveness. Therefore it is necessary to subject the present international political economy (chapter three) to a critical analysis. This will be the topic of the next chapter.

10.4 Summary

In this chapter, the effects of the reform measures described in chapter nine have been addressed. The first section dealt with the effects of the reform measures on the equity principle. It concluded that cost-sharing measures on the demand side of health care have hardly resulted in cost containment, particularly because of the many detailed exemption regulations that came along with the introduction of these measures. As for the supply side of health care, cost containment has caused rationing of different kinds which, together with cost-sharing measures, has started to influence the equity principle negatively.

The second section dealt with the flood of regulatory measures that governments, under the rubric of accountability, have imposed on health care providers. Implementation of these measures, with the numbers of administrative personnel slowly rising to meet the numbers of caring/curing staff, has changed patient/staff ratios in health care considerably.

The third section attempted to draw a general picture of the reforms since the 1980s. It concluded that, despite all the staff, methods, and money that went into quality improvement, the results have not been overwhelming, particularly with respect to the quality of outcomes. Cost containment has been mainly a matter of cleaning up the mess: i.e., that after years of neglect, governments have finally started to do something about the developments in the costs of health care. It is questionable, however, whether governments are capable of real cost containment in the sense of controlling (future) developments. For an innovative sector like health care, this seems unlikely in democracies where the production of goods and services is, in principle, a matter of private enterprise. This conclusion will surely have consequences for the sustainability of collective financing of health care systems. Worded differently, it is precisely the innovation in health care that puts collective financing of health care systems at risk.

Part Three
Reflections

11
The Social Context Reconsidered

Life cannot be captured in mathematical equations. Because of this, in democracies, determining the optimal economic order is not a matter of arithmetic but of political debate. So is decision-making about movement along the continuum. It is also a matter of finding an *acceptable balance* between the government and the market.

When liberalism, as defined by Adam Smith, deteriorated at the end of the 19th century into the belief that government should interfere in economic life as little as possible, this created an imbalanced society, leaving many people behind and, in turn, causing social unrest.

In order to restore the balance, we started to reassess the role of government in the economic process, which resulted in moving to the left side of the continuum. In this respect, the third quarter of the 20th century was particularly important when, thanks to a period of strong economic growth, national economic orders were able to establish their welfare states. Based on economic conditions, cultural characteristics, and political constellations, some did so earlier, some later; some were rather limited, some were more extensive; but regardless, the government was in a leading position based on democratic decision-making. These welfare states were based on the belief that society was manageable through market socialism, and that governments could look after their citizens from the cradle to the grave.

This also added two new imperatives to the notion of civilization. Firstly, economic policy and social policy came to be seen as interrelated. Secondly, social security became a collective good and not something which was intended only for the poorer citizens of society. In order to achieve these objectives, welfare states established extensive bureaucracies. The result was, again, an imbalanced society, financially and organizationally. Not only did bureaucracies come to be seen as too expensive, but they also were recognized as an impediment to individual initiative and personal responsibility. In addition to this, society itself was changing; a change which can be summarized by saying that the world is becoming smaller and more complicated. Furthermore, human endeavor created increasing externalities beyond national frontiers which had to be coped with through international cooperation. As a consequence, national economic orders had to broaden their perspective to successive economic orders at the level of, for example, the European Union or even the globe. Consequently, the idea of society's manageability became even more utopian than it had already been during the heyday of market socialism.

In order to redress the new imbalance, the market was rehabilitated, with price-making as the instrument for coordination, while governments started to withdraw from the economic process through privatization and deregulation. So, from the start of the final quarter of the 20th century, we have begun to move to the right side of the continuum again, trying to find a new balance. The difference from earlier attempts to restore the balance between government and the market is that, thanks to the developments in the third quarter of the 20th century, citizens are now used to being looked after. This makes reforming the welfare state a delicate matter because it may harm solidarity, which is assumed to be what holds society together. Formulated neutrally, the challenge of finding a new balance is not to create a new imbalance in process.

11.1 Normative Economics

As was argued in section 1.1.2, there is no right or wrong answer to the question of which side of the continuum is preferable. Choosing a position on the continuum, i.e., a specific combination of government interference and market operation regarding the economic process is, therefore, a matter of normative economics. Normative economics implies taking a personal position regarding social arrangements in society. That is what the first section of this chapter is about.

My personal view, based on the information which I have presented in the first two parts of this book, is that since the final quarter of the 20th century, the developed world, by accepting ever-increasing inequalities, is on its way to a new social imbalance. To me, the way we are moving to the right side of the continuum is threatening society's solidarity.[1] In order to restore the balance again, I fully agree with Stiglitz that it is time to take up the challenge of rebalancing the state with the market.[2] Admittedly, economies can suffer from an over-intrusive government. But they can also suffer from a government that does not do the things that governments are there for, like regulating financial markets, providing a decent basic safety net for each and every citizen, or promoting a form of competition which is conditioned by protecting the environment.[3] A government that takes these tasks seriously would deal differently with the currents trends toward privatization and deregulation. Furthermore, I believe it to be nonsensical to assume beforehand that government ownership of public utilities like the water supply, hospitals, and public transport is an impediment to increasing efficiency. The recent history of privatization initiatives delivers several examples of governments that had to take regulatory measures because greater efficiency had not been achieved or, more often, because customers appeared to be worse off. The efficiency of publicly owned utilities depends on controlled managerial freedom. That freedom is poorly served by the bodice of rules and regulations that public managers have to live with.[4]

All in all, it is time to give up market fundamentalism, assuming that markets are stable and efficient. Believing so is an ideology, a matter of faith. I fully agree with Stiglitz, once again, that market fundamentalism does not rest on an acceptable economic theory, because the underlying assumptions of perfect information and perfect competition do not match economic reality.[5] It is, like the neo-liberals and the believers in planning, modeling again. But, once again, life cannot be caught in mathematical equations.

In order to prevent any misunderstanding, however, let it be clear that I am not against reforming the welfare state, provided that we maintain a certain level of decency, because that belongs to what I call a civilized society. Furthermore, I am not a supporter of an egalitarian society, because I realize very well that creating prosperity demands initiative, innovation, and differentiation. Therefore, I have nothing against people in responsible positions being remunerated substantially more than those who are not. But also here, it is the balance that counts. In summary, I realize very well that "at the heart of every successful economy is the market, but successful market economies require a balance between the government and the market."[6] It seems to me that such a balance is at stake.

There is something fundamentally wrong in a world which suffers from what I call "social stagflation," i.e., increasing wealth, associated with increasing individualism, resulting in an increasing split between people who benefit from growing wealth and those who do not, or who even become worse off. To me, it is morally improper that a few hundred billionaires earn almost half of the world's income. To me, it is morally objectionable that, in the United States, 97% of increases in income over the past 20 years have gone to the richest 20% of households, leaving 36.5 million people, i.e., 13.7% of the population, living in poverty.[7] To me, it is morally discreditable that, in the United Kingdom, the number of households living below the poverty line increased in the 1980s by no less than 60%.[8] To me, it is morally unacceptable that, according to a recent report, in a rich welfare state like the Netherlands, some 300,000 children of families of low socio-economic status do not get fresh vegetables, fruit, or a hot meal daily for financial reasons.[9] And, finally, it is immoral to me that CEOs of corporate businesses, on top of their huge salaries, receive bonuses in cash or stock options that to normal-thinking people cannot be related to their efforts. All the more so since these salaries and bonuses "are often quite unrelated to the performance of the company concerned, and are sometimes actually inversely correlated with company performance."[10] And to me, it is even more immoral if these extras are granted because these top managers have succeeded in realizing massive redundancies in the short-term interests of shareholders.[11]

Present-day conduct is not only immoral, it is also dangerous. Why shouldn't the paramount rule of the Old West—that you must pay a price when you abuse your own people (quoted by President Clinton in 1996 while addressing the American public on the sanctions in Iraq)—not apply to those currently abusing their fellow citizens?[12] In section 1.1.2 I referred to various scholars who have warned governments about the increasing tensions which may result in society from increasing inequality. Although these authors mainly focus on the developed world, social tensions can also be expected worldwide. The following statistics underline this argument: (a) until recently, the assets of the world's 84 richest people were higher than China's GDP; (b) over 60% of the Indonesian stock market value is owned by the 15 richest families (for the Philippines and Thailand the figures are 55% and 53%, respectively); (c) the income gap between the 20% of the world's population who live in the richest countries and the 20% who live in the poorest countries grew from 30:1 in 1960 to 74:1 in 1998; (d) unless we are able to address the challenge of inclusion, the world will have 5 billion people living on less than $2 a day by the year 2030; and (e) around the same time, over 3 billion people around the globe will suffer from anemia, 80 million of whom will be living in industrialized countries.[13]

In 1992 a United Nations Development Program study already warned that "a prolonged and ferocious class war is under way" and added that "you cannot hide the poorest behind national boundaries."[14] In line with this, Legrain warns that "if the poor stay poor, we must not only live with our consciences but also in fear of the hatred that envy and despair breed."[15] One has to realize that social progress and democratic rights are never acquired definitively but are continuously at risk in a confrontation with supporters of an economic system which is, in fact, self-destructing. As Galbraith said, naked capitalism is extraordinarily cruel. It is only because of social corrections enforced by, among others, the unions, that capitalism is made socially and politically acceptable.[16] In American society, poverty and social exclusion have gradually led to a "run-down democracy."[17] This is all the more reason for Europe to be very careful if it wants to reduce the benefits of the welfare state.

Terms like *underclass revolt* and *social explosion* describe a scenario in which the "have-nots" revolt against the growing inequality in society. That danger is clearly present in the United States. It is emerging in Europe. Galbraith takes the possibility of an "underclass revolt" seriously,[18] and Peterson calls on the American government to prevent an "explosion."[19] Robert Reich, the Secretary of Labor in Clinton's first administration, expresses himself in similar terms;[20] while Dawson points to the major political threat posed by the effects of economic insecurity on large numbers of highly educated students. Finally, Lasch warns that disaffection in the American society is bound to increase "if things continue to fall apart at the present rate". To him, "conditions in American cities begin to approach those of the Third World."[21]

And, in fact, many armed conflicts around the world, though presented ideologically as religion- or race-based, have much to do with poverty and can be blamed on oppressive and corrupt regimes.[22] The "have-nots" may not have much effective power, since they can be easily repressed, but they are a danger to social and political stability, since they could opt for "inflaming the masses against the super-rich and their defenders."[23] In this respect, a CIA report published in 2000 warns that people who feel that they are being left behind economically are inclined to political, ethnical, ideological, or religious extremism which will result in violence.[24]

Meanwhile, "underclasses" have already constructed trans-world solidarities outside the labor movement.[25] In this respect, Pilger speaks of the universal "invisible revolution." This revolution connects people against "the union of totalitarianism and capitalism, and the stillbirth of democracy."[26] During the mid-1990s it was present in the United States with 858 active militia movements,[27] training people for a decisive confrontation with the government.[28] It is present in Latin America and Africa, in East Asia and in Russia, in East Timor and the United Kingdom, on the Indian subcontinent and in Brazil.[29] Everywhere, exploited people are protesting "bandit capitalism"[30] and trying to restore democratic control over corporate power which, apparently, international politics cannot do. Increasingly, discontented people are organizing to regain their dignity. Furthermore, there are inspiring examples of women's movements which have developed the courage and conviction to challenge the market forces that threaten their lives.[31] In addition, it should be noted that poor people are easy victims for populist demagogues who endanger democracy.

The present-day international political economy also affects EU health care systems. The previous chapter delivered several examples of decreasing solidarity. Meanwhile, despite all the reforms that have been made, difficulties regarding efficiency, rising costs, and equity of health care delivery and finance have remained the same. In general, these difficulties, as summarized by the OECD almost 15 years ago, were and still are (1) continuously growing health expenditure, whether or not as a consequence of popular pressure; (2) concerns about excessive or unnecessary care; (3) worries about inadequate care and a lack of responsiveness by providers; (4) growing queues and waiting times; (5) inexplicable variations in medical activities and costs; (6) inadequate coordination between health care providers; and (7) persistent inequities in health between different socioeconomic groups, as well as in access to health care facilities.[32] Consequently, if the past 25 years have made one thing clear, it is that problems of rising costs, inadequacies and inequities regarding health care are very difficult to remedy. In this respect, it is unrealistic to assume that collective financing of health care systems can be upheld by continuously increasing efficiency and effectiveness. This is particularly the case since health care has its own immanent dynamics (chapter six), leaving governments with finance as the only effective instrument of control. If we add to this the facts that (a) in democracies, citizens expect their governments to provide health care equally to all according to their needs; and (b) scientific and technological developments will increase health care opportunities which, in turn, will (c) make health care more expensive, then, in the context of the present-day international political economy, democratic governments face an insoluble dilemma. On the one hand, including each new health care opportunity, drug, or procedure in a collectively financed coverage package will make health care unaffordable in the longer term. On the other hand, leaving new health care opportunities out will contribute to the economic split in society, since those who can afford to pay will buy these new opportunities privately on the health care market.

Admittedly, this is a rather pessimistic perspective. However, it is a perspective based on the present-day international political economy. Therefore, it is important to deal with the underlying assumptions of this political economy. Reviewing the social context from this perspective may cause us to change our minds. That is what the next section will deal with. I will argue that there is every reason to be critical about the assumptions described in chapter three which underlie the current international political economy. Firstly, it seems to me that neo-liberalism and the theory of public choice, together the foundations of the present-day international political economy, have to be modified, because these dogmas are neither in accordance with the reality of human decision-making nor with what motivates people. Secondly, I will criticize the argument that in a globalizing economy, employers are forced to reduce the costs of labor in order to remain competitive. I will argue that, so far, it is not so much the economy but the neoliberal ideology which is central to the present-day international political economy. This ideology rules because politics appears not to be able to control the developments sufficiently. The chapter will conclude by going back to the European Union which, under certain conditions, may contribute to upholding as long as possible the values of the members' welfare states, i.e., solidarity with the vulnerable people in society.

11.2 Modifying the Dogmas

In section 3.2.2, I dealt with the theory of public choice, which I labeled as a new morality or dogma, having as its point of departure the idea that rational people, out of self-interest, only pursue the maximization of their personal utility. This is also a central point in neo-liberal views on economics. In these views, personal-utility-maximizing individuals are assumed to participate in the market economy where they will rationally try to satisfy their individual preferences, with price as the decisive coordinating mechanism. It would not be necessary for governments to play a role here other than as indicated before, because the market would reach a natural competitive equilibrium.

Of course, the question of whether the theory is right is an interesting one. In this respect, we could be satisfied by concluding with the economist Pen that the proponents of public choice arouse the suspicion that they are bad people who have constructed a theory about other bad people.[33] But there is more.

First of all, a long time ago already, Polanyi regarded the neo-liberal view as a-historical. In *The Great Transformation*, he says, "Economic history reveals that the emergence of national markets was in no way the result of the gradual and spontaneous emancipation of the economic sphere from government control. On the contrary, the market has been the outcome of a conscious and often violent intervention on the part of government which imposed the market organization on society for non-economic ends." To him, therefore, the idea of a self-regulating market was a "utopian experiment."[34] In the 19th century, similar views can be found: the German economist Friedrich List, for example, argued that history shows that "everywhere does the State consider it to be its duty to guard the public against danger and loss, as in the sale of necessaries of life, so also in the sale of medicine, et cetera."[35]

Secondly, it is utopian to assume, as the supporters of public choice and neo-liberalists do, that people decide on their preferences rationally and consistently. Instead, decision-making appears to be "context-dependent, unstable, and often reflect[s] non-economic motivations."[36] Some 50 years ago, this led Herbert Simon to publish his ideas on "bounded rationality." Furthermore, decades of experimental economics demonstrate inconsistencies and asymmetries in individual preference setting.[37] In line with this, Ormerod, who for years worked as an economic forecaster, argues that economics' understanding of the world "is similar to that of the physical sciences in the Middle Ages."[38] There is also sufficient evidence that economic model-building, either by supporters of a centrally planned economy or by prophets of the free market, is too inadequate a basis for a practical political economy. Here, referring to numerous research findings, Ormerod convincingly rebuts present-day neo-liberal supporters of the free market. Their idea that an as-free-as-possible market, with the price as the coordinating mechanism, would, in the long run, automatically result in a natural competitive equilibrium with Pareto optimality, has been shown by Stiglitz and Newbery to be too "extremely restrictive" to be of any practical use.[39] Furthermore, free marketers' assumption of rational expectations by market players has proven not to be consistent with data produced by American and British scientists.[40] In addition, American macro-economic forecast studies over the period 1981–1991 showed that, out of 75 forecast series, only two satisfied the conditions of rationality.[41] Therefore, Ormerod concludes that "the appropriation of the word 'rational' to describe the basic postulates of orthodox economy was a propaganda coup of the highest order."[42] All in all, the present-day neo-liberal economic model of competitive general equilibrium is premised on an entirely faulty view of the modern world. That world is considerably more than economics.[43]

Just because of this, today's "third way" politicians should realize that economic success can be achieved "within a broader and more beneficial framework than that driven by the pure, individual rationality of the economics textbooks."[44] Retrospectively, Reagan and Thatcher used free market economics to underpin their ideological preconceptions like deregulation, privatization, and flexibility, all themes flowing from the logic of the theory of competitive equilibrium. This created a world of increasing inequality, leaving many people behind and thus endangering social cohesion. Today's supporters of the "third way" should learn from that. To begin with, they should realize that the price mechanism is not an infallible solution to all problems.[45] Neither is a government that is kept as small as possible. Moreover, it is a comforting thought that the size of a government as such has no clear effect on economic growth.[46] In this connection, Stiglitz points out that there is no reason to assume that market economies from which the sharp edges have been removed lead to worse results than market economies in which freedom of trade is greater.[47]

Thirdly, the ideas of neo-liberals and supporters of the theory of public choice are not only out of line with market history and reality, they also misinterpret what motivates people.

On the strength of research, Lewin, for example, concludes that the voting behavior of Americans cannot be determined exclusively by their economic self-interest but also must take into account their belief in the alternative which they consider to be best suited to the country as a whole. Research among voters in Europe leads to comparable conclusions. The British Commission on Social Justice, for example, concludes that "people are essentially social creatures, dependent on one another for the fulfillment of their needs and potential, and willing to recognize their responsibilities to others as well as claiming their rights from them."[48] The thesis, also based on research, that politicians are led entirely by their own self-interest, is equally untenable. And finally, this also applies to those whom we define by the term *bureaucrat*.

Anyway, it cannot be maintained that people in contemporary Western societies want to wage a war of all against all;[49] nor can it be maintained that the general interest is the sum total of all the individual self-interests. It appears that people "are also motivated by values, purposes, ideas, goals and commitments that transcend self-interest and group interest."[50] Individuals, therefore, are not only motivated by a subjective utilitarianism, but also by "moral commitments" in their relations with others, based on internalized moral values or, as Edgerton argues, "people are also predisposed to co-operate, to be kind to one another, and sometimes even to sacrifice their interests for the well-being of others."[51] It seems as if they are also guided by convictions about what they regard to be beneficial for society as a whole. This induced Etzioni to develop a new paradigm based on the principle of co-determination.[52] In this regard, he uses the term "responsive community." Such a community is continually searching for a balance between two forces: that of the individuals and that of the community to which they belong. But the community is more than the sum total of the individuals. The individuals and the community need each other: "The I's need a We to be," or in the terms of a Schopenhauer aphorism, "Porcupines freeze to death if they get too far apart, but they suffocate each other if they get too close to each other."[53] The same reasoning can also be found in Jung, by the way.[54] In a responsive community, individuals are not exclusively guided by subjective utilitarianism, but also by "moral commitment" to others.[55] Contrary to what the proponents of public choice believe, these mitigating views undermine the basis of utility-maximizing. Supporters of public choice are completely indifferent to the redistributive aspects of their views and neglect rights and freedoms which have nothing to do with utility-maximizing. In the words of Sen, it is reasonable to bear happiness in mind, but not everyone wants to be a happy slave. Utility-maximizing can work out very unreasonably for those who persistently experience a lack of freedom to pursue opportunities, like the underdogs in layered societies, or exploited workers in the sweatshops of developing countries.[56]

In this connection, it may be regarded as striking that, although the proponents of the theory of public choice rely on Adam Smith's *An Inquiry into the Nature and the Causes of the Wealth of Nations* as the foundation of the neo-classical paradigm, they seem to forget that Smith focused on a *national* free market system in which nations were supposed "to sell abroad what was not needed for home consumption and buy abroad what could not be produced at home."[57] They also seem to forget the same author's *Theory of Moral Sentiments*, which was published 17 years earlier. Reading the opening sentence of this book, which Smith himself considered to be the foundation for his *Wealth of Nations*,[58] ought to at least give them something to think about: "How selfish so ever man may be supposed, there are evidently some principles in his nature, which interest him in the fortune of others, and render their happiness to him, though he derives nothing from it except the pleasure of seeing it."[59] Notorious supporters of public choice will probably object that, in this case, "the pleasure of seeing it" is the determining self-interest. What is more important, however, is that, as mentioned before, for Smith, *The Theory of Moral Sentiments* and *An Inquiry into the Nature and the Causes of the Wealth of Nations* principally belonged together, i.e., "the concept of morality to that of the pleasure utility and the concept of community to that of competition."[60] Hirsch goes even further. He points out that the *Wealth of Nations* "rested to a substantial extent on Adam Smith's social analysis in *The Theory of Moral Sentiments*."[61] The message Smith's two books together hold is, in fact, that ethics should precede economics.[62]

The aforementioned concept of "moral commitment" suggests active involvement based on internalized moral values. It is more than passive compassion, because it presupposes a willingness to change. Therefore, one could also call it solidarity.[63] The conclusion is that there is insufficient proof for the assumption that people are continuously and exclusively engaged in looking after their self-interest. That assumption is not only depressing but also at odds with reality.[64] The danger of this line of reasoning is that solidarity or social cohesion and individualism are approached as two opposite concepts. Regarding this, the Dutch Scientific Council for Government Policy points to the fact that, with such an approach, individualism is associated incorrectly with fragmentation, hedonism, the inexorable functioning of the market, and the detriment of the consultation culture. In short, in this line of reasoning, individualism would be responsible for the loss of cohesion in society. The council, however, points to scholars like Tocqueville and Durkheim who, in their work, have drawn attention to a kind of associative individualism which is actually in agreement with solidarity and social cohesion, or in the words of a contemporary German philosopher: "*Ohne Ich, kein Wir!*" ("without me, no us": author's translation).[65] Therefore, the "I and We" paradigm is not an antithesis of the theory of public choice, but a supplement to it. Individuals are influenced in their actions by two simultaneous factors: self-interest and moral commitment. Their self-interest, according to Adam Smith, is that of honorable people who, in a process of socialization, have a morally internalized self-control. Therefore, he recognized that "government had a function in [. . .] caring for the needy, in building public works, in education and public health, and in preventing merchants from conspiring against the public interest."[66] There is a polar relation here, which is that both factors, self-interest and moral commitment, can be identified as impulses existing next to each other.[67] The extent to which one factor or the other prevails may differ depending on historical, social, or personal circumstances.[68] This conclusion is not without interest where social provisions, such as a system of social security, are involved. Such a system is the product of a combination of self-interest and moral commitment. This product, like the whole idea of the welfare state, is "a national compromise in policy areas which are particularly sensitive to conflict."[69] The appearance of that compromise at any given moment in time depends on the current combination. In a certain sense that product is manageable. Therefore, if moral commitment prevails in society, it may have a positive impact on the extent of a social security system. If the emphasis is on self-interest, the reverse may be the case. Regarding the latter, the question is whether Western civilization has created enough public support to prevent self-interest from turning into egoism.[70] All this leaves unaddressed the fact that the relationship between self-interest and moral commitment is partly determined by historical, social, and personal circumstances. One could assume that if social and personal circumstances are favorable for the sum total of the individuals in society, for instance, in the growth of individual prosperity and widespread employment, this would lead to an increase of moral commitment which would find expression in, among other things, a wider acceptance of the welfare state, which would ensure that those who do not benefit from the favorable developments would continue to share in them. The same favorable developments would also lead to less emphasis being placed on the operating of the market mechanism. In this connection, Etzioni comments that "when moral commitments are prominent, they in effect create non-markets in some areas, and rather poor ones in others."[71] However, if we follow Hofstede, this is arguable. On the basis of research, it is more plausible to him that increasing wealth causes individualism. When a country's wealth increases, its citizens have access to the means that permit them to do their own thing. Countries that appear to have realized a relatively rapid economic development have also experienced a shift in the direction of more individualism. Japan, for instance, where care for the elderly used to be an obligation for relatives, is now forced to establish state facilities because these relatives no longer want to fulfill their traditional obligations.[72] Here, the implicit message is that particularly with growing wealth, governments have to exert extra efforts to maintain social cohesion in society.

11.3 Globalization and Politics

In section 3.1, I provided an overview of the differing opinions on and approaches to the process of globalization. It showed that "the only consensus about globalization is that it is contested."[73] Nevertheless, the phenomenon can be summarized in ten categories: (1) technological (the third industrial revolution), (2) financial (the liberalized capital market), (3) economic (corporate power on a global market), (4) social (labor as a commodity), (5) ecological (increasing degradation of the natural environment), (6) political (loss of national sovereignty and a shift of power from politics to corporate business), (7) military (the bipolarity of the Cold War being replaced by a single military hegemony), (8) cultural (the penetration of foreign cultures and educational institutions), (9) ideological (liberalization, privatization, deregulation, and short-term thinking), and, finally, (10) philosophical (considering human beings and nature as utilitarian).[74]

Apart from those who, for quantitative reasons, believe that concerns regarding the effects of globalization are overdone, the phenomenon has its supporters and its opponents. Supporters, however, mostly formulate their views in a rather conditional way. To them, globalization is a blessing to the world "provided that," et cetera. Resistance against globalization is spread over a motley collection of interest groups. They are (1) labor unions (working conditions), (2) environmentalists (ecological costs), (3) women's movements (poverty becoming increasingly female), (4) Third World movements (trying to change North–South relations to the benefit of the South), (5) peace movements (opposing military hegemony), (6) farmers' movements (claiming that agriculture and food safety cannot be left to the market), (7) indigenous people (defending their culture and traditions), (8) human rights movements (opposing oppression), (9) consumer organizations (defending consumer interests), (10) small political parties from the left (resisting liberal capitalism), (11) small political parties from the right (believing their traditions and values to be threatened by globalization), (12) church and humanistic institutions, as well as other religious groups (opposing the excesses of present-day capitalism, and believing that materialism should not be the criterion for everything), and (13) critical minds from academic, media, and cultural spheres (criticizing the postulates of the international political economy).[75]

All in all, there are many characteristics of and much opposition to the phenomenon of globalization. Contemporary globalization has brought about important benefits, but it has also, in various ways, undermined human security, social equity, and democracy.

Notwithstanding the differing opinions on and the effects of the globalization phenomenon, the reality of the present-day international political economy is that, in the framework of increasing global competitive forces, the costs of labor have to be reduced. In this respect, producers in industrialized countries in particular are forced to rearrange their affairs by relocating their production processes to low-wage countries, by reducing their share in the financing of social security systems, and by downsizing their labor force. These producers appear to be supported by politics at national and international levels, as well as by globally operating institutions like the World Bank and the International Monetary Fund.

Since these ideas regarding global competition have reigned for some decades now, one would be inclined to consider them to be true, i.e., maintaining a welfare state would correlate negatively with economic growth. And, following this line of argument, one would assume that a general reduction in social security spending has been carried out. Neither is true.

As for the first assumption, a recent study by Lindert is rather revealing.[76] It shows that "nine decades of historical experience fail to show that transferring a larger share of GDP from taxpayers to transfer recipients has a negative correlation with either the level or the rate of growth of GDP per person. The average correlation is essentially zero."[77] Similarly, Turner concludes that, although the European Union should liberalize its product, capital, and labor markets, it is not necessary to reduce taxes and government spending to American levels. Consequently, liberalization will not make EU welfare states unaffordable.[78] Even American states like Connecticut, New Jersey, and California, which have relatively generous welfare systems, have not experienced negative effects on growth of state production per capita.[79]

So, despite all the rhetoric, there has been no general rollback of the welfare state, though there have been some cutbacks in some categories of welfare spending in some countries. In this respect, Lindert mentions that only 3 out of 21 leading OECD countries have reduced spending on health care as a share of GDP; two have cut spending on public pensions; four, on welfare; and three, on unemployment.[80] His overall conclusion is that, in the long run, changes in social spending are a consequence of shifting political power between income groups, age groups, and ethnic groups.[81] Similarly, Castles, analyzing the developments in the same 21 OECD countries, concludes that there is no "race to the bottom" regarding welfare standards. Instead, "while there are real signs of a slowdown in expenditure growth [since the 1980s] compared with a previous era of welfare state expansion, there are equally no signs of a consistent trend to welfare retrenchment or diminishing welfare standards."[82] Likewise, Pierson, based on research regarding developments in four advanced welfare states, did not find radical changes during the period 1975–1990. All in all, what stands out is the relative stability of the welfare state, caused by its widespread popular legitimacy.[83] Politicians who want to change this status quo may face serious electoral defeat.

Three things should be kept in mind, however.

Firstly, the figures presented by Lindert and Castles are at an average aggregate macro-level, which implies that specific countries may have, indeed, reduced the extent of their welfare states. In this respect, research by Gough found that, as regards compatibility of state welfare and competitiveness in the 1980s, inclusion or exclusion of specific countries made a big difference in the outcomes.[84] Furthermore, although social expenditure as a percentage of GDP may have increased during the period 1980–1998, as was the case in all 21 OECD countries except for Ireland (–3.1%) and the Netherlands (–3.4%),[85] it may well be that a welfare state's "generosity ratio"[86] has decreased. In other words, in order to accommodate an increasing dependency level (increasing from 17.8% of the population in OECD countries in 1980 to 22.8% in 1998), eligibility standards may have been tightened. This is what has indeed happened to a limited extent in about half of the EU countries. Only in Sweden, Belgium, and the Netherlands, with changes in the generosity ratio of –0.37, –0.20, and –0.20 respectively, has the generosity decrease been rather substantial.[87] But then, these countries were among the highest welfare spenders.

Secondly, measuring the size of the welfare state in terms of social spending as a percentage of GDP is not uncontested, because it fails to take into account changes in welfare needs. In this respect, Clayton and Pontusson focus on the allocation of welfare state resources among individual programs, thus not only exploring welfare state retrenchment but also welfare state restructuring. They found that, for many wage earners in advanced capitalist societies, inequality has increased, while employment and income security has diminished.[88]

Thirdly, it should be noted that the non-social components of public spending (general public services, housing, education, defence, culture, et cetera) have, in aggregate, experienced a downward pressure. So, apparently, there is a trade-off between total public expenditure and aggregate social spending or, in the words of Castles, during the 1980s and 1990s, "new welfare demands could only be satisfied by cutting private consumption or by making trade-offs against other public spending programmes."[89] After all, money can be spent only once. Nevertheless, so far, according to the figures, it cannot, in general, be maintained "that increasing exposure to the international economy has fuelled a general trend towards declining welfare standards."[90] Policies, in this respect, seem to be more an expression of (neo-liberal) political opinions on how society should be arranged than an inescapable consequence of a globalizing economy.

Furthermore, as regards the employers' argument that, in order to stay competitive, the costs of labor should be reduced, it would be correct to include labor productivity. In this respect, it may be true that Europeans work fewer hours per year, have longer paid holidays, and enjoy more generous social security (section 1.2.1), but GDP per hour worked, a good measure of labor productivity, is not that bad at all. Between 1990 and 1995, productivity growth was higher in 12 EU countries than in the United States. And although since then the American growth rate has been higher (1.9%) than that of the EU (1.3%), seven EU countries still grew faster, whereas despite the surge in American productivity in 2002, six European countries still achieved higher productivity levels. For Europe as a whole, the productivity gap with the United States had virtually closed in 2002 when labor productivity per hour worked was 97% of the American level.[91] This leads Lindert to conclude that "so far, any negative feedback from social programs to productivity levels, or productivity growth, remains well hidden."[92]

The implicit message from these facts for the countries of the European Union is that increasing the number of working hours will probably contribute to maintaining their social security systems.[93]

Once again, there was nothing wrong with restructuring systems of social security by limiting eligibility criteria for benefits, by reducing the level of employee insurance, by coupling wages and benefits, and so forth (section 1.2.1). Indeed, the trees of wealth do not grow into heaven. But now that these matters have been put in order, according to the available figures to 1998, so far the general idea of the welfare state has hardly been touched. The best one can say is that (14) EU countries are converging somewhat with respect to welfare standards, with generosity modestly declining.[94] In general, the idea that the 1990s were an era of massive welfare retrenchment is "quite incompatible with the available evidence."[95]

Meanwhile, we have moved on a decade. And although figures such as those used by Lindert and Castles are not yet available for more recent years, we do know that neo-liberalism still unreservedly rules the international political economy, connecting globalization with marginalization due to a lack of political control. This also applies to global organizations like the World Bank, the IMF, and the WTO. Illustrative of this policy is an IMF bulletin of 1994, which reads, "It should not be that European governments, because of the anxieties that have arisen from the fact that they have lost control over income distribution, stop carrying out courageous and profound reforms with respect to the labor market. A flexible labor market results from a revision of the benefit system, the legal minimum income and the regulations concerning employment protection" (author's translation).[96] We also know that, in the industrialized world, inequalities are still increasing, and the number of people living below the poverty line continues to grow. In the United States, the family savings rate is sinking further, prisons are ever more overcrowded, and unofficial unemployment is approaching the EU level.[97] Similar developments can be observed in the countries of the European Union.

As for health care, EU governments continue to pursue policies directed at introducing the market. Several examples, in this respect, were presented in chapter nine. As a consequence, we now see phenomena such as an increased number of people who have difficulty paying their medical bills and who seek fewer medical consultations for financial reasons, which effectively rations health care in favor of the better-off in society. A final example of decreasing equity in health care is the fact that the number of uninsured people is increasing. In the Netherlands, although still small in absolute figures, their number more than doubled during the period 1995–2004.[98]

Furthermore, since Lindert's and Castles' analyses, the European Union was enlarged by the entrance of ten relatively poor countries in 2004. This fact may have consequences for some of the welfare states in the EU. In this respect, I refer, once again, to Article III-103 of the draft European Constitution, in which it is assumed that the functioning of the European internal market will promote a harmonization of systems of social security (section 1.3.3). Regarding this harmonization, the EU will have to cope with the fact that the new member states have lower wage levels, lower payroll levies for social security, and lower levels of social benefits. Furthermore, their unemployment rate is higher and their agrarian sector is oversized. Even now, governments of the original 15 members have adopted restrictive measures to prevent mass migration from East to West.[99] Because of this, I do not exclude the possibility that in the framework of European "market making," the more extended welfare states of the former 15 EU members will carry through (temporary) reductions in their generosity ratios to the benefit of the less extended welfare states of the ten newcomers, if only because, for the sake of a continuously stable European Union, social differences between the 25 member states should not be too large. But carrying through such reductions demands delicate political maneuvring. Regarding this, Calleo rightfully argues that "EU countries are stable collectively insofar as they willingly accept and fulfill common or converging policies."[100] As long as these policies (also) serve national interests, problems will probably be minor. However, it is not necessarily true that national interests of the new member states are similar to those of the old members.

Because of this, quick and heavy subsidising of the new members "could prove disruptive to cohesion and morale, and hence harmful to transformation."[101] If EU politicians can solve this dilemma, probably by pursuing policies of incremental change, the money saved by decreasing the generosity ratios could be used for investments in the new member states in order to improve their economies so that westward migration, border tensions, and ethnic hatreds can be prevented. In fact, we are talking here about an intra-European Marshall plan.[102] Admittedly, when Portugal, Spain, and Greece (then also poor countries) joined the EU, this did not cause unrest.[103] But then again, in those days, globalization was not the buzzword it is now.

At the turn of the century, this buzzword has become "a modern mythology, a secular religion informed by neo-liberal beliefs deeply implanted in Western cultures, and ardently promoted by the political, economic, intellectual and cultural interests served by it."[104] Because of this, some argue that globalization "more often than not reflects a politically convenient rationale for implementing unpopular orthodox neo-liberal economic strategies." They may even interpret this rationale as the revival of 19th century capitalism from before the start of the welfare state.[105]

Based on this rationale, and as underlined in chapter three, governments of the Western world, including those of the European Union, are pursuing specific macroeconomic policies of convergence which are directed at the creation of a level playing field for business life. This boils down to improving businesses' competitive position in a globalizing economy by reducing the costs of labor. In fact, employer organizations publicly demand that governments arrange for this convergence. Furthermore, it has been made clear that the European Commission has also taken this road. And since social security systems are financed to a large degree through corporate taxation, a future downward convergence in more extended EU welfare states also cannot be excluded.[106] After all, there is a limit to finding trade-offs between total public expenditure and aggregate social spending.

Finally, to the extent that Lindert concludes that, in the long run, changes in social spending are a consequence of shifting political powers, voters have every interest in participating in political elections. That seems to be the only effective way to unmask the present international political climate, on the basis of which it is constantly argued that for reasons of global competitive power the costs of labor (a source of finance for social security) have to be reduced. Through this, it can be made clear that globalization is not an autonomous affair which has to be accepted. Those, like Thatcher, who hold the belief that there is no alternative, characterize the globalization process as a politically neutral force, springing from developments in its boosters, i.e., technology, free trade, and liberalized financial markets.[107] This is a rather depressing view, I would say, because it leaves the future of humanity to the whims of these boosters. Consequently, it would also be a dangerous way.

Contrary, it seems more productive to start to realize, together with Scholte, that "globalization is not inherently good or bad; its outcomes are largely the result of human decisions that can be debated and changed," or "globalization is very much what we make of it."[108] Similar reasoning can be found in Legrain, who stipulates that the explosion in cross-border links is also the result of governmental decisions regarding the removal of restrictions on free trade, foreign investment, and capital flows, and not just a consequence of better transport and communications.[109] To both authors, decision-making is the central point. Consequently, the outcomes of globalization are not the result of a natural course of things. They follow from human decision-making or from the lack of it.

In fact, all critics and supporters of globalization call on governments to control the phenomenon. Implicitly, this means that it is not correct to blame globalization for its negative consequences. Neither is it correct to blame technological developments. Furthermore, it would be rather naïve to blame business for creating opportunities or taking advantage of opportunities offered by others or by changing external circumstances. Therefore, the only level of society which can rightfully be blamed for the negative consequences of globalization is the political level. The blame is that the globalization process would be left politically uncontrolled. In democracies, this implies that, ultimately, voters have to blame themselves by not participating in political elections. In this respect, more than 40 years ago, Myrdal had already pointed to the laxity and aloofness of voters who, by refusing to live up to their responsibilities as citizens of democracies, have themselves to blame for uncontrolled developments. The lack of citizens' participation in public affairs, he argues, is one of the most important problems welfare states have to deal with. These welfare states should educate their citizens continuously to take part in state activities.[110] Lack of participation is the other side of a malfunctioning democracy.[111]

However, governmental control of the globalization process would be nothing new from a historical perspective. Throughout history, governments have not only provided the essential impetus and support for notable innovation from a wealth perspective (electricity, chemistry, automobiles, and aerospace), but they also had to deal with negative social, economic, and political side effects. Especially during the Industrial Revolution, governments had to cope, "as a matter of course," with rising social and economic inequality.

Governments seem to have lesser influence these days. The disturbing fact, however, is that, just now, their interference is urgently needed. If indeed, as predicted, a great scientific revolution in molecular electronics (genomics, biotechnology, robotics) occurs, governments will certainly have to deal with the question of who will benefit from these developments: the wealthy elite or the public in general? Moreover, the coming technology boom will also raise ethical questions regarding health care that governments will have to deal with (cloning, life extension, genetic manipulation). Again, the question is, who will benefit? Given this future, "it is difficult to argue that the effects of technological innovation, from interchangeable parts to the microprocessor, have outweighed the impact of government power and preferment," according to Phillips.[112] As throughout history, so also now, even more than ever, political control is necessary in order to prevent developments getting out of hand. Referring to what has been said in the first chapter, it seems a logical consequence of present developments in the economic order to try to exert this control at the level of the European Union.

Now, what should be done? To begin with, it should be realized that "what matters most in shaping international politics are the capabilities of states and not globalization."[113] Freely translated, this means that, nationally as well as internationally, politics can control globalization if there is the will to do so. Neither international trade nor global institutions like the WTO, the World Bank, or the IMF are obstacles to addressing concerns regarding increasing inequalities, child labor, exploitation, or pollution, if there is the political will to do so.[114] This also implies that governments have to realize that reforming the welfare state cannot be sold categorically as an inevitable consequence of globalization with, as a linked argument, an inescapable erosion of binding norms and values in society. Therefore, the biggest challenge for the world economy of today is to make globalization compatible with social and political stability,[115] because, in the words of the Secretary-General of the United Nations, Koffi Annan, "If we cannot make globalization work for all, in the end it will work for none."[116] However, Annan refers to a global political level which does not exist. Moreover, on that global level, it is predominantly self-interested American politics which determines the course of things. Because of this, there is no reason to be optimistic regarding a change in the global political economy. An alternative could be to try to make globalization compatible with social and political stability at the supra-territorial level of the European Union. Such a European approach could take into account the deeply imbued sense of general duty to assist the needy in society (chapter one). It is not clear in advance whether such an approach, instead of a free-trade world as promoted by the WTO, would have a negative effect on economic developments in the countries of the (enlarged) European Union. That is the topic of the final section of this chapter.

11.4 The European Union in a Globalizing Economy

Almost 40 years ago, the Frenchman Servan-Schreiber wrote his famous book, *The American Challenge*.[117] In no time, this book became an enormous success, was translated into several languages, and was praised by politicians across the political spectrum. In his book, Servan-Schreiber delivered, in fact, a summary of the reasons that in competitive terms the European Community of those days, being made up of only six countries, was increasingly losing ground scientifically, technologically, and industrially vis-à-vis the United States. He concluded that this was not because of American capacities but of European incapacities. These incapacities were caused by rigid educational structures, by inflexible methods of organization, and by a lack of real cooperation between member states. Consequently, the United States was far ahead in many spheres of activity that matter for the development of wealth. In the beginning of the 1960s, the productivity of American industrial workers was 40% higher than in Sweden (then second in the world ranking), 60% higher than in Germany, and 80% higher than in the United Kingdom.[118] Furthermore, the United States spent almost four times as much on scientific research and development per capita than the European Community.[119] Finally, compared to what the American government did to support industrial developments financially, EU governments only handed out a pittance. The government's share in the financing of the chemical industry, for example, was 20% in the United States and 2.5% in France. For the automobile industry, the figures were 24% and 0.5%, respectively.[120] American corporations were furthermore very active on the European continent. Figures, in this respect, were impressive. In 1963, American companies controlled 40% of French oil distribution, 65% of agricultural machinery, 65% of materials for telecommunication, and 45% of synthetic rubber. And, in particular, in the then most promising area of business activity, electronics, American companies completely controlled developments in Europe. Fifteen percent of the durable consumer goods market (radio, television, tape-recorders), for example, was American controlled. For semiconductors, calculators, and integrated circuits, the figures were 50%, 80%, and 95%, respectively.[121] Meanwhile, American activities in Europe were 90% financed by Europeans through the Eurodollar.

Altogether, the overall picture one gets from reading Servan-Schreiber's account of Europe in the 1960s is that of a dull, sluggish, and sleeping continent, lacking the talent to organize economic life, missing the entrepreneurial spirit, caught in bureaucratic rigidities, and lacking the resilience to oppose American domination. Furthermore, the European Community suffered from a lack of federal power. Consequently, industrial annexation by the Americans, i.e., making Europe an American satellite with its industry in the role of a subcontractor, could be a realistic prospect unless Europe was capable of combining its talents, concentrating its powers, and promoting scientific research. Thus said Servan-Schreiber.[122]

Meanwhile, we are 40 years down the road. During the days of Servan-Schreiber's publication, the term *globalization* had yet to be invented; Japan had started to industrialize very rapidly; the Asian tigers, with annual growth figures of 8% during the 1960s and 1970s,[123] had never been heard of; and China was a mysterious country of 700 million people, enmeshed in a cultural revolution.[124]

Today, countries like India and Bangladesh, and to a lesser extent Indonesia, Malaysia, and the Philippines, have joined the Asian tigers; Japan has grown into a mature economic world power; and China is expected to grow into the world's second largest exporter and importer by 2020, with its consumers having purchasing power larger than all of Europe's, and it is expected to rival most industrialized countries regarding the use and supply of capital.[125]

As for the European continent, the communist-ruled Soviet Union has disappeared. Eight of its former members have joined the European Union, while others have applied for membership. In the long term, say 25 years, some even speculate that Russia may become a member of the European Union.[126] After all, it is difficult to deny Russia's shared history with the rest of Europe, culturally and otherwise.[127] In this respect, it is good to remember that even in the 1950s, Charles de Gaulle defined Europe as a union existing from Portugal to the Ural mountains, whereas Gorbachev spoke of a "Common European Home."[128] Others believe, however, that Russia is too big to become a member of the EU, arguing that the country is a continent on its own. Besides, although Russian membership would enlarge the EU by only one country, its population would increase by 30%, which would disturb internal EU relations.[129] In the longer term, therefore, a tri-polar Pan-Europe, as described by Calleo, seems more likely. Such a Pan-Europe would distinguish between the EU, Russia, and the United States as three distinct but articulated poles. These poles would cooperate closely, to be sure, but at the same time, remain sufficiently distinct from each other to prevent undermining their own cohesion.[130]

As it is, over the past decades an enlarged and (economically) more integrated European Union has not become an American satellite but an economic superpower in itself. The Eurodollar has disappeared, and in several economic spheres the European Union has surpassed the United States. This can be illustrated with many facts. The EU has the largest internal single market in the world. It is the world's largest trader in goods and services, running a positive trade balance.[131] In 2003, EU GDP exceeded that of the United States. Furthermore, of the 140 biggest companies of the Global Fortune 500 rankings, 61 are European. Royal Dutch/Shell and BP are in the top five of the world's biggest companies. Nokia is the world's biggest producer of cell phones, controlling almost 40% of the world market. Vodafone is the first or second wireless operator in the 12 biggest markets in the world, including the United States. After TimeWarner and Walt Disney, the German company Bertelsmann is the third largest media company.[132] In addition to this, since Servan-Schreiber's research, direct foreign investment patterns have been reversed. Instead of American companies investing in the EU, EU companies heavily invest in the United

States. In 2000, a total of 65% of all foreign investment in the United States was provided by Europeans.[133] These investments cover a wide range of economic activities. British Petroleum is the owner of the American gasoline company Amoco; the Holiday Inn chain belongs to the British company Six Continents; Ben & Jerry's belongs to Unilever; and kings of American fiction like Tom Clancy, and John Grisham are published by European-owned companies.[134] Of course, there is also direct American foreign investment in Europe. Car brands like Volvo, Jaguar, and Land Rover are owned by the Ford Motor Company, and American labels like Gap, Tommy Hilfiger, and Levy can be found in most European cities as can McDonald's and Starbucks. But, on balance, European direct investment in the United States in 2000 was 45% higher than American direct investment in Europe.[135]

Furthermore, the number of applications filed with the Pan-European patent office has increased by 75% since the beginning of this century. The number of PhDs has increased at about the same rate. In several high-tech consumer goods areas (wireless communication, smart cards, interactive television, automated vending, et cetera), Europe is well ahead of the United States, whereas in several state-of-the-art markets (cell phones, passenger jetliners, et cetera), the most innovative products are coming from Europe. Finally, Europe's top universities stand roughly equal with those in the United States in technological fields like chemistry, physics, mathematics, and biology.[136]

Altogether, in many of the world's key industries, European companies dominate business and trade.[137] The possible future that Servan-Schreiber described did not become reality. Instead, the world today holds three competing economic blocs: Asia, the United States, and the European Union, while others (South American) are emerging.

As a consequence, it is no longer a compelling necessity for the European Union to agree with the United States. Such is the new world order.[138] In this new world order, the European Union can and does draw up its own plans and may possibly disregard American views. There are even Europeans who predict a future of Europe as a world power,[139] or who favor a policy of becoming a "civilian superpower" because they believe that the United States is losing ground.[140]

Of course, this change in outlook and attitude is not the outcome of a sudden decision that was taken over night. It is the outcome of a long maturation process within the European Union. This maturation not only finds expression in economic terms. People living in the different member states increasingly also start to *feel* "European." At present, 92% of European leaders see their "future identification as mainly or partly European, not national," according to the World Economic Forum.[141] Furthermore, without losing their national identities, two-thirds of EU citizens (also) feel "European," whereas 60% say they feel fairly or very attached to Europe. As for young EU citizens (between the ages of 21 and 35), over 30% "now regard themselves as more European than as nationals of their home country."[142]

So it seems as if, next to national identities, some kind of "EU identity" is slowly arising, an identity which will probably be enhanced if the fruits of prosperous economic developments are fairly redistributed among EU citizens. This incipient "EU identity" may explain why, in 2004, a total of 77% of EU citizens supported an EU Constitution.[143] Apparently, therefore, the European Union experiences some type of double maturation: economically and culturally. Together they can contribute to EU "nation" building, while maintaining the existing diversities between the member states. In an ongoing EU integration, this combination of EU "nation" building, while maintaining existing diversities, will certainly be a slow process with many obstacles and drawbacks to overcome. And likewise it will demand political *tours de force* (see section 11.2). But it will also change the attitude of the European Union regarding its relations with the "outside" blocs, i.e., with Asia and the United States.

As for the latter bloc, a growing "EU identity" will make EU citizens increasingly aware of the feelings, things, and ideas they have in common with the United States. But they will also become increasingly aware of the things from the other side of the Atlantic that they do not like. This makes our relation with the United States a rather ambivalent one. On the one hand, EU citizens owe a lot to the United States. In this respect, one first of all has to think of the liberation from the German Nazi regime and the reconstruction money distributed under the Marshall plan,[144] but there is also much to appreciate regarding American society. To this day, many scientific and technological innovations have their origins in the United States. Many Europeans like the American open-mindedness, determination, and flexibility. They furthermore enjoy American entertainment and culture. On the other hand, there is the present-day reality of cultural and social differences between the two continents, as well as differing views on how the world should be organized.[145] These social and cultural differences have been pointedly summarized by (the American!) Rifkin. He argues that, in contrast to Americans, Europeans emphasize (a) community relationships over individual autonomy, (b) cultural diversity over assimilation, (c) quality of life over the accumulation of wealth, (d) sustainable development over unlimited material growth, (e) deep play over unrelenting toil, (f) universal human rights and the rights of nature over property rights, and (g) global cooperation over the unilateral exercise of power.[146]

Regarding these differences, it seems as if the gap between the EU and the United States is widening. This is particularly so in the context of a globalizing economy, which is assumed to be dominated by an "over-armed and overambitious" United States.[147] In its foreign policy, it is said, the country only pursues its own interests, even being prepared to defend these by deploying its military power.[148] The reality is, that throughout history, including the years after the fall of communism, Americans have always succeeded in justifying interventions which, despite the rhetoric, had nothing to do with self-defense but everything to do with self-interest and ambition.[149] But the reality is also that, on several occasions (Indonesia, East Timor, Iraq, Burma, et cetera), other Western powers, particularly France and the United Kingdom, took part in these interventions with the support of corporate business. It is rather hypocritical, therefore, to assume that American self-interest is the cause of alienation between the European Union and the United States. EU countries are equally self-interested. For an explanation of this alienation, in addition to the fact that at present the European Union is an economic power on its own, we can look to two other factors.

First of all, the end of the Cold War was a relevant factor. During that war, freedom and democracy, regained after fascism had been defeated, were the ideas, or the rhetoric, which kept the United States and Europe together in a Western alliance against communism.[150] Members of the alliance cooperated with each other for the first time in world history because that was thought to be necessary for survival. Consequently, parochial interests were subordinated to alliance unity. International economic institutions like the World Bank and the International Monetary Fund were an expression of that unity. That unity even allowed members of the Western alliance to interfere in independent countries all over the world if developments in those countries were at odds with their interests.

The second factor could be that the United States has willfully turned away from multilateralism. Particularly since the Bush administration of 2000, the country is unilaterally trying to impose its economical, political, and cultural views on the rest of the world, based on reports of ultra-right-wing conservative think tanks which have spread the idea that entering into multilateral global treaties, alliances, and commitments would not serve American interests.[151] Americans can easily maintain this attitude since they are the most powerful country in the world, economically and militarily.[152] America is the only "hyper-power," and has dominated world politics since the fall of communism.[153] This attitude has had a number of negative consequences.[154] It has created "a reservoir of bitterness and anger,"[155] and it has increased global fear and loathing of the United States.[156] In line with this, Sardar and Davies hold the view that, worldwide, people outside America hate "the political [American] entity based on authoritarian violence, double standards, self-obsessed self-interest, and an a-historical naïveté that equates the Self with the World."[157] Because the United States is the richest and most powerful country on earth, it is perceived not to be concerned about what the rest of the world looks like. The tragic events of September 11, 2001, did not change this attitude. The country is "still untouchable in its self-esteem, shameless in its double morale, always ready to shoot but never to listen,"[158] according to Hertsgaard (author's translation). Consequently, the United States is suffering a crisis of international legitimacy.[159]

Meanwhile, it also seems as if global institutions like the World Bank and the IMF, "originally cast as liberal custodians of a global public interest, [. . .] have become de facto agents of the US Treasury in its quest to sustain American financial hegemony and policy prescriptions irrespective of the consequent contradictions and strains."[160] The same applies for the WTO.[161] Critics also claim that the WTO is mainly a defender of American interests, which makes its performance, like American foreign policy, an example of hypocrisy.[162] In fact, the literature is full of reproaches that all three institutions operate as a continuation of American foreign policy, creating a Bill of Rights for capital.[163] They are perceived to be "interchangeable masks of a single [American] governance system."[164] Others hold the view that they create the rules of the new global economy largely "on behalf of the most powerful corporate and financial interests," with the United States in a leading role.[165]

Leaving aside this Americanization of globalization (as "the only game in town"), these global institutions perform their task from the neo-liberal perspective. The World Bank and the IMF do so by demanding structural adjustment policies (cutting public spending, privatization, liberalization of financial markets), and the WTO does so by pursuing the elimination of barriers to free trade. For the rest of this section, the focus is on this latter point.

As for free trade, there appear to be considerable differences between theory and practice. Where theoretically the advantages of worldwide free trade promise growing wealth for all, practice continuously has to overcome a reality which shows that "the doctrine of trade protection [which may be very costly for that matter[166]] continuously resurfaces in new guises."[167]

While the American government demands that other countries stick to the WTO free trade rules, which forbid subsidising farmers and industries, the American agricultural business is subsidised with billions of dollars without a blink of the eye. Moreover, when in the second half of the 1990s the European Union stuck to its earlier decision not to allow hormone-treated meat on the European market, the Americans responded with a customs surcharge of 100% affecting hundreds of products.[168] And, finally, although these same free trade rules forbid the imposition of tariffs on foreign steel, the Americans did so anyway. In 1998, President Clinton opposed "unfairly" cheap steel imports by imposing anti-dumping duties and offering a $300 million subsidy package for the American steel industry. In addition to this, after strong lobbying by this industry, the House of Representatives passed a bill in 1999 imposing quotas on foreign steel producers,[169] while the Bush administration raised tariffs on imported steel by 30% (again) in 2002.[170] Likewise, the European Union announced a tariff schedule for a broad range of American products in 2004 (textiles, paper, citrus fruits, et cetera).[171] Furthermore, it successfully filed a formal complaint with the WTO regarding American legislation which provided billions of dollars in subsidies for American export firms.[172] Further, it restricted the import of American genetically modified goods, which can cost American companies $4 billion yearly.[173] Finally, in 2005, the European Union, with the support of the United States, filed a formal complaint with the WTO regarding cheap textile imports from China.[174] Many more examples could be given.[175] The examples illustrate that, notwithstanding the WTO, protectionism is the leading principle for all countries which, individually or in combination with others, participate in world trade. Politicians may even openly take pride in being protectionists.[176] This leads Hettne and Söderbaum to argue that "the patterns of economic interdependencies tend to be exploitative rather than cooperative and mutually reinforcing, often resulting in hostile protectionism, trade wars, beggar-thy-neighbour policies, relative gain-seeking and various strategies to isolate the 'national' economies from the negative effects of the larger regional (and, of course, global) economic system of which they form a part, while at the same time trying to exploit the opportunities of the same system(s)."[177] To put it bluntly as a first conclusion, free world trade is very much a theoretical construction. In practice, most governments remain mercantilists.[178] Increasingly, they follow inward-looking protectionist policies,[179] either on their own or in cooperation with others. Regarding the latter point, in 2002, "free" world trade recognized no less than 170 regional arrangements, with a further 70 in the making. Half of these regional trade arrangements have been concluded since the beginning of the 1990s. Because they are meant to deliver mutual advantages to the countries concerned, these regional trade arrangements "make a mockery of the notion of a single global economy."[180]

As a second conclusion, a closer look at world trade patterns shows that globalization does not bring about a "planetary economy."[181] In contrast, Rugman's figures from 1996 demonstrate that most trade is between three currency blocs or triads (dollar, yen, and euro). As for the European Union, "there is overwhelming evidence that European trade is internal, and that only just over 10% goes to other triad members."[182] For the United States, 90% of what Americans consume is produced in the United States, 90% of Americans work for American companies, and American savings are mainly invested on Wall Street.[183] As for regional trade arrangements, 90% of Canadian and Mexican exports are within NAFTA (the North American Free Trade Agreement concluded between the United States, Canada, and Mexico in 1990).

Furthermore, regional arrangements appear to influence trade figures positively between the countries involved. Since the establishment of NAFTA, Mexico has replaced Japan as America's second-biggest export market. Mexico and Canada together now account for 36% of American exports, up from 28% in 1990.[184] Similarly, the United Kingdom's exports to the rest of the European Union are now 58.8%, up from 35% in 1973 when it joined the Union.[185] Likewise Spain, Portugal, and Greece saw growing trade relations with other members after joining the EU.

Intensifying trade as a result of preferential deal arrangements between countries gives the impetus to extend these arrangements. The present Bush administration, for example, has endeavored to enlarge NAFTA into FTAA (Free Trade Area of the Americas).[186] As for the European Union, it may be expected that the enlargement of May 2004 will positively influence trade between the member states, particularly when the new members have started to use the Euro.[187]

Apart from the fact that there is reason to challenge the idea that globalization has resulted in more integrated global markets for goods, services, and other factors of production,[188] protectionism and regionalization put a different complexion on the phenomenon of globalization. As a third conclusion, regionalization instead of globalization seems to be a better label for the developments in world trade.

In this free trade world of protectionism and regionalization, the (enlarged) European Union "would have the capacity to contribute to building a more harmonious and prosperous world."[189] This is particularly the case because, first of all, it has regional arrangements with the broadest mandate, including a wide range of legal instruments. Secondly, it is the world's largest trading bloc with a market size which is difficult to neglect in the development of international trade policies.[190] There are even those who speculate that EU business regulations could become the world's business regulations.[191]

However, for its contribution to a more harmonious and prosperous world, the European Union would have to reject Americanism as "the only game in town." It would have to turn away from the individualist American libertarian market approach and, instead, take up the challenge of building a powerful economy while upholding longstanding commitments to social and economic justice for all its citizens (as is characteristic in the European states).[192]

At issue in the relations with the United States are not so much competing interests but competing values. After all, the social models of the two blocs are considerably different. Two examples serve to underline these differences. First of all, EU countries spend far more on health care through collective financial arrangements than does the United States. Data from 2001–2002 show that countries like the Netherlands, France, Sweden, and the United Kingdom spent 8.5%, 9.4%, 8.0%, and 6.7% of GDP on health care, respectively. In contrast, the United States spent 13%. For the four EU countries mentioned, government spending on health care was 70%, 77%, 84%, and 84%, respectively. The US government spent 45%.[193] As it is, EU countries have higher life expectancy, lower infant mortality, and lower rates of heart disease and cancer.[194] Secondly, EU countries are (still) more inclusive. In the United States, around 20% of adults live in poverty. In

France, Germany, and Italy the figures are 7.5%, 7.6%, and 6.5%, respectively. Replacement ratios for comparable families, i.e., replacing a worker's former income through benefits, are 86%, 83%, 74%, and 90% in France, the United Kingdom, Germany, and Sweden respectively. For the United States, the overall figure is 50%.[195]

Although the differences are still considerable, EU living standards are, in general, threatened by libertarian American ideas regarding the global market. Furthermore, EU political leaders are following the American views. If these leaders, however, fail to protect the living standards of EU citizens, they may easily be replaced by less conventional political forces.[196] In order to prevent such a development, therefore, it seems wise for the European Union to oppose the libertarian free trade religion by turning to protectionist measures, simply by introducing import levies for goods and services from outside the EU. Protectionism on a collective EU scale, therefore,[197] with EU living standards threatened by globalization, under present circumstances seems desirable.[198]

As it is, over the past decades the European Union has become more autonomous and less willing to follow the American lead. It now has the biggest single market in the world, with 450 million citizens. It has a single currency, it speaks increasingly with a single voice, and it is gradually emerging as an effective economic counterweight to the United States.[199] It has, therefore, reached a position where it is no longer necessary for it to trade according to the rules imposed by international organizations. With 90% of EU trade already being intra-European, a figure which will probably rise as a consequence of trade with the new entrants of 2004, and with, so far, no clear correlation between economic growth and the level of transfer payments, it is difficult to see the need to continue structural reforms regarding the welfare states of the European Union, including the collective financing of health care systems.

11.5 Evaluation

In the first part of the book, I argued that the most important question in any society is the one concerning decision-making regarding the production and consumption of goods and services. Here, two extreme theoretical constructions have been distinguished. On the one hand, these decisions can be left completely to the market, with every individual pursuing personal objectives based on personal preferences and plans. All these individuals meet in the neutral marketplace where coordination of all the individual plans comes about through the use of the price mechanism. On the other hand, decision-making regarding the production and consumption of goods and services can be left completely to the government. Here, the government is responsible for designing the plans, their execution, and the inspection of the results.

In order to do so, that government needs a more-or-less extended bureaucracy for assistance.

One can think of a continuum between these two extremes and argue that any real society, country, or economic order can be located somewhere on this continuum. That position is not permanent, however, since the economic order is a dynamic phenomenon, which implies that countries may move along the continuum from left to right and vice versa. Moreover, moving to the left or to the right side of the continuum may be influenced by developments beyond the level of the national economic order. Regarding this, it appears for the countries of the European Union that decision-making regarding the production and consumption of goods and services is increasingly being lifted from the level of the nation state to a higher level, i.e., the EU level or the global economy. Consequently, political economy is increasingly becoming an international affair.

Reviewing the past 100 years of international political economy shows that combining market forces with government responsibility has been a regular topic for discussion all over the Western world. The 20th century started with a widespread belief in the blessings of the market. A greatly uneven distribution of wealth created an unstable economy in those days. Growing social unrest and a changing economic tide, culminating in the Great Depression of the 1930s, resulted in a change in attitude, and governments began to consider how the price system could be supplanted by a planned economy without loosing the efficiency of the market. The basic assumption of this new approach was that government intervention in the economic process was needed, not only to neutralize the negative effects of market operation, but also because of new externalities and economies of scale brought about through new methods of production. In particular, the idea of counter-balancing shortfalls in private investment through counter-cyclical government policies, directed at creating effective demand, caught on well. This led to a long period of Keynesian economics after the Second World War, during which governments were pointedly present in the economic process. Societies started to move to the left side of the continuum. Moreover, a long period of strong economic growth, which started in the beginning of the 1960s, with democracies growing to full stature, created the belief that society was, indeed, manageable. Consequently, the government's role was extended beyond neutralizing the negative effects of market operation. The government was also expected to look after its citizens from the cradle to the grave. And so, gradually and almost self-evidently, two new imperatives were added to the notion of civilization in the wealthier countries of the EU. First of all, economic policy and social policy came to be seen as interrelated. Secondly, social policy became a public good and not something intended only for the poorer members of society. The extension of the welfare state in these wealthier countries was a logical consequence of these imperatives. In general, EU societies became more egalitarian, benefits became more generous, and eligibility criteria expanded in societies imbued with government presence in many aspects of life. In short, the wealthier countries of the EU were living in a dream. This dream was cruelly interrupted by the oil crisis of 1973. For several EU countries, however, it took a second oil crisis, the one of 1979, and a new economic phenomenon, called stagflation, to really wake up.

Waking up meant that, roughly halfway through the 1970s, EU countries started to move to the right side of the continuum again. Government interference came to be seen as an impediment to sound economic development, and welfare states were thought to be overdeveloped. Privatization and deregulation became the new mantras, together with an increasing emphasis on citizens' personal responsibility for the course of their lives. Restoring fiscal balance, reducing costs for corporate business, eliminating labor market rigidities, and loosening bureaucratic trammel became explicit political objectives at the EU level. In short, the market was re-labeled, and still is labeled, the most efficient instrument for the pursuit of individual wealth. As a consequence, governments started to reconsider the terms of their welfare states, initially within the established structures, then through fundamentally reforming their systems of social security. And, again, governments face the negative effects of these reconsiderations. Inequalities are on the increase, causing an ever-widening gap between the "haves" and the "have-nots" in society, while leaner labor terms and working conditions, in particular for low-skilled workers, make employment increasingly insecure.

Health care is no exception to this revival of the market. However, the idea of solidarity in health care which, one way or another, is central to all health care systems of the countries of the European Union, particularly impedes unscrupulous government policies in this area. Therefore, the reality of moving to the market in health care is that of incremental, trial-and-error decision-making with built-in correction mechanisms and continual adjustments. And although all these "market measures" by themselves may not be that shocking, taken together over a longer period of time they reveal that also in health care there is a widening gap between those who have the means to receive the treatment they need or want at the time that suits them, and those who do not. Consequently, solidarity in health care, i.e., equal access according to need, is decreasing, which implies that EU health care systems as we know them, i.e., considerably financed collectively, are at risk. And this is particularly the case for the following reasons.

First of all, despite all the reform measures which have been carried out during the past decades, the costs of health care have not been contained.[200] To the extent that they have been affected, this has hardly been more than cashing in "onetime savings," either by squeezing out "organizational slack" on the health care providers' side, or by carrying out organizational reforms. Furthermore, cost-containment on the demand side has been rather meaningless in general, due to the many exemption regulations that have been applied. Besides, one can hold the view that measures which have been taken on the demand side have only shifted the financial burden from public to private sources, which has nothing to do with containing costs. Nevertheless, a few decades of reforms have taught health care providers to think about efficiency and effectiveness of health care delivery. But from this it by no means follows that it will be possible to contain future cost developments. This has everything to do with the following reasons why EU health care systems are at risk.

Health care is a very innovative sector of society. New technologies, procedures, and pharmaceuticals appear frequently in daily health care practice, all meant to treat a growing number of patients more effectively. And although not every item which comes onto the market makes health care more expensive, in general, innovations tend to cause an upward pressure on health care costs.

Furthermore, upward pressure on health care costs results from the fact that people are inclined to spend more on health care as they become more wealthy.

Finally, an aging population also causes the costs of health care to grow.

In the context of present-day international political economy, all these reasons together will set limits to financing the costs of health care collectively.

In that context, two arguments are used to stipulate the necessity of pushing back collective arrangements in society. First of all, it is argued that the phenomenon of globalization forces employers to reduce the costs of labor and loosen labor terms and conditions for reasons of competitiveness in a global economy. Politicians at the EU level go along with this argument. However, trade appears very much to be concentrated in trading blocs with geographically contiguous countries. The challenges facing the developed world, therefore, do not so much result from a globalizing economy, but from domestic developments like rising inequality, the need for flexibility, and the demand for key public services, which are far more difficult issues than global competition.[201] Furthermore, the economy shows that there is no convincing correlation between economic growth and spending on social security, and that, so far, globalization delivers no motive to reduce the costs of labor. We appear to have more freedom to choose the arrangements for society than we are told these days. Therefore, there is no economic necessity to reduce the EU welfare states to the American level.[202] Globalization is, indeed, "a modern mythology."

Secondly, in the present-day international political economy, two dogmas together seem to function as a kind of catechism. The first is the neo-liberal dogma that the market is very much the best way to satisfy consumer needs. Therefore, that market should be as free as possible. Furthermore, the role of government should be a limited one. Privatization and deregulation should be carried through, and members of society should be held individually responsible for the pursuit of their personal objectives. The second dogma, the new morality, centers on the view that individuals participating in the market do so only for the pursuit of personal interests. Personal utility maximizing, ignoring the interests of others, would be the guiding principle for market behavior.

The two arguments have together ruled the international political economy since the final quarter of the 20th century. Starting with the Reagan and Thatcher administrations in the United States and the United Kingdom, the whole developed world has been conquered by the new dogmas. In summary, the effect of this rule is a decreasing social cohesion all over that same developed world, which also affects health care. The European Union is no exception. All the protests from different organizations have not changed the tide. Nevertheless, combating these dogmas through political action seems to be the only way to change the international political economy. In contrast to Levine, I do not believe that "in the real world of politics, the pendulum is sure to swing back."[203] One has to work on it, as was done in earlier centuries.

12
On Managing Health Care

I suggested in chapter ten that the methods used by EU governments to clean up the mess resulting from excessive health care spending from the past, i.e., the period 1960–1980, may have laid the foundations for the creation of another mess in the near future. Methods such as detailed exemption regulations on the finance side to exclude certain groups of vulnerable citizens from copayments, a forest of regulatory measures to get control over the supply side, as well as an increasingly intense involvement of several stakeholders in the health care process, all cause upward pressure on health care costs. These methods also hinder the transparency of health care arrangements in society. Health care managers increasingly experience limitations in their managerial freedom; there is an increasing "burn-out" problem among medical specialists;[1] and there is a slowly but steadily changing staff ratio to the disadvantage of direct care/cure personnel.[2] These are developments which may negatively influence the image of health care. That image has been damaged already by the negative labeling which has become rather customary over the past decades. Health care delivery is considered to be ineffective and inefficient, doctors' incomes are assumed to be too high, hospital directors are said to have joined the ranks of overpaid managers from the business community, patients are treated like dirt, hospitals are assumed to be places where one dies very easily, patients' safety is compromised, insurers charge their clients too much, supervisory boards do not act when necessary, et cetera: these are all expressions of distrust and suspicion regarding the performance of the medical profession in its broadest sense. Although each of these aspects of criticism may be true to some extent and in some cases, it is certainly unjust and unfair to generalize in this respect. Just as there are (in)effective and (in)efficient lawyers and industrial companies, so also there are (in)effective and (in)efficient individual health care providers and hospitals. Besides, if acute care in hospitals is so inefficient, how is it that figures for the period 1960–1980 show a decrease in the average length of stay of approximately 25% for countries like Finland, Germany, and the Netherlands? What is so ineffective if countries like Greece and Spain, over the same period, saw their investment expenditures on medical facilities increase well over 30- and 50-fold respectively—after these countries turned to democracy?[3] What is so ineffective and inefficient about hospital care which is increasingly being delivered through outpatient clinics and day care facilities instead of in hospitals? What about ineffectiveness and inefficiency in hospital care when, in the United States, almost half of all surgery took place on an outpatient basis by 1989, up from 16% in 1980?[4] We do not declare a whole industry inefficient if one of its specific companies goes bankrupt. Similarly, we should not blame the whole health care sector for mismanagement that occurs at some places. Just as in the "normal" world, health care has good and bad managers. As in the "normal" world, health care managers, as well as individual health care providers, are constantly working on their organizations, trying to improve the effectiveness and efficiency of their operations. They do not deserve to be labeled squanderers of public money. Nevertheless, this seems to be the mentality underlying government regulation regarding health care these days. This is not only unjust and unfair, it is also unwise. It is unwise, first of all, because it discourages those who are involved in the health care process on a daily basis. After all, we all know that discouraged people (health care managers and providers) are very difficult to motivate and reluctant to cooperate. Secondly, it is also unwise for governments that want to control future developments in health care costs. As stated previously, trying to control these developments has started only recently, since the mess was cleaned up; and, in fact, it still has to be proven that governments are capable of doing so by means other than by imposing financial constraints. Because of the immanent dynamics of health care, this seems unlikely. Therefore, governments should realize that cooperation between all parties involved is a prerequisite for any control attempt to be successful. Governments and insurers may blame individual health care providers and health care organizations for performing ineffectively and inefficiently, for squandering money, for not being client-friendly, and so on; but at the same time governments have to realize that they cannot do without them. This being so, it is important to point out that controlling developments in the costs of health care is not served by a climate of institutionalized mistrust, which is the current situation. Instead, a climate of open communication between the parties involved about the pros and cons of policy alternatives may provide opportunities to improve effectiveness and efficiency, which, in turn, will contribute indirectly to maintaining the solidarity principle. This type of communication is conditional on a change in the attitudes of governments, health care professionals, and managers. Reviewing their role in the health care process in a climate of open communication is the topic of this final chapter, which will be concluded with some lessons for all three parties.

12.1 The Role of Governments

The role of governments in a climate of open communication is, first of all, conditional on a change of mind regarding society's appreciation of health care. The following serves to explain this.

During the 1960s, medical care was believed to contribute to the growth of wealth. It was accepted that this required substantial expenditures, because it was thought that inadequate medical care might cause even still greater costs.[5] With the reforms that have been carried out since the 1980s, however, the euphoria about medical capabilities has disappeared and has been replaced by criticism regarding expenditures. Instead of being seen as an area of investment, which could contribute to making the world a healthier and better place, health care came to be seen as an item of public social spending, which was to be treated in a similar way as, for example, unemployment benefits or disability payments. After all, in their effects on overall public expenditure, there is no difference between copayments for health care consumption and restrictions regarding eligibility criteria for social benefits. Nevertheless, for two reasons it is a twisted argument to treat expenditures on health care in the same way as expenditures on benefits. Firstly, although one may argue that both are paid for through premiums or payroll taxes, expenditure on health care is not an item of social support, but it is the consequence of a service delivered. Secondly, and contrary to social benefit expenditures, the quality and extent of this service is affected by scientific and technological developments.

A second consequence of the criticism regarding health care spending has been that the benefits of increasing health care expenditure are less clearly seen than the costs that come with it. In short, a focus on the joys of good health care has been replaced by emphasizing its burdens. In this respect, one may wonder why a growing health care sector is mainly considered from the perspective of costs, while the growth of the business community is viewed as a contribution to national income and employment.[6] Apparently the idea is that, while the business community contributes to growing wealth, health care does not. This is wrong. Firstly, it is wrong because the health care sector is a significant source of employment. Depending on the way one calculates it, that sector's share of total employment is easily over 10%.[7] Secondly, the contribution of the health care sector to the economy, measured in production value and added value, is considerable. Regarding this, a recent pilot study for France and Austria, covering the period 1984–1993, indicated annual nominal growth rates of 7.4% (production value) and 7.1% (value added) for France. For Austria the figures were 8.0% and 8.2%, respectively.[8] Furthermore, a British report of 2001 calculated that (a) British production capacity annually loses 47,000 man-years due to heart problems; (b) taking all diseases together, this figure is 250,000 man-years; (c) short-term illnesses cause trade and industry to lose £10 billion per year; (d) poor health conditions cause considerable productivity loss; (e) back problems result in 119 million days of absenteeism from work, 12 million visits to the general practitioner, and 800,000 bed-days in hospitals; and (f) 8.25% of the working population receive disability payments totaling £12 billion annually.[9] It is difficult to think of a stronger argument in favor of considering health care as a productivity factor. Therefore, governments who want to control health care costs should take account of these facts. They should realize that "good health is a prerequisite for economic development." The two must go "hand in hand and together form part of the glue necessary to build [. . .] harmony."[10]

Thirdly, a climate of open communication between health care parties requires a bureaucracy, which is based on the concept of stewardship regarding the government's role in health care.[11] According to the WHO 2000 World Health Report, governments' stewardship should cover six elements, all of which are necessary for oversight regarding its main task of improving their populations' health. Among these elements are system design, performance assessment, priority-setting, regulation, and consumer protection. One would assume that for policy-making at the macro-level a rough insight into the details of these elements would suffice. As it is, however, collecting data and making detailed rules regarding these elements seems to have become an end in itself, a development which is typical for a world where public funds are limited. In such a world, the emphasis on rules, data, and regulatory oversight enjoys an elevated status.[12] However, it also creates problematic certainties, with regulators believing that a problem will be solved with the introduction and implementation of a new specific rule. As a consequence, deviation from the rules leads to further regulation, thus creating a tunnel vision where there is no room for reflection on future health care needs.[13] Next to this, it may lead to simplifying, "one size fits all" regulations that treat all health care providers and organizations as if they were the same.[14] Consequently, and before we realize it, "the tyranny of controls"[15] has arrived.[16] This tyranny may be reinforced by the way the regulators interpret their task. Regarding this, Walshe distinguishes between a deterrence-oriented approach, on the one hand, and a compliance-oriented approach, on the other. The latter approach focuses on improvement through learning and sharing good practice. It seeks to encourage regulated parties to cooperate instead of seeking ways to evade the rules.[17] The former approach is inspection-oriented, with the scope to expose malpractice, deal out fines, and even take health-care providers to court. It seems that, along with reforming health care, regulators are moving away from a compliance approach toward a more deterrence-oriented approach.[18] This is certainly not conducive to a climate of open communication. On the contrary, it will probably lead to a hardening in points of view, it will intensify the search for ways out, it will increase inventiveness to hide mistakes, and it will certainly impede innovation. Regulators who want to prevent these negative developments from happening through further regulation are completely misguided. Further regulation creates a downward spiral. Instead, a climate of open communication is better served by "responsive regulation," which is based on a number of concepts.[19] First of all, it recognizes the differences between the organizations that have to be regulated. In so doing, it makes the nature of the regulatory regime contingent on the behavior of the individual organization. Secondly, responsive regulation tailors the regulatory interventions to the needs of the regulated organization, ranking these interventions according to their degree of seriousness. Thirdly, responsive regulation leaves room for the regulators to exercise discretion or judgment; and fourthly, responsive regulation is based on tripartism, thus providing a mechanism for regulators to take account of information from and judgments of other stakeholders. Furthermore, responsive regulation is based on parsimony, which implies the idea that "regulatory regimes should be designed to use the least intrusive and cheapest possible regulatory interventions to achieve their objectives."[20] Finally, responsive regulation aims at empowering organizations to perform well. It is not limited to setting minimum expectations which may become accepted norms in the course of time. In summary, responsive regulation is in line with the ideas on new public management which came into fashion during the 1980s. In this framework of ideas, regulators do not primarily act on the basis of their institutional power. Instead, the relation between the regulators and those who are regulated is derived from "principal-agent" contracts.[21] Such contracts are not based on generalized guidelines regarding the level of discretion in public administration, because such guidelines do not exist.[22] Instead, they are an expression of the will to cooperate together in the pursuit of effectiveness and efficiency.

12.2 Medical Authority Reconsidered

Even during "the glory days of medicine" described in chapter eight, doctors' performance was not as impeccable as its social appreciation suggested. There is an example of a London-based legal insurance company which reported a doctors' conduct record over the period 1962–1979, showing that 482 swabs were left inside the body after surgery. Including other articles (instruments, needles, et cetera), this number increased to 946. In those same glory days, 290 out of 815 patients from a hospital in Boston suffered from the effects of their treatment, i.e., iatrogenesis; 76 suffered seriously and 15 were killed by it.[23] In the glory days of medicine, these facts regarding medical performance were not made available to the public at large. People were not expected, nor did they dare, to complain about their doctor's professionalism or behavior. Things are different nowadays. Medical malpractice is regularly exposed. For example, a year 2000 report from the United States concluded that errors in health care organizations were the eighth most common cause of death, killing around 70,000 people each year in the United States. A British report reached similar conclusions for the United Kingdom. Based on these studies, it was estimated that (a)between 4% and 10% of inpatient admissions suffered some kind of adverse event, of which (b) around half were preventable, and (c) for which the annual health care costs amounted to £2 billion,[24] plus £2.4 billion in potential liability for negligence claims and £1 billion for hospital-acquired infections.[25] Medical errors are not exclusively a hospital affair, however. General practitioners also make mistakes. For the Netherlands, for example, it has been calculated that, on average, general practitioners make more than four mistakes per year with negative consequences for the patients concerned. Once in 7.5 years the consequence is that a patient will die.[26]

The difference from the glory days of medicine, however, is not only that nowadays medical practice is exposed regularly, but also that medical errors are no longer considered to be acceptable. Furthermore, the occurrence of errors has brought safety matters regarding health care to the forefront. And, most importantly, the openness about medical malpractice has caused an "erosion of trust, confidence, and satisfaction amongst the public and health care providers."[27]

These developments have also placed medical knowledge in a critical perspective. Medicine and its practitioners are not as infallible as their image long suggested. Openness about medical malpractice has made it clear that the doctor may *not* know best. Furthermore, medicine appears not to be the science that its practitioners want us to believe. If medicine were truly scientific, there "ought to be norms" for service provision.[28] Instead, the practice of medicine is the application of skills and techniques which have been learned during a long period of vocational training. Doctors are craftsmen, therefore, and like any other craft, there are good ones and bad ones.[29] And as in any other craft, one medical craftsman may be satisfied with the quality-level he delivered, while another may not. These differences are reflected, for example, in variations in the use of procedures that cannot be explained by demographic characteristics of the populations concerned. Even tenfold variations in the use of procedures (or resources) are no exception. In this regard, research shows large practice variations in the United States as well as in Europe. To give an example: according to a recent study, the percentage of American heart-attack patients receiving beta-blockers after discharge varied between hospitals from under 10% to over 90%.[30] Such differences suggest that some craftsmen are doing something wrong, but we do not know for sure who is to blame. High-utilization craftsmen may overuse medical services; low-utilization craftsmen may miss promising treatment opportunities.[31] Both approaches reflect "divergent schools of thought," resulting in different practice styles.[32] Some evidence suggests that these differences in the use of resources stem from uncertainty about appropriate care.[33] And there is far more uncertainty about appropriateness or effectiveness than is generally imagined. In 1995, the OECD reported that 80% of medical procedures and around 65% of medical goods have never been evaluated with respect to their effectiveness or costs.[34] Similarly, there is "steadily increasing evidence from the international research community that a significant proportion of health care activity is ineffective, inefficient, inexplicable, or simply unevaluated."[35] This has several consequences.

First of all, at the macro-level, it justifies why governments are becoming increasingly reluctant to finance a growing demand for health care collectively. After all, governments want value for their money, but whether they actually receive this has become doubtful, since "the growing field of health services research has accumulated extensive evidence inconsistent with the assumption that the provision of health care is connected in any systematic or scientifically grounded way with patient 'needs' or demonstrable outcomes."[36] Governments, therefore, are rightfully critical of accommodating expanding health care demands. In addition to this, the burden of illnesses, disabilities, and distress in society appears to be less and less sensitive to extensions of health care. Some, therefore, believe that we are reaching the limits of medicine.[37]

Secondly, at the level of the individual patient, it may increase the demand for a second opinion. In addition to patients' emancipation, distrust regarding doctors' professional capabilities plays a role here. Besides, the probability that a second opinion will lead to a different diagnosis should not be neglected. In this respect, research in the Netherlands showed that in 25%–30% of second opinion cases, the outcome differed from the initial advice given.[38]

Quite often, doctors react defensively to critical comments regarding their professionalism or behavior.[39] They may deny shortcomings or choose to counterattack, arguing that complainants are after revenge and/or compensation money. However, research has shown that non-material goals (such as getting an explanation, preventing mistakes from happening again, or simply voicing grievance) are far more important motives for people to complain than receiving compensation money or getting revenge.[40] When a complaint is made, medical technicalities are usually not an issue. Instead, feelings of disappointment and anger, and a lack of communication skills on the doctor's side in relation to the patient (as well as among doctors), are far more often the reasons.[41]

Altogether, all is not well with the current state of medical practice. Mistakes are made regularly, iatrogenesis causes a considerable number of deaths, and formal complaints about doctors are increasing.[42] This leads naturally to the question of whether the concept of professional autonomy should be reconsidered. In this regard, it would be wise for the medical establishment to realize that professional autonomy in medicine is not so much a right as an historic privilege for self-control and regulation that society has entrusted to it.[43] Meanwhile, the reality is that this privilege is increasingly undermined. First of all, the way a patient will be treated is no longer for the doctor alone to decide. He or she has to live up to guidelines, protocols, and standards. Medical performance is regularly audited, and complications, infections, and mistakes have to be reported; moreover, financial conditions also have to be met. Secondly, patients have become emancipated through legal arrangements which simultaneously impose obligations on doctors. Furthermore, patients may have access to data regarding the individual performance of medical practitioners, as is the case in the United States, where a National Practitioner Data Bank has operated since 1990.[44] In short, health care has experienced a cultural change and unquestioned trust in medical knowledge no longer exists. Instead, the present social climate regarding health care is one of constantly checking the quality of (individual) medical performance.[45]

In line with this development, one can question if it is wise for medical practitioners to maintain the practice of self-regulation.[46] Self-regulation only works if those who practice medicine are trusted, i.e., if people are confident that health care professionals are competent, performing at state-of-the-art levels, and prepared to correct malpractice among their members. But if trust has been replaced by criticism and doubt, some other way of regulation has to be found. In this regard, the British inquiry into the Bristol children's heart surgery clinic scandal concluded that "an effective system of professional regulation must be owned collectively," suggesting the establishment of some kind of regulatory agency, independent of both the medical establishment and the government.[47] Since that inquiry, the British NHS has come to know an "increasingly crowded regulatory landscape,"[48] consuming around £115 million annually. Auditing the performance of individual practitioners, the development of clinical guidelines and, in general, ensuring a consistently high standard of patient care, are among the tasks that the five new regulatory agencies, which have been set up, have been charged with.[49]

The existence of regulatory agencies like these contributes to the erosion of professional autonomy. A further erosion of this autonomy may be expected when medical practitioners are forced to abide by appropriate norms of care, as formulated in clinical guidelines, protocols, or examples of "best practice medicine," which simultaneously could lead to cost reduction and outcome improvement.[50]

The latter development would certainly please governments, insurers, and even (non-medical) hospital directors, because of its implicit suggestion of being in control. After all, imposing guidelines or protocols means that medical performance is subjected to the authority of a hierarchical organizational (hospital) structure, i.e., there is a "power of office" which sets the rules of professional conduct, with line managers in a position to enforce these rules. In Mintzberg's language, through the imposition of guidelines and protocols, medical performance is embedded in a machine bureaucracy, a structural organizational configuration which generates its own standards.[51] The only particularity is that these medical standards are delivered by an external agency. That agency is the professional bureaucracy, which has the "power of expertise," i.e., the development of operational standards in self-governing associations having similar expertise. Imposing guidelines and protocols, therefore, may also be considered as an internalization of external rules; or, alternately, imposing guidelines and protocols means incorporating the "power of expertise" into the "power of office." However, there is a third element, which makes things more complicated.

In this respect, it should be realized that all health care starts with a diagnosis, i.e., categorizing "the client's need in terms of a contingency, which indicates which standard program to use."[52] Here, uncertainty remains an important characteristic,[53] with mistakes made regularly.[54] Phrased differently, one might say that knowing what to do (the therapy) is preceded by knowing what is wrong (the diagnosis). Whereas the first matter may increasingly be caught in prescribed lines of action, the latter remains a matter of craft. And craft needs freedom to maneuver, scope for personal interpretation, and an innovative attitude, aspects which are difficult to foster with any form of standardization. Diagnosing, therefore, requires a third structural configuration, which Mintzberg calls the adhocracy. Such a configuration refers to a highly organic structure with little formalization of behavior, with reliance on liaison devices for support, and with medical specialists joining forces in multidisciplinary teams outside the formal authority lines. In short, the adhocracy configuration refers to an organizational climate where it is possible to break away from established patterns, and where there is room for innovative chaos and creativity. In such a climate, individual professionals have room to develop their talents to the benefit of the organization. The positive effects this can have for the organization as a whole, particularly in terms of innovative developments and quality, should not be underestimated, since "there is plenty of reason to suppose that individual talents count for a good deal more than the firm [i.e., the hospital] as an organization."[55] The problem with these individual talents is that they cannot be controlled through the imposition of rules and procedures and the application of management information systems.[56] Consequently, managing innovative medical professionals (in hospitals) means dealing with ambiguities. On the one hand, there is the certainty of following prescribed lines of action. On the other hand, there is the uncertainty of giving room for innovation. Managing hospitals means finding a balance between the two. I will return to this matter in the next section.[57]

12.3 The Health Care Manager

In 2020, a researcher looking back at health care management history will certainly conclude that, since the 1980s, health care has experienced turbulent times during which all its dimensions have been subjected to fundamental change. Whether one deals with the financial or the quality aspects, with the structural characteristics of the systems, or with the position of patients in the health care process, radical changes have been carried out. These changes cannot simply be summarized as the consequence of a transition process from a closed system into an open one with, consequently, providers being accountable to a range of stakeholders. Accountability alone does not cover what is going on. It is more. Health care has become the property of these stakeholders. They want to codetermine the developments. However, as argued in section 5.2, health care is like a wheelbarrow full of frogs, which makes it impossible to come to a generally accepted policy line. Every alternative will always have its supporters and opponents. Therefore, in democracies, it is the task of governments to distill some kind of policy out of the melting pot of differing, or even conflicting, health care interests.

Since the start of the 1980s, a decisive and determinative characteristic of the health care policy of EU governments and "Brussels" has been the introduction of market principles, while at the same time trying to uphold the solidarity principle. Based on this new characteristic, several health care markets have come to the fore. This is illustrated in the following pyramid[58]:

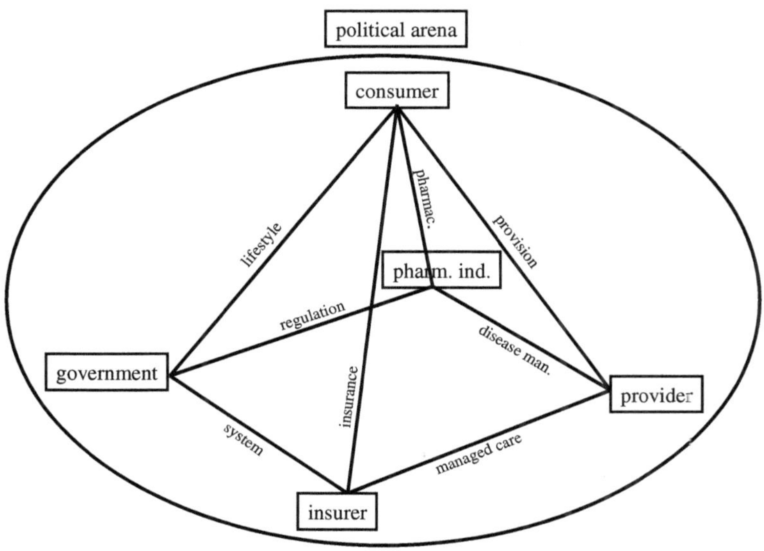

Source: Koning, P. C. J. de, Vries, P. G. de: Ketenvorming; samen de Schouders eronder, in: ZM-Magazine, nr. 5, May, 1998, pp. 16–21.

The pyramid covers the involvement of five health care parties. It is no coincidence that the consumer is positioned at the top. After all, in the market, the customer is always right. He or she can move freely, trying to find the best quality at the lowest price. At the base of the pyramid, we see four other players in the health care arena, i.e., the government, insurers, providers, and the pharmaceutical industry.

In these future health care markets, the government will have a limited role. It will increasingly focus on conditioning and correcting, particularly in relation to matters of quality. Furthermore, the government will try to influence its citizens' life-styles through prevention policies (anti-smoking, healthy nutrition, et cetera). Finally, the government will oversee the operational aspects of the health care system. However, the core business of health care will be left to the other parties.

Insurers and providers will meet in the purchasing market. Here, insurers will no longer function simply as an intermediary, passing on money from the consumer to the provider. In contrast, they will play a central role as regards demand, supply, and quality of health care, including the financial aspects. These days, we tend to call this "managed care," a term which also covers the efficiency and effectiveness of medical performance.

Insurers and consumers will meet in the insurance market. In that market, competition will not be limited to price and quality. It will also include exclusivity and extras regarding the health care services delivered.

Health care providers will bid for the consumers' favors on the provision market. Here, coherence of health care provisions, short waiting lists, efficient and effective treatment, client friendliness, adequate information, et cetera, will be important.

As for the pharmaceutical industry, including the manufacturers of medical devices and appliances, it is predicted that they will increasingly operate as managers of the health care process. They will design diagnostic and therapeutic procedures that are tailored to their products. Even now, one can observe the assistance of representatives from manufacturers in the operating theatres of hospitals. In other words: the pharmaceutical industry will increasingly be involved in disease management.

This possible future will surely have consequences for health care managers, a point of view that I will elaborate for top managers of hospitals.[59] More than ever, their contribution to a hospital's success will result from their capability to operate successfully in the context of different health care markets. They will have to observe the developments regarding these markets and demonstrate that they are capable of formulating and applying strategic options following from their observations to the advantage of the hospital organization. To put it simply: the successful top manager is the one who is "making money" for the hospital outside the hospital.

However, it is not only the top manager's ability to deal with the external environment that is critical to a hospital's success. To ensure success, a manager must also be able to manage the hospital organization. In a market environment, that organization must be such that one can easily take advantage of increasing complexity and adequately react and anticipate to changing external conditions. In general, the hospital's organizational structure should contribute to its flexibility. Here, a decentralized organization based on a distinction in three levels of decision-making is recommended.[60] First of all, there are strategic decisions. These refer to the organizational objectives (for example, what patient categories do we treat by what methods? and will there be a future need in this respect? et cetera, are questions that have to be answered here). The second level deals with decision-making regarding organizational structures. These decisions focus on the organizational framework which is necessary for operational decision-making (the third level). Establishing job descriptions and the authorities that go with each job, as well as information and communication procedures, are examples. Finally, there is operational decision-making, which concerns the day-to-day procedures necessary to do each job (hospital admission and discharge, as well as the distribution of medicines, are examples).

Taking account of this distinction, decentralization can be defined as laying operational and structural decision-making competences at lower organizational levels in order to stimulate employee involvement, as well as to increase the organization's decisiveness, while at the same time taking account of centrally formulated guidelines and conditions. Such a decentralized hospital organization not only presupposes the existence of clear job descriptions, including the formulation of competences and responsibilities, it also demands stimulating leadership at all organizational levels, starting with the top manager. What matters for the hospital organization in an environment of health care markets, therefore, is a clear organizational blueprint which does not frustrate the creativity and innovativeness of the members of the organization.

It is not only the top manager's responsibility to design and implement such an organizational structure, it is also a necessity, since observing and dealing with the hospital's external environment and taking advantage of this environment is a demanding job, which is difficult to combine with detailed attention to the hospital's day-to-day worries. In Covey's words, the hospital's top manager should demonstrate leadership not by working *in* the system, but *on* the system.[61] Creating a decentralized organization gives top managers the opportunity to operate where they should, i.e., on the edge of the hospital organization, where they can oversee the hospital's external and internal environment, limiting their attention mainly to strategic decision-making. This can be illustrated with a simple diagram.

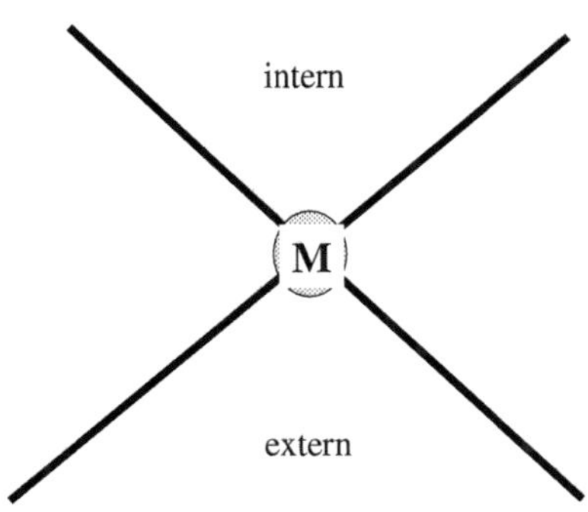

At the intersection of the hospital's internal and external environments, the top manager will have to function as an interpreter. In this role, on the one hand, he or she will have to translate to the members of the hospital organization what the external environment (governments, insurers, patients, et cetera) expects regarding the hospital's performance. As discussed, the top manager must also be able to formulate strategic options resulting from his or her observations regarding the external environment. On the other hand, he or she must be able to translate to the external environment what in all fairness may be expected from the hospital organization. After all, a hospital is not only an instrument for a specific service delivery. It is also a labor organization, with all the obligations and problems that go with it.

It will be clear from what has been said so far that a bookkeeping type of person is unfit to deal with the present-day dynamics of hospital care. Such a person would probably perform poorly as regards the three most important tasks of a hospital's top manager. The following serves as an explanation.

First of all, the hospital's top manager must know the outside world very well and be capable of interacting with that world. Therefore, that top manager has to be a *networker*. A top manager who knows the outside world well, but who is unable either to communicate with it or to formulate, in cooperation with the hospital's internal environment, strategic options in order to deal with the external environment, is not fit for the job. Therefore, the top manager must be a good *communicator*. Thirdly, in order to have the time to operate on the edge of the organization, the top manager must retain competent staff members who are capable of dealing with the hospital's daily affairs. Therefore, the top manager must be a good *recruiter*. In addition to this, the position of top manager demands specific personality characteristics. First of all, he must know the difference between being right and getting right. Secondly, he must be wise enough not to settle for a 100% score only. Quite often, it is sensible to accept 70%, keeping in mind that the other 30% may be gained in a further round. Thirdly, in the complex hospital environment, the top manager would be wise to look for coalition partners among the other stakeholders. In short, the top manager needs to be a *negotiator*, a *compromiser*, and a *coalition-maker*.[62]

12.4 Some Lessons To Be Learned

In the introduction to this chapter, I suggested that the methods used by EU governments to control the health care developments may have negatively influenced the image of health care as a sphere of activity to work in. Detailed administrative regulations, limitations in managerial freedom, and, in general, negative labeling of medical performance have created an atmosphere of institutionalized mistrust, with the supply side on the defensive. This may have counterproductive effects if we want to control the health care developments. Exercising control is not served by imposing regulations or by putting the medical world in the pillory. Control starts with the recognition that cooperation between all parties involved is needed. Governments cannot do this alone. Neither can insurers or health care managers. What is needed is a climate of open communication, based on trust between the stakeholders. With regard to the three stakeholders in this chapter, some lessons will be drawn which could contribute to the restoration of trust. After all, trust "is a vital precondition for entrepreneurship, as organizations are more innovative and function more effectively on the basis of trust and confidence than on the basis of suspicion."[63]

As for the government, it should be realized that health care has its own immanent dynamics, of which scientific and technological developments are determining factors. In democracies where the production of goods and services is a matter of private enterprise, governments can condition and correct. But it starts with tolerating the developments. Nevertheless, the government has several ways to contribute to a climate of open communication based on mutual trust. In this respect, I mention three lessons to be learned.

1. Instead of mainly considering health care as an item of public spending, governments should (re)appreciate its contribution to the economy. Health care delivers important services to the economy in that it (a) creates a considerable number of jobs, directly and indirectly and (b) adds to a healthy society, which, in turn, has a positive effect on society's productive capacity, which, in turn again, (c) contributes to the growth of wealth. In short, it is time that governments revalue health care as an item of investment in society.

2. Since controlling health care has turned into "the tyranny of controls," governments should reconsider the effectiveness of one-size-fits-all regulations. Attempts to restore a climate of open communication, which rests on mutual trust, are served by a regulatory regime which is tailored to the specific circumstances of individual organizations. The starting point for this tailor-made regulation should be the will to cooperate in the pursuit of efficiency and effectiveness through mutual learning and sharing good practice. Tailor-made regulation leaves room for discretion by the regulators. Organizations which perform relatively well need less regulation than those which do not. However, tailor-made regulations require a specific type of regulators. They must not only know the rules; they must also understand "the business."[64] In this respect, it could be worthwhile to offer older hospital CEOs (say, after the age of 55) positions as regulators. They will probably be qualified to balance regulation with entrepreneurialism in daily health care practice.[65]

3. Governments should realize that incentives have more effect on entrepreneurial behavior than does punishment.[66]

As discussed, professional autonomy in medicine is not a right but an historic privilege. This privilege has been undermined, not only because there is an erosion of trust, confidence, and satisfaction regarding doctors' capabilities among the public at large, but also because the way a patient is treated is no longer exclusively for the doctor in charge to decide. Therefore, showing some modesty about their capacities would be to doctors' credit. After all, there is still much uncertainty about the appropriateness and effectiveness of medical interventions. Clinical guidelines may be of help in this respect. On the one hand, they may increase the "certainty" of medical performance. On the other hand, they may impede innovative activities. Between the two, a middle course has to be found. Both result in some lessons for medical practitioners.

1. Medical practitioners should openly communicate about the limitations of their trade. After all, there is nothing wrong with some modesty.
2. Since communication between doctors and their patients appears to be a regular item of complaint, training in communication skills should be included in the respective training programs.
3. Medical professionals working in hospitals should be obliged to practice in conformity with clinical guidelines, unless they have permission to work in other ways. Exceptions should be permitted only by the hospital's first medical officer, who should be the hierarchical superior of the medical staff. The first medical officer should be appointed for a certain period of time with the possibility of reappointment. The fact that medical professionals increasingly work part-time in hospitals (particularly female medical specialists) provides an extra reason to establish a hierarchical work environment.

Finally, let us return to the top manager of the hospital. He or she is appointed by the hospital's board of governors. To begin with, these governors should take to heart the old English piece of wisdom which says that perfect intentions do exist, but perfect men do not. Unfortunately, when a new top manager has to be recruited, the board of governors is often looking for the impossibly perfect candidate. He or she must have a vision regarding the health care business, must be able to manage and structure a complex professional organization, must show stimulating leadership, must be decisive, must be able to create an innovative environment, must have a participative attitude, must be a representative personality, et cetera—these are all qualifications which can be found on a board's wish list. Although the services of an assessment agency may be of help in this respect, I add a few simple extra points:

1. The top manager should be appointed because of his or her qualifications and personality characteristics to do the job, and not because of his or her political views.

2. In a recruitment procedure, particular attention should be paid to matching the potential top manager with other members at the top of the hospital organization.
3. Top managerial appointments should be limited to a certain contractual period of time with the possibility of continuation only after evaluation.

Epilogue

The history of the international political economy over the past 100 years is one of societies moving along a continuum from left to right, and vice versa, alternately choosing for more or less governmental interference in the economic process through democratic decision-making procedures. By doing so, these societies are exchanging the market for the government, or the government for the market. Apparently, the government and the market are each other's correction mechanism. When the market produces excesses, excluding too many people from prosperous developments, the government is there to correct it, in order to uphold social cohesion. When the government has too strong a grip on society, thereby frustrating personal freedom and development, the market is there to reward individual initiative to undertake new ventures.

Since 1975, the countries of the developed world, including those of the European Union, have been moving toward the market again. They do this wholeheartedly and without obstruction, in particular since the far worse alternative of communism is no longer a threat. Nevertheless, there needs to be a balance between government and the market. That balance will be disturbed if the government is too intrusively present in economic life. This may cause social suffocation, leading to resignation and apathy among citizens. The balance can also be disturbed if the government is too absent, leaving too many people out when it comes to sharing wealth. However, the problem is that nobody can be sure when too great an imbalance becomes manifest. But what is certain is that both extremes can create unrest in society. People who feel that the government is too much involved in their personal lives are sensitive to the appeal to "get government off our backs." On the other hand, people who feel that they have been let down by the government are sensitive to popular political appeals. Behind all this lies the question of what kind of society we want. For the answer, one has to take account of the spirit of the times. Years ago, when the political economy remained a national affair, and a country's borders could, to a certain extent, exclude external ideas and affairs, the answer was determined by national circumstances and political opinions. Today, however, the question as to what kind of society we want has to be answered in the international context of globalization. Here, Friedman's matrix is helpful[1]:

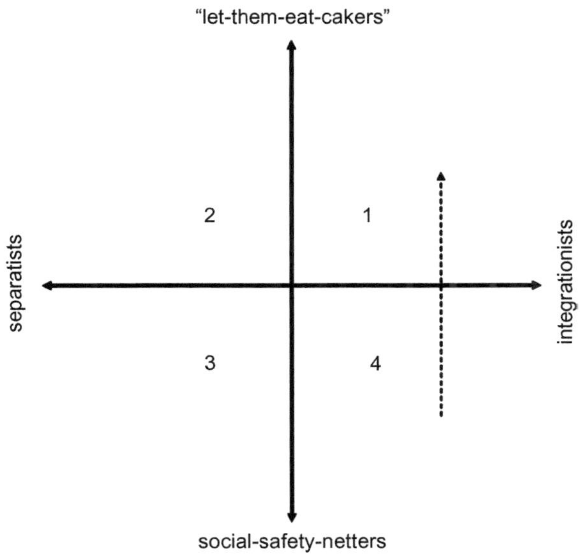

Source: Friedman, Th. L.: *The Lexus and the Olive Tree*, Anchor Books, 2000, p. 438.

In this matrix, the author distinguishes between four basic political identities that people can adopt in a globalizing world. They first have to determine their position regarding the process of globalization; i.e., they have to decide whether they want to be integrationists or separatists. Choosing the first identity means welcoming globalization because it is thought to be good or inevitable, while accepting all that comes with it. Choosing to be separatists implies that one fears the dangers of globalization, like widening income gaps, homogenized culture, and the control of life by faceless market forces.

The vertical line is the distribution axis. Here, the "social-safety-netters" (at the bottom) are those who believe that globalization can only be sustainable if it is democratized in an economic and political sense. They want the government to pursue policies of inclusion, helping those left behind to acquire the tools to participate in the global economy. Their opposites are the "let-them-eat-cakers" at the top. They believe that globalization is essentially a winner-take-all phenomenon. They want to reduce government and taxes, and they want the losers to take care of themselves. Combining the two lines results in four quadrants, which represent four political identities.

Although Friedman had the American society in mind when he developed this matrix, his approach can easily be adapted to the European

Union. Then the question becomes, What kind of European Union do we want? The analysis presented in this book suggests that EU governments and "Brussels" are pursuing economic policies of moving from quadrant four to quadrant one (the direction of the dotted arrow); i.e., they are playing the globalization game while accepting that an increasing number of people are left behind. It is believed that policies in line with quadrant four are no longer tenable because of the forces of global competition. "There's no alternative," said Thatcher in this respect. The reality is not so bad, however. So far, global competitive forces appear not to have had the predicted devastating effects, and EU trade is mainly an intra-European affair. Furthermore, research has shown that spending on social security has not affected economic growth in the countries of the developed world. It is even the case that, although there are signs of a slowdown in the growth of public spending on social security, welfare states are not involved in a "race to the bottom." True, cutbacks in some areas have been carried through, but, in general, welfare states appear to be relatively stable. The ones that have somewhat reduced their "generosity level" are those who were relatively big spenders. However, although welfare state retrenchment has not been so bad, there is reason to be worried about welfare state restructuring, which has caused increasing inequality and insecurity among wage earners. In the longer term, it may also be worrying that social security spending has been upheld at the expense of the non-social components of public spending. After all, there is a limit to making trade-offs in this respect. So far, however, it is a gross exaggeration to argue that global competitiveness would force EU governments to move from quadrant four to quadrant one of the matrix. Policies in this respect are more an expression of (neo-liberal) political opinions on how society should be arranged than an inevitable consequence of a globalizing economy.[2] Nevertheless, there are at least three reasons to be more reticent about future developments.

First of all, creating employment for low-skilled workers will demand tremendous efforts by EU governments in order to prevent social disintegration. In this respect, it is important to realize that in a market economy, the service sector cannot endlessly continue to serve as a labor pool for low-skilled workers. Consequently, as in agriculture and industry, the demand for low-skilled workers in the service sector may soon dry up in a market economy.[3] In order to prevent social disintegration from happening, governments could pursue policies of inclusion, i.e., policies through which unemployed low-skilled workers nevertheless continue to feel recognized as equals (see section 1.1.2 above). In this regard, long-term health care particularly delivers promising opportunities for a trade-off between unemployment benefit payments and creating low-skilled jobs in health care. Long-term health care can, indeed, absorb many low-skilled workers who have become unemployed.

Secondly, it should be realized that the enlargement of the European Union in 2004 could make things more complicated, if only for reasons of size. It will certainly demand political leadership and wisdom to steer this enlargement in the right direction. If the original 15 members are prepared to invest for a longer period of time in the new member states, the European Union could, after China, become one of the strongest economies in the world, which could afford—relatively easily—to uphold its own social policy agenda. In this respect, it is a comforting thought that, despite prophecies of fear to the contrary, earlier enlargements of the European Union (then the EEC) intensified trade among its members to the benefit of all. The same is already happening with the new entrants. As it is, the new entrants are achieving higher growth figures compared to the original 15 countries. In 10 to 20 years, they may have reached a comparable level of wealth. That growing wealth will result in higher wages.[4] Consequently, it will become less attractive to relocate industrial activities to the low-wage countries of the European Union. The complications of the recent enlargement, therefore, may considered to be friction problems, which will be solved in due time.

The third reason for reticence is provided by China, the fastest-growing economy in the world. Here, the costs of labor are 10% to 20% of the level of the wealthier original members of the EU. But, here too, there are "friction" problems. China already experiences tensions between the rapidly developing areas along its coastline and the inland areas which lag behind. Growing wealth in China will result in a demand for higher wages, thus narrowing the gap between this country and the countries of the EU. Such a development is already occurring in India. Here, a real wage increase of 7.3% is predicted for 2006.[5]

Finally, let us return to health care. Here too, a matrix can be of help. In this regard, in 1994, a Dutch research team devised a simple framework regarding possible future developments of the Dutch health care system.[6]

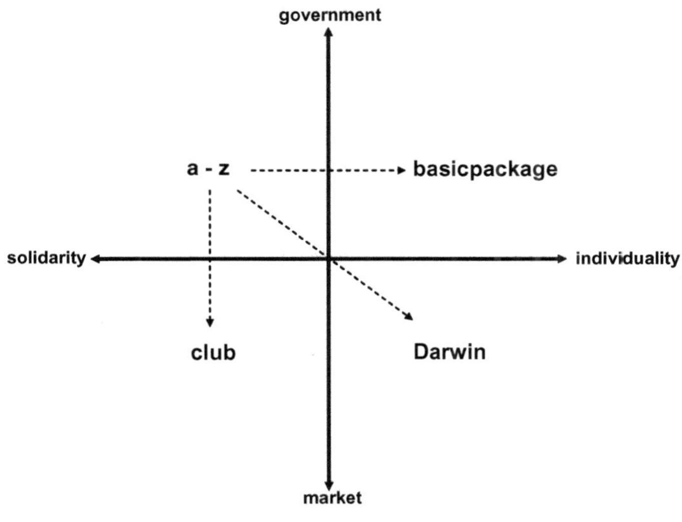

The horizontal axis represents the social-cultural dimension, with complete solidarity and complete individuality at the extremes. The vertical axis stands for the structural dimension, with the market at one end and the government at the other end. The four quadrants represent four types of health care systems. The "A–Z" scenario includes all possible health care, accessible to all, and of high quality. Here, the government leads, taking responsibility to look after all citizens. In the "basic package" scenario, individual responsibility for one's health has a central position. The government guarantees access to this basic package. The "club" scenario differs from the "A–Z" scenario in the sense that the market players, not the government, determine the concepts of solidarity, accessibility, and quality of health care. Market parties are self-regulating, and membership in the club is conditional. Finally, in the "Darwin" scenario, as the name implies, the fittest survive. The market rules, and the price coordinates. If you cannot play the market game, then too bad.

The dotted lines that I have included in the matrix indicate possible future developments of health care systems. As for the "Darwin" scenario, I believe EU countries to be too civilized for it to develop. So, there remain two options for moving away from the "A–Z" scenario. The analysis presented in this book shows that both are slowly happening. The arguments are similar and, therefore, similarly controversial so far.

Notes and References

Preface

1. That same issue of *The Times* further described a patient who had to wait 12 months for an MRI scan, but got it done in a few weeks by paying £400.
2. The scope of this book is mainly limited to the countries of the European Union from before May 2004.
3. Eucken, W.: *Die Grundlagen der Nationalökonomie*, Achte Auflage, Springer-Verlag, Berlin, 1965. Subsequently, Milton Friedman took a similar approach.
4. Scrivens, E.: *Quality, Risk and Control in Health Care*, Open University Press, 2005, p. 2.
5. Fanu, J. Le: *The Rise and Fall of Modern Medicine*, Abacus, 2004, p. 271.
6. Cyert, R. M. and March, J. G.: *A Behavioral Theory of the Firm*, Prentice Hall, 1963, pp. 36–38
7. It seems to me that the Dutch and French "no" to the treaty on a European Constitution in 2005 was not an anti-European expression, but a sign of people feeling disappointed in politics.

Chapter 1

1. I define a health care system as a social infrastructure, i.e., the organization, financing, and delivery of health care, which is purposely set up by governments for their citizens.
2. Swaan, A. de: *Zorg en de Staat. Welzijn, Onderwijs en Gezondheidszorg in Europa en de Verenigde Staten in de Nieuwe Tijd*, Amsterdam, 1993.
3. Sparrow, M. K.: *License to Steal: How Fraud Bleeds America's Health Care System*, Updated Edition, Westview Press, 2000, p. vii.
4. That is, before the enlargement of May 1, 2004.
5. Samuelson, P. A., and Nordhaus, W. D.: *Economics*, International Edition, McGraw-Hill, Inc., 1995, p. 6.
6. It is no surprise that the economic order has been an ongoing topic of study. The relevant literature sufficiently addresses the following themes: definitions of the concept of the economic order, attempts to classify economic orders, and descriptions of the development of economic orders (See, for example, Hartog, F.: *Economische Stelsels*, Groningen, 1970; Bergsma, S.:

De Vermaatschappelijking van de Onderneming, Deventer, 1965, chapter 1; Popta, S. van: *Inhalen en Voorbijstreven*, Rotterdam, 1971; Doel, J. van den: *Konvergentie en Evolutie*, Assen, 1971; Zijlstra, J.: *Economische Orde en Economische Politiek*, Leiden, 1956, chapter 2).

7. Eucken, W.: *Die Grundlagen der Nationalökonomie*, Achte Auflage, Springer-Verlag, 1965. It should be noted that in Eucken's view, a central authority does not necessarily have to be a government as we know it. It may also be a tribal chief or the boss of a sheikdom. Regarding the first basic type (*Zentralgeleitete Wirtschaft*), the author distinguishes between three variations: (a) the totally centrally controlled economic order (*Total Zentralgeleitete Wirtschaft*) which knows no freedom of exchange between individuals, and where the use of productive resources and the distribution of production and consumption are completely centrally controlled; (b) the centrally controlled economic order where consumers are free to exchange the goods that have been allocated to them (*Zentralgeleitete Wirtschaft mit freiem Konsumguttausch*); and (c) the centrally controlled economic order with complete consumer freedom (*Zentralgeleitete Wirtschaft mit freier Konsumwahl*). As for the second basic type (*Verkehrswirtschaft*), the author describes 25 market forms, based on the two determining characteristics of the idea of the market, i.e., supply and demand, with the price as the regulatory mechanism. Supply and demand know five variations: competition (*Konkurrenz*), partial oligopoly (*Teiloligopol*), oligopoly (*Oligopol*), partial monopoly (*Teilmonopol*), and monopoly (*Monopol*) (Eucken, W.: ibid., pp. 80–112). If we add to this the distinction between open and closed market forms from both the supply side and the demand side, or from an open demand side and a closed supply side (and vice versa), the number of market forms will be 100 (Meijer, G.: *Neoliberalisme: Neoliberalen over Economische Orde en Economische Theorie*, Assen, 1988, p. 72).
8. In organizing economic activity, prices perform three functions, namely, (1) transmitting information, (2) optimizing efficiency, and (3) determining income distribution (following Friedman, M. and Friedman, R.: *Free to Choose: The Classic Inquiry into the Relationship between Freedom and Economics*, Harvest Books, 1990, p. 14).
9. Later on, Friedman adopted a comparable approach, arguing that, fundamentally, there are only two ways to coordinate the economic activities of millions of people. One is central direction, involving the use of coercion, or "the technique of the army and the modern totalitarian state." The other is voluntary co-operation of individuals, or "the technique of the marketplace." (Kuttner, R.: *Everything for Sale: The Virtues and Limits of Markets*, The University of Chicago Press, 1999, p. 33.)
10. The terms "*market economy*" and "*command economy*," as alternatives to Eucken's "*Verkehrswirtschaft*" and "*Zentralgeleitete Wirtschaft*," are from: Samuelson, P., and Nordhaus, W. D.: ibid., p. 6.
11. Dyson, K.: *The Politics of the Euro-Zone. Stability or Breakdown?* Oxford University Press, 2000, p. 227. This has been the case throughout European history. In this respect, De Swaan points to the fact that even charitable work has not changed that much: "visiting the sick, teaching the ignorant, and feeding the poor. In modern terms: health, education and welfare," are still a fundamental characteristic of European culture (Swaan, A. de: Dutch Welfare in Europe XL, in: Gier, E. de, Swaan, A. de, and Ooijens, M., (eds.): *Dutch Welfare*

Reform in an Expanding Europe: The Neighbours' View, Het Spinhuis, 2004, p. 3).

12. Vathorst, S. van de: *Your Money or My Life: Justice, Solidarity & Responsibility in Dutch Health Care*, dissertation, Free University of Amsterdam, 2001, p. 54.
13. The philosopher Van der Wal distinguishes between three levels of meaning regarding the solidarity principle. First, there is the descriptive level. This is "the actual realisation of solidarity [. . .] which exists between people and the resulting preparedness to share existence with others, in particular where the dark sides are involved" (author's translation). The second level, the analytical level of the solidarity principle, involves "the central notion of a theory of society" (author's translation). At the third level, solidarity is "a yardstick to promote the quality of interpersonal relationships" (author's translation): Wal, G. A. van der: Solidair, Hoe en Waarom? Over de Betekenis van Solidariteit bij de Bekostiging van de Gezondheidszorg, in: Jacobs, F. C. L. M. and Wal, G. A. van der, (eds.): *Medische Schaarste en het Menselijk Tekort*, Ambo, Baarn, 1988, pp. 85–87).
14. Leijnse, F.: *Verzorgingsstaat: Last of Lust?* Rotterdam, 1994.
15. Gooijer, W. J. de: *On Solidarity in Changing Health Care Systems: Europe in Search of a New Balance*, Leuven, 1996.
16. For a discourse on different types of solidarity see, for example, Beer, P. de: Insluiting en Uitsluiting: de Keerzijden van de Verzorgingsstaat, in: Entzinger, H., and Meer, J. van der, (eds.): *Grenzeloze Solidariteit: Naar een, Migratiebestendige Verzorgingsstaat*, De Balie, 2004, pp. 26–42.
17. Loo, H. van der and Reijen, W. van: *Paradoxen van Modernisering*, Bussum, 1997, p. 103. This does not imply that systems of social security are a mainstay of equal importance in other societies. Asian countries, for example, differ from the countries of the Western world in the sense that pursuing personal ambitions, and striving for economic productivity, are thought to be mainstays of society (among other things). In these countries, social security is, to a large extent, thought to be the responsibility of family circles.
18. Rifkin, J.: *The European Dream: How Europe's Vision of the Future Is Quietly Eclipsing the American Dream*, Tarcher/Penguin, 2004, p. 282.
19. The government is not necessarily the only preserver of the quality of society's cement. Throughout history, the church, for example, played an important role in looking after the sick and vulnerable members of society. Also, unionized labor has contributed much to improving the faith of the less well-off. Nowadays, voluntary organizations, particularly in the United States and Great Britain, are important instruments for maintaining "civil society." Therefore, the withdrawal of government from the economic process may be compensated for by other members or organizations of society. Nevertheless, in whichever direction a country chooses to move along the continuum, in democracies, governments are always expected to act as the guardian of the "general interest" or "common good," no matter how fictitious these concepts may be (in this respect, see Kleerekoper, S.: *De Fictie van het Algemeen Belang*, Deventer, 1963, and Schumpeter, J. A.: *Capitalism, Socialism and Democracy* (Dutch Translation), Hilversum, 1963, pp. 213–228).
20. Eucken, however, provided some examples which not only demonstrated that one should be careful about taking definite positions in this respect, but also

that it is disputable whether it is possible to distinguish between irreversible series or stages in the development of economic orders. History shows that there have been severe regressions, with people falling back to a preceding economic order again. For example, the well-known scheme of the development from a "natural" economy, via a "monetary" economy, to a "credit" economy, which had already existed in the Eastern Mediterranean countries during the 300s BC, was reversed from a "credit" economy, via a "monetary" economy, to a "natural" economy again when these countries were impoverished under the Roman Empire. Comparable things happened around the same time in Egypt. The fact that, during the 300s BC, the Hellenistic states had reached the stage of a "national" economy, did not prevent them from falling back to a "natural" economy five centuries later. During the third century AD, the use of coins as the circulating medium was confined to some sectors of the economy, with the rest using a barter or "natural" economy (Eucken, W.: ibid., pp. 70–75). It is equally wrong to assume that the extensive national economies (*Volkswirtschaft*) of Europe developed directly out of the medieval city economies (*Stadtwirtschaft*). The long-distance traders of those days, who were the engines of economic development, had the whole of Europe as their field of economic activity. Craft industries not only worked to meet local requirements. It was a free-trade "European Union" ahead of its time (in this respect, see Bauer in: Eucken, W.: *Die Grundlagen der Nationalökonomie*, English Translation, Springer Verlag, 1950, p. 73). Around the end of the sixteenth century, this union fractured as a consequence of the power plays of state creation. In the 1500s, Europe had more than 500 states, many of which were no larger than a city (Zakaria, F.: *The Future of Freedom: Illiberal Democracy at Home and Abroad* (Dutch Translation), Contact, Amsterdam/Antwerpen, 2003, p. 31). These were states that saw the world as "a battle arena where import prohibitions, prohibitive tariffs and other weapons of mercantilist policy might be employed" (Eucken, W.: *Die Grundlagen der Nationalökonomie*, English Translation, ibid., p. 74). As a consequence, the economic order did not advance from a city economy to a regional (European) economy. Instead, it resulted in the breaking-up of the pre-existing European unity, very much to the disadvantage of the various small countries on the European continent. According to Eucken, it may therefore be concluded that a higher form of economic order does not necessarily result from a gradual transition from a lower one. History has shown several times that the opposite may also happen.

21. Kahn, H. and Wiener, A. J.: *The Year 2000: A Framework for Speculation on the Next Thirty-Three Years*, Macmillan, New York, 1967, table 18.
22. Krugman, P.: Competitiveness: A Dangerous Obsession, in: *Foreign Affairs*, March/April, 1994, pp. 28–44.
23. For several reasons, one can argue with Eucken's ideas regarding possible regressions in the development of economic orders. Firstly, his examples of regression from before the beginning of our era cover very long periods of time, even up to five centuries. And, as we know, in the light of eternity, everything is relative. Secondly, one queries whether it is accurate to underline one's point of view with examples from troublesome times. The regression in the Eastern-Mediterranean countries occurred in the centuries after the Roman Empire had conquered the area, and the period from 1550 to 1650 involved several religious wars on the European continent (such as the war between the

Low Countries and Spain from 1568 to 1648, the war of the Huguenots, and the Thirty Years War from 1618 to 1648). Troublesome times may lead to shock reactions, which are not normative for general developments. Likewise, after the Second World War, the natural economy was reborn, with barter trading under special circumstances. In Germany, cigarettes replaced money as the medium of exchange for some time after the war (Urwin, D. W.: *A Political History of Western Europe Since 1945*, Fifth edition, Longman, 1997, p. 29). The collapse of the Russian economy after the fall of communism led to a return of barter trading in several Russian regions for some time (Todd, E.: *Après l'Empire: Essai sur la décomposition du système américain* (Dutch Translation), Prometheus, 2003, pp. 171–172). Nevertheless, we do not speak of a "regression" in these circumstances. The increasing information and communication of modern times has led some fundamentalist religious groups to conclude that it is better not to take part in these developments. Consequently, they withdraw, closing themselves off, or they choose to oppose modernity. But again, this is not normative for a general development of the economic order. Therefore, it is difficult to see the error in distinguishing between different consecutive developmental stages of the economic order, provided these stages are not considered too rigidly.

24. Cowles, M. G., et al., (eds.): *Transforming Europe: Europeanization and Domestic Change*, Cornell University Press, 2001.
25. Conant, L.: Europeanization and the Courts: Variable Patterns of Adaptation among National Judiciaries, in: Cowles, M. G., et al.: ibid., chapter 6.
26. This is not to say that we have reason to be satisfied with the way these institutions work.
27. The most famous representative from the left side of the continuum and a fierce critic of the market economy was Karl Marx. He was convinced that the productive powers of capitalism, markets and competition, needed to be controlled in order to prevent them from causing depressions and misery for workers. For Marx, the best way to do so was government ownership of the means of production, together with the power to enforce decisions regarding their use. Marx's influence is difficult to overestimate. At its peak, almost one-third of the world was ruled by the Marxist doctrine (Samuelson, P. and Nordhaus, W. D.: ibid., p. 7), organized in left-leaning political parties that supported a socialist or communist economic order. However, Marx himself did not intend to interpret the world and capture it in a doctrine ["*Moi, je ne suis pas Marxiste*"]. Instead, Marx believed that government ownership of the means of production would make the world a better place by rooting out the many abuses of the Industrial Revolution. Therefore, Marxism can only rightfully be approached as a doctrine if one is prepared to do so from the perspective of an entity of tensions, resulting from economical, political, sociological, philosophical, historical, and ethical motives (Banning, W.: *Karl Marx: Leven, Leer en Betekenis*, Utrecht/Antwerpen, 1960, pp. 57–59).

The most famous representative from the right side of the continuum and a strong supporter of the market economy was Adam Smith. The ingredients of his market economy were private ownership of the means of production, with the price mechanism as the coordinating instrument for all the individual plans of economic subjects. In Smith's line of reasoning, the role of the government is twofold. First of all, it has to protect its citizens against *external* aggression.

This legitimizes a defense system. Secondly, individual citizens have to be protected from attacks by other citizens against their lives, health, freedom, and private ownership. This legitimizes the police, a judiciary, and legislation; in short: *internal* legal protection (Meijer, G.: ibid., chapter 2). However, two important matters should be taken into account regarding Smith's liberalism. First of all, he and fellow thinkers expected their ideas on the economic order to provide liberation from the pressures of mercantilism of the preceding era. This liberation was expected to bring increasing wealth. Secondly, it should not be forgotten that *An Inquiry into the Nature and the Causes of the Wealth of Nations* (1776), the manual for a liberal economic order, had been preceded by Smith's *The Theory of Moral Sentiments*, 17 years before. If one is to understand the philosopher Adam Smith, these two books should be read together, i.e., he believed that people dealt with "built-in restraints derived from moral, religion, custom and education when they strive towards self-interest" (Hirsch, F.: *Social Limits to Growth*, London, 1995, pp. 137–138). The two studies together envisage a balanced approach to self-interest. Smith uses the term "*sympathy*" in this respect. To him, this is a feeling of compassion with others, which he regards as the only element of ethical behavior, and which imposes a moral obligation to take one's fellow citizen into account (Handy, C.: *The Empty Raincoat* (Dutch Translation), Amsterdam/Antwerpen, 1994. pp. 22 and 83), from the perspective of a "personal responsibility for making the world a better place (Green, D. G.: *From Welfare State to Civil Society: To Welfare that Works in New Zealand*, New Zealand Business Round Table, Wellington, 1996, p. 12). Consequently, "the marketplace of Adam Smith did not exist in some imaginary land of autonomous, amoral individuals, but within an interdependent social fabric in which virtue was extolled and a moral conscience constrained individual actions" (Wight, J. B.: *Saving Adam Smith: A Tale of Wealth, Transformation and Virtue*, Prentice-Hall, Inc., 2002, pp. 199–200). From this it follows that, to Smith, the market was not the neutral instrument for allocating efficiency that some present-day supporters of neo-liberalism assume it to be. It never has been. Instead, the idea of a self-regulating market is a "utopian experiment" (Polanyi, K.: *The Great Transformation: The Political and Economic Origins of our Time*, Beacan Press, 1957, p. 250). Polanyi would have regarded the neo-liberal view as a-historical. In *The Great Transformation,* he says in this respect, "Economic history reveals that the emergence of national markets was in no way the result of the gradual and spontaneous emancipation of the economic sphere from government control. On the contrary, the market has been the outcome of a conscious and often violent intervention on the part of the government which imposed the market organization on society for non-economic ends." Although Smith had, and still has, many supporters, this does not mean that his ideas have never been contested. Even in 1885, List argued strongly that there may be good political reasons for governments to interfere in the economic process (List, F.: *The National System of Political Economy*, Augustus M. Kelley Publishers, Reprints of Economic Classics, New York, 1966). Essentially, both Marx and Smith wanted to make the world a better place. In order to achieve that, both focused on the market. Marx wanted to eliminate it completely, because of the morally and ethically reprehensible excesses it produced in his days. Apparently, he was not confident that the market would provide a situation of checks and balances in society. In contrast, Smith wanted to regulate the market in order to prevent it from producing these same excesses. Apparently, he feared that an unregulated market would destroy an existing situation of checks and balances in society.

28. Samuelson, P. and Nordhaus, W. D.: ibid., p. 6.
29. Friedman, M. and Friedman, R.: ibid., p. 284.
30. Urwin, D. W.: ibid., p. 126.
31. Myrdal, G.: *Beyond the Welfare State* (Dutch Translation), N. V. De Arbeiderspers, Amsterdam, 1963, pp. 34, 73, and 90.
32. Keynes, J. M.: *The General Theory of Employment, Interest and Money*, The Easton Press, Collector's Edition, Norwalk, Connecticut, 1995.
33. Mueller, D. C.: *Public Choice II: A Revised Edition of Public Choice*, Cambridge University Press, 1995, pp. 2–3.
34. Besides, this was the time of a mechanistic economic worldview, which led economists to become social technocrats who developed planning instruments laid down in econometric models, which were meant to serve as anchors of security in a world of crises, wars, and ideological conflicts. In this respect, Klein's ideas on "statistical significance," Samuelson's "proofs on paper," and Tinbergen's belief in a "manageable society" are examples which, according to McCloskey, were all attempts to create an atmosphere of independence which was not susceptible to conflict (McCloskey, D. N.: *The Vices of Economists—The Virtues of the Bourgeoisie* (Dutch Translation), Amsterdam University Press, 1997).
35. Despite the "neo," neo-liberalism did not come out of the blue. In the 1920s and 1930s, scholars like Von Hayek, Eucken, and Von Mises argued for a different design of the economic order, motivated by the shortcomings of liberalism in practice. These shortcomings can be captured by the term *rigidity*. Laissez-faire, as intended by Smith some hundred years before, had evolved into the dogma that the government should, in all circumstances, abstain from interfering in the economic process. Consequently, the outlook of the economic order became almost completely determined by individual economic subjects. Through this, liberalism became the defender of the vested interests in society, with supporters such as Spencer from Great Britain, Bastiat from France, and the Manchester business school.
36. Hayek, F. A.: *The Road to Serfdom*, University of Chicago Press, 1994.
37. This may seem new, but it is not. As early as 1933, Oppenheimer, a neo-liberal, published his "*Weder so noch so. Der Dritte Weg.*" Furthermore, Röpke, Proudhon, and others have used the term, together with labels like "revisionist liberalism," "liberal revisionism," "liberal conservatism," and "constructive liberalism." These authors all rejected the rigid development of laissez-faire liberalism after Smith, as well as socialism (Meijer, G.: ibid., pp. 2 and 30). In this respect, laissez-faire liberalism can be distinguished as the "first way" capitalism. It ruled during the time of the Industrial Revolution, with the "robber barons" in power. It was replaced by the "second way," state capitalism, which shifted power to public-sector bureaucrats.
38. Gates, J.: *Democracy at Risk: Rescuing Main Street from Wall Street*, Perseus Publishing, 2001, p. 23.
39. Gates, J.: ibid., pp. 92–94.
40. Gusmorino, P. A., III: "Main Causes of the Great Depression," in: *Gusmorino World* (May 13, 1996), available from: http://www.gusmorino.com/pag3/

great_depression/index.html. It reads, "According to a study done by the Brookings Institute, in 1929 the top 0.1% of Americans had a combined income equal to the bottom 42%. That same top 0.1% of Americans in 1929 controlled 34% of all savings, while 80% of Americans had no savings at all. [. . .] This maldistribution of income between the rich and the middle-class grew throughout the 1920s. While the disposable income per capita rose 9% from 1920 to 1929, those within the top 1% enjoyed a stupendous 75% increase in per capita disposable income."

41. Honesty requires me to say, however, that the dawning of the Second World War restored the economy again.
42. In this respect, see: Urwin, D. W.: ibid., chapter 3.
43. Calleo, D. P.: *Rethinking Europe's Future*, Princeton University Press, 2001, p. 180.
44. Stiglitz, J.: *The Roaring Nineties: Seeds of Destruction*, Allen Lane, 2003.
45. The theory of a general (Pareto) equilibrium for the economy proved not to apply, due to the extensive statistical data that were needed to solve the many equations. Even the Chinese economist Li Yining has lost his belief in the planning capacities of the government and has become a strong supporter of the establishment of local private businesses.
46. McCloskey, D. N.: ibid. To this author, these economists have been doing nothing more than playing in a sandbox, an activity, which is very different from operating in the real world.
47. The fact that we would be on our way to the end of history, with one universal homogeneous state, does not imply that history will not, temporarily, repeat itself. In this respect, Fukuyama's use of the term *isothymia* is important. It refers to the desire of people to be recognized as equal to others (Fukuyama, F.: *The End of History and the Last Man* (Dutch Translation), 4th edition, Olympus, 1999).
48. Rawls in: Sen, A.: *Development as Freedom* (Dutch Translation), Amsterdam/Antwerpen, 2000, p. 135.
49. Fukuyama admits, however, that the end of history may be a dull time, leading people to get history started again from a powerful nostalgia for the time when history still existed (in: Wheen, F.: *How Mumbo-Jumbo Conquered the World*, Harper Perennial, 2004, pp. 68–70).
50. Albert, M.: *Capitalism versus Capitalism* (Dutch Translation), Amsterdam, 1992; Dawson, A. D.: *The Two Faces of Economics*, Longman, 1996; Galbraith, J. K.: *A Journey through Economic Time: A Firsthand View* (Dutch Translation), Baarn, 1995; Handy, C.: *Beyond Certainty: The Changing World of Organisations*, London, 1996; Huntington, S. P.: *The Clash of Civilizations and the Remaking of the World Order*, New York, 1996; Peterson, W. C.: *Silent Depression: Twenty-Five Years of Wage Squeeze and Middle-Class Decline*, Norton and Company, 1995; Reich, C. A.: *Opposing the System*, New York, 1995; Thurow, L. C.: *The Future of Capitalism.* London, 1996; Buchanan, P. J.: *The Great Betrayal: How American Sovereignty and Social Justice are Being Sacrificed to the Gods of the Global Economy*, Little, Brown and Company, 1998; Kelly, C. M.: *Class War in America: How Economic and Political Conservatives are Exploiting Low- and Middle-Class Americans*, Fithian Press, 2000.
51. NRC/Handelsblad, February 17, 1996.
52. Fukuyama, F.: *The End of History and the Last Man*, ibid., p. 162.

53. Mestrum, F.: *Globalisering en Armoede: Over het Nut van Armoede in de Nieuwe Wereldorde*, Berchem, 2000, p. 24.
54. Gates, J.: ibid., p. xxxvii.
55. Offe, C.: Contradictions of the Welfare State, Keane (ed.), the MIT Press, Massachusetts, 1993, p. 147.
56. Self, P.: *Rolling Back the Market: Economic Dogma and Political Choice*, MacMillan Press Ltd., 2000, p. 89.
57. Handy, C.: *Beyond Certainty: The Changing Worlds of Organisations*, ibid., p. 21. Looking back, one can wonder how unexpected the end of the communist dream was. Although Henry Kissinger, from the perspective of power politics, as United States Secretary of State declared in the 1970s that communism would never disappear, Fukuyama presents a list of 13 events in China and the Soviet Union that indicated that communism was on the way to its end, starting in the 1980s (Fukuyama, F.: *The End of History and the Last Man*, ibid., pp. 51–53). Regarding the dangers that threaten present-day capitalism, Lacher remarks that "the gravediggers of Marxism are many, alone the corpse will not lay still" (Lacher, H.: "Making Sense of the International System: The Promises and Pitfalls of Contemporary Marxist Theories of International Relations," in: Rupert, M. and Smith, H., (eds.): *Historical Materialism and Globalization*, Routledge, 2002, p. 147).
58. Berman, P.: *Terror and Liberalism*, W. W. Norton & Company, 2003, p. 162.
59. Becker, U.: *Europese Democratieën: Vrijheid, Gelijkheid, Solidariteit en Soevereiniteit in Praktijk*, Het Spinhuis, 1999, p. 23. One could also argue that communism was instrumental in keeping capitalism alert in maintaining a fair society. With the end of communism, however, capitalism has been thrown back upon its own characteristics. In this respect, it may be reassuring that each economic system demands a certain ethical behavior. Capitalism is no exception to that. In the longer term, its success not only depends on self-interest, but also on a complex and subtle system of values and norms with ingredients like dependability, trust, and honesty. Consequently, a solid system of values and norms, reaching beyond the market economy, is instrumental to an effective capitalist economic order. To put it more strongly; from its origins, the basic ethics of behavior have enormously contributed to the success of capitalism. The challenge for present-day neo-liberal capitalists is to take these origins to heart, by maintaining elementary social provisions of fairness and justice as additional elements of a market economy (Sen, A.: ibid., pp. 141, 252, 256, and 268). In Gates' words, free enterprise has to be "guided by rules that put some limits on greed so that more of us can afford to give expression to that innate yearning for connectedness" (Gates, J.: ibid., p. 3). This will make the difference between an economic order that is directed at economic growth and one that pursues development (Sen, A.: ibid.).
60. Wilkinson, R. G.: *Unhealthy Societies: The Afflictions of Inequality*, Routledge, 1996, pp. 223–224. I do not want to suggest that the Asian tigers represent a more preferable society. After all, countries like Malaysia and Thailand know much poverty. Nevertheless, while moving to the right side of the continuum in search of a new balance, it is good to remember how these Asian countries used political means to become, indeed, economic tigers.
61. Popta, S. van: *De Gemengde Economische Orde en de Christelijk-Sociale Gedachte*, Kampen, 1974, p. 5.

62. Myrdal, G.: ibid., p. 87.
63. The economic orders positioned relatively more on the left side of the continuum are irrelevant for the purposes of this study. Moreover, it is not the intention of this book to provide a discourse on democracy. The meaning of democracy is assumed to be known.
64. Gooijer, W. J. de: *Beheersing van Technologische Vernieuwing*, Alphen a/d Rijn, 1976.
65. An assumption which is highly debated these days.
66. Some countries, like the United Kingdom, have a liberal tradition; France is known for its Parisian *dirigisme*; the Netherlands, Belgium, Luxembourg, Germany, Austria, and the Scandinavian countries favor a democracy of mutual consultation; and the political process in Italy shows characteristics which are difficult to combine with democracy. Moreover, if we look at the institutional frameworks, countries like Belgium, Germany, and Austria are federations, whereas other democracies have a central government. Some countries are monarchies and others are republics. Electoral systems may be based on constituencies or on proportionate representation. In short, a study of European democracies would show an enormous complexity, which in turn would contribute to explaining the difficulties of European integration (Becker, U.: ibid.). In order to bring some structure to this complexity, Becker distinguishes between four typologies of the political process. The first is the typology of *arena politics*. This is the most pluralistic model, with many participants in the decision-making process who can, to a certain extent, operate autonomously. Participants compete and check each other. In the context of arena politics, innumerable organizations try to influence the policy areas of their interests. Politics is a market here, but it is a market that also knows compromise and deal-making. The second typology is that of *state imposition*. Here, centrally formulated policies are dictated to the members of society by an elected majority government that feels entitled to do so. Negotiating is less developed here, and consultation is rather elitist and selective. The third typology relates to a situation where the political process is channelled through an *institutionalized framework of consultation*. Here, the objective of social integration is paramount. Therefore, consensus-building is characteristic for this typology. The alternative name for this typology is *corporatism*. Finally, the fourth typology is *clientelism*, which refers to a relationship "of personal dependence, unrelated to kinship, which links two persons who control unequal resources, the patron and the client, for a reciprocal exchange of favours." Central in this typology are hierarchy, service, favors-in-kind and personal dependence relations. All democracies show features of these typologies (Becker, U.: ibid., pp. 138–140).
67. Regarding movement along the continuum, the focus is particularly on the economic dimension. I do realize, however, that this dimension is greatly influenced by cultural and political conditions. One may even argue that the present economic situation of what we call "the developed world" has its origins in a threefold cultural premise from around four centuries ago. The first premise is that democratic development conditions economic development. Consequently, a country will stay economically behind if it is organized in a top-down structure with citizens living in fear of their leaders. China has been a longstanding example of this until recently. As it shows, however, the country is

very well capable of realizing a strong economic growth without a democratic form of government. The second premise is that a country will develop economically only if it has both a middle class, which is characterized by an entrepreneurial spirit, and if society is characterized by gender equality. The third premise is that, through personal observation and experience, individuals can succeed in wresting themselves from dictated dogmas, which is the basis for scientific development. In combination, these premises condition democratic economic development. Consequently, there is every reason to be critical of linking development aid to political democracy. (For the influence of cultural aspects on economic development, see Landes, D. S.: *The Wealth and Poverty of Nations: Why Some Are So Rich and Some So Poor* (Dutch Translation), Het Spectrum, 1998).

68. Becker, U.: ibid., p. 11. More specifically, democracy in the countries of the developed world means "liberal democracy," i.e., a political system which is not only characterized by universal suffrage, but also by the existence of a constitutional state, the separation of powers, and the protection of constitutional rights like freedom of speech, religion, and property. This type of democracy dates to around 1950 (Zakaria, F.: ibid., pp. 13, 45).
69. For an extensive discussion in this respect, see: Hartog, F.: *Overheid en Economisch Leven*, Alphen a/d Rijn, 1965, chapters 5–8.
70. Hoffman, L.: Sector-Structuurbeleid, in: *Economisch Statistische Berichten*, 23-5-1973, p. 441.
71. Pen, J.: *Harmonie en Conflict*, Amsterdam, 1962, p. 5.
72. Kalma, P.: *De Illusie van de "Democratische Staat,"* Kluwer, 1982.
73. Kalma, P.: ibid., p. 20.
74. Regarding this, the Dutch seem to be envied for their so-called "polder model," which is characterized by time-consuming negotiations between employers, the unions, and the government (*The Economist*: Model Makers: A Survey of the Netherlands, 4 May 2002, p. 3). Nonetheless, this model is immediately renamed the "Dutch Disease" whenever the economy slows down. This "polder model" is assumed to have contributed to improving the Dutch competitive position in the international economy, thanks to social-economic stability and an agreed-upon wage restraint. However, there is reason to modify the benefits of the Dutch model to a certain extent. First of all, wage restraint in the Netherlands in the 1980s did not result in increased employment in industry. Furthermore, although exports in the Netherlands increased during that time , this was not the effect of wage restraint, but of investments in quality and increased productivity, both of which were facilitated by the strong Dutch guilder (Delsen, L.: *Exit Poldermodel? Sociaal-Economische Ontwikkelingen in Nederland*, Second edition, 2001).
75. These countries (still) consider social security to be an investment in society that contributes to political stability, the latter being an indispensable factor for economic growth, according to Dornbusch (Dornbusch, R.: *Agenda voor Economische Groei*, Economisch-Statistische Berichten, 22-2-1992. pp. 708–711).
76. Dyson, K.: *The Politics of the Euro-Zone: Stability or Breakdown?* Oxford University Press, 2000, p. 4.
77. Sennett, R.: *The Corrosion of Character: The Personal Consequences of Work in the New Capitalism*, W. W. Norton and Company, 1998, p. 53.

78. Vos, P. J.: Overleeft het Rijnlandse Model? in: Toren, J. P. van den and Vos, P. J., (eds.): *Overleeft het Rijnlandse Model? Perspectief op Arbeidsverhoudingen*, Nationaal Vakbondsmuseum, 1997, p. 10.
79. Braybrooke, D. and Lindblom, C. E.: *A Strategy of Decision*, New York, 1970.
80. Kirschen, E. S., et al.: *Economic Policy in Our Time*, Vol. I, II and III, Second edition, Amsterdam, 1968.
81. In this respect, Urwin adds greater productivity and better social security to the policy objectives of governments (Urwin, D. W.: ibid., p. 126).
82. Meadows, D. L.: *The Limits to Growth: A Report for the Club of Rome Project* (Dutch Translation), Utrecht/Antwerpen, 1972.
83. Beek, W. J.: Het Eco-Circus is serieus te nemen, in: *De Ingenieur*, Volume 88, no. 8, February 1976.
84. Urwin, D. W.: ibid., p. 126.
85. Becker, U.: ibid., pp. 93–94.
86. Pierre, J. and Guy Peters, B.: *Governance, Politics and the State*, MacMillan Press Ltd., 2000, p. 81.
87. Pierre, J. and Guy Peters, B.: ibid., p. 1.
88. Pierre, J. and Guy Peters, B.: ibid., pp. 4–5.
89. Pierre, J. and Guy Peters, B.: ibid., p. 9.
90. Pierre, J. and Guy Peters, B.: ibid., p. 194.
91. Marks, G., et al.: European Integration from the 1980s: State-Centric v. Multi-Level Governance, in: Nelsen, B. F. and Stubb, A., (eds.): *The European Union: Readings on the Theory and Practice of European Integration*, Second edition, Palgrave, 1998, p. 292.
92. Marks, G., et al.: ibid., pp. 273–293.
93. If we include the applicant countries, this number would be 480 million.
94. The World Economic Forum's 1999 competitiveness ranking, for instance, shows that they remain far behind the United States. The United States ranks second (after Singapore); and the United Kingdom, France, Germany and Italy only hold the 18th, 23rd, 25th, and 35th positions, respectively. In addition, the World Competitiveness Yearbook 2000 ranks the United States first for five consecutive years, with Germany in the 18th place and Italy in the 30th. Reports of the European Commission present a comparable picture. They show that the European Union lags 20% behind the United States in terms of productivity levels and employment rates. Moreover, the European Union has created only ten million new jobs since 1960, which is less than 20% of the jobs created in the United States. Finally, when it comes to investments, in the European Union there was a sharp decline from 2.5% in the 1980s to 0.8% during the 1990s, compared with an average annual increase of 5.4% in the United States during the 1990s, up from 2.4% in the 1980s (Lee, S.: Discovering the Frontiers of Regionalism: Fostering Entrepreneurship, Innovation and Competitiveness in the European Union, in: Breslin, S., Hughes, Ch. W., Phillips, N., Rosamond, B., (eds.): *New Regionalism in the Global Political Economy: Theories and Cases*, Routledge, 2002, pp. 163–164). In a globalizing economy, these are alarming differences.
95. In this respect, it is sufficient to note that, from 1850 onward, national European governments, mainly in the industrializing world, started to assume a growing responsibility for the management of social affairs within their territory through the development of "complex surveillance systems to monitor

social conditions, including those that might lead to instability, and to confront problems" (Dunkerley, D., Hodgson, L., Konopacki, S., Spybey, T., and Thompson, A.: *Changing Europe: Identities, Nations and Citizens*, Routledge, 2002, p. 27). In those days, the permanent foundations were also laid, on a national scale, for compulsory and collective social security systems in capitalistic democracies in Europe, to the advantage of the great majority of wage laborers. Since then, systems of social security in Europe have been extended, refined, professionalized, and bureaucratized, creating the "equanimity of the welfare state" (Swaan, A. de: ibid., p. 158; author's translation). Although there are differences in the timing and scope of the development of these systems, they all contributed to social stability. Nonetheless, these developments imply that the relational tensions between the privileged and the poor continued to exist. In this respect, De Swaan argues that, on the one hand, laborers had to develop a sense of collective solidarity. After all, what had happened to others today might happen to them tomorrow. On the other hand, the privileged would have to start to realize that mass poverty among industrial labourers could also threaten their own existence. What was required, therefore, was an understanding of the "general interdependence of people in an industrial society, a social consciousness" (Swaan, A. de, ibid., p. 160; author's translation).

96. As for the origins of social security, there is an acknowledged distinction between Bismarck and Beveridge. Bismarck introduced employee insurance against industrial and other diseases, accidents, invalidity, and old age in Germany around 1880. The objective was, on the one hand, to promote the political and social integration of the working class into society, and on the other hand, to prevent social unrest and class struggle. In the period between the two World Wars, the circle of insured parties was extended to include higher incomes, family members, and senior citizens. At the dawn of the Second World War, all the countries of Western Europe had social insurance against these four risks. In addition to social integration and the prevention of social unrest, stabilization of the economy also became an objective, inspired by Keynes, who regarded social insurances useful because of their anti-cyclical effect on the economy. The Beveridge model was introduced in the United Kingdom in 1942. This involved a universal insurance system, which gave all citizens the right to health care and protection. In contrast to Bismarck, the Beveridge model is not related to income (Einerhand, M., et al.: *Sociale Zekerheid: Stelsels en Regelingen in Enkele Europese Landen*, Den Haag, 1995, pp. 27–29). For other approaches to models of social security see, for example, Jallade, J-P., (ed.): *The Crisis of Redistribution in European Welfare States*, Stoke-on-Trent, 1988; Geleijnse, et al.: *Tussen Ministelsel en Participatiemodel: Een verkennende Studie naar Stelselvarianten in de Sociale Zekerheid*, Sociaal en Cultureel Planbureau, Rijswijk, 1993; Alber, J.: Some Causes of Social Security Expenditure Developments in Western Europe 1949–1977, in: Loney, M., Boswell, D., Clarke, J., (eds.): *Social Policy and Social Welfare*, Open University Press, Philadelphia, 1993, pp. 156–170; Lee and Raban, in: Jones, L.: *The Social Context of Health and Health Work*, London, 1994, pp. 59–60; Einerhand, M., et al.: ibid., pp. 29–35; Goudswaard, K. P.: *Sociale Convergentie*, Leiden, 1996; Esping Andersen, in: Schuyt, K. and Veen, R. van der, (eds.): *De verdeelde Samenleving: Een Inleiding in de Ontwikkeling van de Nederlandse*

Verzorgingsstaat, Houten, 1995, pp. 6–7; Dent, M.: *Remodelling Hospitals and Health Professions in Europe: Medicine, Nursing and the State*, Palgrave, 2003, chapter 2.

97. Sandmo, A.: Introduction: The Welfare Economics of the Welfare State, in: Andersen, T. M., Moene, K. O., Sandmo, A., (eds.): *The Future of the Welfare State*, Blackwell Publishers, 1995, p. 1.
98. Thinking about welfare, however, had already started a few hundreds years earlier, as can be seen from Thomas Paine's writings (Pierson, Chr. and Castles, F., (eds.): *The Welfare State Reader*, Polity, 2003, pp. 1–2).
99. In his *Citizenship and Social Class* (1950), T. H. Marshall gave a well-known syntheses of the development of modern citizenship. According to him, the concept of citizenship is linked to the development of three sets of rights over the past few centuries. The 18th century saw the development of *civil rights*. They concerned individual freedom and justice, with a judicial system for their enforcement. In the 19th century, *political rights* were added, which meant that citizens became entitled to political participation and decision-making procedures. Finally, the 20th century saw the emergence of *social rights*, providing entitlements to an appropriate quality of life linked to education and welfare services. Marshall argued that "the modern drive towards social equality is the latest phase of an evolution of citizenship which has been in continuous progress for some 250 years" (in: Dunkerley, D., Hodgson, L., Konopacki, S., Spybey, T., Thompson, A.: ibid., p. 11). From this perspective, the welfare state is a logical and irreversible next step in a process of civilization. A comparable approach can be found in Vasak, who distinguishes between three types of revolution: (1) the French revolution of 1789, which brought *classical rights*; (2) the socialistic revolutions of around 1848, resulting in *social rights*; and (3) the revolutions as a consequence of the process of decolonization after the Second World War, which brought *collective rights* (in: Cliteur, P.: *Tegen de Decadentie: De Democratische Rechtstaat in Verval*, De Arbeiderpers, Amsterdam/Antwerpen, 2004, p. 169).
100. Urwin, D. W.: ibid., p. 130.
101. Calleo, D. P.: ibid., p. 166.
102. De Volkskrant, 5 September 2003.
103. Geleijnse, L., et al.: ibid., pp. 7–8.
104. Urwin, D. W.: ibid., p. 123.
105. Here, we have an important difference with the United States. Citizens' expectations about what the government should or should not do are essentially lower in the United States than in Europe. Research from the 1990s, for instance, shows that twice as many Europeans as Americans expected their governments to decrease income inequality. In addition to this, almost three times as many Europeans as Americans expected their government to provide a guaranteed minimum income (Becker, U.: ibid., table 5.5, p. 125).
106. Increasing unemployment, combined with increasing inflation and declining economic growth.
107. As for the latter, around 24% of German businesses with works councils, for instance, had corporate-level pacts by 1998, concluding concessions on pay and working hours in return for employment guarantees. German Chancellor Schröder tried to extend this practice to the national level in the form of an

"alliance for jobs," aiming to relate job creation to issues of taxation, welfare state reforms, wages policy and working time.

108. Dyson, K.: ibid., pp. 19 and 38.
109. Becker, U.: ibid., p. 157. For the United States, Friedman proposes an even more rigorous change. After concluding that most of the American welfare programmes should never have been enacted, because they make people dependent and de-motivated to work, he suggests a transitional programme that would have two essential components. Firstly, the many different specific programmes, including the huge accompanying bureaucracy, would be replaced by a single comprehensive programme of cash income supplements, paid through a negative income tax linked to the positive income tax. This single programme would also provide a safety net for every American, so that nobody would have to suffer from dire distress. Secondly, he suggests unwinding social security (although meeting existing commitments), and simultaneously (but gradually) requiring people to make their own retirement arrangements (Friedman, M. and Friedman, R.: ibid., p. 120).
110. The relative increase of government expenditure over the first period of fifteen years is 35.9%, 83.0%, and 78.7% for the United States, the European Union and Japan, respectively. Starting from almost the same position of 27.0% and 28.2% in 1960, by 1985 the expenditure of the governments of the European Union and Japan appears to have been more than twice as high as that of the United States. The relative increase of the European Union and Japan does not differ much, whereas the difference in starting position between Japan and the other two continents can probably be related to cultural differences. The tremendous increase in public spending within the European Union is a reflection of European Union countries' establishing their welfare states or extending an existing welfare state. Countries like France, the United Kingdom, the Netherlands, the Federal German Republic, and Luxembourg were already "big spenders" in 1960 (the countries that spent more than 30% of GDP in 1960, according to the table mentioned in footnote 105, are labeled "big spenders"). Here, citizens expected their governments to make their dreams come true. For countries like Ireland, Spain, Portugal, and Greece, growing prosperity and the fact that they benefitted from the European Union budget, as well as, for all but one, the transition to democracy, made it possible to make up for budgetary arrears. On the revenue side (either via taxation or premiums), the money raised was sufficient for the European Union to realize a slightly positive balance of 0.3% of GDP in 1960, compared to 2.4% for Japan. The United States had a small deficit of 0.7%. Fifteen years later, however, the balance showed a deficit of 5.6% of GDP for the USA, 5.9% for the European Union, and 1.5% for Japan.
111. The figures for 1960 and 1985 are from Mueller, D. C.: ibid., p. 322, table 17.2.
112. Figures from the OECD Economic Outlook, OECD website, December, 2002.
113. It is also possible to repair some of the damage inflicted on the welfare state during the reform phase. For example, around the turn of the century, the Dutch government allowed its health care system to be further extended.
114. In this respect, Pakaslanti distinguishes between four groups of countries (see Theofilatou, M. A.: ibid.: pp. 151–152). The French and the Germans, with budget deficits in 2003 of 4% and 3.8%, respectively, are thus in trouble.

115. In the United Kingdom, an Anglo-American country, 20% of the working population worked at least 60 hours per week in 2002. Currently, 25% of Canadians work more than 50 hours per week, up from 10% in 1991 (Honoré, C.: *In Praise of Slow: How a Worldwide Movement is Challenging the Cult of Speed* (Dutch Translation), Lemniscaat, Rotterdam, 2004, p. 148).
116. In 1997, Americans worked 1,966 hours per year, compared to, for example, 1,399 for Norway, 1,552 for Sweden, 1,643 for Switzerland, 1,689 for Denmark, and 1,679 for the Netherlands (Phillips, K.: *Wealth and Democracy: A Political History of the American Rich*, New York, 2002, p. 165). In the United States, there has been a trend reversal. Back in the 1950s and 1960s, Americans worked fewer hours than their colleagues elsewhere. In 1999, however, "the typical American worked 350 hours more per year than the typical European, the equivalent of nine work weeks," according to the American Bureau of Labor Statistics (Phillips, K.: ibid., p. 115).
117. In this respect, German statistics from 2000 reveal that a German four-person household living on social security received 73% of the wage earnings of a comparable working family. For the United Kingdom, France and Italy the figures were 68%, 56%, and 48% respectively (Miegel, M.: *Die deformierte Gesellschaft: Wie die Deutschen Ihre Wirklichkeit verdrängen*, Propyläen, 2002, p. 105).
118. Rifkin, J.: *The End of Work: The Decline of the Global Labor Force and the Dawn of the Post-Market Era*, New York, 1995, pp. 202–203. See also Luttwak, E.: *Turbo Capitalism: Winners and Losers in the Global Economy*, London, 1998, p. 106. The importance of these differences is illustrated by empirical research from Alesina and Perotti. They found that if taxation on labor would increase by 1% of GDP, the costs of each labor unit in countries with average institutional labor relations would increase by 2.5% (in: Rodrik, D.: *Has Globalization Gone too Far?*, Washington, 1997, p. 45).
119. Fairlamb, D.: Too Few Cradles and too Few Graves, in: *Business Week*, European Edition, 29 March 2004, p. 56.
120. In: Komter, A. E., Burgers, J. and Engbersen, G.: *Het Cement van de Samenleving. Een verkennende Studie naar Solidariteit en Cohesie*, Amsterdam University Press, 2000, p. 20. In this respect, Habermas speaks of the "welfare state compromise," which has characterized post-war capitalist societies. This compromise emerged to fill up the "functional gaps" of the capitalist economy caused by the economic disequilibria of "crisis-ridden growth" (business cycles and poor infrastructural investments) (Scambler, G.: *Health and Social Change: A Critical Theory*, Open University Press, 2002, p. 47).
121. Offe, C.: Some Contradictions of the Modern Welfare State, in: Pierson, Chr. and Castles, F., (eds.): ibid., p. 70.
122. Komter, A. E., Burgers, J. en, and Engbersen, G.: ibid., chapter 1.
123. Klein, N.: *Fences and Windows: Dispatches from the Front Lines of the Globalization Debate*, Picador, USA, 2002, p. 182.
124. Komter, A. E., Burgers, J. and Engbersen, G.: ibid., p. 21
125. Schnapper, D.: The French View of the 'Dutch Miracle, in: Gier, E. de, Swaan, A. de, Ooijens, M., (eds.): *Dutch Welfare Reform in an Expanding Europe: The Neighbours' View*, Het Spinhuis, 2004, p. 52.
126. Castells, M.: *End of Millennium*, ibid., p. 129.
127. Luttwak, E.: ibid., p. 203.

128. In support of this view, for example, is the way the United Kingdom's government handled the privatization of UK prisons, with the American Wackenhut company becoming the British prison privateer, despite its higher-cost bid and its negative public image (murder, sexual abuse of prisoners, illegal use of gas in prisons) (Palast, G.: *The Best Democracy Money Can Buy*, London, 2003, pp. 310–314).
129. Regarding this, the Dutch economist Teulings correctly argues that a monopolist in public hands also behaves like a monopolist, with political control and responsibility remaining publically symbolic. With this experience, the search for more efficient control mechanisms has a rational basis. Regarding this, Teulings refers respectfully to the initiatives of Prime Minister Thatcher, who was responsible for the privatization of British public utilities like water, electricity and telecommunications. They resulted in such productivity increases that a 40% increase was not exceptional (Teulings, C.: Hoe de Beursgang van een Staatsmonopolist de Welvaart dient, in: Dalen, H. van and Kalshoven, F. (eds.): *Meesters van de Welvaart: Topeconomen over Nederland*, uitgeverij Balans, 2002, p. 118). In line with this, Mueller produces a list of 50 studies showing that privatization of public services resulted in efficiency gains in all examples but two (Mueller, C.: ibid., pp. 262–265). Though the United Kingdom was the forerunner of privatizations, corporate businesses in the United States were quick to smell the potential profits. As an example, the Californian lobby for the deregulation of electricity was very successful, not the least because of the promise that deregulation would cut consumer prices by 20%. However, after deregulation, normal households experienced a price increase of 379% in 1999, compared to the 1998 level. In addition to this, Californian plant owners started to behave like "power pirates" by manipulating the available capacities. This was exposed on the first hot Californian summer day after deregulation, when the electricity price per unit of power increased by no less than 30,000% (!) above the old regulated price of about $30. The electricity producers chose not to use all available generators, thus creating shortages through "physical withholding" and "economic withholding." Between May and November 2000, this is reported to have occurred no less than 98% of the time. It is not difficult to guess who suffered most from this outrageous behavior of "revaluating capitalists" (Palast, G.: ibid., pp. 125–129). As for the role of Enron in this matter, see Stiglitz, J. E.: *The Roaring Nineties: Seeds of Destruction*, ibid., chapter 10.
130. Feigenbaum, H., et al.: *Shrinking the State: The Political Underpinnings of Privatisation*, Cambridge University Press, 1999.
131. In this respect, Palast shows that, due to privatization, water bills in the United Kingdom shot up to 250% of the USA price, whereas company stock prices quintupled. In some parts of England, you could even be arrested for watering your lawn (Palast, G.: ibid., p. 130).
132. Yergin, D. and Stanislaw, J.: *The Commanding Heights: The Battle between Government and the Marketplace that is Remaking the Modern World*, New York, 1998, p. 121. An illustration of the necessity for government regulation has been provided, sadly enough, by the railway accident in London some years ago, which led to the decision to make quality control of the railroad network a task for the government again.
133. Yergin, D. and Stanislaw, J.: ibid., p. 380.

134. Barber, B.: *Fear's Empire: War, Terrorism and Democracy* (Dutch Translation), Ambo/Manteau, 2003, p. 170.
135. For instance, a strike in late 1995, intended to prevent intervention in the social security system and originally supported by two-thirds of the population, crippled public life in France (NRC/Handelsblad, 6 December 1995). Next, the Juppé social security renovation plan of 1995, submitted to the French national assembly as a bill of only one page long, elicited no less than 5,277 amendments from the opposition (NRC/Handelsblad, 11December 1995). It is, for that matter, no exception that legislative proposals are substantially amended. In 1995, an Education Bill in the United Kingdom was amended 981 times (Alexander, R.: *The Voice of the People: A Constitution for Tomorrow*, London, 1997, p. 60). Furthermore, in Germany in 1996, the unions fought for continued full sickness payments, even though the German parliament had proposed only very limited adjustments to the existing regulation. In Spain, 100,000 people went on strike in Cadiz, refusing to accept that the government subsidy for the local shipbuilding wharf was to be cut. Finally, at about the same time, many Italians went on strike because they saw their pension rights under threat.
136. Hooghe, L.: A House with Differing Views: The European Commission and Cohesion Policy, in: Nugent, N., (ed.): *At the Heart of the Union: Studies of the European Commission*, 2nd edition, MacMillan Press Ltd, 2000, p. 99.
137. Zonneveld, M.: *Kermis in de Politiek: Waarom de Nederlandse Kiezer op Drift raakte*, Van Gennep, 2002, p. 98. Recently, a former leader of the Dutch federation of labor unions also criticized the model by stating that it is too dull; the 2006 minister of finance claimed that it is too slow and lacks dynamics, and comparable developments can be observed in the other countries of the European Union.
138. As an example that the corporatist social-economic infrastructure is coming under pressure, for eight years the Kok administration in the Netherlands tried to confine the competencies of the Social Economic Council, to reduce the influence of private broadcasting corporations in favor of the Netherlands Broadcasting Authority, and to make the execution of social security arrangements, so far something done by social partners, a government affair.
139. Becker, U.: ibid., pp. 160–161.
140. Rodrik, D.: ibid., p. 6. In this respect, it should not be forgotten that the welfare state has not been the result of the natural course of things, but has, instead, been achieved through a long-lasting struggle for a fair society. Though this welfare state may, indeed, promote "a sense of dependence": "it is either naïve or cynical to lead the public to think that dismantling the welfare state is enough to ensure a revival of informal cooperation," because "market mechanisms will not repair the fabric of public trust. On the contrary, the market's effect on the cultural infrastructure is just as corrosive as that of the state" (Lasch, C.: *The Revolt of the Elites and the Betrayal of Democracy*, W. W. Norton & Company, 1995, pp. 82 and 100–101). In this respect, also see Myrdal, G.: ibid., p. 219.
141. 1997 research of The Economist Intelligent Unit showed that the Netherlands was first in a ranking of 58 countries for international corporations, based, among other things, on its solid social-economic infrastructure (The Economist Intelligence Unit, Press Release, May 15, 1997).

142. In this respect, the World Economic Forum, a private not-for-profit foundation, headquartered in Geneva and supported by more than 1,000 member companies, uses a weighted composite index, including open markets, lean government spending, low tax rates, flexible labor markets, a stable political system, and an effective judiciary (Mittelman J. H.: *The Globalization Syndrome: Transformation and Resistance*, Princeton University Press, 2000, p. 39).
143. Scholte, J. A.: *Globalization: A Critical Introduction*, Palgrave, 2002, p. 265.
144. In 1958, 73% of interviewed Americans answered that the government "mostly" or "almost always" made the right decisions. In 1994, this figure had decreased to no more than 15%. Also in 1958, 23% of Americans "never" or "sometimes" trusted the government. In 1995, this figure was around 80% (Fukuyama, F.: *The Great Disruption: Human Nature and the Reconstruction of Social Order* (Dutch Translation), Amsterdam/Antwerpen, 1999, pp. 62–63). In 2003, over a hundred million Americans, almost 40% of the population, did not participate in the elections (Moore, M.: *Downsize This: Random Threats from an Unarmed American*, Pan Books, 2003, p. 23). Research in Great Britain has shown that the number of people having "much or reasonable confidence" in parliament decreased from 54% in 1983 to 10% in 1996. Research in Britain in 1998 among youngsters between the ages of 16 and 21 showed that 71% held the opinion that voting (or not voting) would not make a difference to their lives. In France, research in 1990 revealed that 60% of those interviewed did not trust the political parties, whereas the presidential elections of April 2002 showed that almost 30% of the population abstained from voting in the elections, a figure that was 22.5% five years earlier. This decreasing interest of the public in politics has become increasingly manifest over the past 20 years. This also applies to the countries of Middle and Eastern Europe. In Poland, voter participation dropped from 64% in 1989 to 49% in 1997. In Czechia, voter participation was 93% in 1990 and 77% in 1998. In Hungary, the figure dropped from 76% in 1990 to 60% in 1998 (Hertz, N.: *The Silent Takeover—Global Capitalism and the Death of Democracy* (Dutch Translation), Amsterdam/Antwerpen, 2002, pp. 122–123). Finally, a recent Eurobarometer reveals that confidence in public institutions, i.e., the civil service, the national government, the national parliament, and political parties, is low in both the "old" and the "new" member states. In particular, political parties do not enjoy high esteem. They appear to be trusted by only 13% of a region's population (European Commission: Applicant Countries Eurobarometer 2001, ibid., p. 23).
145. To Levine, democracy is a plutocracy "in which moneyed elites, not undifferentiated citizens, endeavour to control the political process" (Levine, A.: *The American Ideology: A Critique*, Routledge, 2004, p. 121).
146. This is in line with the identification of three levels of power in post-war America by the sociologist C. Wright Mills. To him, the virtually powerless citizen-voters compose the lowest power level. Above that level comes organized labor, together with medium-sized corporations and other organized interests. Major decisions affecting national policy, however, are reserved for the "power elite" and state leaders. Wright Mills' approach would suggest a relationship of co-operation between corporate business and the political scene. It is assumed, however, that it is no longer politics that controls corporate business, but that it is corporate business that tells politics what to do.

147. Beck, U.: ibid., p. 3. Corporate business would make decisions that completely disregard nation states, while "displaying contempt for the political system" (Bové, J. and Dufour, F.: *The World is not for Sale: Farmers against Junk Food*, Verso, 2001, p. 187). In the words of Palast, "investing in politicians has a consistently higher rate of return than investing in plants or products" (Palast, G.: ibid., p. 129). In this respect, Beck speaks of the "jubilant mass suicide" of politicians who sing the praises of the market and thereby undermine their own position (in: Fox, J.: *Chomsky and Globalization*, Icon Books, p. 21).
148. Barber, B. R.: *Jihad versus McWorld: How Globalism and Tribalism are Reshaping the World*, Ballantine Books, 1995, p. 117.
149. In this respect, it is rather convincing to quote Richard Goodwin, the speechwriter for former United States President John F. Kennedy, who said, "The principal power in Washington is no longer the government or the people it represents. It is the Money Power. Under the deceptive cloak of campaign contributions, access, and influence, votes and amendments are bought and sold. Money establishes priorities of action, holds down federal revenues, revises federal legislation, shifts income from the middle class to the very rich. Money restrains the enforcement of laws written to protect the country from abuses of wealth—laws that mandate environmental protection, antitrust laws, laws to protect the consumer against fraud, laws that safeguard the security markets, and many more" (Phillips, K.: ibid., p. 320).
150. Phillips, K.: ibid., p. 324. Regarding this, there is hardly any difference between Republicans and Democrats. Both political parties, though in different measures, share "a contempt for the electorate's will" (Palast, G.: ibid., p. 80). During the 2000 presidential election campaign, Bush managed to raise no less than $191 million, the highest amount in American history, whereas Gore had to settle for $133 million. These campaign moneys are almost completely contributed by the richest 4% of the population (Hertsgaard, M.: *The Eagle's Shadow*, (Dutch Translation), Cossee, 2002, p. 164). No wonder that a Republican candidate for the presidency denounced the campaign finance system as "an elaborate influence-peddling scheme with both parties conspire to stay in office by selling the country to the highest bidder" (Phillips, K.: ibid., p. 325). In this respect, Hutton reveals that, for the last 20 years, every presidential election has been won by the candidate who raised the most money (Hutton, W.: *The World We're In*, Little Brown, 2002, p. 172). Furthermore, Kelly argues that "it's obvious to almost everyone that wealthy individuals and corporations have purchased the government of the United States" (Kelly, C. M.: ibid., p. 181). "The corporations don't have to lobby the government anymore. They *are* the government," said a former American politician in this respect (Palast, G.: ibid., p. 86). All in all, American "money-responsive" politics has become "a commercial parody of itself [. . .] along with mediocre political candidates" (Gates, J.: ibid., pp. xxiii and 14). It is sufficient to note further that Palast estimates that candidates for the American federal election cycles invested a total amount in G. W. Bush's election campaign of $447 million (Palast, G.: ibid., p. 83).
151. Former German Chancellor Kohl encountered big difficulties when it came into the open that corpoarte business had lined the purse of the Christian-Democratic party. France had her Elf/Totalfina affair, and Italy saw politicians convicted for bribery.

152. Beck, U.: ibid., p. 4. A more moderate position is taken by Legrain. He agrees that money and politics should be kept as separate as possible and that government should be conducted far more openly, but he also believes it not to be true that governments simply do companies' bidding (Legrain, Ph.: *Open World: The Truth about Globalisation*, Abacus, 2002, pp. 147–150). To him, it is untrue that global competition prevents governments from taxing, spending and regulating. He also believes it to be untrue that globalization harms the poor and is a danger to democracy. To Legrain, ideas like these are dangerous, because they encourage frustration, apathy, and anger. They invite people to take the street, instead of thinking creatively about what kind of globalization we want (Legrain, Ph.: ibid., pp. 21–22). Companies, Legrain argues, are constrained by competition law (Microsoft versus the United States government, General Electric versus the European Commission), and companies have to abide by extensive legislation from workers' rights to health-and-safety procedures and environmental protection. As examples he refers, among other things, to former United States President Clinton's decision to raise the minimum wage and to Prime Minister Blair's decision to introduce such a wage (Legrain, Ph.: ibid., pp. 19–20). This, however, is the weak point of his reasoning, because he apparently does not know that British and American employers do not live up to the minimum wage law without this having consequences regarding the majority of violations discovered.
153. Deakin, N.: *The Politics of Welfare: Continuities and Change*, London, 1994. For the American situation in this respect, Moore uses the term "Republicrats" (Moore, M.: *Downsize This*, ibid., p. 26). Gates observes a *de facto* merger of the principal political parties (Gates, J.: ibid., p. xi).
154. Instead, a new world is emerging. In this world, pragmatism will replace ideals and consumption will be more important than convictions. This transformation makes "leaders who lead" an antique phenomenon. Instead, markets and corporate CEOs lead, with prime ministers and presidents listening (Palast, G.: ibid., pp. 297–299).
155. Lasch, C.: ibid., p. 80. Regarding this, former Prime-Minister Kok of the Netherlands, a social-democrat, declared in 1995 that the Labor party had definitively said goodbye to the ideology of socialism and to "the ideological ties with other descendents of the traditional socialist movement" (Vroonhoven, L. van: *De Al-Ene Mens: Op zoek naar het Individu*, Damon, 1999, p. 11; author's translation). According to Lasch, both left- and right-wing ideologies "are now so rigid that new ideas make little impression on their adherents" (Lasch, C.: ibid., p. 80).
156. Bové, J. and Dufour, F.: ibid., p. 173.
157. Zonneveld, M.: ibid., p. 62.
158. Schoo, H. J.: De Jaren Zestig in de Herkansing, in: *De Volkskrant*, 11 May 2002.
159. Gunsteren, H. van: Fortuyn gaf de Democratie Leven, in: *De Volkskrant*, 11 May 2002. If one looks at daily political practice, the correctness of these observations is hard to deny. In France, it was the social-democrat Mitterand (the term *socialist* is hardly used anymore) who started to reform the French social security system. After winning the elections in 1981, Mitterand promised to end with capitalism. This was a promise he had to break after a right-wing victory in the national assembly a few years later. In the Netherlands, former

Prime Minister Lubbers, a Christian-Democrat, invented the term "no-nonsense" policy; Mike Harris from Canada introduced the "Common Sense Revolution" (Klein, N.: *Fences and Windows*, ibid., p. 113); German Chancellor Kohl is responsible for limiting social security and health care arrangements, for reducing corporate taxation, for privatizing public utilities, and for amending the trade unions and trade disputes legislation to the advantage of employers (Hertz, N.: ibid., p. 36). In addition, there is a large difference between Tony Blair's writings before he was elected and what he is actually doing in Downing Street. It was his initiative to delete Article IV from the Labor statutes (Hertz, N.: ibid., p. 39). According to Pilger, Britain has become "a single-ideology state with two principal, almost identical factions, so that the result of any election has a minimal effect on the economy and social policy. People have no choice but to vote for political choreographers, not politicians" (Pilger, J.: *Hidden Agendas*, Vintage, 1999, p. 98).

160. In this respect, Peter Mandelson, one of Blair's confidants, publicly said that "the era of representative democracy might come to an end" (Cameron, S.: *The Cheating Classes: How Britain's Elite Abuse their Power*, Simon and Schuster, 2002, p. 8).
161. Cameron, S.: ibid., p. 8.
162. People would exist for the rulers of the system instead of the other way around. If one reads Cameron's *The Cheating Classes*, one can wonder if this is not the case already (Cameron, S.: ibid.). Governments do not seem to realize that political colorlessness may endanger democracy, since democracy without pluralism cannot exist (Forrester, V.: *Une étrange Dictature* (Dutch Translation), Amsterdam, 2001, p. 19), and democracy without critical opposition loses its resilience (Gunsteren, H. van: ibid.). True democracy should embrace diversity. "True democracy is messy and fractious, if not outright rebellious," says Klein in this respect (Klein, N.: *Fences and Windows*, ibid., p. 189).
163. Regarding this, research done by the Dutch employers' organization VNO/NCW in 1999 showed that two-thirds of the members of the Dutch parliament did not understand anything of economics, and only 20% of those members could make a fair estimation of the amount of public spending. Therefore, it is appropriate to conclude that the most important safety mechanism for a democracy, being parliament, should be improved. One way to do this could be to increase the support of members of parliament, in order to decrease the leeway they have in their relation with the government (Dalen, H. van and Kalshoven, F., (eds.): ibid., pp. 11 and 22). In this respect, Kalma proposes to increase the countervailing power of members of parliament against the executive power of the government by, among other things, extending parliament's administrative apparatus (Kalma, P.: ibid., p. 102).
164. Urwin, D. W.: ibid., pp. 263–264.
165. Phillips, K.: ibid., p. 318.
166. In this respect, British participation in the war on Iraq (whether it is deemed correct or incorrect) is an example. Long before President George W. Bush, with support of Prime Minister Blair, started the war on Iraq, the argument to do so (that is, the presence in Iraq of weapons of mass destruction) was refuted from several sides, including Scott Ritter, a former UN weapons inspector (Ritter, S. and Rivers Pitt, W.: *War on Iraq: What Team Bush Doesn't Want You to Know*, Profile Books, 2002). For the Netherlands, information regarding

noise pollution as a consequence of the enlargement of Schiphol airport is an example.

167. Kelly goes even further and suggests that [American] politicians deliberately neglect the interests of uneducated ordinary people, because capitalism has become plutocratic. Plutocratic capitalism, he argues, is designed "to benefit the educated and powerful, at the expense of the uneducated, poor and powerless." Democratic capitalism, as it existed from the 1930s to the beginning of the 1980s, was designed by politicians who believed in realistic equal opportunities for all citizens to live healthy, productive, and rewarding lives. That kind of capitalism does not exist anymore (Kelly, C. M.: ibid., pp. 712–173). Only 7% of Americans believe that their government most often responds to the public's wishes in this respect (Gates, J.: ibid., p. 87).
168. Regarding this, Klein refers to young Czechs who have come to conclude that communism and capitalism have something in common: "they both centralize power in the hands of a few and they both treat people as if they are less than fully human. Where communism saw them only as potential producers, capitalism sees them only as potential consumers" (Klein, N.: *Fences and Windows*, ibid., p. 35). Regarding this, voting for extreme right-wing parties (not left-wing parties, since communism has proven not to be an attractive alternative), may partly be considered to be more a declaration of dissatisfaction with the political elite, than an expression of a genuinely increasing resistance against ethnical minorities or a generally increasing xenophobia.
169. Widening income gaps, however, "could turn out to be globalisation's Achilles' heels," says Thomas Friedman in this respect (Friedman, Th. L.: *The Lexus and the Olive Tree: Understanding Globalization*, Anchor Books, 2000, pp. 318–319).
170. Regarding this, Judt expresses his unrest by observing that European populist political parties like that of Haider from Austria, Jean-Marie Le Pen from France, Bossi from Italy, or De Winter from Flanders "attract more votes from unemployed young people and insecure elderly than from employed people in the prime of their lives" (Judt, T.: *A Grand Illusion: An Essay on Europe* (Dutch Translation), Erven Bijleveld, 1997, p. 105; author's translation). Meanwhile, we are not speaking solely of a European phenomenon. The electorate of Pauline Hanson, the leader of a provocative anti-Aboriginal/anti-immigration platform in Australia, had one of the highest unemployment rates. More than half of all Australian young people cannot find a job (Pilger, J.: *Hidden Agendas*, ibid., p. 233). Altogether, the increasing split in society is one of the most serious dangers to democracy. According to Handy, to prevent this from causing society to fall apart, we have to close the "hole in the heart of capitalism" (Handy, C.: People and Change, in: Radice, G. (ed.): *What Needs to Change: New Visions for Britain*, Harper Collins Publishers, 1996, p. 27). This hole exists because, contrary to communism, which had a cause without an effective mechanism, capitalism has an effective mechanism but no cause. The cause should be that through democratic political decision-making, capitalism shows a proper concern for others in the sense of Smith's "sympathy." If politics is not capable of achieving this cause, the end of democracy may not, contrary to Hertz, be caused by corporate business, but by politics itself.
171. Commission on Global Governance: *Our Global Neighborhood*, Report, Oxford University Press, 1996, p. 11.

172. Hertz, N.: ibid., p. 232.
173. Zonneveld, M.: ibid., p. 75.
174. Kuttner, R.: *Everything for Sale*, ibid., p. 29.
175. Unionised labor has a weakened position in bargaining for higher wages, because labour markets have increasingly become worldwide, and governments have been reluctant to regulate the free movement of capital since the end of Bretton Woods in 1973.
176. Scholte, J. A.: *Globalization: A Critical Introduction*, ibid., p. 136. To Scholte, sovereignty has been replaced by supraterritoriality. This being so, one can distinguish between five general changes in the position of the state. First of all, states have to face the fact that supraterritoriality has changed the meaning of the concept of state sovereignty, since many current worldwide problems (for example, global warming, ozone depletion, and pollution) have to be solved by joint action between states. Consequently, as a second change, states have to reorient themselves to serve supraterritorial interests in order to serve territorial interests. Thirdly, due to worldwide changing labor terms, states have to cope with the problem of downward pressures on public-sector welfare state provisions. Fourthly, states have to take part in the process of redefining warfare, and, finally, territorial interests have to be balanced with an increased reliance on multilateral arrangements. These demonstrations of the spread of supraterritoriality have "tended to create a different kind of state" (Scholte, J. A.: *Globalization: A Critical Introduction*, ibid., p. 135), but that does not mean that globalisation and the state are inherently contradictory. The difference with the pre-supraterritorial sovereign state is a relative decline in relative primacy, which has mainly transpired in two ways. First of all, supraterritoriality has promoted downward shifts (local and provincial) as well as upward shifts (suprastate governance at regional or transworld level) of regulatory competences. Secondly, globalization has promoted increasing regulatory activities through non-official bodies (Scholte, J. A.: *Globalization: A Critical Introduction*, ibid., chapter 6), i.e., an outward shift of state power.
177. The term is from Scholte, J. A.: *Globalization: A Critical Introduction*, ibid..
178. Hitiris, Th.: *European Union Economics*, Prentice Hall, 4th edition, 1998, p. 54.
179. Dunkerley, D., et al.: ibid., p. 121.
180. Dunkerley, D., et al.: ibid., p. 132.
181. First of all, this was based on the belief that economic integration and cooperation would contribute to ending the history of regular warfare on the European continent. Creating a European Union was perceived to be "a road constructed out of consent and consensus rather than upon military conquest" (Urwin, D. W.: ibid., p. 4). It was assumed that such a union would create "a more civilized political framework" (Dyson, K.: ibid., p. 205). In addition to this overall political objective, "the idea of free trade has always been the key to integration" (Jørgensen, J. G., Lüthje, T., and Schröder, Ph. J. H.: Trade: The Workhouse of Integration, in: Hansen, J. D., (ed.): *European Integration: An Economic Perspective*, Oxford University Press, 2001, p. 138). Furthermore, the European Union was meant to establish a place of dignity for Europe in a post-war world that was dominated by the two superpowers, the United States and the Soviet Union. Finally, two further motives for integration were raising the standard of living for the member states and encouraging political unifi-

cation by economic coordination and harmonisation of national policies (Hitiris, Th.: ibid., pp. 345–346).

182. It should be noted that this process shows that, despite all its "messy diversity" (Calleo, D.: ibid., p. 8), economic integration and cooperation are moving forward. The dynamics of this process were further underlined in the early 1990s when the European Commission included a "functioning and competitive market economy . . . [and] an adequate legal and administrative system in the public and private sector" as a further objective (Croft, S., et al.: *The Enlargement of Europe*, Manchester University Press, 1999, p. 61).
183. Eyden, T. van der: Betrouwbare Grenzen van de Europese Rechtsunie, in: Kaars Sijpesteijn, E. J., (ed.): *Het Volk en Europa—Grenzen aan Europa*, Vereniging Democratisch Europa, Amsterdam, 2004, p. 68.
184. Croft, S., et al.: ibid., pp. 67–68.
185. I refer, instead, to Dyson, who ably describes several legitimacy problems that the European Union has to solve in order to prevent it from falling apart (Dyson, K.: ibid., chapter 7). It should be noted that these legitimacy problems may increase as a consequence of enlargement. Moreover, the fact that the European Union has admitted political "dissidents" (the United Kingdom, Denmark) may have critical implications for its future development, particularly if the number of obstructionists increases through enlargement. In other words, enlargement may generate centrifugal forces (Croft, S., et al.: ibid., p. 81). In this regard, since the beginning of European integration, the United Kingdom has been a regular "dissident." In this respect, Winston Churchill is known to have said long before the Second World War that "We see nothing but good and hope in a richer, freer, more contented European commonality. But we have our own dream and our own task. We are with Europe, but not of it. We are linked, but not compromised. We are interested and associated, but not absorbed." (Urwin, D. W.: ibid., p. 74). This quotation illustrates the relation between the United Kingdom and the other member states throughout the history of the European Union. For that matter, this quotation is completely in line with his famous speech at the University of Zurich in 1946, where he promoted a United States of Europe under the leadership of France and Germany, with the United Kingdom as a *friend* and *sponsor* (italics mine), together with the United States and, possibly, the Soviet Union (Nelsen, B. F. and Stubb, A., (eds.): ibid., p. 11). He advocated being with Europe, but not being part of it, because the United Kingdom had its own dream and its own task. It is intriguing to know what is behind this attitude. Two historical arguments seem to be important. The first argument has to do with a shared history between the United Kingdom and the United States. Both nations speak the same language, inherited the same cultural history, stem from the same liberal tradition, and share the same political beliefs, all of which led to the Anglo-American approach regarding social arrangements and comparable dealings with unionized labor (Carew, A.: *Democracy and Government in European Trade Unions*, Allen & Unwin Ltd., London, 1976, p. 16). Similarly, Huntington quotes Vaughan who, referring to the original English settlers in the United States, argues that "almost everything was fundamentally English: the forms of landownership and cultivation, the system of government and the basic format of laws and legal procedures, the choices of entertainment and leisure-time pursuits, and innumerable other aspects of colonial life" (Huntington, S.

P.: *Who are We? America's Great Debate,* Free Press, 2005, p. 60). The second argument has to do with the United Kingdom's history as a colonial world power. In the years after the Second World War, these colonies were converted into the Commonwealth. The United Kingdom's own dream and its own task probably have to do with both historical arguments. They turn up regularly in the history of the establishment of the European Union. This can be illustrated with several examples. First, they led to different answers to the question of whether people desired a European community or a broader Atlantic community, including the United States. During the Cold War, choosing for the latter had delivered an effective bulwark against the communist superpower. Because of this, supporters of the Atlantic option were not only British. However, when as a result of a certain balance of power between the United States and the Soviet Union, the threat of communist rule in Western Europe was softened, countries like France and Germany, instead of being dominated by outsiders, favored the union of the European countries in order to flourish in a new global environment. In contrast, the British "continued to rely on importing an external hegemon," that is, the United States (Calleo, D. P.: ibid., p. 27). In this respect, Prime Minister Thatcher, in her speech to the College of Europe in Bruges in 1988, called on Europe to preserve the Atlantic Community in the sense of "that Europe on both sides of the Atlantic" (Nelsen, B. F. and Stubb, A., (eds.): ibid., p. 54). "This disjuncture of historical imagination and sympathy between the British and the French runs throughout post-war European politics and continues to bedevil the future of the whole European project" (Calleo, D. P.: ibid., p. 27). In fact, there are two aspects that continue to be a problem in respect of further European integration (including Britain). The first aspect is the sympathy the British have for the United States. In this respect, it is worth mentioning that, as recently as March 2000, an American congressional delegation visited the United Kingdom in order to discuss with British Euroskeptics the option for the United Kingdom to leave the European Union and to join NAFTA instead (Wallace, H.: Europeanisation and Globalisation, in: Breslin, S., Hughes, Ch. W., Ohillips, N., and Rosamond, B., (eds.): ibid., p. 139). These Euroskeptics were strongly supported by Thatcher, who insisted, that "British values and essential interests do not lie with Europe" (Hutton, W.: *The World We're In,* ibid., p. 15). One should not be mistaken about the influence the Euroskeptics have in Great Britain; for example, in the mid-1990s, almost half of the British people opted for complete withdrawal from the European Union (Norris, P.: Global Governance and Cosmopolitan Citizens, in: Nye, J. S. and Donahue, J. D., (eds.): ibid., p. 157). The second aspect has to do with the country's readiness to accept the transfer of sovereignty to a supranational level. Here, throughout the process of European integration, the United Kingdom has shown relatively more reluctance than any of the other member states. Instead, the country favors a loose intergovernmental structure for the European Union. This was already the case in the early days of European integration when, for instance, the European Coal and Steel Community was established. Though the country was invited to take part in this undertaking, "Britain refused an invitation to join the new organization, being unwilling to accept beforehand the principle of a new and binding supranational authority" (Urwin, D. W.: ibid., p. 83). The same applies to examples from more recent times, like the country's choice to stay outside the fixed exchange rate cooperation within the European Community, its refusal to sign the Social Protocol of the Maastricht Treaty, its non-participation in the European currency, and its rejection of the establishment of the European Central Bank. As early as the 1950s, Charles de Gaulle, who favored keeping the United States at a comfortable distance and vetoed an earlier British attempt to join the European Community, labeled Great Britain as a "European maverick" because of its sympathy for the United States (Urwin, D. W.: ibid., pp. 274–275). For reasons of balance, it should be mentioned that in the late 1950s, the United Kingdom declared itself to be against a Union of the Six with agreement to an external tariff wall. The British opposition can even be said to have been threatening to the Six, if one believes Charles de Gaulle in this respect. Referring to a meeting de Gaulle had with the then British Prime Minister, Harold MacMillan, on 29 June 1958, the latter is quoted to have said, "The Common Market is the Continental System all over again. Britain cannot accept it. I beg you to give it up. Otherwise, we shall embark on a war which will doubtless be economic at first *but which runs the risk of gradually spreading into* other fields" (italics mine) (Nelsen, B. F. and Stubb, A., (eds.): ibid., p. 41). Britain has also been described as "the problem child of the EC" (Urwin, D. W.: ibid., pp. 274–275) and "a reluctant European" (Dunkerley, D., et al.: ibid., p. 143). For reasons of sympathy and sovereignty, "in view of the past it is not surprising, and in view of the future it is significant, that Britain still preferred to remain aloof from Europe and to consider itself the link *par excellence* between the continent and the United States" (Urwin, D. W.: ibid., p. 78). This preferred link between the United Kingdom and the United States is important for the theme of this book, because it implies a preference for the confrontational "winner-takes-all" style of the "majoritarian" liberal democratic social-economic infrastructure, known as the Anglo-American model. This contrasts to the consensual form of "non-majoritarian" negotiated democracy, known as the continental European Rhine model. The difference between the two models is about more than differences in power sharing between employers, unions and the government. The fact that the Anglo-American model is characterized by less government interference in the economic process and a smaller state-provided safety net, is also an expression of cultural and historical differences between the United Kingdom/United States and the countries of the European continent. These differences become manifest in matters like choosing shareholder or stakeholder capitalism, deciding whether to conclude social pacts with the unions, preferring "external" or "internal" flexibility, appreciating the Charter of Fundamental Social Rights, and so on. In a globalizing economy, choosing between these alternatives makes a difference. The Anglo-American approach clearly is the neo-liberal view of subordinating social policy objectives to economic objectives, for the simple reason that, thanks to a globalizing economy, "there is no alternative way," according to Thatcher (Phillips, K.: ibid., p. 339). The Rhine model is struggling to maintain social cohesion while at the same time playing the game of global competition. Nevertheless, the latter model is slowly caving in. Figures regarding the non-wage costs per employee in the United Kingdom illustrate the differences between the models: in 1996, non-wage costs were cut to £18 per £100 spent by employers on wages. At the same time, these figures were £32, £34, £41, and £44 for Germany, Spain, France, and Italy, respectively.

Though this gives the United Kingdom a competitive advantage in a global economy, it is at the expense of social cohesion in the British society. This latter point is illustrated by the increasing proportion of the population living on less than half of the average national income, after allowing for the costs of housing, being 9% at the start of the first Thatcher government in 1979, growing to 25% or 14.1 million people in 1992 (Lee, S.: Discovering the Frontiers of Regionalism: Fostering Entrepreneurship, Innovation and Competitiveness in the European Union, in: Breslin, S., Hughes, Ch. W., Phillips, N., Rosamond, B., (eds.): ibid., p. 176). Also, when it comes to measurable working hours, Britain is top of the European league. In 1999, the average male working week in the United Kingdom was 45 hours, 7 hours more than in Belgium and 5.5 more than in Germany. The application in 1999 of the EU directive on Working Time to Britain, stipulating a maximum of 48 hours a week for certain occupations, demonstrated that an estimated number of 4.5 million Britons exceeded that number, 600,000 more than in 1992 (Frank, S.: *Having None of It: Women, Men and the Future of Work*, Granta Books, 1999, p. 69). Finally, in Britain, only a third of people capable of gainful employment were fully employed, in the classical sense of the term, around the beginning of the new millennium, compared to 60% in Germany. Twenty years ago, the figure was over 80% in both countries (Beck, U.: ibid., pp. 58–59). This is typical of the development of the Anglo-American model since Thatcher came to Downing Street and Reagan moved to the White House. The differing preferences between the two models explain why the United Kingdom was conspicuous by its absence when the Social Protocol of the Maastricht Treaty, eventually annexed to the treaty as an addendum, was signed (Council of the European Communities, Committee of the European Communities, Treaty of the Union, Brussels/Luxembourg, 1992, p. 197. Also see: Corbett, R.: *The Treaty of Maastricht*, Longman Group, United Kingdom, 1993, p. 464). Springer points to the fact that the integration of the United Kingdom into the European Community in 1972 made European policy-making especially difficult for two reasons. Firstly, the economy of the United Kingdom, based on ties with former colonies, "was not easily aligned with the more rapidly growing economies of the original members. In addition, the legal system differed significantly from that of continental countries." As a consequence, "the writing of EC laws became more complex. The entire decision-making process became tedious" (Springer, B.: *The Social Dimension of 1992: Europe Faces a New EC*, New York, 1992, p. 4). According to Hay, this opting-out of the Social Protocol should be seen as "an attempt to construct a niche for Britain on the periphery of the European market as a low-wage, low-skill, flexi-time, sweatshop economy—an assembly plant for non-European products that wish to penetrate the European market" (Hay, C.: *Re-Stating Social and Political Change*, Open University Press, Buckingham, 1996, p. 173). Hay argues that, in fact, the United Kingdom was forced not to sign the Social Protocol in order to stay competitive in a globalizing economy. A reasonable question behind all this is whether the United Kingdom feels more American than European. In the words of Hutton, the British themselves will not only have to answer how European they are, but also what they have in common with an America that is "increasingly in thrall to a very particular conservatism" (Hutton, W.: *The State We're In*, ibid., pp. 1–2). In a compelling discourse, Hutton strongly argues that it is not just geography that defines Britain as a European country. It is "a value system born of sharing the same essential history." British history mirrors that of the rest of Europe. Catholic feudal Europe, for instance, of which Britain was part, demanded that wealth and property were associated with reciprocal social obligations. This ethical view partly inspired socialism when advocating, among other things, respect for the rights of workers. Despite the fact that Christianity and socialism have lost much of their meaning for society, the ethical basis has survived. As an example, Hutton argues that no single European country shares the American majority view that governments should not redistribute income. In Britain, 63% of the population are in favor of income redistribution. In the United States, this figure is only 28%. To Hutton, this difference is part of a complex system of values that are deeply entrenched (Hutton, W.: *The State We're In*, ibid., p. 43). All in all, it seems as if history can be manipulated to serve particular interests. Those in favor of the Anglo-American model use it to detach the United Kingdom from the European Union; those against this model focus on the negative sides. Meanwhile, there remains a difference in the continental European approach and the Anglo-American approach, which is an important obstacle for further integration.

186. Furthermore, I will not go into the patchwork of different cultures, religions, languages, and views, because many others have ably dealt with one or more of these aspects. Accepting that the concept of "Europe" means different things to different people, because "there is no identikit" (Croft, S., et al.: ibid., p. 9), I also will not deal with the advantages and disadvantages of the pluralist, the functionalist, the neo-functionalist, or the federalist approach to integration (Hitiris, Th.: ibid., pp. 39–41; for further information on theories on community policy-making, see: Theofilatou, M. A.: *The Emerging Health Agenda: The Health Policy of the European Community*, dissertation, Maastricht University, 2000, chapter 4). I will also not address schools of thought regarding institutionalized forms of cooperation within the European Union, like neo-realism, neo-liberal institutionalism, or social constructivism (Croft, S., et al.: ibid., chapter 1). After all, this book is not about the question of what the most preferable type of European integration would be and how this preferred situation could or should be achieved. It is about decision-making at the level of the European Union regarding policies which effect the direction in which it and its member states move along the continuum. I take the patchwork of different cultures for a fact, accepting that this has always been the case and always will be. Given the existence of the European Union and the large political and economic differences between the member states, it is no surprise that the developments intended to achieve the aforementioned objectives progressed slowly. The large cultural differences made the establishment of the European Union itself no less than a miracle (Hofstede, G.: *Culture and Organizations: Software of the Mind* (Dutch Translation), Amsterdam, 2002). Patience, therefore, is a necessary precondition for further integration (Cini, M. and McGowan, L.: *Competition Policy in the European Union*, London, 1998, p. 23). It has taken some 25 years to formulate a more or less crystallized European competition policy. The genesis of a European currency took approximately the same time (for the difficulties regarding the introduction of the Euro, see: Haas, B. de and Lotringen, C. van: *Mister Euro: Een Biografie van Wim Duisenberg*, Business Contact/Het Finaciële Dagblad, 2005). But now,

more than 50 years since the Coal and Steel Community of 1952, followed by the Common Market of 1956, and with subsequent enlargements of the Single European Act of 1985 and the Single Market of 1992, the framework exists for an integrated Europe, being "the most extensive economic cooperation project among sovereign nation states" (Jørgensen, J. G., Lüthje, T., and Schröder, Ph. J. H.: ibid., p. 115).

187. Dyson, K.: ibid., p. 215. To the author, "power and policy gravitate around the Council—that is, governments—and the ECB, not the European Parliament."
188. Beck qualifies the European Union as a "negotiation state" (in: Rifkin, J.: *The European Dream*, ibid., p. 229).
189. Christiansen, Th.: European and Regional Integration, in: Baylis, J. and Smith, S.: ibid., p. 517. Transferring national decision-making powers to the higher level of the European Union "leaves the nation-state both as the main focus of expectations, and as the initiator, pace-setter, supervisor, and often destroyer of the larger entity" (Hoffmann, S.: Obstinate or Obsolete? The Fate of the Nation-State and the Case of Western Europe, in: Nelsen, B. F. and Stubb, A., (eds.): ibid., pp. 168–169).
190. Dyson, K.: ibid., p. 279. As a consequence, member states will continue to cause economic integration and cooperation to be "a series of pragmatic bargains among national governments based on concrete national interests, relative power, and carefully calculated transfers of sovereignty" (Moravscik, in: Dyson, K.: ibid., p. 110) This occurs in accordance with the intergovernmental approach of integration, based on the pillars of the sovereignty of member states, focusing on grand bargains, while using international institutions as instruments (Pierson, P.: The Path to European Integration: A Historical Institutionalist Analysis, in: Nelsen, B. F. and Stubb, A., (eds.): ibid., p. 320). Sovereignty once transferred, however, implies that the power to decide has been shifted to the supranational level of "pooled sovereignty" (Held, D., McGrew, A., Goldblatt, D., Perraton, J.: *Global Transformations: Politics, Economics and Culture*, Polity Press, 1999, p. 76), including the extensive bureaucratic competencies, unified judicial control, and capacities to modify policy that go with it (Pierson, P.: ibid., p. 321). This transfer of sovereignty may include decision-making regarding the *what*, the *how*, and the *for whom* of the production and consumption of goods and services. Depending on the subject of decision-making and their economic and political situation, member states may be willing or reluctant to transfer sovereignty. In this respect, Dyson developed an "interest-based" model, using two distinctive criteria for member states: on the one hand, the wish to avoid economic vulnerability for their citizenry, and, on the other hand, minimizing the domestic costs of economic convergence (Dyson, K.: ibid., pp. 110–114). Brought together in a diagram, his approach results in four types of member states: pushers, draggers, intermediates, and bystanders. Pushers are member states that strive for deepening integration. In contrast, draggers oppose this development. Intermediates have incentives to integrate, but have to face the fact of high convergence costs. Finally, because of low convergence costs, bystanders can take a more ambitious position, but they have little to gain directly. The problem with classifications like these, however, is their general applicability. Dyson notes that the model is static and partial. France, for example, generally termed as a pusher, demonstrates behavior of a dragger when it comes to centralizing monetary policy with the Euro-

pean Central Bank. France and Germany are pushers on the subject of harmonization of corporate taxation. In contrast, countries like Belgium, Ireland, and the Netherlands are disposed to be draggers or intermediates on this subject, because they would face higher costs. Nevertheless, the model is instrumental to illustrating the differing interests of the member states. Their position in the diagram may change in accordance with the subject that has to be dealt with. Behind all this is the everlasting question of what type of integrated Europe we want. Do we want a kind of European "governance," thus accommodating a more active and independent role for supranational European institutions? Or do we want a "state-centric" principal-agent model, with supranational European institutions having limited power? (Dyson, K.: ibid., chapter 3). In this respect, Calleo distinguishes between four basic models, i.e., (a) America's Atlantic Europe; (b) Jean Monnet's federal Europe; (c) De Gaulle's confederation of European states, and (d) an anarchic Europe of states (Calleo, D. P.: ibid., p. 135). Here, opinions differ, which in turn explains why economic integration proceeds slowly and why the outcome of decision-making at the level of the European Union is not always clear. Differing opinions imply that one will face dilemmas in collective decision-making, taking into account that, at the level of the European Union, decision-making is "extremely complex, with a multiplicity of governmental and non-governmental actors at national and European Union levels interacting with one another through a multiplicity of channels" (Nugent, N., (ed.): ibid., p. 11) Apart from the distinction in unanimity, qualified majority and simple majority voting, this complexity also appears in the outcomes of the decision-making processes. In this respect, one can distinguish between three kinds of decisions (Leibfried, S. and Pierson, P., (eds.): *European Social Policy: Between Fragmentation and Integration*, Washington, DC, 1995, pp. 25–26). Firstly, there are the "lowest common denominator" and "packaged" policies. Here, one compromises either the proposals of the least ambitious participant in the decision-making process, or one handles "side payments" to buy off potential opponents. Secondly, the decision-making process can result in the "incorporation of institutional protections," where one indulges the wishes of member states to remain their own masters. This kind of decision-making is a breeding ground for "rigid policy designs." The third type of decision-making is "the search for escape routes," which means that member states are looking for alternatives because they are not satisfied. The picture that results from this distinction is one of a fragmented and poorly co-ordinated decision-making process, which is "well suited to finding compromises that avoid sharp conflicts and long-standing grievances among the member states" (Calleo, D. P.: ibid., p. 281). However, if compromises cannot be found, this decision-making process will probably cause disputes about competencies, which, in turn, is likely to limit the possibilities to reach generally accepted conclusions. Consequently, decision-making at the level of the European Union is very complicated, a fact that will probably impede the design of further integration. Furthermore, the dilemmas in decision-making become clear if one studies the political balance within the European Commission. In this respect, MacMullen developed a seven-point political left-right scale, with one representing state intervention/collective provision and seven representing laissez-faire/individualism. Over the period 1952–1995, the mean score for Commissioners appears to be 3.9, almost in the centre (MacMullen, A.: European Commissioners National Routes to a European Elite, in: Nugent, N., (ed.): ibid., p. 41). So it seems that, in terms of the continuum, the European Union showed a rather balanced situation until 1995. This undoubtedly influenced decision-making on moving to the left or to the right side of the continuum, combined with compromising and negotiating regarding the dilemmas. The problem with MacMullen's approach, however, is the length of the time span. For approximately 30 of the 42 years considered, global competitive forces were hardly perceived to be a problem. This potentially made it easier to come to some agreement on the middle of intervention/collective provision and laissez-faire/individualism. Given the more recent policies of the European Union, further outlined in this chapter, I would not be surprised if comparable research over the period 1980–2000 would result in a mean score that is considerably more in the direction of laissez-faire/individualism. This disregards the fact, however, that McDonald rightfully observes that the European Commission "is required to face and to negotiate daily the structural contradictions and the complex moral and political baggage, the tensions and the compromises, of Europe and nation and of unity and difference that stand prominently at the heart of the European Union, and which pervade any discussion of its history and its future, its shape and its 'added value', and its very *raison d'être*" (McDonald, M.: ibid., p. 72). Nevertheless, though things proceed slowly and incrementally, there is progress, because meanwhile, aspects of decision-making regarding specific items, like competition and environmental policy or defence, may be and are transferred to the European Union level. And it is not unlikely that the European Union's sphere of influence will be broadened to policy items that are not yet an item of a common approach. In other words, sovereignty has already been transferred, and will continue to be so. Consequently, Brussels produces a lot of legislation and directives. The officials of DGXI alone, which is responsible for environmental policy, had produced 12,000 pages of legislation by 1993 (Cini, M.: Administrative Culture in the European Commission: The Cases of Competition and Environment, in: Nugent, N., (ed.): ibid., 81).

191. Theofilatou, M. A.: ibid., p. 40.
192. Yergin, D. and Stanislaw, J.: ibid., p. 306 ff.
193. Cini, M. and McGowan, L.: ibid., pp. 32–33.
194. Lawton, Th. C.: "Uniting European Industrial Policy: A Commission Agenda for Integration," in: Nugent, N., (ed.): ibid., p. 133.
195. Castells, M.: *End of Millennium*, ibid., p. 355. In this view, the European Union is part of an open world with three main players in the game of global competition. Each of these players will be forced to monitor continuously what is going on in the other two regions. Also, each region will try to achieve comparative advantages on the global playing field. In this environment, it will be very difficult for the European Union to differ much from the other two regions with respect to their institutional and macro-economic frameworks (Castells, M.: End of Millennium ibid., p. 129). In this respect, Castells anticipates "a relative equalization of working arrangements" between the three regions (Castells, M.: End of Millennium ibid., p. 324). One may argue that looking at the European Union as a defensive construction is a rather negative approach, because it makes the Union dependent on what is going on within the other two regions. However, the other side of the coin is that this kind of

dependence may create realism, alertness, and innovative capacity. In other words, a European Union that, due to the process of globalization, is forced to be alert, may also discover new opportunities. To Axford, for instance, the defensive strategy that has led to the establishment of the European market is based on the recognition that the European economies have lagged behind, compared to the more dynamic, expansionary, and technologically more efficient economy of Japan and the large economies of scale in the United States (Axford, B.: *The Global System: Economics, Politics and Culture*, Cambridge, 1995, p. 121). Once this lagging behind has been recognized, one can initiate actions directed at creating a level playing field in relations with the other two regions. According to the World Economic Forum, for this ambition to become reality, the European Union has to overcome the present situation of being outperformed by the United States and other OECD countries regarding all but one of the strategic objectives that are relevant in a globalizing economy. These objectives are (1) the creation of an information society, (2) a European area for research and innovation, (3) completion of the Single Market, (4) increasing efficiency and integration of financial markets, (5) strengthening of entrepreneurship through a reduction of regulations, (6) sustainable development, and (7) social inclusion through bringing people back to work, upgrading skills, and modernizing social protection (World Economic Forum: The Lisbon Review, 2002). The final strategic objective is the only one where the European Union has the lead.

196. World Economic Forum: The Lisbon Review, 2002.
197. Cowles, M. G.: The Transatlantic Business Dialogue and Domestic Business-Government Relations, in: Cowles, M. G., et al.: ibid., pp. 159–179. The author speaks of a Europeanization of business–government relations in the common commercial policy area to which national industrial organizations would do better to adjust. During the 1980s, the coordination of research and technological development, for instance, became "the central pillar of EC industrial policy, with knowledge creation and dissemination coming to be seen as central to innovation" (Lawton, Th. C.: ibid., p. 135). Consequently, European Union support for research funding increased from 500 MECU in 1982 to 12,300 MECU in 1998, with priorities for information and communication technologies, industrial and material technologies, and life sciences and technologies, together rising from 22% of the total available amount in 1982 to 57% in 1998 (Theofilatou, M. A.: ibid., table 2, pp. 177–178).
198. Lawton, Th. C.: ibid., p. 136. This spirit of unity was something new, since during the first 20 years of the European Union's existence, business was kept largely outside policy decisions at the European level (Lawton, Th. C.: ibid., p. 145). Regarding this, it could be that the change of attitude of the political scene was enforced by European industrial leaders who played a strong political card by intimating that the very existence of the European Union would be questioned by the business community, if the European Commission did not try to assist industry in times of stiff international competition. Supportive of this view is Dyson's observation that, around the turn of the millennium, "the field was opened for a breed of internationally oriented corporate entrepreneurs to effect major changes in national economic structures and policies within the Euro-zone." These corporate actors "displayed a new willingness to seize the initiative," where traditional political and banking elites were reluctant to do

so (Dyson, K.: ibid., p. 192). Consequently, states experience "an increasingly assertive policy-pushing corporate sector" (Dyson, K.: ibid., p. 278). As an example, the development of a liberalized pan-European telecommunications infrastructure was the result of a strong alliance between the European Commission and large European industrial firms like Siemens, Philips, Alcatel, and Olivetti (Schneider, V.: ibid., pp. 60–78). Close cooperation between European industrial leaders and politicians at the level of the European Union, whether or not enforced by corporate business, might raise the suggestion that, as a consequence of this particular type of bilateralism, individual member states are at the mercy of "Brussels"; whereas, in turn, the European Union would be in the hands of the United States and Japan. In other words, there would be "state denial" (Weiss, L.: *The Myth of the Powerless State: Governing the Economy in a Global Era, Cambridge*, 1998, p. 2). According to Weiss, there is no reason to fear such a development, because governments have "transformational capacities," which allow them to develop domestic strategies for industrial change (Weiss, L.: ibid., p. 15). According to Weiss, central to the capacities is the idea of "governed interdependence," which is based on cooperation with business life, in the course of which governments have a coordinating role. Such cooperation is a "negotiated relationship," which, though giving autonomy to public and private participants, is ruled by broader objectives and which, therefore, is monitored by the governments (Weiss, L.: ibid., p. 38). Though Weiss does not speak of Europe, her approach can be considered the Dutch "polder model" on a European Union level. Its weakness is implied in the term "negotiated relationship." What scope is there for corporate business to negotiate, when it has to survive in an environment of fierce global competitive forces? A European "polder model" will also have to face these facts. Therefore, less government interference in the economic process, a reduction in time-consuming corporatist procedures of consultation, and the demand for flexibility, "Europe's big headache in the last quarter of the twentieth century," would simply be lifted to the level of the European Union. Moreover, in a relation of "governed interdependence," the only interest of corporate business is survival (Olsen, F. and Skak, M.: Labour Markets: "Europe's Big Headache," in: Hansen, J. D., (ed.): ibid., p. 34). However, it is not just employer organizations that try to influence the European political scene. On the contrary, the internal market program has caused an explosive growth of lobbying in Brussels by a large number of interest groups. Even in 1985/1986, a total of 659 federations, ranging from consumers, environmentalists, labor representatives, public health promoters, and many others, had a representation in Brussels, together with 6,000 lobbyists. This leads Theofilatou to conclude that in "each specific area of Community activity, policy-making is controlled, to a large extent, by special interest coalitions." Not each and every one of them is taken equally seriously, however. On the contrary, "the concept of equal access of interest groups to the policy-making machinery in Brussels is a myth." Priorities lie with agricultural and economic policy (Theofilatou, M. A.: ibid., p. 88).

199. Frankel, J.: Globalization and the Economy, in: Nye, J. S. and Donahue, J. D., (eds.), ibid. The author refers to research by Rose, who found that adopting a common currency multiplied trade between the respective countries by an additional 3.5 times. This may somewhat compensate for the fact that a multitude of languages is one of the reasons that economic integration within the

European Union is far from complete. In this respect, Frankel reveals that trade between countries that speak the same language is 50% more than between two otherwise similar countries (Frankel, J.: ibid., p. 54).

200. Hansen, J. D. and Olesen, F.: Monetary Integration: Old Issues—New Solutions, in: Hansen, J. D., (ed.): ibid., p. 167.
201. In order for the Euro to be an "anchor of stability," the new currency, according to the then president of the German Bundesbank, had to be "depoliticized," i.e., monetary policy should "be kept as much as possible away from daily political influences, short-term calculations and fashion as well as from political compromises" (Tietmeyer, in: Dyson, K.: ibid., p. 129). Therefore, after much political debate, the European Central Bank "was deliberately created by governments so that it would evade such [political] control and be able to set and pursue its own preferences" (Dyson, K.: ibid., p. 110). Setting its own preferences does not mean, however, that the European Central Bank is completely out of political control forever, because "ultimately, governments have the final power to dispose of central banking rules as they feel fit" (Dyson, K.: ibid., p. 181). Central to these preferences, and most welcomed by the International Monetary Fund, the G7, the OECD, the Bank for International Settlements, the United States government, and multinational corporations, appears to be the pursuit of a "sound money" policy, i.e., commitment to price stability. All in all, the introduction of the Euro and the establishment of the European Central Bank caused the "denationalization of money," together with the relevant monetary policy instruments.
202. Dyson, K.: ibid., p. 157.
203. The International Monetary Fund, the G7, the OECD, the Bank of International Settlements, the United States Government, and multinational corporations.
204. Axford, B.: ibid., p. 102.
205. Yergin, D. and Stanislaw, J.: ibid., p. 321.
206. Soros, G.: *The Crisis of Global Capitalism: Open Society Endangered*, London, 1998, p. 185. Castells also stipulates the necessity of homogenizing the macroeconomic conditions of the different European economies, in particular fiscal and budgetary policy (Castells, M.: *End of Millennium*, ibid., p. 319. Also: Castells, M.: *The Power of Identity. The Information Age: Economy, Society and Culture*, Volume 2, Oxford, 1997, p. 245).
207. Lamy, P. and Pisani-Ferry, J.: The Europe We Want, in: Jospin, L.: ibid., p. 118.
208. Hansen, J. D. and Olesen, F., in: Hansen, J. D., (ed.): ibid., p. 188.
209. Hansen, J. D. and Jørgensen, J. G.: Industrial Structures: Specialization, Efficiency, and Growth, in: Hansen, J. D., (ed.): ibid., p. 105. This type of harmonization will also take considerable time, because the member states have largely differing systems regarding the tax base, the tax type, and the tax rate, as well as tax compliance and tax enforcement (Hitiris, Th.: ibid., p. 116). The rate of value-added tax, for instance, ranged from 15% in Germany to 25% in Sweden in 1995. In 1996, company profits tax was 39.6% in Portugal and 28% in Finland, whereas in the same year personal income tax was 60.6% in Belgium and 40% in the United Kingdom (Hitiris, Th.: ibid., pp. 126 and 135).
210. The French and German governments, for instance, favor harmonization of corporate taxation and of taxation on income from savings, whereas the Dutch and the Irish have reservations in this respect because of the effects that tax

harmonization may have on employment and competitiveness (Dyson, K.: ibid., p. 18). Furthermore, Ireland would oppose tax harmonization since it would harm its competitive position in attracting multinationals. The United Kingdom blocked a directive from Brussels regarding taxation of the savings balance because the City of London would suffer from it. Moreover, corporate business appears to be capable of blackmailing governments that want to increase corporate taxation.

211. Dyson, K.: ibid., p. 245.
212. In this respect, we have to realize, however, that the further shaping of the European Union will be the result of a politically dynamic process during which "integration often creates a need for further integration" (Hansen, J. D. and Olesen, F.: From European Economics towards a European Economy? in: Hansen, J. D., (ed.): ibid., p. 239) The creation of the European Union's customs union, for instance, led to measures directed at removing visible trade barriers, such as tariffs and quotas. In turn, this increased invisible trade barriers like discriminatory public procurement, national technical standards, and abuse of tax systems for national protectionism, which, in turn, led to the creation of the Single Market (Hansen, J. D. and Olesen, F.: ibid., p. 239). Consequently, "interdependence rises with integration," according to Hitiris. To him, the final profundity of the dynamic integration process knows only two stable forms, being (a) a free trade area or (b) complete economic integration. All other forms are simply intermediate and temporary stages (Hitiris, Th.: ibid., p. 3). Politics at the level of the European Union is directed at the second form. It includes fiscal harmonization. The importance of this aspect of economic integration has been continuously realized since the early days of the formation of the European Union. For example, the Werner Report of 1970 argued for a simultaneous harmonization of economic, fiscal, and budgetary policy (Urwin, D. W.: ibid., p. 279). In 1963, the European Economic Community installed the Neumark Committee, followed by the Van den Tempel Committee in 1970 and the Ruding Committee in 1992 (Hitiris, Th.: ibid., p. 136). In one way or another, all these committees delivered proposals regarding the harmonization of fiscal policy.
213. Worded differently, the question is not whether member states of the European Union can remain their own master, but if they can continue to fund collectively social policy arrangements in a Europe where economic growth is the binding ideology of further integration (Judt, T.: ibid., p. 45), and in which decreasing the costs of labor in a globalizing economy is the dominating objective of the economy.
214. Dunkerley, D., et al.: ibid., p. 21.
215. One of the reasons for this reality is probably "that areas dealing with the 'cultural' or the 'social,' whilst seen to give a 'human face,' have to battle for their credibility" (McDonald, M.: Identities in the European Commission, in: Nugent, N., (ed.): ibid., p. 54). To Caporaso and Jupille, therefore, social policy is "something of a poor cousin to the more fundamental economic aims of the European Community" (Caporaso, J. and Jupille, J.: The Europeanization of Gender Equality Policy and Domestic Change, in: Cowles, M. G., et al.: ibid., p. 21).
216. As an example: the policy of becoming "the most competitive and dynamic knowledge-based economy in the world by 2010, capable of sustainable

growth," as declared during the Lisbon Summit of 2000, was conditioned by the addition of "more and better jobs and greater social cohesion." Another example of interrelatedness has been provided by the European Commission which, in trying to trace the causes of the European Union's relatively poor economic performance, referred to suboptimal macro-economic management resulting from the levels of public expenditure, particularly in the social field. These had become "unsustainable and [had] used up resources which could have been channelled into productive investment" (Lee, S.: ibid., p. 170). This picture of ambiguities is broadened if we include differing political views regarding social policy. To Tony Blair, for instance, the Community Charter of Fundamental Social Rights is "simply a statement of policy . . . [not] something of a binding nature" (Dunkerley, D., et al.: ibid., p. 105). To Lionel Jospin, however, it "deserves to be considered the keystone of the European edifice" (Jospin, L.: ibid., p. 16). In this respect, Theofilatou correctly points to the fact that the Social Charter "reflects fairly accurately the disagreements characterizing the development of active Community intervention in social security, including the health (care) sector and also demonstrates the lack of willingness (and determination) of discontented interest groups to carry their appeal to a wider forum" (Theofilatou, M. A.: ibid., p. 131).

217. Leibfried, S. and Pierson, P., (eds.): ibid.
218. There are differences in taxation, in policies of redistribution, in contributions to the social security system, and so on.
219. No wonder, therefore, that harmonization of fiscal policy has been an ongoing subject of analysis since (almost) the start of the integration process. In this respect, tables presented by Hitiris clearly demonstrate the difficulties that have to be overcome. If we assume that the government, through policies of redistribution, remains the most important player in the pursuit of social policy objectives, the necessary tax collection (indirect taxes, direct taxes, social security and other receipts) as a percentage of GDP ranged from 36.6% in Ireland to 61.5% in Sweden in 1996. Within the different tax components, the Danes contributed only 2.8% of GDP to social security, compared to 19.9% for the Germans. The latter, however, paid only 10.5% of GDP in direct taxes, whereas the Danes had to cough up 32.1%. Comparable differences are apparent in the contributions to social security by employers, employees, the government, and other sources in 1995. The ranges are remarkable. Employers appear to have contributed to social security between 6.9% in Denmark and 52.9% in Spain. For employees the range went from 5.1% for Denmark to 41.7% for the Netherlands, whereas government contributions were 21.6% for Belgium and 81.6% in Denmark (Hitiris, Th.: ibid., table 5.1, p. 123, and table 10.1, p. 263). If we add to this the differences in value-added tax and corporate tax rates, harmonization of fiscal policy, if feasible at all, will prove to be an enormous job.
220. Leibfried, S. and Pierson, P., (eds.): ibid., 434.
221. Lee, S.: ibid., p. 169. In this respect, Theofilatou points to the fact that it is apparently easier for member states to reach agreement on the economic aspects of integration than to deal with the budgetary consequences of tackling the distributional and redistributional repercussions they may have for social welfare. Here, a lack of solidarity as well as the absence of a sense of European citizenship are assumed to be the most important obstacles (Theofilatou, M. A.: ibid., pp. 133–134).

222. Dyson, K.: ibid., p. 213. In this respect, it is important to note that, recognizing the interrelatedness of economic and social policy objectives, the European Commission asserted a direct correlation between economic and social cohesion and industrial and economic performance which "could 'add strength to each other' on the basis of the externalities generated by cohesion for infrastructure, especially in health, education and research" (Lee, S.: ibid., p. 172). Apparently, the idea of economic returns from investing in human capital still appealed to the European Commission (Dyson, K.: ibid., p. 227). Thus, social policy could be seen as a matter which contributed to productivity (Jospin, L.: ibid., p. 37).
223. Leibfried, S. and Pierson, P., (eds.): ibid., p. 28.
224. Streeck, W.: From Market Making to State Building? Reflections on the Political Economy of European Social Policy, in: Leibfried, S. and Pierson, P., (eds.): ibid., p. 412.
225. One may think that this perspective is too pessimistic, because one might, like Touraine, assume that employers know their social responsibility (Castells, M.: *End of Millennium*, ibid., p. 325. Regarding this, Handy gives examples which support Touraine's views). This remains to be seen, however. The appeals of Senator Kennedy and other Democrats in the United States about a decade ago, to act against the "corporate killers," responsible for massive redundancies, have not succeeded to date. Massive redundancies are still carried out regularly in the United States, as well as on the European continent.
226. Hansen, J. D. and Olesen, F.: in: Hansen, J. D., (ed.): ibid., p. 242. This is completely in line with Delors' vision that "the creation of a vast economic area, based on the market and business cooperation, is inconceivable without some harmonization of social legislation." To him, the ultimate aim should be "the creation of a European social area" (Hutton, W.: *The World We're In*, ibid., p. 298).
227. Meij, A. W. H. and Zimmeren, E. van: *Ontwerp-Verdrag tot Vaststelling van een Grondwet voor Europa*, Europocket, supplement bij de dertiende druk, Kluwer, 2003, p. 76. It should be kept in mind that the numbering of the articles in this draft treaty differs from the one on a later website (http://www.grondweteuropa.nl/9326201/v/indexalt.htm).
228. This might happen after the 2004 enlargement. In this respect, see: Swaan, A. de: *Dutch Welfare in Europe XL*, ibid., p. 7.
229. Miegel, M.: ibid., p. 33.
230. Leibfried, S.: Towards a European Welfare State? in: Pierson, Chr. and Castles, F., (eds.): ibid., p. 194.
231. Dunkerley, D., et al.: ibid., p. 7.
232. Schröder, Ph. J. H.: Eastern Enlargement: The New Challenge, in: Hansen, J. D., (ed.): ibid., p. 193.
233. Direct payments to Hungary, Poland, Slovakia, and Czechia alone will cost the European Union some ten billion Euros per year, which was more than the amount paid to Greece, Portugal, Spain, and Ireland when these countries joined the European Union. In 1992, only Germany, the United Kingdom, France, and the Netherlands contributed to the budget of the European Union. Ireland, Greece, Belgium, Portugal, Denmark, Spain, Italy, and even Luxembourg were beneficiaries. Though the countries that have become members since then (Sweden, Finland and Austria) are potential contributors, they have

relatively small economies. It is almost certain that all future members will be beneficiaries for many years.

234. Judt, T.: ibid., pp. 95–96.
235. Dunkerley, D., et al.: ibid., p. 7.
236. Judt, T.: ibid., p. 95. Comparable fear existed when Greece, Spain, and Portugal became members, because their accession increased the European Union's GDP by only 10%, but its population increased by 22% and its employment in agriculture increased by 57% (Hitiris, Th.: ibid., p. 247). However, the consequences of that fear did not materialize. Given the differences in figures, fear may be more realistic with respect to the 2004 enlargement. These figures show that, for instance, if GDP per capita of the initial 15 member states is rated at 100, the equivalent for the ten new members is a mere 30. If we limit the comparison to the four initial member states with the lowest GDP per capita, the outcome is still the double of that of the ten new entrees (Dunkerley, D., et al.: ibid., p. 146), whereas after the latest enlargement, 36% of the European population live in regions with a GDP per capita of less than three-quarters of the European Union's average (Lamy, P. and Pisani-Ferry, J.: ibid., p. 78). To give some concrete illustrations of the differences, in 1999 GDP per capita was \$25,372 in Germany, compared to \$14,266 in Spain, \$11,763 in Greece, \$10,782 in Portugal, \$4,802 in Hungary, \$3,983 in Poland, and \$3,536 in Estonia (Calleo, D. P.: ibid., p. 278).
237. Jospin, L.: ibid., p. 30.
238. An Impact Study of the European Commission is very clear about these expected future advantages: "Economic benefits from enlargement are expected to follow from the expansion of the Single Market, from the overall integration process, as well as from the strengthening of the Union's position in global markets. The Union's human potential will be considerably enriched, not least in qualified and highly qualified labor. Acceding countries have significant natural resources (agricultural land, some minerals, biodiversity, etc.). Their geographic position will be an asset with respect to transport, energy transit and communications. The integration of these countries into the Union will be a powerful stimulus to their economic development. Major investments related to the radical modernisation of the new countries' economies and their catching up with European Union living standards will boost demand across the Union and strengthen competitiveness" (Dunkerley, D., et al.: ibid., p. 147).
239. Thurow, L.: *Head to Head: The Coming Economic Battle among Japan, Europe and America*, Warner Books, 1993, p. 110. In 1999, the European Union, having a population of approximately 290 million, produced a GDP of \$6 trillion, \$2 trillion smaller than the United States with 270 million people, but \$2 trillion more than Japan with a population of 125 million people (Gilpin, R.: *The Challenge of Global Capitalism: The World Economy in the 21st Century*, Princeton University Press, 2000, p. 196).
240. Lamy, P. and Pisani-Ferry, J.: ibid., p. 92. The reason for this may simply be that they don't know what enlargement of the European Union is all about. In this respect, a survey among members of the Dutch parliament, carried out only five months before ten new countries became full members, revealed that one-third of them had no idea about the number of new members, and two-thirds could not tell the size of the European Commission or the Union's budget (De Volkskrant, 6/7 December 2003).

241. Less than 50% of the European citizens took part in the elections for the European parliament of 1999. Two years earlier, this figure was 57%.
242. Although attempts to prevent this deficiency by declaring that the European Union will "continue the process of creating an ever closer union among the peoples of Europe, in which decisions are taken as closely as possible to the citizen," have resulted in some improvements (such as more direct influence of the European Parliament and the appointment of a European ombudsman), the enlargement of the European Union has thus far been an elite movement of political leaders, businessmen and the bureaucracy in Brussels (Gilpin, R.: ibid., p. 215). Regarding this, a recent Eurobarometer revealed that in the 13 applicant countries prior to May 2004, 69% of the population felt "not very well" or "not at all" informed about the enlargement process. For the 15 member states, the figure was 78% (European Commission: Applicant Countries Eurobarometer 2001. Public Opinion in the Countries applying for European Union Membership, March 2002, p. 97). It will not be easy to change this: it is reported that 98% of the citizens do not feel a connection with the European Union as a supranational body (Dunkerley, D., et al.: ibid., p. 40). This supranational body has yet to emerge as a contender for the loyalties of European citizens (Dunkerley, D., et al.: ibid., p. 120). Consequently, much missionary work still has to be done to create some idea of a European "nation." Promoting the perspective suggested by Thurow could be instrumental. European governments apparently do not realize that promoting a strong economic future could also counterbalance the already-existing, small but growing fires of regional separatism within the European Union (Judt, T.: ibid., p. 115). An example is Catalonia, which in 1993 produced 19% of Spanish GDP and 32% of Spanish exports, and where income per capita was 20% above the Spanish average. Another example is Italy, where "the aversion of the people of the North to have to share the country with the parasitical South is as old as the country itself" (author's translation) (Judt, T.: ibid., p. 117). Or consider Belgium, where the Flemish have benefitted in recent decades from the decline of Walloon industry. One can easily find more differences between rich and poor regions within the Union, where the rich regions, from a kind of "we-are-Europe" attitude, bypass national governments in order to promote their particular interests in Brussels and evince no concern for the less privileged regions. Hettne and Söderbaum call this phenomenon "micro-regionalism," which is related to macro-regionalism "in the way that the larger regionalization (and globalization) processes create possibilities for smaller economically dynamic sub-national or transnational regions to gain direct access to the larger regional economic system, often bypassing the nation-state and the national capital, and sometimes even as an alternative or in opposition to the challenged state and to formal state regionalisms" (Hettne, B. and Söderbaum, F.: Theorising the Rise of Regioness, in: Breslin, S., Hughes, Ch. W., Phillips, N., Rosamond, B., (eds.).: ibid., p. 42). Contrary to this view, however, Börzel paradoxically observes a tendency of regions that have the necessary resources to exploit direct channels of access to the European policy arenas, to increasingly "rely on cooperation with the central state government to project their interests in the European policy-making process" (Börzel, T. A.: Europeanization and Territorial Institutional Change: Toward Cooperative Regionalism? in: Cowles, M. D., et al.: ibid., p. 157). Regardless of which scholar is correct in this

respect, these examples are based on economic motives. They have to be distinguished from separatism that is rooted in ethnicity, language, or religion, which results in demands for recognition of identity or even independence. To some scholars, the strengthening of regional identity is a logical consequence of "an erosion or reorganisation of nation-states" (Hettne, B. and Söderbaum, F.: ibid., p. 40). This type of pursued separatism seems to be on the increase (Hofstede, G.: ibid., p. 24).The European map of some 100 years ago is becoming realistic again. Furthermore, the widening gap between different income classes in Europe will demand government action directed at preventing an unsound nationalism. It should be noted, however, that it is very difficult to distinguish between economic motives and motives of identity in this respect. If there is a relation between the two, it seems to me that prosperous economic conditions will mitigate feelings of identity, whereas poor economic conditions will exacerbate them. This, however, should not be interpreted as a general conclusion. Therefore, added to the problems sketched above, in order to maintain social stability in Europe, governments will have to display political *tours de force*.

243. Myrdal, G.: ibid., pp. 160 and 238.
244. In this respect, Lasch refers to referenda on the unification that have revealed "a deep and widening gap between the political classes and the more humble members of society." The latter fear that the Union will be dominated by bureaucrats and technicians "devoid of any feelings of national identity or allegiance." In their view, a European government will be "less and less amenable to popular control," whereas "the international language of money will speak more loudly than local dialects" (Lasch, C.: ibid., p. 46).
245. McGrew, A.: Power Shift: From National Government to Global Governance? in: Held, D., et al: *A Globalizing World? Culture, Economics and Politics*, Routledge/The Open Unversity, 2000, p. 141.
246. However, some, like Elias, believe that these modern times of globalization will automatically lead to a global unification into a world state with a world government. Such a world state would resemble the welfare states as we know them now. So far, however, there are no signs that such a development will take place. On the contrary, separatism and demands for greater autonomy are on the increase (Loo, H. van der and Reijen, W. van: ibid., pp. 285–288).
247. McGrew, A.: ibid., pp. 140–141.
248. Consequently, we see an explosive growth in the number of global platforms. For example, the number of intergovernmental organizations grew from 37 in 1909 to almost 300 in 1999. Next to this, global governance has resulted in a multiplicity of expert groups, summits, conferences, and congresses. Their coming together amounts to around 4,000 meetings annually (McGrew, A.: ibid., p. 138).
249. Two examples demonstrate these devastating effects. The first example regards the liberalized exchange of capital flows, one of the boosters of the globalization process. Financial disasters since the 1990s in Mexico, Indonesia, Russia, Malaysia, South Korea, Argentina, and also the demise of Long Term Capital Management in the United States, which forced the Federal Reserve Board, "the cockpit of world finance" (Phillips, K.: ibid., p. 138), to save a group of American Banks (Hertz, N.: ibid., p. 44) with a \$3.6 billion rescue package (Scholte, J. A.: *Globalization. A Critical Introduction*, ibid., p. 119), have demon-

strated how unstable financial markets can be. As a consequence of the financial crisis, Indonesia's economy, which expanded by 8% and 5% in 1996 and 1997 respectively, contracted by no less than 13% in 1998. South Korea's economic growth sank by 7% in 1998 after having grown by 7% in 1996 and 5% in 1997 (Legrain, Ph.: ibid., p. 281). Consequently, unemployment in the South Asian region soared, with the number of people living in poverty increasing by 90 million (Werner, K. and Weiss, H.: *Schwarzbuch Markenfirmen* (Dutch Translation), Rijswijk, 2002, p. 194). As for Mexico, the privatization of Mexican banks in the 1990s created 28 billionaires, leaving ordinary Mexicans paying the price of the economic damage (Phillips, K.: ibid., p. 229). Contrary to the proponents of neo-liberal market fundamentalism, financial markets do not tend to reach a natural market equilibrium (Soros, G.: *Soros on Globalization*, ibid., p. 160). Instead, Soros says, "they need supervision and regulation" (Soros, G.: *The Crisis of Global Capitalism: Open Society Endangered*, Little, Brown and Company, 1998, p. 194). There are a few indications that the G8 countries are starting to realize this. Meanwhile, global financial experts hope that financial markets will become less volatile when good quality relevant macro- and micro-economic information is available. In this respect, it is helpful that the IMF established a Special Data Dissemination Standard in 1996 and a General Dissemination System in 1997, which are freely available on the Internet. In addition to this, the IMF, together with the World Bank and the International Federation of Accountants, launched an International Forum on Accountancy that aims to build accounting and auditing capacity (Scholte, J. A.: *Globalization: A Critical Introduction*, ibid., p. 217). These and other initiatives (Scholte notes the International Organization of Securities Commissions, the International Association of Insurance Supervisors, the OECD Committee on Financial Markets, the BIS Committee on Payment and Settlement Systems, et cetera: Scholte, J. A.: *Globalization: A Critical Introduction*, ibid., p. 218) are meant to increase stability in global finance. To a large extent, worldwide capital flows have to do with speculation. According to Phillips, only 2–3% of the daily 1.5 trillion dollars (Mittelman J. H.: ibid., p. 21) of currency trade in the global market in the late 1990s, which was an eightfold increase since 1986 (Gilpin, R.: ibid., p. 140), had to do with actual trade in goods and services (Phillips, K.: ibid., p. 138). Others give speculation estimations of 90% (for example, according to Scholte, the proportion of foreign exchange dealings that relate to transactions in real goods fell from 90% in the early 1970s to less than 5% in the early-1990s: Scholte, J. A.: *Globalization: A Critical Introduction*, ibid., p. 218). Consequently, "total turnover in currency markets alone, is inflated far beyond the underlying economic realities," says the Independent Commission on Population and Quality of Life in this respect (*Report of the Independent Commission on Population and the Quality of Life: Caring for the Future*, Oxford University Press, 1996, p. 281). Concurrently, new stock exchanges were opened in 70 countries in recent years, including the African continent, Eastern Europe and Russia (Scholte, J. A.: *Globalization: A Critical Introduction*, ibid., p. 117). Commercial banks take part in this speculation. In 2000, a group of just 24 commercial banks made a profit of around €5 billion in just three weeks on the Brazilian commodities and futures market. The major part of these earnings, €800 million, went to American Citibank, whereas Deutsche Bank was among the top ten winners with €200 million (Werner, K.

and Weiss, H.: ibid., p. 195). In addition to this, the three types of democratization described by Friedman have made it possible for individuals to take part in the capital-market gambling game. In 1980, a total of 4.6 million American households owned shares in mutual funds. By 2000, "more than half the U.S. population was investing in the stock market, either through equities they purchased themselves or through mutual funds or through their pension-retirement plans" (Friedman, T. L.: ibid., p. 125). This represented, by and large, a tenfold increase in 20 years. Illustrative of this gambling game is the fact that many individual shareholders hold their shares no longer than four to five days (Gates, J.: ibid., p. 144). The Internet plays a facilitating role here. Cheap online trading caused 10 million Americans to opening online accounts between 1996 and 2000 (Levitt, A.: *Take on the Street: What Wall Street and Corporate America Don't Want You to Know; What You Can Do to Fight Back*, Pantheon Books, 2002, p. 29). To many authors, this is the most destabilizing force in a globalizing world. Soros, for example, believes that the globalization of financial markets has superseded the welfare states that were created after the Second World War, since people who need a social safety net cannot leave their country, whereas the capital that governments used to tax, easily can (Soros, G.: *Soros on Globalization*, ibid., p. 19), because "money has no flag" (Buchanan, P. J.: ibid., p. 54). However, it is assumed that this is not the fault of corporate business. To Burton-Jones, liberalized exchange of capital flows is one of the forces that are beyond the control of firms. In his opinion, "firms have as much control over these forces as a farmer has over the weather" (Burton-Jones, A.: *Knowledge Capitalism*, Oxford University Press, 1999, p. 230). Nevertheless, there is a destabilizing factor here, as the examples given earlier demonstrate. World leaders are compelled to design a policy that limits monetary speculation. In this respect, it is worth mentioning that the G8 called for "a new financial architecture" during its meeting in 1998. One of those G8 leaders, Tony Blair, urged a new Bretton Woods conference, with the aim of rewriting international financial rules (Gates, J.: ibid., p. 198). Furthermore, the Commission on Global Governance formulated the view that "systemic financial stability; a stable monetary system, a capacity to deal with major systemic slumps and shocks, and prudential regulation of international financial markets" would be among the basic international public goods that global governance should provide (Report of the Commission on Global Governance: *Our Global Neighborhood*, Oxford University Press, 1996, p. 150). This demands a revision of the Bretton Woods agreement (1944–1971). After all, "if markets are global, their regulators must also be global" (Kuttner, R.: The Role of Governments in the Global Economy, in: Hutton, W. and Giddens, A., (eds.): *On the Edge: Living with Global Capitalism*, Jonathan Cape, London, 2000, p. 153). Regarding this, the Commission on Global Governance suggests the establishment of an Economic Security Council which aims: "(a) to continuously assess the overall state of the world economy and the interaction between major policy areas; (b) to provide a long-term strategic policy frame work in order to promote stable, balanced and sustainable development; (c) to secure consistency between the policy goals of the major international organisations, particularly the main multilateral economic institutions, the Bretton Woods bodies and the [then] (proposed) WTO, while recognising their distinct roles; (d) to promote consensus-building dialogue between governments on the evolution of the international economic system, while providing a global forum of the new forces in the world economy—such as regional organisations" (Report of the Commission on Global Governance: ibid., p. 156). Indeed, a Bretton Woods-like regulatory system seems more appropriate than ad hoc interventions by the great powers in order to, for instance, prevent the yen from crashing in 1998, stabilise the dollar against the yen (the Louvre Accord of 1988), or produce a period of coordinated reduction in interest rates (the Plaza Accord of 1985) (Kuttner, R., in: Hutton, W., and Giddens, A., (eds.): ibid., pp. 162–163). Moreover, there is no certainty that currency rates will produce optimal outcomes under free flows of capital. Several mainstream economists have challenged this thesis (Kuttner, R., in: Hutton, W. and Giddens, A., (eds.): ibid., p. 161). A Bretton Woods-like regulatory system, for that matter, would be in line with the intentions that the architects of Bretton Woods, Harry Dexter White and John Maynard Keynes, had in 1944. They not only proposed gradually to liberate international trade, but also to control speculative capital tightly (Legrain, Ph.: ibid., p. 104). One could also consider levying taxes on capital flows. After all, one can wonder why governments raise value-added taxes on physical transactions but not on financial ones (Soros, G.: *Soros on Globalization*, ibid., p. 84). The magnitude of capital flows is beyond human imagination. On a single day in April 1998, the turnover in the currency markets was $1.5 trillion, which is around a hundred times more than the trade in goods and services. (Today's *net* capital flows, however, are far smaller as a share of GDP than were pre-First World War net flows out of Britain to countries like Argentina, Australia, and Canada [Frankel, J.: ibid., p. 57]). If we calculated a year of 240 working days, with governments imposing a tax of 0.01%, which would hardly influence the financial markets, this would produce considerable revenues for governments (Report of the Independent Commission on Population and Quality of Life: ibid., p. 282). Related to this are the so-called "Tobin tax" proposals of 1994, named after the Nobel Prize winner James Tobin, which entailed a 0.05% taxation on all foreign exchange dealings. It is estimated that such a taxation would yield over €100 billion annually on a worldwide basis. This represents a considerable amount of money that could be used for combating poverty and unemployment, while those who pay these taxes would hardly notice it (Werner, K. and Weiss, H.: ibid., p. 199). In this respect, Soros would like to see such tax revenues channelled to international institutions in order to finance the provision of public goods like combating infectious diseases and education (Barrez, D.: *De Antwoorden van het Antiglobalisme Van Seattle tot Porto Alegre*, Mets & Schilt, 2001, p. 110). Further, one could devise an international tax treaty or impose stronger reserve requirements on bank lending to discourage rash loans (Self, P.: ibid., pp. 199–200). Regarding these ideas, The Independent Commission on Population and Quality of Life suggested that the United Nations and the Bretton-Woods institutions could install a small group of experts to study and report on the possibilities of a global transaction charge on financial activities (Report of the Independent Commission on Population and Quality of Life: ibid., p. 284). All these suggestions could be carried through rather quickly, if politicians such as the leaders of the G8 could agree on a common line and had the courage to implement them. The second example may cause a profound impact in the near future. It concerns the growing worldwide inequality. The relevant question is whether we can prevent present-day capitalism, since communism has been defeated, from becoming its own worst enemy by making it politically acceptable through social corrections. In this respect, it is worth mentioning that during the World Economic Forum and G7 summits of 1999 and 2000, "much was made of the apparent trade-off between international competitiveness and the social and political priorities of democratic systems. Privatization and deregulation in welfare provisions, especially, were recognized to have contributed to rising levels of domestic inequalities, and the "logic" of international restructuring to have fed into an increasingly painful differentiation between rich and poor countries. Social injustice came during this time to be associated with the absence of effective economic regulation, or at the very least with the process of deregulation which most countries were engaged in engineering for much of the 1990s" (Phillips, K.: ibid., p. 71). Consequently, in economic and political circles, the objectives of neo-liberal market economies are thought to be in need of re-evaluation. Part of this re-evaluation should deal with the fact that privatization and deregulation have nothing to do with globalization. American airlines, for instance, have been deregulated. Nevertheless, foreign airlines are not allowed to fly domestic American routes, nor has the United States airline industry been opened to international competition. The same applies to the privatization of British Airways, Air France, and Lufthansa, which do not face American competition on European routes. Conversely, globalization need not imply deregulation or privatization. The pharmaceutical industry is a good example. Although they compete in a global playing field, pharmaceutical companies are strictly subjected to regulation (Legrain, Ph.: ibid., p. 6).

250. Commission on Global Governance: ibid., pp. 61 and 137.
251. Kapstein, E. B.: *Sharing the Wealth: Workers and the World Economy*, Norton and Company, New York, 1999, p. 111.
252. In this respect, one can agree with Kaplan that "there are no universal truths on how to organise society or to improve it" (Kaplan, R. B.: *The Coming Anarchy: Shattering the Dreams of the Post Cold War*, Random House, New York, 2000, p. 176).
253. It is impossible to consider the World Bank, the IMF, and the WTO in a completely isolated way, because their activities are closely tied up with the foreign policy of the developed world, especially American foreign policy, as is illustrated by the fact that within the IMF, the ten most industrialized countries have over 50% of the votes, of which the United States has 18% (Hobden, S. and Jones, R. W.: Marxist Theories of International Relations, in: Baylis, J. and Smith, S., (eds.): ibid., p. 213). The IMF has 183 members; the WTO 145. The WTO was established in 1995. Its members have a right of veto. The organization employs 550 people and has a yearly budget of $80 million, half of which is spent on the translation of documents (Legrain, Ph.: ibid., p. 183). Since its inception, the International Trade Organisation (ITO) and the General Agreement on Tariffs and Trade (GATT, 1947) represent the "embryonic trade ministry of a world government" (Buchanan, P. J.: ibid., p. 313). To Legrain, however the WTO is a simple forum where governments hammer out trade rules and have an umpire in trade disputes (Legrain, Ph.: ibid., p. 178). It faces difficulties in administering a series of rules, and in governing international trade and its related areas, in order to achieve its objectives of

(1) non-discriminatory treatment in international commerce, (2) the pursuit of a reduction and possible elimination of barriers to trade, and (3) the pacific settlement of disputes (Wilkinson, R.: *Multilateralism and the World Trade Organisation: Architecture and Extension of International Trade Regulation*, Routledge, 2000).

254. Within the IMF, the ten most industrialized countries have over 50% of the votes, of which the United States has 18%.
255. Stiglitz, J.: *Globalization and its Discontents* (Dutch Translation), Utrecht, 2002.
256. Klein, N.: *Fences and Windows*, ibid., p. 21.
257. Mestrum, F.: ibid., p. 21. In this perspective, combating poverty, for example, is not additional to but an alternative for social security. This kind of social security is not meant to protect people against market failures. Instead, it is an incentive and an obligation to participate in that market. This means that, in order to survive, poor people must participate in the market in accordance with neo-liberal views. Consequently, organizations like the IMF and the World Bank criticize systems of social security, because egalitarian access to the advantages of social security would not respond to the demands of a market economy.
258. Mestrum, F.: ibid., pp. 75, 77, 126, and 137.
259. Democracy, however, cannot be enforced by foreign institutions. Neither can it be valued as an export article of the developed world, for the simple reason that civil rights cannot be imported. Democracies grow inside-out and bottom-up in a long-term process. For such a process to succeed, it is more productive to take indigenous traditions and rules as the point of departure, than imitating exogenous constitutions and political instruments (Barber, B.: *Fear's Empire*, ibid., chapter 8). Hofstede, therefore, rightfully observes that introducing democracy as a pre-condition for material help will not change the political traditions of developing countries. Besides, one cannot expect participation in democracy from people who are hardly fed and who do not have the chance to be educated (Hofstede, G.: ibid., p. 57; also, Myrdal, G.: ibid., p. 130). On the contrary, forcing underdeveloped nations to introduce political democracy may work "like a razor in the hands of a child" (author's translation) (Lichtveld, in: Jansen van Galen, J.: *Het Suriname-Syndroom. De PvdA tussen Den Haag en Paramaribo*, Bert Bakker/Wiardi Beckman Stichting, 2001, p. 27). In 1959, Lipset proved that there is a strong correlation between, on the one hand, a country's democratic stability and, on the other hand, its level of economic development (Fukuyama, F.: *The End of History and the Last Man*, ibid., p. 135). Research by Przeworski and Limongi over the period 1950–1990 indicated that democracies in countries with a per-capita income of less than \$1,500 lasted on average eight years; with per-capita income between \$1,500 and \$3,000, democracy lasted on average 18 years; and at an income level of more than \$6,000 per capita, democracy appeared to be stable (in: Zakaria, F.: ibid., p. 63). And if, on top of this, those same people are forced to accept harsh adjustment measures as a pre-condition for financial support from the IMF/World Bank, this may endanger the assumed coexistence of democratisation and structural adjustment (Fukuyama, F.: *The End of History and the Last Man*, ibid., p. 135). This co-existence was already made critical by the IMF/World Bank in stating that a minimum wage of less than \$1 per day was "excessive" (Mittelman, J. H.: ibid., pp. 104 and 107). One wonders then, how

these international institutions define poverty. To provide some balance, however, Sen's observation that the generation and enforcement of a democratic system is an essential element in a process of development is worth mentioning, because, to him, democracy has three separate advantages. Firstly, it has an intrinsic value. Secondly, it plays a role in creating a sense of standards in society. Thirdly, and most importantly, democracy is a means in the process of decision-making regarding the objectives of society. If governments can be criticized by their citizens, it may be that those in power will listen to hear what people want (Sen, A.: ibid., p. 155). Though all of this may be true for developing countries, one can doubt if Sen's advantages apply to the so-called mature democracies of the Western world. Here, the continuously decreasing participation in elections makes me hesitant about citizens' perceptions of the intrinsic value of democracy. Furthermore, one can argue that increasing demands for personal safety in the countries of the Western world are the result of a decreasing general attachment to an accepted sense of standards on what is right or wrong. Finally, the fact that a growing number of people have come to believe that politics no longer matters implicitly means that they no longer have the idea that they can influence political decision-making. Therefore, I tend to agree with Hofstede and Lipset. After all, the well-being of people begins with a full stomach and good health. The wish to be taken seriously by those in power comes after that.

260. Ironically, the IMF, established exactly because markets do not always work perfectly, has become a strong promoter of market superiority.
261. Chalmers Johnson: *Blowback: The Costs and Consequences of American Empire*, Little, Brown and Company, 2000, p. 80.
262. Since 1985, the IMF and the World Bank have controlled Tanzania's economy. When taking over the country, with its diseases and debts, no time was lost in cutting trade barriers, reducing public spending and selling state industries. Fifteen years later, GDP per capita had dropped from $309 to $210, literacy had fallen, and the rate of abject poverty had jumped to 51% of the population (Palast, G.: ibid., p. 148). Meanwhile, settling the country's debts demanded an amount of money that was six times as high as what the country spent on health care (Ellwood, W.: *The No-Nonsense Guide to Globalization* (Dutch Translation), Lemiscaat, 2003, p. 57). An Economic and Rehabilitation Programme for Mozambique in 1988, sponsored by the IMF and the World Bank, further squeezed the already-low social provisions in the country. The privatization of health care drove up the price of medical services. As a result, attendance at local clinics and hospitals, particularly by women, dropped immediately by 50% to 80%. In addition to this, the IMF/World Bank conditions accelerated the already-downward spiral of inadequate nutrition (Mittelman, J. H.: ibid., p. 83). This policy of squeezing social provisions resulted in a dramatic decrease in public spending on health care and education. Per-capita spending on health fell from $4.70 in 1982 to $0.90 in 1989, whereas spending on education in 1989 was only one-third of that in 1982 (Mittelman, J. H.: ibid., p. 97). In South Africa, "apartheid based on race has been replaced with apartheid based on class." According to Trevor Ngwane, a former ANC municipal council member, this was caused by the restructuring programme that was imposed by the IMF and the World Bank and executed by the South African government. The results have been devastating. Since 1993, a total of 500,000 jobs have been lost, wages

for the poorest 40% have dropped 21%, the price of water has gone up 55%, and the price of electricity has increased 400% (Klein, N.: *Fences and Windows*, ibid., pp. 108–109). In Indonesia in 1998, the IMF eliminated food and fuel subsidies for the poor in a framework of "market-based pricing" of food, water and domestic gas. The same happened in Bolivia in 2000, where the population suffered water price hikes (Palast, G.: ibid., p. 153). Here, the American-owned International Water Limited secured from the Bolivian government a guaranteed 16% return on investment, which accounted for a 35% price increase. Protest organizers knew that just over the border in Argentina, the privatization of water supplies had eliminated the jobs of 7,500 people. Brazil provides a good example of how the IMF and the World Bank serve the interests of the developed world. As Palast reveals, Cardoso's re-election to the presidency in 1998 was dependent on his ability to maintain the high value of the *real*, the Brazilian currency. The IMF and the World Bank offered a loan of $41 billion that would not be handed over before the elections. Thirteen days after Cardoso had been re-elected, publicly supported by Peter Mandelsohn, Blair's favorite, "the U.S. Treasury gave the nod, a trap door opened and Brazil's currency plunged through, dropping 40%." This appeared to be very convenient, because in order to be able to pay its new multi-billion dollar debts, Brazil held a fire sale. The Texan companies Enron and Houston Industries purchased the electricity companies of Rio de Janeiro and São Paolo, and a pipeline, for peanuts, and British Gas received São Paolo Gas Company for a song (Palast, G.: ibid., pp. 303–304). For most underdeveloped and developing countries that have received loans from the IMF/World Bank, annual interest payments are higher than combined spending on health and education. Interest payments leaving many African countries are three times as high as aid money coming in. Situations on other continents deliver a comparable picture. Pakistan, for instance, spent just 0.05% of its budget in 2000 on health, 2.2% on education, and 60% on repaying debt (Neale, J.: ibid., p. 39). As a condition for an IMF loan, the government of Ecuador was ordered to raise the price of cooking gas by 80% from November 2000. Furthermore, 26,000 government jobs had to be eliminated, and for the remaining staff, real wages had to be cut by 50% in four steps in accordance with a timetable delivered by the IMF. Finally, by July 2000, and in order to serve the interests of the developed world, ownership of Ecuador's biggest water system had to be transferred to foreign operators, while British Petroleum was granted the right to build and own an oil pipeline over the Andes (Palast, G.: ibid., p. 145). As for the recent crisis in Argentina, the World Bank ordered the government, in its secret "Country Assistance Strategy" report of June 2001, to increase labor flexibility by cutting works programs, smashing union rules, and slicing real wages. All of this satisfied the conditions for a $20 billion emergency loan package, together with "stand-by" credit from the IMF. At the time of the deal, Argentina already owed $128 billion in debt. For this debt, $27 billion in interest and premiums had to be paid annually. Consequently, the Argentinian population did not get one penny from the so-called bailout loan (Palast, G.: ibid., p. 160). Meanwhile, the population revolted over massive cuts in social spending, almost $8 billion in three years, as a condition to qualify for the IMF loan (Klein, N.: *Fences and Windows*, ibid., p. 49). Moreover, since cutting social spending was not enough to meet the financial obligations, a big hunk of the water system was sold to the French, who promptly raised the price of water in some cities by 400% (Palast, G.: ibid., p. 162). Finally and most revealingly, in 2001, two weeks before the G8 came to Genoa, in Papua New Guinea three students were killed while protesting a World Bank privatization scheme (Klein, N.: *Fences and Windows*, ibid., p. 151). It would be wrong, however, to assume that the IMF and the World Bank's neo-liberal strategy is only applied to the underdeveloped and developing countries. On the contrary, the "one size fits all" strategy is implemented worldwide. In this respect, the following quotation from an IMF bulletin of 1994, regarding the developed world, is of interest. It reads: "It should not be that European governments, because of the anxieties that have arisen from the fact that they have lost control over income distribution, cease carrying out courageous and profound reforms with respect to the labor market. A flexible labor market results from a revision of the benefit system, the legal minimum income and the regulations concerning employment protection" (author's translation) (Forrester, V.: *L'horreur économique* (Dutch Translation), Amsterdam, 1997, p. 109). This is the IMF which, like the World Bank, is part of the United Nations, but nevertheless operates like "self-righteous surgeons, skilfully removing the remnants of political control over market forces" (Castells, M.: *The Power of Identity*, ibid., p. 269). Meanwhile, these tax-free salaried surgeons saw their remuneration increase by 38% in 1992–1993, with a further budgeted increase of 22% for 1994 (Ormerod, P.: *The Death of Economics*, Faber and Faber, 1994, pp. 3 and 124).

263. Gray, J.: *False Dawn: The Delusions of Global Capitalism*, London, 1999, p. 272.
264. Hutton, W. and Giddens, A., (eds.): ibid., p. 93. Perhaps this explains why there seemed to be a change in policy during the Asia crisis of 1997–1999, when the IMF and the World Bank departed from their traditional fiscal conservatism, advocating public sector deficits in order to protect food security, primary health care, basic education, and employment. Similarly, since 1996, the World Bank, through its Structural Adjustment Policy Review Initiative, has joined with civic associations to explore possible connections between neo-liberal economic restructuring and poverty (Scholte, J. A.: *Globalization: A Critical Introduction*, ibid., p. 215). In this respect, the African country of Chad, by exploiting its extensive oilfields, delivers an example of the World Bank's policy change. In Chad, the government had to accept a legal regulation guaranteeing that 80% of oil incomes will be spent on health, education, and rural infrastructure; 5% for the population living near the oil fields; and 10% as a reserve for coming generations. So, only 5% can be spent in accordance with what the government wants (Zakaria, F.: ibid., p. 147).
265. Recent American manipulations of temporary members of the Security Council of the United Nations (Angola), and conditioning financial help to support in a then possible war against Iraq (Turkey) show that, in fact, nothing has changed. Meanwhile, the United States continues to claim moral superiority in a way that no other country can (Hertsgaard, M.: ibid., p. 75).
266. According to Wheen, the IMF, the World Bank and the WTO have been created and are directed by "a small elite conclave of capitalist cardinals" (Wheen, F.: ibid., p. 239).
267. Scholte, J. A.: *Globalization: A Critical Introduction*, ibid., p. 272.

268. In this respect, the Meltzer committee proposes to reshape the World Bank into a World Development Agency, instead of just lending money on severe terms (Soros, G.: *Soros on Globalisation*, ibid., p. 115).
269. Bové, J. and Dufour, F.: ibid., p. 158.
270. As for the latter, it is possible to argue that the WTO is worse than its predecessor the ITO, since the Havana Charter of 1948 required members to "take fully into account the rights of workers under inter-governmental declarations, conventions and agreements" (Wilkinson, R.: ibid., p. 57). Now, however, the only thing the WTO asks from its members is to conduct their commercial relations "with a view to raising standards of living, ensuring full employment, and a large and steadily growing volume of real income and effective demand" (Wilkinson, R.: ibid., p. 58). This seems to be more rhetorical than substantial, given the fact that, contrary to the Havana Charter, the WTO has no formal relations with the International Labour Organisation (ILO), nor does it want to have such relations. Moreover, the WTO managed to resist pressures from a number of members in this respect. France, for example, did not succeed in establishing a permanent working party between the ILO and the WTO (Jospin, L.: ibid., p. 38).
271. Pilger, J.: *Hidden Agendas*, ibid., p. 73. In this respect, one can wonder if there is an essential difference between present times and the nineteenth century, when imperialism and globalization went hand in hand. Legrain would call this neo-Marxist claptrap, because nowadays countries are no longer forced to open their borders but, instead, can choose to do so (Legrain, Ph.: ibid., p. 100). However, one can criticize the meaning of free choice in a context where the terms of trade are determined by the developed world, be it directly or indirectly via international organizations like the WTO, the IMF, and the World Bank. Figures demonstrate that, through their policies, developing countries are becoming more dependent on an ever-increasing free trade world. It has always been like this. At the start of the nineteenth century, the richest country was three times richer than the poorest one. A century later this was ten times. Now the richest country is sixty times better off (Legrain, Ph.: ibid., p. 90). New to the current day, however, is the fact that, according to Bhagwati, the idea of free trade has been "hijacked by the proponents of capital mobility" (Chalmers Johnson: ibid., p. 205). O'Rourke and Williamson, however, warn that we should take a more balanced view regarding the effect of free trade on Third World countries' increasing dependence (O'Rourke, K. H. and Williamson, J. G.: *Globalization and History: The Evolution of a Nineteenth-Century Atlantic Economy*, The MIT Press, 2000).
272. Jospin, L.: ibid., p. 7.
273. Gates, J.: ibid., p. 255.
274. He reveals an internal WTO memo, which he claims to have held in his hands, that in March 2001, the WTO would design a system to replace democracy with something that one day might be seen as the post-democratic Magna Carta. "At its heart was a bold plan to create an international agency with veto power over individual nation's parliamentary and regulatory decisions. The memo begins by considering the difficult matter of how to punish nations that violate a balance between two potentially conflicting priorities: promoting trade expansion versus protecting the regulatory rights of governments." Both seem

to have been thought out in the preparations for a General Agreement on Trade in Services (GATS), and have found expression in Article VI.4. Once countries have signed this article, they will be subject to the so-called "Necessity Test." This test demotes parliaments and regulatory agencies, in effect, to advisory bodies, because "final authority will rest with the GATS Disputes Panel to determine if a law or regulation is 'more burdensome than necessary.' And the GATS panel, not any parliament or congress, will tell us what is necessary" (Palast, G.: ibid., pp. 165–166). If one reads things like this, one does not believe one's eyes. Admittedly, Palast refers to an internal WTO memo. Nevertheless, it is disturbing that WTO staff give expression to ideas like these. And it is likewise disturbing that trade ministers, "in the course of secretive multilateral negotiations, agreed that, before the GATS tribunal, a defence of 'safeguarding the public interest . . . was rejected.' In place of a public interest standard, the secretariat proposes a deliciously Machiavellian 'efficiency principle' " (Palast, G.: ibid., p. 167). Finally, Palast wonders where the trade ministers got these ideas, and he answers: "There are conspiracy cranks and paranoid antiglobalizers who imagine that the blueprints for WTO supranational control are designed in secret meetings between the planet's corporate elite and government functionaries, with media leaders attending to adjust propaganda as ordered. They're right. One of these quiet groups is the LOTIS committee, which stands for Liberalisation of Trade in Services" (Palast, G.: ibid., pp. 170–173).

275. Legrain, Ph.: ibid., pp. 200–202.
276. Bové, J. and Dufour, F.: ibid., p. 165.

Chapter 2

1. Doel, J. van den: ibid., p. 2.
2. Worldwide there are less than 200 governments but approximately 60,000 major trans-national companies, 10,000 single-country non-governmental organizations (NGOs), 250 intergovernmental organizations (IGOs), and 5,800 international non-governmental organizations (INGOs) (Willetts, P.: Transnational Actors and International Organizations in Global Politics, in: Baylis, J. and Smith, S.: ibid., (eds.) p. 357). All of these organizations may try to influence political outcomes, including moves along the continuum. Willetts divides them, rather arbitrarily, into two broad categories: (a) interest groups who seek to influence economic policy, like corporate businesses and unions, and (b) pressure groups who promote their own values (Willetts, P.: ibid., p. 369). At least three objections can be raised against this approach. The first is that pressure groups may try to influence economic policy precisely by promoting their values. Environmentalism is an example. Secondly, not all those who promote their values are representatives of pressure groups. The church is an example, as are those who criticize the way the Western world defines concepts like economic growth and gross domestic product. Thirdly, it is questionable whether unions should be considered to be seeking to influence economic policy. It seems to me that unions primarily seek to serve the interest of their members, i.e., the improvement of wages and working conditions (Bendiner, B.: *International Labour Affairs: The*

World Trade Unions and the Multinational Companies, Clarendon Press, Oxford, 1987, p. 34). That this may, in turn, influence economic policy is a different matter.

3. In: Klein, N.: *No Logo*, Flamingo, 2001, p. 340.
4. Hertz, N.: ibid.
5. Kaplan, R. D.: ibid., p. 80
6. Lasch, C.: ibid., pp. 192, 193. In this respect, Reich reveals that a growing proportion of university payrolls in the United States depends on grants and research funded from outside the university. Since outside support is unpredictable, universities have to rely increasingly on contract workers whose jobs and pay vary accordingly. This may explain why professors and graduates are turning to the unions for help in protecting their salaries and benefits and for assistance in negotiating job security (Kelly, C. M.: ibid., p. 94). Consequently, part-time faculty members in the United States increased from 22% in 1970 to over 40% by the end of the 1990s (Reich, R. B.: *The Future of Success: Working and Living Conditions in the New Economy*, Vintage Books, 2000, p. 99). Similar developments can be observed in the United Kingdom, where in 1995–6, 40% of teaching, academic, and research staff were on temporary contracts (Frank, S.: ibid., p. 93).
7. One might argue that this is nothing new. Already by 1890, "the fight to control big business had become the leading problem of American politics" (Phillips, K.: ibid., p. 307). In that same year, Mary Ellen Lease, a populist firebrand, told her audience that: "Wall Street owns the country. It is no longer a government of the people, by the people and for the people, but a government of Wall Street, by Wall Street and for Wall Street" (Phillips, K.: ibid., 308), whereas historian Arthur Schlesinger Sr., looking back at the 1930s, concluded that the United States "had become a government of the corporations, by the corporations and for the corporations" (Phillips, K.: ibid., p. xvi). Observations like these illustrate that American corporate history continuously repeats itself. Abraham Lincoln "worried greatly about the dangers to democracy implied by the money-myopic nature of the corporate entity and its potential corrupting influence." Similar worries were expressed by Jefferson and Madison (Gates, J.: ibid., p. 250).
8. Bendiner, B.: ibid., p. 184.
9. Phillips, K.: ibid., p. 148, and Hertz, N.: ibid. p. 17. Legrain, however, points to the fact that a company's size is not as important as is often assumed. He strongly opposes the idea of comparing a company's sales with a country's GDP, like Klein and Hertz do. Alternatively, he suggests that a company's added value should be compared with a country's added value. Such an approach would reveal that the value added by the 50 largest corporations represents only 4.5% of the 50 largest GDPs (Legrain, Ph.: ibid., pp. 138–141). In this alternative approach, however, Legrain wrongly assumes that a country's GDP is equal to its added value, since a country's GDP covers more than only its added value because of different taxes.
10. Hertz, N.: ibid., p. 17.
11. Gates, J.: ibid., p. 157. At present, the ten biggest corporations in the field of telecommunications control 86% of the market. For the computer sector, the figure is 70%, and for pharmaceuticals, it is 35% (Ellwood, W.: ibid., p. 62).

12. In this respect, Buchanan claims that "it is an amoral institution that exists to maximize profits, executive compensation and stock dividends" (Buchanan, P. J.: ibid., p. 55).
13. In addition to this, there are many top executives who, after retirement, show compassion for the poor, become philanthropists, and try to influence political agendas in order to improve living conditions for the underprivileged (Hertz, N.: ibid., chapter 8).
14. Though the research is 25 years old, it is worth mentioning in this respect that the percentage of Americans crediting business with pursuing a fair balance between profits and the public interest dropped from 70% to 15% over the period 1968–1977 (Phillips, K.: p. 147).
15. Though corporate business may have formulated so-called "codes of conduct" regarding the way it does business in underdeveloped countries, these are codes it has freely imposed on itself. Checking to ensure that it lives up to those codes is also its own business. Independent agencies that do this are the exception rather than the rule. In this respect, the Thai sociologist Yimprasert concludes that codes of conduct are only in the interest of the corporations that formulated them (Werner, K. and Weiss, H.: ibid., p. 182), whereas the American economist Sethi estimates that possibly 10% of Western corporations accused of nasty practices have done something useful to improve labor conditions (Werner, K. and Weiss, H.: ibid., p. 180).
16. Hertz, N.: ibid., chapter 10.
17. "The Global Compact is not a regulatory instrument or code of conduct, but a value-based platform designed to promote institutional learning. It utilises the power of transparency and dialogue to identify and disseminate good practices based on universal principles," says its website (Legrain, Ph.: ibid., p. 205).
18. According to Hertz, the main task of governments seems to be to offer attractive conditions for corporate business (Hertz, N.: ibid., chapter 6).
19. Moore, M.: *Stupid White Men . . . and Other Sorry Excuses for the State of the Nation* (Dutch Translation), Amsterdam/Antwerpen, 2003, p. 79–83.
20. In this respect, the Cato Foundation from Washington has estimated that, next to some $60 billion a year in industry-specific tax breaks, the American federal government provided business some $75 billion subsidies a year, whereas the broader social costs of corporations that go unreimbursed, i.e., corruption, injury, stress, lobbying, pollution, waste, and overcharges, are hypothesised by Estes to have been $2.6 trillion in 1994. These costs were born by the community, employees, customers, and society at large (Phillips, K.: ibid., p. 149.
21. Examples are $278 million in government technology subsidies to General Electric, AT&T, IBM, and others, and nearly $300 million in tax deductions to Exxon over the settlement of the Exxon Valdez disaster (Moore, M.: *Downsize This*: ibid., pp. 43–45).
22. Hertz, N.: ibid., chapter 6.
23. Phillips, K.: ibid., p. 150.
24. If one adds to this the monetary value of leases to ski resorts, bargain sales of minerals on public lands, irrigation subsidies, and bailouts for corrupt savings and loan operators, the amount would be closer to $1.5 trillion, according to Gates (Gates, J.: ibid.).

25. Beck, U.: *What is Globalization?* Polity Press, 2001, p. 6.
26. Hertz, N.: ibid., pp. 66–67.
27. Pilger, J.: *Hidden Agendas*: ibid., p. 89.
28. Castells, M.: *The Rise of the Network Society. The Information Age: Economy, Society and Culture*, Volume 1, Blackwell Publishers, 1996, p. 276. Also: Castells, M.: *End of Millennium. The Information Age:* ibid., p. 129.
29. Self, P.: ibid., p. 158.
30. Hertz, N.: ibid., pp. 321–232.
31. Although one has to be careful not to exaggerate or to generalize, apparently this was the perspective of CEOs like Carl Gerstacker from Dow Chemicals and Philip Condit from Boeing, who, respectively, would like "Dow to have its headquarters on an island owned by no nation" or to get rid of the corporation's American image (Phillips, K.: ibid., p. 148). Apparently, these gentlemen would prefer a situation where shareholders would be their only accountability context.
32. Werner, K. and Weiss, H.: ibid.
33. As for the latter, the ICFTU (International Confederation of Free Trade Unions), which knows only the tip of the iceberg, revealed that almost 3,000 union members were tortured and 210 murdered in 2000 (Mestrum, F.: ibid., p. 217).
34. Moore, M.: *Downsize This*: ibid., p. 116. The author reports that 99% of the 90 million shoes that Nike sells each year are produced in Asia by a contractor workforce of over 75,000.
35. Scholte, J. A.: *Globalization: A Critical Introduction*: ibid., p. 78.
36. Mittelman, J. H.: ibid., p. 86.
37. These zones, with low-paid female labor as a prime component may function as an engine of economic growth, as was the case in the Philippines in the 1990s (Mittelman, J. H.: ibid., p. 77). In the Philippines, around 90% of the workforce employed in EPZs are women between 17 and 29 years old, of whom 40% receive less than the legal minimum wage, compared to 17% of the men. These young women routinely work and live in the factory compounds for a few years, sleeping in dormitories and saving as much money as possible for their dowries which, for that matter, is not a new phenomenon. Comparable circumstances existed in Japan in the 1930s (Allen, G. C.: "Japan," in: Smith, E. O., (ed.): *Trade Unions in the Developed Economies*, Croom Helm, London, 1981, pp. 74–75). Furthermore, Scholte reveals that the number of women employed in 200 EPZs in the South alone increased from 1.3 million in 1986 to 4 million in 1994 (Scholte, J. A.: *Globalization: A Critical Introduction*: ibid., p. 251). Meanwhile, the number of these EPZs is rapidly increasing: from 79 in 1984 to 200 in 1989, across 35 countries. Their location is no longer limited to countries in Southeast Asia but now includes several countries on the African continent (Mittelman, J. H.: ibid., p. 157). According to Mittelman, 100 more EPZs were established in 2000 (Mittelman, J. H.: ibid., p. 42), and Scholte reveals that, including in former communist-ruled countries, 850 EPZs were in place worldwide at the turn of the millennium. In the words of Kelly, "the woman in Bangladesh took the job [making T-shirts] from the woman in Korea, who took the job from the woman in Taiwan, who took the job from the woman in South Carolina, who took the job from the woman in America's Northeast" (Kelly, C. M.: ibid., p. 200). Bendiner provides a comparable example from

some 15 years earlier. He calculated that the difference in wages and living standards between countries meant that an American had to work 28 hours to buy a refrigerator, whereas, across the border, a Mexican had to work 416 hours, and an Indian worker had to work 1,069 hours for the same refrigerator (Bendiner, B.: ibid., pp. 184–185). In line with this, one could also compare the purchasing power of workers engaged in a similar job classification within a single trans-national corporation, as suggested by the world company councils that have been set up by international trade unions. As an example, one could develop a common market basket "for a General Motors headlight assembler (one kilogram of meat, one white shirt, one month's rent, etc.) and dividing the costs of these commodities in local currency by the worker's hourly wage. The resultant figure (number of minutes of work needed to purchase a certain commodity) indicated the comparative remuneration of the headlight assembler and provided a crude international comparison of wages within a transnational." (Busch, G. K.: *The Political Role of International Trades Unions*, The MacMillan Press Ltd., 1983, pp. 194–195).

38. Mestrum, F.: ibid., p. 153.
39. Klein, N.: *Fences and Windows*: ibid., p. XXII.
40. Kuttner, R.: *Everything for Sale*: ibid., p. 96.
41. *De Volkskrant*, 7 May 2002, p. 17.
42. Scholte, J. A.: *Globalization: A Critical Introduction*: ibid., p. 258. Meanwhile, corporate business is finding different ways to brush up its image, varying from innocent public relations strategies, pressure on political parties and lobbying, to fully fledged intelligence operations with groups of fake activists and on-line detective agencies (Lubbers, E.: *Battling Big Business* (Dutch Translation), Amsterdam, 2002). With the support of the International Chamber of Commerce (ICC), even the events of September 11, 2001, are used to counter protest movements. In this respect, the ICC's Secretary-General stated on the organization's website that a lack of progress regarding the further development of the WTO would be acclaimed by all the enemies of free trade and investment, which include those who were responsible for the attacks on the World Trade Center and the Pentagon. This is in line with the view of the chairman of the American Coalition of Service Industries, a member of the ICC, who claims that we have to defeat the powers of terror and anti-globalization in order to be able to extend global trade and investment (Lubbers, E.: ibid., p. 99).
43. *De Volkskrant*, 7 May 2002, p. 17
44. Consumption seems to be the new "erotic dysfunction" (McIntosh, A.: *Soil and Soul: People versus Corporate Power*, Aurum Press, 2002, p. 106), which leads to freedom because "to buy is to be" (Klein, N.: *Fences and Windows*: ibid., p. 174). Here, according to Klein, the end of the Cold War was an important turning point (see section 1.2.1). After the Cold War, a new ideology had to be invented, because without an ideology, shopping would just be shopping. That ideology was "lifestyle branding": "an attempt to restore consumerism as a philosophical or political pursuit by selling powerful ideas instead of mere products" (Klein, N.: *Fences and Windows*: ibid., p. 182). One might also say that, after the Cold War, disoriented Americans started "seeking comfort in the security of great brands" (Hutton, W.: *The World We're In*: ibid., p. 173).Consequently, modern consumers do not buy products, but feelings and images (Loo, H. van der and Reijen, W. van: ibid., p. 183). Through branding,

i.e., the way producers try to differentiate their product from the competition, Benetton sweaters have become the symbol of fighting racism, Ikea furniture stands for democracy, and computers symbolize revolution. The new ideology worked tremendously well, and branding became "the high point of seller-centric narcissism" (Mitchell, M.: *Right Side Up: Building Brands in the Age of the Organized Consumer*, HarperCollinsBusiness, 2002, p. 7), and "the chief cultural activity in the United States" (Kuttner, R.: *Everything for Sale*: ibid., p. 57). Consuming is in the genes of Americans. "Shop till you drop," so it seems (*De Volkskrant*, 23 December 2003). This may explain why President Bush, in an attempt to calm down the nation after the dreadful events of September 11, 2001, advised his fellow Americans to visit the shopping malls in order to overcome their fear (Barber, B; *Fear's Empire*: ibid., p. 230). Consuming has become a new American religion. In 1999, the country spent \$535 billion on amusement alone, which is more than the GDP of the 45 poorest countries in the world (Hertsgaard, M.: ibid., p. 40). Around the turn of the century, American consumer debt was just under \$5 trillion, virtually the same amount as the federal debt (Moore, M.: *Downsize This*: ibid., p. 137). It should be noted, however, that consumerism is not an exclusively American phenomenon. In Germany, for example, the individual savings quota, which was still 14.6% in the mid-1960s, had decreased to less than 10% in 1999 (Miegel, M.: ibid., p. 148).

45. Beigbeder, F.: *99 Francs* (Dutch Translation), Breda, 2000, p. 49. According to this author, who worked as a copywriter with one of the world's largest advertizing agencies, the influence of brand leaders is so penetrating that, in time, the saints on the Roman Catholic calendar will be replaced by 365 logos (Beigbeder, F.: ibid., p. 147). Therefore, his conclusion is that "the brands have won the Third World War against humanity" (Beigbeder, F.: ibid., p. 31; author's translation). It is no longer advertizing that imitates life, but it is life that imitates advertizing. And it is also advertizing that has taken over the role of those who previously gave meaning to life, like schools, the church, and cultural institutions (Werner, K. and Weiss, H.: ibid., p. 36). The Netherlands has an internet site for personal advertisements which only uses brand names to characterize potential partners for men and women who are surfing the internet to find one. Apparently, known Dutch brands are more characteristic than qualifications like sympathy, friendliness, and warmth (Berenschot BV: *Beelden van Bestuur: Berenschot Trendstudie*, Lemma, 2002, p. 116).
46. Scholte, J. A.: *Globalization: A Critical Introduction*, ibid., p. 114.
47. Mitchell, M.: ibid., p. 47.
48. Hutton, W.: The World we're in: ibid., p. 173.
49. They do not stem from necessity but from vanity or what Rousseau already called "amour-propre" (Fukuyama, F.: *The End of History and the Last Man*: ibid., p. 108). The so-called Frankfurt School of sociology even argues that mass consumption is the new expression of repression by the capitalistic culture industry. By creating false needs, consumerism intoxicates the class-consciousness of the working class (Loo, H. van der and Reijen, W. van: ibid., pp. 179–180).
50. Klein, N.: ibid.
51. In the 1990s, exclusive contracts between schools and producers of beverages increased by 1,384%, and 240 school districts in 31 states gave exclusive rights

to Coca Cola, Pepsi, and Dr. Pepper (Moore, M.: *Stupid White Men*: ibid., p. 134). The same applies for fast food chains. Taco Bell, Pizza Hut, and McDonald's, among others, are now selling in about 30% of American public high school canteens (Schlosser, E.: *Fast Food Nation: What the All-American Meal is doing to the World*, Penguin Books, 2002, pp. 51–57). During the 1990s, the sponsoring of school programs and activities in the United States increased by 248% (Moore, M.: *Stupid White Men*: ibid., p. 133).

52. Moore, M.: *Stupid White Men*: ibid., p. 137. Meanwhile, creating brand loyalty this way contributes to health care problems for American children. Research in 2003 among school children from New York, for example, found that more than half of them need to lose weight, while 25% suffer from obesity. In this respect, 61% of all Americans are overweight, while obesity results in an estimated corresponding health care burden of $117 billion per year (*De Telegraaf*, 19 August 2003).
53. In 1992, the multinational advertizing corporation Saatchi & Saatchi formed a "Kids Division," targeting children between 2 and 14 years of age. For this service, the company was paid $100 million (Pilger, J.: *Hidden Agendas*: ibid., p. 68).
54. Schlosser, E.: ibid., p. 43.
55. Schlosser, E.: ibid., p. 44.
56. Sennett, R.: ibid., p. 21.
57. Kuttner, R.: *Everything for Sale*: ibid., p. 56. At the age of seven, an American child watches television for, on average, four hours per day, swallowing about 20,000 commercials per year (Hertsgaard, M.: ibid., p. 40). Proposals from the American Free Trade Commission to ban all television advertisements directed at children seven years old or younger, although supported by, among others, the American Academy of Pediatrics, the National Congress of Parents and Teachers, the Consumers Union, and the Child Welfare League, were blocked by the National Association of Broadcasters, the Toy Manufacturers, and the Association of National Advertisers (Schlosser, E.: ibid., p. 3). A known alternative expression for breeding consumerism is the term "McDonaldization." Ritzer defines this phenomenon as "the process by which the principles of the fast-food restaurant (efficiency, calculability, predictability, and control through non-human technology) are coming to dominate more and more sectors of American society as well as the rest of the world" (Ritzer, G.: ibid., p. 7). To him and others, the McDonaldization principles are also applicable to, for instance, theme parks, the police, the courts, the sex industry, and even the family. And in each realm, a fifth principle, i.e., the irrationality of rationality, seems to apply. In regard to the latter principle, Ritzer points to the fact that McDonalized systems tend to have negative effects on the environment and to dehumanize the world, which may result in the inhumane or anti-human activities of modern culture.
58. Krugman, P.: *The Return of Depression Economics*, the Penguin Press, 1999, p. 155.
59. Referring to the Japanese recession in the 1990s, Turner speaks of "demand deflation" as the cause of this recession (Turner, A: *Just Capital: The Liberal Economy*, Pan Books, 2002, p. 159).
60. Krugman, P.: *The Return of Depression Economics*: ibid., p. 157.

61. I know that, in general terms, one can argue whether the unions should be considered as promoters or opponents of the market. For example, what about an enterprise that, with help from its unionized laborers, is polluting the environment? (Zuthem, H. J. van: Verantwoord Bestaan, Agora/Kok, Kampen, 1993).
62. The references provide further information.
63. During this repression, particularly in the second half of the 19th and the beginning of the 20th centuries, several people in the United States were killed during clashes between demonstrators and the authorities. In 1886, for example, a demonstration in Chicago over the introduction of an eight-hour working day ended up in a clash with the police, who killed four demonstrators. During the next day's protests another 11 people were killed, both demonstrators and policemen, and 117 persons were wounded. Several leaders of the demonstration were arrested and executed (Busch, G. K.: ibid., pp. 7–8). Eight years later, in 1894, the same city saw 30 strikers killed by federal troops (Busch, G. K.: p. 17), while in 1892 a group of guards, hired by a robber baron from Homestead, Pennsylvania, killed a number of striking workers (Berman, P.: ibid., p. 34). As for legal repression, the beginning of the 20th century was characterized by "the consistent hostility of American legal culture to virtually any form of labor organization." This legal culture was manifested in several rulings of the American Supreme Court, "condemning unions as an invasion of entrepreneurial rights and dismissing legislative attempts to endorse them as legitimate bargaining agencies" (Tomlins, Chr. L.: ibid., p. 30). The Great Depression of the 1930s temporarily changed this attitude with the passing of the Wagner Act, which implied that "collective bargaining was guaranteed to play a major role in the regulation of employment practices in a wide range of industries" (Tomlins, Chr. L.: ibid., p. 147). By 1947, however, labor relations went considerably back to "normal" again with the passing of the Taft-Hartley Act (Tomlins, Chr. L.: ibid., chapters 7 and 8). A few decades later, Reagan fired striking air-traffic control staff, calling in the army. One may argue without reservation that this was another expression of anti-unionism, which is characteristic of the history of American labor relations. To a certain extent, the history of the union movement in the rest of the world is comparable to that of the United Sates. In Germany, as a consequence of the passing of the Anti-Socialist Act in 1878, unions were driven underground (Owen Smith, E., (ed.): *Trade Unions in the Developed Economies*, Croom Helm, London, 1981, p. 178). Great Britain's turbulent history of those days can aphoristically be captured in terms like "the Tolpuddle Martyrs," "the Derby turn-out," "the Sheffield outrages," "the Junta," or "Black Friday" (Owen Smith, E., (ed.): ibid., p. 123). In industrializing Japan, the authorities suppressed the unions under the terms of the Public Peace Police Act of 1900, whereas Australia experienced the "savagery of the union–employer, union–government collective bargaining conflicts of the 1890s" (Cupper, L. and Hearn, J. M.: Australia, in: Owen Smith, E., (ed.): ibid., p. 13).
64. In this respect, Great Britain adopted the Trade Union Act of 1871 and the Trades Disputes Act of 1906, the French granted freedom of association by law in 1884, while in 1890 Germany withdrew the suppressive anti-socialist legislation of 1878 (Windmuller, J. P., et al.: *Collective Bargaining in Industrialised Market Economies: A Reappraisal*, International Labour Office, Geneva, 1987, pp. 121–122). Also at this juncture, trade unions joined forces by establishing

national federations. Those of Great Britain formed a Trades Union Congress in 1868, the United States saw the establishment of the American Federation of Labour (AFL) in 1886, while the French formed a General Confederation of Labor (CGT) in 1895. Around the same time, social democratic parties were emerging into legitimacy and power all over Europe. Meanwhile, the continuing spread of communism resulted in the establishment of communist unions and communist political parties; these communists felt strongly supported when a revolution in 1917 brought their compatriots to power in Russia. If we add to this the facts of the First World War (1914–1918), the Great Depression (1930s), the Second World War (1940–1945), the start of the Cold War, and several examples of corruption, treason by communist unions, and militant behavior by unionists, which, of course, did not contribute to a positive image of the union movement, then, looking back, it is no exaggeration to say that the first half of the 20th century, and more than a decade after that, was hardly a time of a balanced and welcomed developments of union movements. In this respect, British history from the 1920s reveals that shop stewards acted as espionage agents for Russia, passing on information on production methods. In France, the "Fantomas Affair" of 1932 brought into the open that the Profintern, the international organisation of communist trade unions, had developed a network of over 3,000 "correspondents" who passed information about workplaces, via the Parti Communiste Français (PCF), directly to Moscow. Even worse, during the Second World War, after Germany and Russia had concluded a non-aggression treaty, PCF unionists sabotaged French war production and sought to assist the Nazi occupation (Busch, G. K.: ibid., pp. 22–23). After the Second World War, communist intervention in national affairs in countries of Eastern Europe like Czechoslovakia, Hungary, Bulgaria, and Romania was not the exception but the rule (Busch, G. K.: ibid., chapter 4). As for the United States, it was revealed in 1967 that the AFL-CIO union was acting as a disbursement agent for the CIA, thus funding overseas projects of political interest to the American government (Busch, G. K.: ibid., pp. 189–190). Finally, in the beginning of the 1970s, it appeared that the British Trades Union Congress, closely allied with the Labour Party, was unable to control militant shop stewards who opposed deal-making with the Heath government on a policy of wage constraint (Busch, G. K.: ibid., pp. 215–218). Furthermore, unions did not always limit their activities to their basic function of improving the wages and working conditions of their members (Bendiner, B.: ibid., p. 34). The AFL, for example, competing with the militant Industrial Workers of the World (IWW) to attract new members, was staunchly supported by the American government, who took severe steps to repress militant socialists, anarchists, and communists because they were believed to threaten American policies. In short, the hunt for the American left was on, with the government assisted by vigilantes who organized lynching parties (and got away with it) and an AFL who "supported the government in its crackdown on the left" (Busch, G. K.: ibid., p. 34). In addition to this, labor in America has always been subject to the influence of gangsters who seized control of local union organizations. In this respect, congressional hearings between 1955 and 1960 "disclosed a widespread and unsavoury state of affairs," which led the then AFL-CIO president to comment in 1957, "We thought we knew a few things about trade union corruption, but we didn't know the half of it, one-tenth of it, or the one-hundredth part of it" (Owen Smith, E., (ed.): ibid., p. 161).

65. Almost from their earliest days, as players in the decision-making process regarding movement along the continuum, unions had to think about how they would operate internationally. In this respect, Busch argued in 1983 that "except for the transnational corporation, there has been no international organisation which has been more active or played such an important role in international relations than the international labour movement." To him, the international trade union movement has been and continues to be "a vital tool of governments in the shaping of the political destinies of foreign political parties and states and is an important part of most nations' foreign policy system" (Busch, G. K.: ibid., p. 1). The first platform for international collaboration between unions, the International Trades Secretariat, involved the creation of international clearinghouses, which were meant to disseminate information regarding the introduction by employers of new production methods and techniques that were of mutual concern. After the First World War, and in the context of the establishment of the League of Nations, trade unionists were represented in the commission, which had "to study the problems of labour and social policy" (Busch, G. K.: ibid., p. 20). The commission, with the participation of unionists, advised creating an autonomous organization under the umbrella of the League of Nations. This organization is now known as the International Labour Organisation (ILO). The ILO has a tripartite structure, representing workers, employers, and government officials of the member states. As stated in its constitution, its primary objective is the protection of the fundamental rights of workers all over the world. In addition to this, the organization tries to encourage programs of member states that are directed at achieving full employment, raising the standard of living, increasing health and safety measures in the workplace, and so on. In order to achieve these objectives, its International Labour Code, which is periodically reviewed, defines minimum standards, which are presented to the governments of the member states in the form of recommendations for ratification. Ratification, however, is voluntary (Bendiner, B.: ibid., pp. 57–58). A comparable situation exists in Europe with the Social and Economic Committee of the European Union. Here too, we see a tripartite membership of trade union delegates, representatives from employers, and representatives from respective governments. But, like the ILO, its recommendations are not binding on the European Commission (Bendiner, B.: ibid., p. 60). If one adds to this the fact that there are no formal relation between the ILO and the WTO, one can have serious doubts about the effectiveness of international platforms like these for the pursuit of unionized labor's basic function, being the improvement of the wages and working conditions of their members. Very important for international cooperation is for unionized labor to find ways to cope with the problems resulting from the transnationalization of corporations, i.e., (a) the fractioning of work content; (b) internal international sales operations, with components being sold from a subsidiary in one country to a subsidiary in another; and (c) the opportunity to escape from the constraints of the product cycle by innovating in a highly developed country and starting manufacturing in less-developed areas, taking advantage of tax incentives. These problems demanded that European and American union organizations protect not only

the jobs and welfare of their members, but also to assist trade unionists in the developing world to resist exploitation. Here, the setting up of "corporation councils" was hoped to deliver an effective international countervailing power to that of the transnational corporations (TNCs). The long-term objectives of these councils included collective negotiations with corporate headquarters over matters like job security and retraining and re-employment rights in the event of plant closures. As an example, the European Union of Workers in the Metal Industry have tried to compose international delegations for negotiations on labor terms at national levels (Visser, J.: De Europeanisering van de Arbeidsverhoudingen, in: Toren, J. P. van den and Vos, P. J., (eds.): ibid., p. 95). However, these councils did not obtain employer recognition as an international bargaining agent (Windmuller, J. P., et al.: ibid., p. 27). In addition to this, the idea also failed because of conflicting interests among unions of different countries (Busch, G. K.: ibid., chapter 9).In this respect, Wright observes that the reactions of the trade union movement to the spread of TNCs "has been far from concerted and organised." Those reactions not only reflected the differing impact of TNCs on each national economy, but also "the different ability of trade unions to organize a coordinated response to TNCs within each country and internationally" (Wright, M.: *Transnational Corporations, Trade Unions and Industrial Relations*, Transnational Research Project, Faculty of Economics, the University of Sydney, Working Paper No. 10, July, 1981, p. 56). Alternately, trade unions "have relied heavily on governments to minimize TNCs effects and assistance has been sought in terms of Codes of Practices" (Wright, M.: ibid., p. 59). Those governments, however, were reluctant to constrain the operations of TNCs unilaterally. Instead, they preferred setting up international codes of practice for TNCs by the ILO or the OECD. An example, in this respect, are the OECD's "Guidelines for Multinational Enterprises" of 1976, covering on a voluntary basis matters like the disclosure of information, finance, competition, employment, and industrial relations (Wright, M.: ibid., p. 69). In 1976, the ILO also started to draft a "Declaration of Principles of TNCs and Social Policy", whereas in 1974 the United Nations established a "Commission on Transnational Corporations" (Wright, M.: ibid., p. 73). Nevertheless, all these attempts to offset the impact of TNCs suffered from voluntariness and are, therefore, "inadequate to efficiently counter the TNC challenge" (Wright, M.: ibid., p. 93). However, one can argue that, despite the lack of legislative powers, the ILO has had a positive impact on working conditions worldwide, since it brought unfair and abusive conditions into the spotlight of public awareness, thus pressing for international treaties to ban them (Gates, J.: ibid., pp. 163–164).

66. However, it would be disputable to conclude that unions' strength has increased over this period, because there have been some important developments regarding employment. The first one is the reduction of employment in traditionally well-organized manufacturing industries, and rising employment opportunities in the less well-organized tertiary sector. Secondly, there has been a shift from blue-collar to white-collar occupations, which has had an adverse effect on union density rates. Thirdly, there is a decreasing need to join a union, since protective elements regarding employment also apply to non-union members. Although the increasing number of female employees, as well as increasing unionization among higher-educated employees and civil

servants, facilitated compensation, one cannot conclude absolutely that the unions have strengthened their position as a partner in the social-economic infrastructure. What has happened is that unions have broadened their sphere of activities, but that does not automatically mean that they have gained in strength.

67. To Moore, an important turning point in this respect is the fact that on August 5, 1981, President Reagan fired 11,400 striking air traffic control workers. Particularly in the United States, the argument among economists is that the influence of unions on the level of wages would distort economic efficiency. Unions would be able to keep down the number of available jobs by demanding wage increases and minimum wages.
68. Friedman, M. and Friedman, R.: ibid., p. 246. Clearly, Friedman demonstrates a very simple, but narrow, market view. This view does not provide a perspective for all those workers who, as will be argued later, became victims of downsizing since he published his ideas. Moreover, research by Harvard economists Freeman and Medoff demonstrates that this approach is too limited. Good labor relations and a decent wage level appear to have a positive effect on productivity. A labor market that treats labor as a commodity "does not necessarily yield optimal productivity. Social forces can significantly alter the pattern of wages and benefits that owners would otherwise pay their employees, with no easily predictable or mechanistic effect on economic efficiency" (Kuttner, R.: *Everything for Sale:* ibid., p. 101). Therefore, a policy of wage reductions, although more market-like, does not necessarily result in an optimal outcome (Kuttner, R.: *Everything for Sale*: ibid., pp. 98–101). A comparable moderate viewpoint can be found with the Dutch economist De Galan, who concluded on the basis of research that there is no substantial evidence that employment reacts in the short-term to changes in wages. Time lags appear to be very important. Moreover, the author found that changes in wages may only influence productivity in the long run (Galan, C. de: *De Invloed van de Vakvereniging op Loonshoogte en Werkgelegenheid*, H. E. Stenfert Kroese N. V., Leiden, 1958, p. 180). However, these more moderate views did not prevent unions in the United States from coming increasingly under attack.
69. Bendiner, B.: ibid., p. 1.
70. Owen Smith, E., (ed.): ibid., p. 9. Although unionization is a legal right in this country, employers are fighting it intensely. Employees who are involved in organizing strikes have a fair chance of being fired, although this has been illegal since the 1930s. The number of fired union members increased from 5% in 1950 to 33% in 2000. According to the AFL-CIO, the number of fired union members is estimated to be 10,000 a year (Ehrenreich, B.: *Nickels and Dimes: Undercover in Low-Wage USA*, Granta Books, 2002, p. 210), whereas research by Weiler demonstrates that, nationwide, 5% of workers who signed a union card were fired (Kuttner, R.: *Everything for Sale*: ibid., p. 99).
71. Reich, R. B.: *The Future of Success*: ibid., p. 78. Figures provided by Buchanan show that the United States' union membership losses over the period 1979–1991 were as high as 1,350,000 (Buchanan, P. J.: ibid., p. 38).
72. Visser, J.: ibid., p. 92. One of the reasons has been the Conservatives' commitment to control union activity through legal measures since the mid-1970s (Owen Smith, E., (ed.): ibid., p. 25). Moreover, Britain started to redefine the responsibilities of the government on the one hand and trade unions and

employers' associations on the other. The absence of clarity in this respect "had contributed to damaging dissension" (Owen Smith, E., (ed.): ibid., p. 5).

73. Dutch Ministry of Social Affairs and Employment, 1997.
74. Visser, J.: ibid., p. 92. Although there is a general decrease in union membership, it should be taken into account that the degree of union membership is correlated to the role that unions play in a country's social-economic infrastructure. Regarding this, one can distinguish between three explanatory factors related to union membership: (a) the involvement of unions in unemployment insurance, (b) the presence of an institutionalized social-economic infrastructure at the corporate level, and (c) union participation in the social-economic infrastructure at the national level (Visser and Ebbinghaus, quoted by the Dutch Ministry of Social Affairs and Employment). Union membership appears to be very high if the three factors apply simultaneously. In this respect, an important explanation for the very high degree of union membership in Sweden and Denmark is their involvement in unemployment insurance. If only two explanatory factors apply, then the degree of union membership is still high. Low union membership applies for countries where only one of the factors is important.
75. Information from the Dutch Ministry of Social Affairs and Employment, 2001.
76. Kuttner, R.: *Everything for Sale*, ibid., p. 64.
77. In the Netherlands, for example, the unions operated effectively as a countervailing power during the process of reforming the Dutch social security arrangements. In this respect, see: Vries, B. de: *Overmoed en Onbehagen*, Uitgeverij Bert Bakker, 2005).
78. Barrez, D.: ibid., p. 144.
79. Busch, G. K.: ibid., chapter 9.
80. Kuttner, R.: *Everything for Sale*, ibid., p. 54.
81. Toren, J. P. van den: *Van Loonslaaf tot Bedrijfsgenoot: 100 Jaar Christelijk-Sociaal Denken, Medezeggenschap en Sociale Zekerheid*, Kampen, 1991, p. 12. Although the church formally opposed avarice and usury, and brought money-lenders who charged excessive interest to ecclesiastical courts as "monsters of iniquity" (Tawney, R. H.: *Religion and the Rise of Capitalism*, Pelican Books, 1964, p. 66), it is improbable that the church had the opportunity to enforce the canon law (Tawney, R. H.: ibid., p. 63). Furthermore, the church had an immense vested interest in the economy until the beginning of the 15th century, especially with respect to agriculture and land tenure. Therefore, the church ignored the exploitation of poor peasants by feudal rulers. Apart from a few exceptional individuals, Thomas Aquinas being one of them, the church even participated in serfdom practices. "Ecclesiastical landlords, though perhaps somewhat more conservative in their methods, seem as a whole to have been neither better nor worse than other landlords," says Tawney (Tawney, R. H.: ibid., p. 70). And, although preaching that Christ had made all people free, the church's position regarding peasants' revolts against serfdom in England, France and Germany in the 14th century was dubious, at the very least. That serfdom, which in France disappeared only in the late 18th century, was part of a general economic movement that the church had hardly anything to do with. Nevertheless, the church was a very important, if not the determining, factor for society's arrangements (Toren, J. P. van den: ibid., p. 12).

82. Tawney, R. H.: ibid., p. 71.
83. Tawney, R. H.: ibid., p. 273.
84. Tawney, R. H.: ibid., p. 273.
85. Weber, M.: *The Protestant Ethic and the Spirit of Capitalism*, Routledge Classics, 2002.
86. Weber, M.: ibid., p. 116.
87. Sedgwick, P. *Christian Teaching on Work and Community*, in: CCBI (Council of Churches for Britain and Ireland), London, 1997, p. 225–226.
88. Berg, C. A. van den, et al., (eds.): *100 Jaar Verantwoordelijkheid: Verleden, Heden en Toekomst van Christelijk-Sociaal Denken*, Kampem, 1991, p. 10.
89. For example, Kuyper, a Dutch Protestant church leader, saw the establishment of labour unions as necessary to increase the influence of workers in a liberal market economy. To him, workers' demands for increased wages were no less than reasonable. Employers that rejected such a demand would make it legitimate for workers to use the instrument of a strike (Berg, C. A. van den, et al., (eds.): ibid., p.10).
90. Sedgwick, P.: ibid., pp. 225–226.
91. Barber, B.: *Fear's Empire:* ibid., p.176.
92. A subtle attempt, in this respect, was produced by the American theologian Novak, who, in his writings, tries to reconcile Papal teaching with the working of a global capitalist economy. Novak was closely associated with Reagan. A related view for Great Britain was produced by the lay theologian Griffith, who was an economic advisor to Thatcher for some years (Sedgwick, P.: ibid., p. 228).
93. Meij, A. W. H. and Zimmeren, E. van: ibid., p. 22.
94. Huntington, S. P.: Who are We?: ibid., p. 360. The author informs about the resurgence of religion in the United States in chapter three.
95. Scholte, J. A.: *Globalization: A Critical Introduction*, ibid., p. 154.
96. In this respect, Scholte reveals that the share of ODA from OECD countries channelled through NGOs rose from 4,5% in 1989 to 14% in 1993, whereas NGO involvement in World Bank projects rose from 6% during the period 1973–1988 to over 30% each year during the 1990s (Scholte, J. A.: *Globalization: A Critical Introduction*, ibid., p. 152).
97. Arts, B.: *The Political Influence of Global NGOs: Case Studies on the Climate and Biodiversity Conventions*, International Books, 1998, p. 320.
98. Pilger, J.: *Hidden Agendas*, ibid., p. 144.
99. Neale, J.: ibid., p. 41.
100. Apart from these widely known NGOs, there are thousands of organizations which have taken a stand in favor of widely defined notions of sustainability. Though these organizations are diverse in focus, their statements of principle are remarkably consistent. An appealing example is an American NGO with 54 million people, mobilizing $1 trillion in buying power to command greater quality of life (Gates, J.: ibid., p. 256).
101. In this respect, see: Barrez, D.: ibid.
102. Bové, J. and Dufour, F.: ibid., p. 145. For Chomsky, anti-globalist action illustrated the collision of two fundamental instincts of human behavior: greed and the desire for freedom. These are in dialectical opposition. The first is embodied in the giant corporations. The desire for freedom causes people around the world to resist these giant corporations. In Chomsky's view, therefore, the activ-

ities of anti-globalists symbolise a battle between "the greedy instinct versus the freedom instinct" (in: Berman, P.: ibid., p. 146).

103. Klein, N.: *Fences and Windows:* ibid., p. XV.
104. Regular examples provide proof that pollution even happens deliberately. In this respect, Palast reveals that the Exxon Valdez oil disaster in 1989, covering 1,200 miles of Alaska's shoreline with oily sludge, could have been prevented if top management had only listened to the ship's captain (Palast, G.: ibid., pp. 258–263). Furthermore, with the blessing of the World Bank, we are dumping toxic waste in underdeveloped countries (between 1989 and 1994, "garbage imperialistic" firms made 500 attempts to export a total of more than 200 million tons of waste from OECD countries to the South: Scholte, J. A.: Globalization, A Critical Introduction, ibid., p. 212). In an internal memorandum of 1999, the then chief economist of the World Bank, Lawrence Summers, identified three reasons for "encouraging more migration of the dirty industries to the LDCs (Lesser-Developed Countries)". The first was that the health costs of pollution in high wage countries, measured in income forgone by those who were ill or dying, were higher than in low wage countries. Secondly, Summers suggested that "the under-populated countries of Africa are vastly *under*-polluted." Dumping in those countries would cause relatively small negative increases in health and other consequences. Finally, Summers maintained that higher-income countries would have a greater demand for a clean environment. So, for example, he argued that "an increased risk of prostate cancer as a result of pollution was more likely to be of concern to people in countries where people survive to get prostate cancer than in a country where under-5 mortality is 200 per thousand," arguing that this would be a "world welfare enhancing trade" (Held, D., (ed.): *A Globalizing World? Culture, Economics, Politics*, ibid., p. 19). We even have set up a so-called market mechanism for "emissions-trading", together with an American "stock exchange," which trades 15 million tons of sulphur dioxide each year (Held, D. (ed.): ibid., p. 20).
105. Bové, J. and Dufour, F.: ibid.
106. As an example of the latter, the American store chain Wal-Mart is known to have paid Guatamalan 13-year-old teenage girls $0.30 per hour for making Wal-Mart label clothes, and $0.18 per hour for seamstresses from Bangladesh for an eighty-hour, seven-day week, which is half the local minimum wage and way beyond the legal work-week of 60 hours (Palast, G.: ibid., pp. 208–209). In this respect, Gates reveals that South Asia alone has 134 million children working 16-hour days for $0.08 per day (Gates, J.: ibid., p. 257). Although it is too simple to label the anti-globalists just as agitators, one can argue that the methods they use are more likely to lead to strong reactions from vested interests than to stimulate reflection on the way we deal with worldwide problems. Regarding this, it can be hoped that more influence can be expected from authors like Klein, Hertz, and others. They argue, substantiate their views, point to dangers, and come up with solutions. Their writings, if read by those in power, will probably have more influence than the revolting methods of the anti-globalists.
107. Neale, J.: ibid., p. 60. This puts a different complexion on the forceful reactions of the Italian Berlusconi government to the Genoa protests. If Neale's account of what happened in Genoa is true, the reaction of the Italian police was close

to an expression of fascism, strongly supported by Blair and Bush (Neale, J.: ibid.).

108. First, an example of this is the success of the Pantanal project in Brazil, where local environmentalists succeeded in engaging environmentalists in North America to join them in opposing the initial plans, with the effect that the Inter-American Development Bank, "sensitive to its global reputation, responded by pressuring the local governments sponsoring the project to scale it back and to do a full-blown environmental assessment" (Friedman, Th. L.: ibid., p. 289). Secondly, thanks to anti-globalists' internet activity, Starbuck's coffee chain announced that it would use coffee grown by farmers who earn a living wage (Klein, N.: *Fences and Windows*: ibid., p. 11). Thirdly, the *Financial Times* revealed in 1998 that the use of the internet was the decisive weapon used by those who opposed the WTO's intended Multilateral Agreement on Investments (MAI) (Barrez, D.: ibid., p. 59). Fourthly, and a well-known example, is the fact that 39 pharmaceutical corporations in May 2001 gave up their plans to bring the government of South Africa, which intended to violate patent laws, to court, because they realized that persisting in their case would increase the already widespread damage to their image. The internet played an important role here (Werner, K. and Weiss, H.: ibid., p. 100). On the other hand, Thailand was forced to give up the manufacturing of a cheap AIDS drug after the United States threatened a WTO suit on behalf of the American pharmaceutical industry (Phillips, K.: ibid., p. 231). It was not until the summer of 2003 that a WTO agreement was reached that enabled developing countries, under very strict conditions, to produce a cheap AIDS drug. More examples of using the internet as an instrument of protest can be given (Shell, Unilever, Nike, MacDonalds, Walt Disney, et cetera).
109. Mittelman, J. H.: ibid., p. 172.
110. Klein, N.: *Fences and Windows*, ibid., p. 25.
111. Mittelman, J. H.: ibid., p. 177.
112. As an example, the Rainforest Action Network includes members from 74 countries (Scholte, J. A.: *Globalization: A Critical Introduction*, ibid., pp. 179–180).
113. A very different position, in this respect, is taken by Friedman. To him, all protest movements (ecologists, consumers, organic food, "small is beautiful," "save the wilderness," and so on) are essentially anti-growth. Acknowledging that growth produces negative externalities, to Friedman the solution to this problem is not the establishment of large regulatory bureaucracies regarding food and drugs, pollution, product safety, energy, or whatever. Instead, "market competition, when it is permitted to work, protects the consumer better than do the alternative government mechanisms that have been increasingly superimposed on the market" (Friedman, M. and Friedman, R.: ibid., p. 222). Market competition would have to take externality problems into account, because these would result in price increases. Consequently, in the end, consumers would have to pay for the solutions to externality problems. On the other hand, we could do with considerably less bureaucracy and, through this, save tax revenues. However, only if an increase in prices is fully compensated for by tax reduction, would purchasing power be left untouched. If not, only those with higher incomes would be able to continue their role as consumer. This, in turn, would negatively influence producers' turnover, followed by decreasing stock

values. What I mean to say is that, although Friedman's approach seems logical since there can be no production without consumption, his approach is not as simple as it may seem if one does not want a change in market accessibility (Friedman, M. and Friedman, R.: ibid., chapter 7).

114. Pret à Manger, a new fresh food chain with 110 stores in the United Kingdom, the United States, and Hong Kong; Subway, with almost 18,000 stores in over 70 countries; and Starbucks, with 6,000 stores, are experiencing rapidly growing popularity. The old formulas of McDonald's, Burger King, and Kentucky Fried Chicken are facing fierce competition from these newcomers, which is translated into decreasing profitability. As an example, McDonald's concluded the final quarter of 2002 with a loss of almost $350 million, the first time since it went public in 1965. In 2002, two hundred franchises were closed, with 500 more closed in 2003 (*De Volkskrant*, 1 February 2003, p. 27). According to Levine, however, it is not just the quality of the food, but also the lack of "brand maintenance" that has caused McDonald's reversion. Since it is the largest, most pervasive fast food brand in the world, the company, wrongly and arrogantly, has taken brand loyalty for granted. And they had been warned, since research on customer satisfaction among 175 companies ranked McDonald's at 171st (Levine, M.: *A Branded World: Adventures in Public Relations and the Creation of Superbrands*, John Wiley & Sons Inc., 2003, pp. 100–103).
115. Legrain, Ph.: ibid., pp. 128–129.
116. Ritzer, G.: ibid.
117. As an example: Starbucks coffee chain announced that it would use coffee grown by farmers who earn a living wage (Klein, N.: Fences and Windows: ibid., p. 11).
118. Leadbeater, C.: *Up the Down Escalator: Why the Global Pessimists are Wrong*, Viking, 2002, p. 207.
119. In this respect, he uses the term "creolisation," by which he means that, although generalized global culture may be dominantly and penetratingly present in our lives, the translation of its influences happens within specific contexts in specific ways (in: Loo, H. van der and Reijen, W. van: ibid., p. 52). Comparable modifications can be found in Watson and Legrain (Watson, J. L.: "Transnationalism, Localization, and Fast Foods in Asia", in: Ritzer, G.: ibid., pp. 222–232). Moreover, there are scholars of cultural theory who insist that cultural globalization does not mean that the world is becoming culturally homogeneous. Instead, they stipulate that globalization always also involves a process of localization, a process they term as "glocalization." This "global-local nexus" appears to be central to corporate calculations. Globally operating corporations do not simply build factories in the world, they also want to become part of the local culture, a strategy which is called "localism" (Beck, U.: ibid., chapter 1).
120. Hertz, N.: ibid., p. 172.
121. Werner, K. and Weiss, H.: ibid., p. 37.
122. Klein, N.: *Fences and Windows*, ibid., p. 30.
123. Mitchell, M.: ibid., p. 167.
124. The American retail chain Wal-Mart estimated customer-driven replenishment decisions to be only 26% in 1987. By 1996, the percentage had increased to 90% (Mitchell, M.: ibid., p. 215).

125. Mitchell, M.: ibid., p. 86.
126. Galbraith, J. K.: *The Affluent Society*, London, 1958.
127. Mishan, E. J.: *The Costs of Economic Growth* (Dutch Translation), Het Spectrum, Utrecht/Antwerpen, 1971.
128. Daly, H. E.: *Beyond Growth: The Economics of Sustainable Development*, Beacon Press, 1996, p. 45.
129. Daly, H. E.: ibid., p. 61.
130. Daly, H. E.: ibid., pp. 12–18. Former United States President Clinton established the President's Council on Sustainable Development, which proclaimed 15 principles on the issue. Whether Americans live up to those principles, however, is a very different thing. The following principles apply: "(1) We must preserve and, where possible, restore the integrity of natural systems—soils, water, air, and biological diversity—which sustain both economic prosperity and life itself; (2) economic growth, environmental protection, and social equity should be interdependent, mutually reinforcing national goals, and policies to achieve these goals should be integrated; (3) along with appropriate protective measures, market strategies should be used to harness private energies and capital to protect and improve the environment; (4) population must be stabilized at a level consistent with the capacity of the earth to support its inhabitants; (5) protection of natural systems requires changed patterns of consumption consistent with a steady improvement in the efficiency with which society uses natural resources; (6) progress toward elimination of poverty is essential for economic progress, equity, and environmental quality; (7) all segments of society should equitably share environmental costs and benefits; (8) all economic and environmental decision-making should consider the well-being of future generations, and preserve for them the widest possible range of choices; (9) where public health may be adversely affected, or environmental damage may be serious or irreversible, prudent action is required in the face of scientific uncertainty; (10) sustainable development requires fundamental changes in the conduct of government, private institutions, and individuals; (11) environmental and economic concerns are central to our national and global security; (12) sustainable development is best attained in a society in which free institutions flourish; (13) decisions affecting sustainable development should be open and permit participation by affected and interested parties—this requires a knowledgeable public, a free flow of information, and fair and equitable opportunities for review and redress; (14) advances in science and technology are beneficial, increasing both our understanding and range of choices about how humanity and the environment relate. We must seek constant improvements in both science and technology in order to achieve eco-efficiency, protect and restore natural systems, and change consumption patterns; (15) sustainability in the United States is closely tied to global sustainability. Our policies for trade, economic development, aid, and environmental protection must be considered in the context of the international implications of these policies."
131. In: McIntosh, A.: ibid., p. 35.
132. Wight, Jonathan, B.: ibid., pp. 89–90.
133. Daly, H. E.: ibid., p. 97.
134. Similar ideas were developed by Tobin and Nordhaus in the early 1970s. They constructed a Measure of Economic Welfare (MEW), ascribing value to things

like leisure time, household work, aspects of urbanization, and commuting to work. They found that if these aspects had been taken into account in the measurement of GDP, the averaged yearly growth percentage of GDP over the period 1929–1965 would have been 1.1 instead of 1.7 (Ormerod, P.: ibid., p. 31). Furthermore, more than ten years ago, a human development index was developed at the request of the Human Development Programme of the United Nations. Its concept of economic growth includes aspects like life expectancy, level of literacy, and child mortality (Barrez, D.: ibid., p. 100).

135. Sen, A.: ibid., p. 11.
136. Sen, A.: ibid., p. 21.
137. Sen, A.: ibid., p. 44.
138. Goudswaard, B. and Thung, M. A.: Tweeërlei Plaatsbepaling van de Economie, in: Goudzwaard, B., et al.: *Een Gezonde Economie? Maatschappelijke Dimensies van het Economisch Handelen*, Kampen, 1994, pp. 233–238. Among this group one could, surprisingly, also count James Wolfensohn, President of the World Bank, who supports the idea of "a new form of accounting that would measure a country's health as an emerging society and not just as an emerging market." For this, countries should "be graded on the quality of their governing software, judicial system, procedures for settling disputes, social safety net, rule of law and economic operating systems" (Friedman, Th. L.: ibid., p. 163).
139. Baumol, W. J.: Macro-Economics of Unbalanced Growth: The Autonomy of Workers in Crisis, in: *American Economic Review*, volume 57, number 3, 1967.
140. Among this group one can also count the so-called "downshifters," i.e., people who purposely accept a lower position in the labor market, including the financial consequences, in order to enjoy a more relaxed life-style (Nijkamp, P., in: Dalen, H. van and Kalshoven, F., (eds.): ibid., p. 44). At the start of the new millennium, the number of downshifters in the United States was estimated to be some 28 million (Gates, J.: ibid., p. 95). In Europe, the number of downshifters is expected to be around 16 million in 2007. Downshifters are people who exchange an exciting and fast life for a more relaxed position so that they can really enjoy life. They want to escape the "time-sickness" that results from always being in a hurry. They belong to the so-called "slow movement" (Honoré, C.: ibid., pp. 10 and 44).
141. Zuthem, H. J. van: *De Geloofwaardigheid van onze Economische Orde*, Kampen, 1969.
142. Mitchell, M.: ibid., pp. 44–45.
143. Gatrell, A. et al.: Understanding Health Inequalities: Locating People in Geographical and Social Spaces, in: Graham, H., (ed.): *Understanding Health Inequalities*, Open University Press, 2003, p. 158
144. Brown, L. D., et al.: Globalization, NGOs, and Multisectoral Relations, in: Nye, J. S. and Donahue, J. D., (eds.): ibid., p. 275. Particularly in the United States, philanthropic organizations like the Rockefeller, the Ford, and the Carnegie foundations have contributed to the spread of culture and education among the public at large, including the poor. Moreover, they have set up many hospitals, orphanages, and other charitable institutions (Friedman, M. and Friedman, R.: ibid., pp. 139–140). Scambler suggests distinguishing between two sectors of civil society, namely (a) the enabling sector, which derives its impetus from the private sphere, dealing with issues of potential concern, and

(b) the protest sector, which mobilizes people in networks and campaign groups in pursuit of influence for purposeful change (Scambler, G.: ibid., pp. 56–57).

145. Brown, L. D., et al.: ibid., p. 276. They may also join like-minded associations from other societies and through that try to influence the direction of global governance (Brown, L. D., et al.: ibid., p. 272). In the urban areas of China, voluntary association is even becoming "the main organizing principle for the migrant communities, many of which have set up their own governing and welfare structures outside of the state" (Saich, T.: Globalization, Governance, and the Authoritarian State, in: Nye, J. S. and Donahue, J. D., (eds.): ibid., p. 218). In this respect, Vogel refers to a "new ethic of comradeship" in China as a form of relationship between citizens.
146. A schematic pamphlet, prepared for the 2002 elections in the Netherlands, revealed that all the major politica parties underline the importance of voluntary work.
147. For the United Kingdom, for instance, voluntary work was estimated to equal £11 billion in financial terms in 1999, which is around 10 % of GDP (Frank, S.: ibid., p. 131).
148. Report of the Independent Commission on Population and Quality of Life, ibid., p. 147. In addition to this, the commission suggests that unpaid caring services at home as well as in the community should be measured and valued in parallel accounts established for each country and widely publicized on a regular basis (Report of the Independent Commission on Population and Quality of Life: ibid., p. 90). One might call this benchmarking for voluntary work, thus underlining its importance for society. In contrast to what one would expect, however, it is not the wealthier people who contribute to increasing budgets for voluntary work. In this respect, the United States saw a decline in charitable spending of 65% between 1980 and 1988 by people earning over $500,000 annually, whereas donations from people with yearly salaries between $25,000 and $30,000 increased by 62%. Even more remarkably, the poorest Americans, earning $10,000 or less, gave 5.5% of their income to charity (Wheen, F.: ibid., p. 29).
149. Lasch, however, observes that "it is either naïve or cynical to lead the public to think that dismantling the welfare state is enough to ensure a revival of informal cooperation," because "market mechanisms will not repair the fabric of public trust. On the contrary, the market's effect on the cultural infrastructure is just as corrosive as that of the state" (Lasch, C.: ibid., pp. 100–101).
150. In this respect, a 2003 news bulletin of the Dutch radio revealed that the interest of younger Dutch people to participate in voluntary work decreased from 38% in 1985 to 25% in 2002.
151. Galbraith, J. K.: *The Culture of Contentment*, ibid., p. 27. Nevertheless, permitting policies that favor moving to the right side of the continuum could be considered as an inducement to a (further) revival of informal cooperation, which will mainly be shaped at the local level of society, by implementing taxation measures which are favorable to this revival. Two points still have to be made. The first concerns the United Kingdom, where at several places a Local Employment Trading System (LETS) has been developed. Members of LETS, all unemployed people, work for one another and are paid in "accounting units" instead of money. The numbers of these accounting units can result in

a positive or negative balance. In fact, the LETS system creates a barter economy, parallel with the conventional market economy and the benefit system (CCBI: ibid., p. 74). One of the advantages of such a system is that it may prevent unemployed people from feeling that they are left behind. In terms of the first chapter, they may, despite their unemployment, still feel connected. In other words: a LETS-like system may preserve people's dignity. The second point regards Rifkin's employment ideas on what he refers to as "the third sector." Not having much faith in (American) government ablity to create sufficient employment, he recognizes the need for "community-based organizations." Organizations like these could, on a not-for-profit basis, contribute to meeting social needs and the provision of worthwhile work opportunities at the community level (Rifkin, L.: *The End of Work: The Decline of the Global Labour Force and the Dawn of the Post-Market Era*, G. P. Putnam's Sons, 1996). Financing these initiatives could be done by taxing the higher incomes of the market economy (CCBI: ibid., p. 95).

Chapter 3

1. Following Levine, I use the term "ideology" "to refer to a doctrine or collection of doctrines that enjoy the influence they do, not in consequence of their cognitive merit, but because they help to sustain or otherwise benefit social elites" (Levine, A.: *The American Ideology: A Critique*, Routledge, 2004, pp. 79–80).
2. Examples from the Netherlands: (1) *Economie met open Grenzen: Vervolgrapportage*, brief van de minister en staatssecretaris van economische zaken, vergaderjaar 1991–1992, no. 21670; (2) *Sociale Nota 1995*, brief van de minister van sociale zaken en werkgelegenheid, vergaderjaar 1994–1995, no. 23902; and (3) *Sociale Nota 1996*, brief van de minister van sociale zaken en werkgelegenheid, vergaderjaar 1995–1996, no. 24402.
3. For instance: Sociaal Economische Raad: *Dimensie Europa 1992*, Den Haag, 1990.
4. Example from the Netherlands: Kolnaar, A. H. J. J.: *Sociale Zekerheid en Verantwoordelijkheid: Een discussienota van de CDA-werkgroep Sociale Zekerheid*, The Hague, 1992, p. 22.
5. For instance: (1) Commission of the European Community, *European Social Policy: Options for the Union*, Green Paper, Consultative Document by Mr. Flynn, 17 November 1993, Com (93) 551, Directorate-General for Employment, Industrial Relations and Social Affairs.
6. Krugman, P.: *Competitiveness: A Dangerous Obsession*, ibid., pp. 28–44.
7. To some, globalization is a crisis, is reshaping the world, is a syndrome, a challenge, a myth, a secular religion, or an obsession. Others pretend to understand globalization or to know the truth about it, thinking they can explain why global pessimists are wrong, or feeling that limits should be set to the phenomenon. Trawling through this mound of literature, therefore, leaves the reader confused.
8. Scholte, J. A.: *Globalization: A Critical Introduction*, ibid., p. 39. This is illustrated by the fact that the term *globalization* is used along with terms like *modernization*, *internationalization*, *liberalization*, *universalization*,

Westernization, *deterritorialization*, and *supra-territoriality*—terms which, although with substantially differing emphases, are related and overlapping to some extent.

9. As for the question of when globalization emerged, some authors refer to the journeys of Marco Polo and Columbus' discovery of America, followed by the exploratory expeditions of the Portuguese, the Spanish, and the Dutch. From those days on, international trade became an important aspect of commercial life, organized in, for instance, the Dutch East Indian Company. Pepper, coffee, tea, sugar, oriental silk, gold, silver, porcelain, rubber, and tobacco, became important items of a booming global trade. This trade involved high import levies, however. Because of that, some scholars do not use the term *globalization* here, since to them globalization presupposes free trade (Legrain, Ph.: ibid., pp. 80–86). Mittelman mentions three possible origins of globalization (Mittelman, J. H.: ibid., pp. 18–19). In his view, one can argue firstly that globalization stems from the origins of our civilization, i.e., when groups of people started to interact with one another through conquest, trade, and migration. This would mean that globalization is about 5,000 years old. Urbanization during the Industrial Revolution of the 18th century would be part of this process of intensifying communication and economic relations. A second view is that globalization developed in parallel with the origins of capitalism in Western Europe during the 16th century. In those days, major technological innovations accompanied decisive shifts in the ratio of labor to capital, resulting in new economic and social relations. It was the start of a market orientation directed at profit maximization, of wage labor, and of private ownership of the means of production. Thirdly, one could argue that globalization is the consequence of fundamental changes in capitalism. Here, the 1970s represent an important turning point. Starting with a severe recession, the 1970s saw fundamental reforms having certain characteristic features: the collapse of Bretton Woods system; the restructuring of production processes toward more flexible, capital- and technology-intensive production; decreasing power of the unions; reductions in social expenditure; deregulation, privatization, and enhancing competitive power. Mittelman does not choose between these three possibilities. To him, globalization can best be understood in terms of its continuities and discontinuities with the past. Based on this distinction, he distinguishes between (a) incipient globalization, which is the period before the 16th century; (b) bridging globalization, being the period from the inception of capitalism in the Western world until the early 1970s; and, since then, (c) accelerated globalization, of which hyper-competition, induced by temporal and spatial reorganization of production, is characteristic.
10. The bulk of literature on globalization can be classified in terms of opinions, ideas, convictions, statements, or perceptions. They illustrate, indeed, that globalization is a highly contested concept. Structural analyses of the phenomenon are not that readily available and, in so far as they are available, they differ in approach. Mittelman, for instance, focuses on the systemic dynamics and myriad consequences of globalization, the interplay between globalizing market forces and the needs of society. To him, globalization is not a phenomenon on its own but a syndrome of processes and activities. This syndrome is propelled by changing divisions of labor and power, manifested in a new regionalism and challenged by resistance movements (Mittelman, J. H.: ibid.).

In short, Mittelman gives a holistic and multilevel analysis of the globalization process, combining economics, politics, and culture and concluding that, though globalization offers many benefits to some, a price has to be paid. That price is "a lessening, or in some cases a negating, of the quantum of political control exercised by the encompassed, especially in the least powerful and poorest zones of the global political economy. In addition, the penetration of world markets and increased polarization on a world level erode cultural traditions, giving rise to new hybrid forms" (Mittelman, J. H.: ibid., p. 5). Since the fall of communism, Marxist scholars define globalization as "the current phase of international capitalist accumulation" (Colás, A.: The Class Politics of Globalisation, in: Rupert, M. and Smith, H., (eds.) ibid., p. 191). Robinson distinguishes between four epochs in the history of world capitalism: (1) mercantilism with primitive capital accumulation; (2) competitive or classical capitalism, marking the Industrial Revolution, the rise of the bourgeoisie, and the forging of the nation-state; (3) corporate (monopoly) capitalism, which led to the consolidation of a single world market, organized within the nation-state system; and (4) globalization, which started with the economic crisis of the 1970s (Robinson, W. I.: Capitalist Globalization and the Trans-nationalization of the State, in: Rupert, M. and Smith, H., (eds.): ibid., p. 211). Marxist scholars insist that the potentially emancipatory resources of a renewed and perhaps reconstructed historical materialism are now more relevant than ever before. Rather than viewing global capitalism as a natural force, they try to show that there is a dialectic of power and resistance at work in the present-day global political economy. They believe that this dialectic could create the conditions for new forms of collective self-determination. For modern Marxists, globalization refers to a re-structuring of state-society and inter-state relations, following the economic downturn of the 1970s. They argue that diverse state-society relations, whether classical liberal, corporatist, interventionist-welfare or neo-liberal, "simply represent variations in the degree of re-politicisation and de-politicisation [. . .] of the economy in what are essentially capitalist totalities" (Teschke, B. and Heine, Ch.: The Dialectic of Globalization, in: Rupert, M. and Smith, H., (eds.), ibid., p. 178). To them, states are structurally tied to the power of capital. Because of that, over the past 20 years, states have not been able to harness their power to any other purposes than the interests of capital (Teschke, B. and Heine, Ch.: ibid., p. 182). Though it is interesting to read the Marxists ideas, brought together in a book of 300 pages, one does not find any idea on how these proclaimed new forms of collective self-determination could deal with democratic values, like freedom of speech, or how self-determining collectivities could stimulate individual initiatives and prevent command-and-control bureaucracies. Because these were precisely the ailments of communism, the modern Marxists' approach of globalization is no more than a theoretical exercise having no practical use. Further, with Van der Loo and Van Reijen, one could consider globalization to be a process of modernization, i.e., as a complexity of mutually connected structural, cultural, psychological, and physical changes that have crystallized from past centuries and through this have shaped the world of today, and are still pushing that world in a certain direction (author's translation) (Loo, H. van der and Reijen, W. van: ibid., p. 14). According to these authors, processes like these always produce their own paradoxical counter-movements regarding aspects like differentiation, rationalization, individualization, and domestication. The transition from an agricultural society into an industrial one, for instance, not only changed production processes, but also led to urbanization, secularization, rationalization, individualization, and many other economic, social, political, and cultural changes. Also, to a certain extent, Romanticism can be interpreted as a reaction to the ideas of the Enlightenment. Supporters of Romanticism criticized the optimistic belief in social progress and utilitarianism of the Enlightenment, because to them the society created by the Enlightenment was inhumane and repressive. A similar line of reasoning could be followed with respect to the transition from industrial society into post-traditional society. According to Giddens though, the latter has not made a complete break with traditions; these have become the subject to permanent reflection. A reflection that is fostered by expert systems, i.e., sectors of professionals who have a knowledge monopoly and who are organized according to their own logic. For those who are excluded from these systems, it is impossible to have an insight in their dealings (Loo, H. van der and Reijen, W, van: ibid., pp. 158–159). As for today's modernization processes, one could argue that the globalizing world finds itself in a new transition phase; i.e., we have entered the network society or the information age (Castells, M.: *The Rise of the Network Society*, ibid.). Jihad and fundamentalism in general could be seen as a reaction to that, because they oppose an ongoing modernization and cultivate tradition. They stipulate the importance of family ties and religion. They call for a return to the clarity, security, and simplicity of earlier times; a longing for the better past (Loo, H. van der and Reijen, W. van: ibid., p. 92). They see the benefits of modernity as a threat to their own fundamental viewpoints. Paradoxically, however, although fundamentalists are longing for the better past, they make use of the most sophisticated communication technology to promote their anti-modernity ideas. Finally, one can, like Beck (Beck, U.: *What is Globalization?* Polity Press, 2001, introduction), focus on the meaning of globalization and ask how it can be molded politically. Beck does so from the perspective of differing modernities. The first modernity is a national one, conceived and organized within a particular cultural identity, i.e., a territory and a state. To post-modern philosophers, this first modernity has failed, because the universalism of the Enlightenment can no longer hold, and the cement in society has grown porous through the process of individualization. Therefore, society has lost its collective self-consciousness and, through that, its capacity for political action. Consequently, the collapse of the first modernity is inevitable, and with it the historical Western model of the association between market economy, welfare state, and democracy. In this scenario, neo-liberal ideas were instrumental in terminating the first modernity. Beck opposes this depressing view by distinguishing between globalism, on the one hand, and globality and globalization, on the other. Globalism is the mono-causal and economical neo-liberal theory of the world market that supplants political action, reducing the multidimensionality of globalization to a single economic dimension, conceived in a linear fashion (A completely different interpretation of the concept of globalism can be found in Keohane and Nye: *Governance in a Globalizing World*, ibid.). In other words, all other dimensions like ecology, culture, politics, and civil society are subordinated to the world market system. This ideological core liquidates an essential element of the first modernity, that is, the difference between economics and politics. Consequently, the central task of politics, which is to define the legal, social, and ecological conditions for economic activities, no longer plays a role, thus resulting in the second modernity. As for globalism, Beck argues that we have been living in a world society for a long time already, in the sense that the notion of closed spaces has become illusory. These days, no country or group can isolate itself from others. Consequently, we have colliding economic, cultural, and political systems. Therefore, what we call "world society" is not a homogeneous entity but a totality of social relationships, which are not integrated into or determined by national state politics. When we speak of world society we have to realize that self-perceptions of states or groups play an important role. World society, therefore, is a perceived or reflexive idea. The question as to the extent to which such a society exists may, on the basis of empirics, be rephrased into the question of "how and to what extent people and cultures around the world relate to one another in their differences and to what extent [their] self-perception of world society is relevant to how they behave" (Beck, U.: ibid., p. 10). Altogether, we may conceive the term *world society* as multiplicity without unity, accepting differences and non-integration. According to Beck, "this presupposes a number of very different things: transnational forms of production and labour market competition, global reporting in the media, transnational consumer boycotts, transnational ways of life as well as 'globally' perceived crises and wars, military and peaceful use of atomic energy, destruction of nature and so on" (Beck,U.: ibid., p. 10). These are globality characteristics of the second modernity which cannot be reversed. Globalisation, on the other hand, "denotes the processes through which sovereign national states are criss-crossed and undermined by transnational actors with varying prospects of power, orientations, identities and networks" (Beck, U.: ibid., p. 11). In order to redress this situation, each single autonomous aspect of the logic of globalization [culture, ecology, economics, politics and civil society] must be independently decoded and grasped in its interdependencies. According to Beck, "only in this way can the perspective and the space for political action be opened up. Why? Because only then can the depoliticizing spell of globalism be broken; only with a multidimensional view of globality can the globalist ideology of 'material compulsion' be broken down" (Beck, U.: ibid., p. 11). In other words, a decisive critique of globalism is necessary to provide space for the primacy of politics.

11. The term is from Mittelman, J. H.: ibid.
12. Scholte, J. A.: *Globalization: A Critical Introduction*, ibid., p. 74.
13. Legrain, Ph.: ibid., pp. 107–110. For Chomsky, this type of globalization is very much connected to the start of a new era in world history, which began in the late 1980s and early 1990s, caused by two important things. The first one was the collapse of the Soviet Union. The second one was the continuing development of information technology, which linked the world together in global networks of computers and communications devices, making international trade and speculation faster and easier (Fox, J.: ibid., p. 18).
14. The Group of Lisbon (Petrella, R., Chairman): *Limits to Competition* (Dutch Translation), Brussels, 1994, p. 46 (author's translation). In defining the phenomenon, the group relies on McGrew. In this definition, the globalization phenomenon covers two separate aspects, i.e., reach and intensity. As for its reach, globalization has a spatial meaning. It may relate to processes that encompass

the whole world. Intensity refers to the levels of interaction, mutual connectedness, or interdependence between states and societies worldwide. The spatial aspect is central to Scholte, to whom globalization refers to the spread of supraterritoriality, which entails "a reconfiguration of geography, so that social space is no longer mapped in terms of territorial places, territorial distances, and territorial borders" (Scholte, J. A.: *Globalization: A Critical Introduction*, ibid., p. 16). Gilpin defines globalization as "the increasing linkage of national economies through trade, financial flows and direct investments by multinational firms" (Gilpin, R.: ibid., p. 299). In doing so, he stipulates the importance of the intensity aspect. In each of the three definitions, however, technological progress, the liberalization of capital exchange, and decreasing government interference in economic life, are the engines of the globalization process (Regarding this, see: Gooijer, W. J. de: *On Solidarity in Changing Health Care Systems: Europe in Search of a New Balance*, ibid., pp. 51–57).

15. I have chosen Gilpin's approach somewhat arbitrarily. I could just as easily have used the schools of thought mentioned by Held, et al. They distinguish between *globalism*, *traditionalism*, and *transformationalism*. The first school encompasses those who argue that states are increasingly subjected to worldwide processes of change, which erodes the power of nation-states. Traditionalists resist this view. They believe that present global circumstances are not particularly unique. They point to a reinforcement of state powers in many places. Transformationalists argue that globalization transforms state powers and the context in which states operate (Held, D., (ed.): ibid.). Elsewhere, Held speaks alternatively of *hyperglobalizers*, *sceptics*, and *transformationalists* (Held, D. & McGrew, A., Goldblatt, D. & Perraton, J.: *Global Transformations: Politics, Economics and Culture*, Polity Press, 1999).
16. Gilpin, R.: ibid., p. 298.
17. For example, the Group of Lisbon: ibid.
18. Went, R.: *Grenzen aan Globalisering?* Amsterdam, 1996, pp. 39–40.
19. Forrester, V.: *Une étrange Dictature* (Dutch Translation), Amsterdam, 2001.
20. References to these authors will follow subsequently.
21. In the words of Pettigrew, the Canadian Minister of International Trade, in: Klein, N.: *Fences and Windows*, ibid., p. 130.
22. Leadbeater, C.: *Up the Down Escalator: Why the Global Pessimists Are Wrong*, Viking, 2002.
23. Leadbeater, C.: ibid., p. 350.
24. Leadbeater, C.: ibid., p. 101.
25. Leadbeater, C.: ibid., p. 327.
26. Therefore, the author does not substantiate the subtitle of his book—"*Why the Global Pessimists Are Wrong*!"
27. Legrain, Ph.: ibid., p. 23.
28. Legrain, Ph.: ibid., p. 23.
29. See section 1.4.2.
30. Legrain, Ph.: ibid., p. 21.
31. Legrain, Ph.: ibid., p. 45.
32. Legrain, Ph.: ibid., p. 45.
33. Legrain, Ph.: ibid., p. 322.
34. Legrain, Ph.: ibid., p. 324.
35. In: Axford, B.: ibid., p. 99.

36. Ruigrok, W. and Tulder, R. van: *The Logic of International Restructuring*, London, 1995.
37. OECD: *The OECD Jobs Study: Facts, Analysis, Strategies*, Paris, 1994.
38. Regarding foreign direct investment (FDI), Gilpin observes that it is concentrated highly and distributed very unevenly around the globe. The strong increase in FDI since the mid-1980s mainly took place in the United States, China and Europe, parts of the globe with promising or potentially promising large markets (Gilpin, R.: ibid., p. 24).
39. In: Mittelman, J. H.: ibid., p. 20.
40. Mittelman, J. H.: ibid., p. 45.
41. Dutch Ministry of Economic Affairs, paper AEP95082709, 24 November 1995.
42. Castells, M.: *The Rise of the Network Society*, ibid., p. 95.
43. Axford, B: ibid., p. 100.
44. These people have a point, since international trade over the past 25 years increased annually on average by 13%, whereas it was seldom higher than 3% annually in the preceding decade: Fukuyama, F.: *The End of History and the Last Man*, ibid., p. 118.
45. Scholte, J. A.: *Globalization: A Critical Introduction*, ibid., p. 75.
46. Evans, Ph. and Wurster, Th. S.: *Blown to Bits: How the New Economics of Information Transforms Strategy*, (Dutch Translation), Amsterdam/Antwerpen, 2002, p. 14.
47. http://www.internetworldstats.com/stats.htm, 31 March, 2006.
48. Reich, R. B.: *The Future of Success*, ibid., p. 23.
49. Friedman, Th. L.: *The Lexus and the Olive Tree: Understanding Globalisation*, ibid., p. 140.
50. Authors like Legrain and Frankel refer to studies that show that developing countries that were open to international trade indeed demonstrated a better growth rate than those who shut themselves off from it. However, it is not clear who actually benefitted from this growth (Legrain, Ph.: ibid., chapter 2; Frankel, J.: ibid., p. 61). Frankel rightfully observes that income distribution is determined by many factors other than trade, among which redistribution policies by governments are very important (Frankel, J.: ibid., p. 63). Nevertheless, Legrain and Frankel have strong support from the Secretary-General of the United Nations, Koffi Annan, and the Director of the WTO, Mike Moore, both of whom argue that free trade (in agricultural products, as far as Annan is concerned) will be to the advantage of poor countries. In this respect, the term "poor countries" refers to countries like South Korea, Taiwan, Japan, and Singapore. It is precisely this point that makes Moore's argument suspicious. Firstly, these countries never liberalized their agricultural sectors. Secondly, Taiwan and South Korea carried out land ownership reforms generations ago. Thirdly, like the United States and the European Union, Moore's sample countries protect their agricultural sectors against the influences of the world market. Furthermore, although Moore agrees that, as a consequence of trade liberalization, ending the subsidization of farmers in poor countries would create a minority for whom the establishment of a social safety net would be necessary, he seems to forget that the large majority of farmers live in countries where subsidies are either very limited or completely unknown. Altogether, we are talking of over one billion people who live on $1 a day or less, people who have to live off the results of their agricultural

activities (Barrez, D.: ibid., pp. 85–88). Apart from this, some relativism is appropriate since, despite the "e-society" and the new economy, two billion people do not yet have electricity (Moore, M.: *Stupid White Men*, ibid., p. 22). And despite the strong increase of mobile telephony from a little over 4 million in 1988, to 400 million in 1999, to probably one billion in 2004 (Mayer-Schönberger, V. and Hurley, D.: Globalization of Communication, in: Nye, J. S. and Donahue, J. D., (eds.): ibid., p. 141), half of the world population has never yet made a telephone call (Nijkamp, P.: Schaarse Ruimte, Cyberspace en de Moderne Nomaden, in: Dalen, H. van and Kalshoven, F., (eds.): ibid., pp. 42–43), whereas world telephone density was only 12 telephones per 100 head of population in 1995 (Scholte, J. A.: *Globalization: A Critical Introduction*, ibid., p. 87). Also, the distribution of the internet appears to be very uneven on a global scale (Nua Internet Surveys 1998). For 1998, Nua gives the following distribution figures by region: Middle East, 0,525 million; Africa, 1 million; South America, 7 million; Asia/Pacific, including Australia and New Zealand, 14 million; Europe, 20 million; Canada and the United States, 70 million (in: Mittelman, J. H.: ibid., pp. 226–227). Around the turn of the century, some 25% of the American population used the internet, compared to 0.01% of the population of South Asia (Nye, J. S. and Donahue, J. D., (eds.): ibid., p. 2). So far, therefore, the Internet still is "an elite operation" of the developed world (Pilger, J.: *Hidden Agendas*, ibid., p. 532). Most of this elite, representing about 6% of the world's inhabitants, resides in the United States and Western Europe Europe (Kupchan, C. A.: *The End of the American Era: U.S. Foreign Policy and the Geopolitics of the Twenty-First Century*, Vintage Books, New York, 2002, p. 106). Finally, it will take at least several generations before most of the world's population will have access to digital interactive television (Scholte, J. A.: Globalization: A Critical Introduction: ibid., p. 276).

51. Huntington, S. P.: *The Clash of Civilizations and the Remaking of the World Order*, New York, 1996.
52. Barber, B. R.: *Jihad vs. McWorld: How Globalism and Tribalism are Reshaping the World*, Random House, 1995, p. 4.
53. Huntington, S. P.: ibid., p. 183.
54. Huntington, S. P.: ibid., p. 183. The term *toxification* seems overdone at first sight. However, by the mid-1980s, worldwide exports of American television programming hours were over 40%, of which 44% went to Europe, 77% to Latin America, 70% to Canada, and 47% to sub-Saharan Africa. Conversely, American imports were no more than 1% of its commercial programming and 2% of its public service programming (Held, D., (ed.): *A Globalizing World?* ibid., p. 63). We should not be too surprised that certain non-Western cultures are uncomfortable with these facts. To put it even stronger, the elites in countries representing two-thirds of the world population (Chinese, Russians, Indians, Muslims, Arabs, and Africans), view the United States as "the single greatest threat to their societies" (Gates, J.: ibid., p. 192).
55. Fukuyama, F.: *The End of History and the Last Man*, ibid., p. 71. For the balance: the United States has no less than 37,000 religious denominations (Hertsgaard, M.: ibid., p. 130). Among them are a number of fundamentalists who are as dangerous as fundamentalist Islamies. In this respect, Qutb, the leading thinker of the influential Muslim Brotherhood, recognized the true

enemy of Islam to be the "insidious penetration of cultural influences and ideas" from the West. To him, these influences were threatening to "exterminate" Islam (Berman, P.: ibid., p. 183).

56. Barber, B. R., 1995, ibid., p. 4.
57. Barber, B. R., 1995, ibid., p. 8. In the introduction to a later edition of his study, after September 11, 2001, Barber argues that the dramatic events of that day were an expression of "a global war between modernity and its aggrieved critics," for which the only way out is the globalization of civic and democratic institutions. To Barber, democracy offers the only proper response to Jihad and McWorld. On the one hand, for jihad, democracy could be an instrument for avoiding the choice between sterile cultural monism and a raging cultural fundamentalism. On the other hand, for McWorld, democracy should mean establishing a front not against terrorism per se, but against "economic reductionism and its commercialising homogeneity that have created the climate of despair and hopelessness that terrorism has so effectively exploited."[56] In a later publication, Barber summarized these ideas with the term "preventive democracy," based on the reality of worldwide interdependence. That reality would demand administrative, economic, cultural, and diplomatic activities directed at the drawing-up of treaties, institutions, and agreements which regulate the relations between nations through coordinating organizations. One would assume the United Nations to be the appropriate organization to achieve this. At the same time, however, one would have to conclude that it does not have the power to do so.
58. The term is from Mittelman: ibid.
59. This attitude towards globalization, however, is an example of unnecessary scare-mongering. I will come back to this later.
60. For this subsection, I have relied on Meijer's dissertation on neo-liberalism (Meijer, G.: ibid.).
61. The designation of industrial areas and measures on population density are examples. The necessity for governmental coordination may also be caused by the existence of technical monopolies. To neo-liberals, this particularly applies to public utilities like transport and energy. Competition in these spheres of the economy could lead to a wasteful use of natural resources. Here, coordination could be organized through concessionary policies.
62. The aim, here, is to counter internal financing which, to neo-liberals, disturbs the importance of the capital market. Internal financing could lead to irrational investments, which is not only incompatible with optimal allocation, but which would also be to the advantage of corporate business. Economic policy, therefore, should be directed at rehabilitating the capital market.
63. As for ideas on combating cyclical economic movements as well as unemployment and instability, neo-liberal thoughts go in two directions. On the one hand, there are those who want to neutralize cyclical economic movements through changing the money system. On the other hand, there are neo-liberals who want to maintain the money system while neutralizing its effects through economic policy.
64. It is difficult to divide collective needs into items that can be delivered to individual economic subjects. It is also impossible to charge them to individual consumers. Therefore, in the developed world, the size and composition of collective needs are determined through the democratic process, where the

minority has to accept the wishes of the majority. As soon as it is clear what the majority wants, the market is the instrument for delivery. Price-determining forces under the conditions of perfect competition value the means of production in accordance with marginal money productivity, thus resulting in optimal allocation. In this situation, income inequality is an inevitable consequence of an uneven distribution of productive performance among economic subjects, as well as a necessary accompanying feature of optimal allocation. Optimal allocation will not result if the market for the means of production is characterized by monopoly. Therefore, monopoly has to be opposed. Furthermore, to a large degree, uneven distribution of productive performances is caused by inequality of opportunity. This, according to neo-liberals, has to be countered, firstly, by legal corrections to inheritance and succession, and secondly, by creating equal opportunities for each citizen in training and education. Further inequalities regarding productive performance could be reduced through systems of taxation. A market of perfect competition could include small business as a counterweight to corporate business. Here, complementary and corrective measures to stimulate small business and self-employed people are appropriate. Temporary subsidies for starters are in line with this idea. Expansion of production is not an explicit objective of neo-liberals. It is thought to result automatically from their proposed complementary and corrective measures regarding the functioning of a free market. Neo-liberals oppose a policy of achieving full employment through continuous public investments. In their view, such a policy counters only the symptoms, but not the causes, of a disturbance of free-market equilibrium. Moreover, they believe it will induce inflation. Finally, although neo-liberals favor the free migration of people, they acknowledge that there can be circumstances which make it legitimate for governments to interfere. A threat to a country's cultural and political traditions is an example.

65. The other tasks are (1) to realize and maintain the economic order thought to be necessary for an optimal functioning of the market economy through legislation and administration of justice; and (2) to pursue social and economic policies, if the objectives of economic policy cannot be achieved through adjustment within the institutional framework of the economic order. In the latter case, interference in the economic process may be necessary to neutralize the defects of the market economy, for example, in the case of a discrepancy between individual and social costs.
66. Alternately, neo-liberals expect institutional changes in the economic order which stimulate the coordinating function of the price mechanism to contribute to the achievement of the objectives of the economic order. In this respect, they particularly have an eye on improving market organization, as well as the functioning of the national and international monetary system.
67. In order to realize all of this, governments have an extensive legislative and administrative task regarding matters like industrial ownership, liability, corporate law, taxation, and labor law. Consequently, neo-liberals are against cartels, monopolies, and vertical price fixing.
68. The translation from theory into practice is the weak point, causing neo-liberals to disagree with each other. Nevertheless, they all seek to change reality in the direction of the idealized image of their economic order.

69. In this respect, the difficulties for the implementation of neo-liberal ideas in practice can clearly be distilled from Robbins, who declared more than 50 years ago: "The idea of a competitive order is by no means a simple notion. It involves the systematic revision of the whole apparatus of law and order—the law relating to patents, the law relating to restraint of trade, the law relating to limited liability of corporations, and many other branches of the law—with a view to creating conditions which tend to maintain effective competition, where it is technically possible, and to control monopoly in the public interest where technical conditions make monopoly inevitable. It involves the search for new method of fiscal control, not only for the purpose of stabilizing aggregate demand, but also for the purpose of correcting and supplementing the operation of the incentive of relative prices, where analysis discloses the probability that this incentive works badly. This is no light task. It would be idle to pretend that we yet possess the knowledge or the technique to proceed very far on our way. Much more work needs to be done, not only in the field of pure analysis, but much more in the examination of the actual facts of industrial and commercial structure. Great as has been the progress of economics in other connections in recent years, this part of our subject has remained relatively underdeveloped; the harvest is likely to be great, but the laborers in the field are few. In the excitement of perfecting our instruments of analysis we have tended to neglect the study of the framework, which they assume. There is an urgent need for the best minds of the rising generation to apply themselves to this task of institutional invention in the light of patient realistic investigation" (cited in Meijer, G.: ibid., p. 142).
70. Palast, G.: ibid., p. 142.
71. Classical examples from the 19th century are Tönnies (Gemeinschaft vs. Gesellschaft), Durkheim (mechanical vs. organical solidarity), Weber (communal vs. associative relations), and Simmel (who took the process of structural differentiation as a central point of departure for his considerations). These scholars are the founding fathers of sociology. Also, the philosopher Karl Marx must be mentioned in this respect. Subsequent anthropologists like Malinowski (the principle of give and take), Mauss (free gifts do not exist), and Levi-Strauss have also dealt with the theme. Finally, Lalive d' Epinay (individualism vs. solidarity), Habermas (justice vs. solidarity), Cooke (self-realization vs. solidarity), and Dean (reflexive solidarity) are examples of 20th-century scholars (regarding this, see (1) Komter, A. E., et al.: ibid., chapter 5; (2) Loo, H. van der and Reijen, W. van, ibid.: chapter 1). The founding fathers of sociology were interested in changes in society. Durkheim, for instance, observed that the industrial society of his time was characterized by a process of differentiation and individualization, which led many to believe that society was disintegrating, resulting in a decreasing cohesion. Through his analysis, he showed that this was not necessarily the case. Instead of disintegrating, society was being transformed from an agricultural one into an industrial one (Komter, A. E. et al.: ibid., p. 15). This transformation changed the character of society and introduced industrialization, individualization, rationalization, bureaucratization, urbanization, differentiation, and interdependence (Komter, A. E., et al.: ibid., p. 16). As for individualization, Durkheim feared that through vanishing traditional structures, the individual might no longer be embedded in society, instead pursuing his or her own self-interest and no

longer subject to society's social control. Similar pessimism was demonstrated by Weber with his ideas on a parallel development of a more subjective individual and a more abstract society, whereas Marx's pessimism followed from his analysis of the way people organize their production processes, which determine their way of life and their thinking (Loo, H. van der and Reijen, W. van: ibid., chapter 1).

72. In this respect, Komter et al. observe that the Western world finds itself in a process of economic restructuring "where the modern industries of the 19th century have become the traditional sectors of the late 20th century" (author's translation) (Komter, A. E., et al.: ibid., p. 17), with similar changes as those of the 19th and early 20th century. These changes involved, among other things, material production, mobility, and the functioning of the state (Komter, A. E., et al.: ibid., pp. 16–17). As for material production, economic restructuring caused unemployment for many, which neither quantitatively nor qualitatively could be compensated with new jobs in the service sector. Mobility is shaped by processes of globalization that moved labor-intensive production processes to low-wage countries, thus resulting in unemployment for low-skilled workers in the developed world.
73. This is in line with Hobbes' *Leviathan*, in which he assumes that "man takes refuge in society not because of any natural affinity he bears his own kind, but simply because without it, he is incapable of living in safety" (Wight, J. B.: *Saving Adam Smith: A Tale of Wealth, Transformation and Virtue*, Prentice Hall, 2002, p. 135). Hobbes does not believe that men are morally free to choose. Though they may behave more-or-less rationally, their rationality is only at the service of objectives imposed by nature like, for instance, self-preservation (Fukuyama, F.: *The End of History and the Last Man*, ibid., p. 175). This is also consistent with the way Locke formulated his ideas on liberalism, with its characteristic bourgeois society. Such a society is only interested in individual material prosperity, it knows neither a sense of community nor virtue, and it is not interested in mutual well-being. It is a society of pure egoists. In this respect, the radical American libertarian Ayn Rand speaks of "the virtues of selfishness" and "the evils of altruism" (Gates, J.: ibid., p. xxix). The only common characteristic assumed to be shared among people is that they have equal chances (Fukuyama, F.: *The End of History and the Last Man*, ibid., p. 171).
74. Mueller, D. C.: ibid., p. 1.
75. Mueller, D. C.: ibid., chapter 1.
76. By that neo-liberal rationale, globalization is propelled. From this perspective, Mittelman rightfully observes that "a commitment to reducing poverty can only be displayed by integration into the international capitalist economy. Neoliberalism is thus presented as the antidote to the problem of poverty, instead of also being implicated in generating it" (Mittelman, J. H.: ibid., p. 78).
77. Vroonhoven, L. van: *De Al-ene Mens: Op Zoek naar het Individu*, Damon, 1999, p. 25.
78. Self cynically observes that "parties formulate policies in order to win elections, rather than win elections in order to formulate policies" (Self, P.: *Government by the Market? The Politics of Public Choice*, London, 1994, p. 3).
79. Reich reveals that 128 former members of the American Congress had become paid lobbyists by 2000. Many of them left Congress voluntarily in order to trade

their connections. Similar facts apply to congressional aides (Reich, R. B.: *The Future of Success*, ibid., p. 137).

80. Reich, R. B.: *The Future of Success*, ibid., p. 155.
81. Centraal Planbureau (Dutch Central Planning Bureau): *Scanning the Future: A Long-Term Scenario of the World Economy, 1990–2015*, The Hague, 1992, p. 45.
82. In chapter eleven, I will argue that it is realistic to modify this view.
83. Self, P.: ibid., p. 70.
84. Albert, M.: *Capitalism versus Capitalism* (Dutch Translation), Amsterdam, 1992, p. 142.
85. This element was based on the ideas of the economist Laffer that levying taxes beyond a certain point would result in reduced economic activity and hence lead to a lower income, which, in turn, would lead to a lower taxable income. In consequence, the highest federal tax rate fell from 75% in 1979 to 33% in 1989. Meanwhile, Reagan reduced corporate taxation from 33% to 16% and enlarged the possibilities for depreciation in such a way that many corporations no longer had to pay taxes or even had previously paid taxes refunded (Hertsgaard, M.: ibid., p. 144).
86. Hertsgaard, M.: ibid., p. 143.
87. In this regard, Gilder, one of Reagan's advisors, argued that "the poor need mainly the traces of their poverty if they are to succeed," whereas Murray, a second advisor, considered the ideal to be "the abolition of the complete federal system of social provisions and support for people who are old enough to work."
88. Hertsgaard, M.: ibid., p. 141. Twenty years later, the American government is still the same. O'Neill, Secretary of Finance in the George W. Bush administration, openly declared that the United States did not need a social security system or state-provided health care (in: Moore, M.: *Stupid White Men*, ibid., p. 48).
89. Self, P.: ibid., p. 72.
90. Hertsgaard, M.: ibid., p. 143.
91. Kuttner, R.: *Everything for Sale*, ibid., p. 90.
92. Self, P.: ibid., p. 72.
93. Moore, M.: *Downsize This*, ibid., p. 129.
94. Known promoters of the new monetary policy were Milton Friedman and Edmund Phelps. Their argument rested on the quantity theory of money as well as on the concept of a natural rate of unemployment. Inflation, in this theory, is primarily a monetary phenomenon, caused by the creation of excess money by central banks. As for unemployment, monetarists argue that every economy has an inherent rate of unemployment that, depending on circumstances, may go up or down a little but that will always exist as the upper limit of economic activity. Therefore, monetarists hold the view that, if governments want to decrease the level of unemployment below this natural rate, it will cause higher inflation. Consequently, the role for central banks and governments should be limited to the establishment of rules for steady non-inflationary economic growth. In addition to this, government intervention in the economy, with high taxes, extensive regulation and welfare programs means, according to the supporters of monetarism, a distortion of the market which, in turn, decreases incentives to save, invest and work, thus undermining the growth of productivity. Less frequently mentioned, but nevertheless important

at the micro-economic level, is the doctrine of structural adjustment, which provided the basis of another conservative political ideology. Promoters of this ideology favor deregulation of the economy, reduction of the welfare state, and downsizing the government (Gilpin, R.: ibid., pp. 83–84).

95. Fox, J.: ibid., p. 38.
96. Rifkin, J.: *The European Dream*, ibid., p. 235.
97. Albert, M.: ibid.
98. Etzioni, A.: *The Spirit of Community. Rights, Responsibilities and the Communitarian Agenda*, London, 1995, p. 5.
99. Although these facts deliver a rather disturbing picture, future research should endeavor to find out whether they are a consequence of governmental policy during Reagan's presidency. In this respect, Fukuyama points out that the question is still whether "the American underclass is poor because it lacks economic opportunities or whether there is something that could be called a 'culture of poverty'—dysfunctional social habits like teenage pregnancy and drug addiction—that would persist even if the economic opportunities existed" (Fukuyama, F.: *Trust: The Social Virtues and the Creation of Prosperity*, New York, 1995, p. 38). Fukuyama may be right about the two examples he gives. Drug addiction, for example, is certainly also a problem for wealthy people, but I cannot believe that, in general, people choose to be poor or to be uninsured against the costs of health care for cultural reasons. In this respect, it is worth mentioning that in none of the documents of international organizations, like the World Bank and the United Nations Development Programme, is poverty attributed to inherent cultural characteristics of people, either implicitly or explicitly (Mestrum, F.: ibid., p. 61).
100. Hutton, W.: *The State We're In*, London, 1995, p. 185.
101. Jessop, B.: From Social Democracy to Thatcherism: Twenty-five Years of British Politics, in: Abercrombie, N. and Warde, A., (eds.): *Social Change in Contemporary Britain*, Cambridge, 1995, p. 32. In 1981, the Conservative government was obliged to abandon its intense flirtation with monetarism, because it had severe consequences for the economy and unemployment (Urwin, D. W.: ibid., p. 249).
102. Phillips, K.: ibid., p. 339.
103. *The Mail on Sunday*, 29 September 1996.
104. Hoogerwerf, A.: *Politiek als Evenwichtskunst*, Alphen a/d Rijn, 1995, pp. 144–145.
105. Goodman, A. and Webb, S.: *For Richer, For Poorer: The Changing Distribution of Income in the United Kingdom, 1961–91*, The Institute of Fiscal Studies, London, 1994, p. 66.
106. Commission of the European Communities: *Growth, Competitiveness, Employment: The Challenges and Ways Forward into the 21st Century*, White Book (Dutch translation), Brussels, 1994, p. 17.

Chapter 4

1. The term is used by Todaro, in: Bronk, R.: *Progress and the Invisible Hand: The Philosophy and Economics of Human Advance*, London, 1998, p. 118.

2. Burton-Jones, A: *Knowledge Capitalism*, Oxford University Press, 1999, p. 52.
3. Filer, R. K., et al.: *The Economics of Work and Pay*, sixth edition, Harper Collins, 1996, p. 71.
4. Fukuyama, F.: *The Great Disruption: Human Nature and the Reconstruction of Social Order* (Dutch Translation), Amsterdam/Antwerpen, 1999, pp. 73 and 77.
5. For instance: (1) Galbraith, J. K.: *The Culture of Contentment*, London, 1992; (2) Hutton, W.: *The State We're In*, London, 1995; (3) Peterson, W. G.: *The Silent Depression: Twenty-Five Years of Wage Squeeze and Middle Class Decline*, New York, 1995; (4) Reich, R. B.: *The Work of Nations: A Blueprint for the Future*, London, 1993; (5) United Nations Research Institute for Social Development: *States of Disarray: The Social Effects of Globalisation*, London, 1995.
6. Etzioni, A.: *The Spirit of Community. Rights, Responsibilities and the Communitarian Agenda*, London, 1995, p. 5.
7. Hertsgaard, M.: ibid., p. 139.
8. Hertsgaard, M.: ibid., p. 147.
9. Kelly, C. M.: ibid., chapter 12.
10. Moore, M.: *Stupid White Men*, ibid., p. 81.
11. Lasch, C.: ibid., pp. 31–32.
12. Phillips, K.: ibid., p. 129.
13. Phillips, K.: ibid., p. 114. Government retreat from progressive taxation is not limited to the United States. In OECD countries, top tax brackets fell from an average of 52% in 1985 to 42% in 1990 (Scholte, J. A.: ibid., p. 240).
14. Phillips, K.: ibid., p. 111.
15. Phillips, K.: ibid., p. xviii.
16. Etzioni, A.: *The New Golden Rule: Community and Morality in a Democratic Society*, London, 1997, p. 81.
17. A term used by Harrod, R. F., in: Bronk, R.: ibid., p. 172.
18. A few years ago, over 28 million Americans (that is, more than 10% of the population) lived in "privately guarded buildings or housing departments" (Gray, J.: *False Dawn: The Delusions of Global Capitalism*, London, 1999).
19. Kaplan, R. D.: *The Coming Anarchy: Shattering the Dreams of the Cold War*, Random House, New York, 2000, p. 83. In 1970, the United States had more public police officers than private security guards. Now the ratio of private guards to public police officers is 3:1 (Reich, R. B.: *The Future of Success*, ibid., p. 201). As a result, private security in the United States was among the top-ten service businesses, with a turnover of more than $100 billion some years ago (Rifkin, J.: *The End of Work: The Decline of the Global Labor Force and the Dawn of the Post-Market Era*, New York, 1995, p. 213).
20. Rifkin, J.: *The European Dream*, ibid., p. 194.
21. Lasch, C.: ibid., p. 56.
22. Lasch, C.: ibid., p. 176.
23. Hutton, W.: *The World We're In*, ibid., p. 153.
24. Leadbeater, C.: ibid., p. 27.
25. In 1990, the New Jersey legislature went along with them (Reich, R. B.: *The Future of Success*, ibid., p. 199).
26. Kelly, C. M.: ibid., p. 205.
27. Hutton, W.: *The World We're In*, ibid., p. 116.
28. Moore, M.: *Downsize This*, ibid., p. 141.
29. Kelly, C. M.: ibid., p. 168; Klein, N.: *Fences and Windows*, ibid., p. XXIII.

30. Forrester, V.: *Une étrange Dictature*: ibid., p. 70.
31. Hertz, N.: ibid., p. 58. Apparently, to these epsilons also belong airplane pilots. In this respect, Moore reveals that the starting salary at American Eagle, an American airline, is no more than $16,800 per year. One of those pilots even had to ask for food stamps (Moore, M.: *Stupid White Men*, ibid., pp. 75–76).
32. Hertz, N.: ibid., p. 59. This is in line with the 1998 Human Development Report of the United Nations, which uses a figure of 19,1% (Forrester, V.: *Une étrange Dictature*, ibid., p. 64).
33. Among the latter, were around 850,000 men between 25 and 54 years old who in 1996 lost their jobs but were not looking for a new one for reasons of depression, pride or of inflexibility (Phillips, K.: ibid., p. 164).
34. Phillips, K.: ibid., p. 345.
35. Moore, M.: *Stupid White Men*, ibid., p. 77.
36. Forrester, V.: *Une étrange Dictature*: ibid., p. 63.
37. Kelly, C. M.: ibid., chapter 10.
38. Frank, R. H. and Cook, Ph. J: *The Winner-Take-All Society: Why the Few at the Top Get So Much More than the Rest of Us*, New York, 1995.
39. Phillips, K.: ibid., p. 133.
40. Reich, R. B.: *The Future of Success*, ibid., p. 102.
41. Luttwak, E.: *Turbo Capitalism: Winners and Losers in the Global Economy*, London, 1998, p. 60.
42. Hutton, W.: *The World We're In*, ibid., p. 26.
43. Phillips, K.: ibid., p. 133.
44. Phillips, K.: ibid., p. 221.
45. Phillips, K.: ibid., p. 133.
46. Hertsgaard, M.: ibid., p. 138.
47. Phillips, K.: ibid., pp. 134–135.
48. Hutton, W.: *The World We're In*, ibid., p. 25.
49. Gates, J.: ibid., p. 22.
50. Hertsgaard, M.: ibid., p. 41.
51. Phillips, K.: ibid., p. 113.
52. A similar picture results from reading Shipler's *The Working Poor* (Shipler, D. K.: *The Working Poor: Invisible in America*, Alfred A. Knopf, New York, 2004).
53. Hertsgaard, M.: ibid., p. 137.
54. Ehrenreich, B.: *Nickel and Dimes: Undercover in Low-Wage USA*, Granta Books, 2002. Similarly reprehensible circumstances can be found in, for instance, the three giant American meatpackers ConAgra, IBP and Excel. If one reads Schlosser's account in this respect, one's stomach turns (Schlosser, E.: ibid.).
55. Gates, J.: ibid., p. 115.
56. Reich, R. B.: *The Future of Success*, ibid., p. 120.
57. Ehrenreich, B.: ibid., p. 219.
58. *De Volkskrant*, 7 January 2003.
59. Moore, M.: *Stupid White Men*, ibid., p. 223.
60. Castells, M.: *End of Millennium*, ibid., p. 150.
61. Moore, M.: *Stupid White Men*, ibid., p. 113.
62. Barber, B. R.: *Fear's Empire*, ibid., p. 210.
63. Moore, M.: *Stupid White Men*, ibid., p. 211.

64. *De Telegraaf*, 11 August 2003.
65. *De Volkskrant*, 26 August 2003.
66. Mittelman, J. H.: ibid., p. 88. The latter implies that current globalization is creating a *Fourth World*, a term that is meant to identify those who are excluded from participation in the new global economy (Castells, M.: *End of Millennium*, ibid., p. 150). One can find these people in the big cities of the developed world and in the shanty towns of the world's mega-cities, which are populated "by millions of homeless, incarcerated, prostituted, criminalized, brutalized, stigmatized, sick and illiterate persons" (Castells, M.: *End of Millennium*, ibid., pp. 164–165). It should be taken into account that, apart from the loss of income, unemployment can also result in far-reaching consequences like psychological damage, loss of self-confidence and skills, increasing inequalities in health, disrupted family relations and social exclusion (Sen, A.: ibid., p. 96). This may explain disturbing facts about American society, like a tripling in the number of suicides since 1960 among youngsters between 15 and 24 years of age, more than 65 million official antidepressant prescriptions in 1998 alone, and the one in six children who take stimulants and antidepressants (Gates, J.: ibid., p. 55).
67. Kuttner, R.: *Everything for Sale*, ibid., p. 74.
68. Kuttner, R.: *Everything for Sale*, ibid., p. 77.
69. Phillips, K.: ibid., p. 151.
70. Sennett, R.: *The Corrosion of Character: The Personal Consequences of Work in the New Millennium*, Norton and Company, 1998, p. 49. This corresponds with Hutton, who presents a figure of 39 million Americans who were caught up in corporate downsizing between 1980 and 1995 (Hutton, W.: *The World We're In*, ibid., p. 164). And this was not the end. In 1995, AT&T, General Motors and Boeing fired 30%, 29%, and 37% of their employees respectively (*NRC/Handelsblad*, 5 March 1996). In December 1998, Boeing announced further redundancies of 48,000 employees over the next two years; in June 1999, Proctor and Gamble announced that they would close down ten factories, leaving 15,000 people unemployed; and Citigroup did so for over 10,000 people (Forrester, V.: *Une étrange Dictature*: ibid., pp. 60–61).
71. Saul, J. R.: *The Unconscious Civilization*, Penguin Books, 1997, p. 108.
72. Some of them even have their pictures on the cover of a national American weekly (Reich, R. B.: *The Future of Success*, ibid., p. 83).
73. Hutton, W.: *The World We're In*, ibid., p. 124. The author refers to an intriguing study showing, unexpectedly, that "high CEO pay tends to be followed by weak rather than strong share price performance; between 1993 and 2000 the majority of companies headed by the ten highest-paid CEOs underperformed the stock market average over both one year and three years afterwards" (p. 135).
74. Hammer and Champy defend reengineering by arguing that it is directed at "doing more with less," whereas downsizing and restructuring mean "doing less with less". In: Sennett, R.: ibid., p. 49.
75. Reich, R. B.: *The Future of Success*, ibid., p. 70.
76. Gates, J.: ibid., p. 54. What all this downsizing does not take into account is the negative influence it has on the motivation and morale of the workers who have not (yet) become its victims. In this respect, research by the American Management Association shows that repeated downsizing produces "lower

profits and declining worker productivity," whereas a study by the Wyatt Companies found that, of companies engaged in downsizing, "less than half [. . .] achieved their expense reduction goals; fewer than one-third increased profitability and less than one in four increased productivity" (Sennett, R.: ibid., p. 50).

77. An example, in this respect, is Dunlap who, after two years of downsizing, walked away with nearly $100 million in salary, bonus, stock gains, et cetera (Kelly, C. M.: ibid., p. 103). This, however, is nothing compared to the CEOs of Coca Cola and Disney, who walked away with over $1 billion in stock grants or equity raids (Gates, J.: ibid., p. 140). Regarding this phenomenon, based on a study of 22 companies that announced large lay-offs in 1994, Downs found a strong correlation (.31) between the size of the lay-off and the compensation of the CEOs (Phillips, K.: ibid., p. 151; Kelly, C. M.: ibid., p. 128). Supportive in this respect was that Wall Street institutional investors had calculated that "a single lay-off added $60,000 to future-year bottom-line earnings" (Phillips, K.: ibid., p. 150).
78. Beck, U.: ibid., p. 5.
79. Zakaria, F.: ibid.: p. 214.
80. Stiglitz, J.: *The Roaring Nineties*, ibid.: p. 100.
81. In this respect, it is important to mention the conflicts of interest for accountants who, on the one hand, did the auditing and, on the other hand, performed as management consultants. The latter job appears to have been very rewarding. The American corporation Tyco, for example, paid Pricewaterhouse Coopers $13.2 million in auditing fees in 2001, but nearly $38 million for consulting services. Similarly, in 2001, Motorola paid KPMG $3.9 million for auditing and $62.3 million for other services. Ernst and Young received $2.5 million for auditing Sprint, supplemented with $63.8 million for consulting services (Huffington, A.: ibid., p. 187).
82. In this respect, an investigation at PricewaterhouseCoopers undertaken by the SEC in 1998 exposed 8,000 cases of PWC executives' making investments in companies they audited (Huffington, A.: ibid., p. 192).
83. Phillips, K.: ibid., p. 153.
84. *De Volkskrant*, 29 April 2003, p. 17. Although American CEOs receive remuneration beyond human imagination, apparently it is never enough. In this respect, Petras and Petras present a list of 25 examples of CEO greed—all purchases for personal use, but paid for by the corporations that employ them (Petras, K. and Petras, R.: *Unusually Stupid Americans: A Compendium of All-American Stupidity*, Villard, New York, 2003, pp. 145–147).
85. Wheen, F.: ibid., p. 273.
86. Petras, K. and Petras, R.: ibid., p. 150.
87. Moore, M.: *Downsize This*, ibid., p. 109. To Levitt, a former Chairman of the American Securities and Exchange Commission, stock options represented some 80% of management compensation in 2001, and these increased in value from $60 billion to $600 billion during the 1990s (Hutton, W.: *The World We're In*, ibid., p. 124), thus creating an environment that rewarded executives for managing the share prices instead of the business. They also were an incentive to use accounting tricks, with help of external auditors, to boost the share price on which their compensation depended. Therefore, Levitt concludes that stock options "have created perverse incentives to keep the share price high, even

if it means falsifying the numbers" (Levitt, A.: *Take on the Street: What Wall Street and Corporate America Don't Want You to Know; What You Can Do to Fight Back*, Pantheon Books, 2002, p. 252). And the numbers were falsified on many occasions, caused by the fact that often the auditors were in a conflict of interests. Consequently, stock options made corporate earnings look a lot better than they really were. In this respect, researchers of the American Federal Reserve found that, between 1995 and 2000, the average growth in earnings of the companies in Standard & Poor's 500 index would have been 9.4% instead of 12% had they expensed stock options (Levitt, A.: ibid., p. 111).

88. Forrester, V.: *L'horreur économique* (Dutch Translation), AMBO/Amsterdam, 1997, p. 141–142. This type of "work" has to be distinguished from workers who are placed "on call" during their days off. Workers who are employed this way are quizzed about their whereabouts 24 hours a day, which is very intrusive in one's personal life (Pilger, J.: *Hidden Agendas*, ibid., p. 345).
89. Frank Field, Minister for Social Security in the 1980s, once counted 30 different revisions of the unemployment level in the United Kingdom, of which 29 resulted in a lower official unemployment figure (Frank, S.: ibid., p. 140).
90. Numbering over 800,000 in the Jobless Count 2001. Thanks to the magic and the juggling of employment figures, only one in five non-working persons was classified as unemployed in 1999.
91. Benzeval, M., et al. (eds.): *Tackling Inequalities in Health: An Agenda for Action*, King's Fund, London, 1995, p. 132.
92. Pilger, J.: Hidden Agendas: ibid., p. 104.
93. Gates, J.: ibid., p. 48. The 1997 UN Human Development Report observes that, since the early 1980s, the number of Britons in "income poverty" increased by 60% during Thatcher's government. Meanwhile, an investigation by the House of Commons showed that infant mortality for the rich in the United Kingdom was 4.3 per 1,000 in 1997, compared to 18.5 per 1,000 for the poor. In addition to this, around the same time, the spokesperson on health for the British Medical Association revealed that suicide had become "the big new killer of men," as it had doubled over the past ten years with, presumably, uncertainty at work being the major cause (Pilger, J.: *Hidden Agendas*, ibid., p. 80).
94. Abrams, F.: *Below the Breadline: Living on the Minimum Wage*, Profile Books, 2002, p. 169.
95. Abrams, F.: ibid., p. 183. Despite the minimum wage, 3.5 million working families live in poverty, although the official statistics try to juggle this figure. In addition to this, employers appear to be able to evade the minimum wage regulations with hardly any consequences. Two years after the introduction of the minimum wage, research by the Inland Revenue revealed that out of 6,400 complaints, 3,200 employers were not complying. This resulted, however, in only 349 enforcement notices and 62 penalty notices (Abrams, F.: ibid., pp. 165–184).
96. Pilger, J: *Hidden Agendas*, ibid., p. 80.
97. Pilger, J.: *Hidden Agendas*, ibid., p. 89. By 2001, representing an exception in Europe as a whole, around 2,000 of these ordinary British people were sent to prison annually because they could not pay their debt to the state (Cameron, S.: *The Cheating Classes: How Britain's Elite Abuse their Power*, Simon and Schuster, 2002, pp. 169 and 181).
98. Pilger, J.: *Hidden Agendas*, ibid., p. 91.

99. *De Volkskrant*, 29 July 2003. As an example, the chairman of steel producer Chorus saw his yearly pay more than double to over £550,000 at the end of the millennium, despite the fact that the company experienced a loss of £462 million (Cameron, S.: ibid., p. 211). Also see: Scambler, G.: ibid., pp. 102–103.
100. Forrester, V.: *Une étrange Dictature* (Dutch Translation): ibid., pp. 64–66.
101. Forrester, V.: *Une étrange Dictature* (Dutch Translation): ibid., p. 82.
102. Beck, U.: ibid., pp. 152–153.
103. Hoogerwerf, A.: *Politiek als Evenwichtskunst*, Alphen a/d/ Rijn, 1995.
104. Vries, B. de: ibid., pp. 208, 224–225.
105. Information received from the Hungarian representative in HOPE.
106. *Metro*, 4 November 2002. One might argue that the applicant countries cannot be compared to the original members of the EU. They show, however, that they are quickly embracing the new morality.
107. Regarding private security, for instance, the number of state police staff in the Netherlands remained the same over the period 1990–1998, whereas private security increased by around 50% (Berenschot BV: *Beelden van Bestuur: Berenschot Trendstudie*, uitgeverij Lemma, 2002, p. 66).
108. Regarding this, Forrester gives figures of between 50,000 and 60,000 for the final two months of 1998, followed by 11,000 in July 1999 as a result of the merger between Axa and Rhone-Poulenc, 4,200 resulting from the merger between Elf and Totalfina, and 10,000 with Ericsson in Sweden (Forrester, V.: *Une étrange Dictature*: ibid., pp. 60–61).
109. To give an example; on September 9, 1999, Michelin announced a 17% increase in profits over the first half-year, while at the same time announcing that 7,500 employees would be fired in the next three years. On the same day, the value of Michelin's shares increased by 10.56%, followed by a further increase of 12.53% two days later (Forrester, V.: *Une étrange Dictature*: ibid., p. 103). Exactly the same thing happened in Germany in 1995 when the Deutsche Bank announced the elimination of more than 10,000 jobs, while at the same time announcing that profits over the first half year were $1.75 billion (Thurow, L.: *The Future of Capitalism*, London, 1996, p. 28). In 2000, Unilever announced the staggered redundancy of 25,000 employees over the next five years. Ericsson revealed in April 2002 that another 20,000 employees would be fired, and FIAT announced the layoff of 8,100 workers in October 2002 (*De Telegraaf*, 10 October 2002).
110. Reich, R. B.: *The Future of Success*, ibid., p. 81. According to an estimation by the United Nations, the world labor pool of 2.8 billion people in the early 1990s included 800 million unemployed, of whom 120 million were officially registered as such, and over 700 million underemployed (Scholte J. A.: *Globalization: A Critical Introduction*, ibid., p. 219).
111. According to Wrist, "intellectual capital will go where it is wanted and it will stay where it is well treated" (Frank, R. H. and Cook, Ph. J.: ibid., p. 28).
112. Today's circumstances are not comparable with, for instance, immigration in the United States at the beginning of the 20th century or immigration in the 1970s.
113. Regarding this, see: Stephen, John D.: The Scandinavian Welfare States: Achievements, Crisis and Prospects, in: Esping-Anderson, G., (ed.): *Welfare States in Transition: National Adaptations in Global Economics*, London, 1997, p. 57.

114. Research by Shaiken, for instance, shows that the productivity of workers in Mexico in the *maquiladoras* trading zones along the American border, employed by the American automobile industry and Japanese consumer electronics manufacturers, was not lower than that of their colleagues in the United States and Japan. Their wages, however, were only a fraction of those paid in the United States and Japan for the same job (Castells, M.: *The Rise of the Network Society*, ibid., p. 128). Meanwhile, there were 1,938 *maquiladora* factories, employing 400,000 Mexicans in 1990 (Mittelman, J. H.: ibid., p. 42). In 2000, this number had increased to 3,600 factories employing 1,300,000 people, of which 68% were women (Reich, R. B.: *The Future of Success*, ibid., p. 77). Total exports in electrical and electronic goods, clothes, car parts, and accessories amounts to $80 billion annually, of which $18 billion is Mexican added value (Legrain, Ph.: ibid., p. 321). In this respect, it should be mentioned that Mexico, in exchange for American financial support and partnership in NAFTA, was forced to adopt the neo-liberal economic ideas of the Chicago School of Economics. Consequently, a whole range of liberalizing reforms were carried out, including reductions in taxation and public spending as well as privatization, the latter meaning that, between 1982 and 1991, around 75% of state-owned companies were sold (Fukuyama, F.: *The End of History and the Last Man*, ibid., p. 131).
115. Hackman calculated that, for the United States in 1995, it would take 3% of GDP per year spent on education and training in order to reduce the extreme differences in wages to the level of 1979.
116. Juhn and Murphy, for instance, conclude that the growth percentage of the total demand for labor has not changed considerably since the 1940s. What did change is that the demand for labor is concentrated at the level of highly-skilled workers (Miles, J.: When Markets Fail: Social Welfare in Canada and the United States, in: Esping-Anderson, G., (ed.): ibid., p. 133).
117. Friedman, Th. L.: ibid., p. 51.
118. Reich, R. B.: *The Future of Success*, ibid., p. 77.
119. Phillips, K.: ibid., p. 270.
120. Reich, R. B.: *The Future of Success*, ibid., p. 77. An example is Wipro, India's biggest software-services Company, with 50 of America's 500 top companies among its clients, which was valued at $6 billion in 2000 with pre-tax profits of 7.7 billion rupees (Legrain, Ph.: ibid., pp. 76–77). Also, because of the democratization of technology, in 15 years Thailand became the world's second largest producer of pickup trucks and the fourth-largest maker of motorcycles (Friedman, Th. L.: ibid., p. 51).
121. Kelly, C. M.: ibid., p. 79.
122. To illustrate: the multinational Philips recently announced that it plans to relocate its R&D activities to China (*De Telegraaf*, 20 December 2002). A further worrying aspect in this ongoing process of globalization is economic and industrial espionage, as well as bribery and piracy. Regarding this, the American International Trade Commission estimates that, in 1998, the United States lost $43 billion and a million jobs due to espionage. As for bribery, the United States' government documented 100 cases in one year (1995–1996), with a consequential loss of $45 billion in contracts for American firms. "Influence in Washington is just like in Indonesia. It's for sale," says the *Japan Economic Journal* in this respect. Finally, the America Manufacturing Policy Project puts

the piracy rate of American intellectual property in China at 98%. Three days after Microsoft introduced Windows 95 in the United States for $89.95, copies were available throughout Asia for $4 or less (Buchanan, P. J.: ibid., pp. 49–50, 113, 306).

123. Held, D., et al.: *Global Transformations*, Polity Press, 1999, pp. 184–186.
124. Drucker, P.: *Management Challenges for the 21st Century*, Harper Collins Publishers, 1999, p.157. Meanwhile, the entry-level offers to new college graduates in the American information and technology sector stagnated during the 1990s, whereas demands for salary increases resulted in threats to shift production to low-wage areas (Phillips, K.: ibid., p. 264). These threats have to be taken seriously, since the Indian government reported in 2001 that several hundred American technology firms already had foreign operations in Bangalore, while in 2000 approximately 75,000 Indian engineers were working in the United States (Phillips, K.: ibid., pp. 270–271). In this regard, Huntington states that since the 1960s Indian engineers have run more than 750 companies in Silicon Valley. Furthermore, a 2002 survey found that many of the Indian (and Chinese) high-skilled technocrats and entrepreneurs had "set up subsidiaries, joint ventures, subcontracting arrangements, or other business operations in their native countries" (Huntington, S. P.: *Who are We? America's Great Debate*, ibid., p. 288). Meanwhile, China is booming. Per capita income in this country almost doubled over the period 1980–2000 and is now $4,000. In China, exports by the dynamic provinces on the coast increased from $17 million in 1981 to over $30 billion at present (Zakaria, F.: ibid., p. 75). The influence of countries like India, Taiwan, and China in the information age is so penetrating that one can wonder if the Western world might have missed this boat already. In this respect, Phillips presents revealing figures, demonstrating the influence of South-East Asia in the field of information technology. It appears that of the 400–500 top internet, telecom, chips, and networking firms in the world, dozens had CEOs from India, China, or Taiwan, and Silicon Valley is home to many executives and engineers from these countries. An economist from Berkeley counted 750 local companies run by Indians; and at the Cisco headquarters in San Jose, 45% of the workforce was Asian. Moreover, the Taiwanese computer industry, tied to the United States, produced 39% of the world's disk drives in 2000, as well as 54% of all monitors, 93% of all scanners, 53% of all laptops, and 25% of all personal computers. Meanwhile, the Taiwanese are moving production to China for the simple reason that the price of labor on the mainland is only 25% to 35% of the Taiwanese level. At the same time, China produces 145,000 new engineers each year, while its computer market is growing 40% annually (Phillips, K.: ibid., pp. 289–290). In this respect, Gilpin observes that the extraordinary population decline in the industrialized world and the explosive population growth in China and other parts of Asia will alter the global distribution of economical and military power (Gilpin, R.: ibid., p. 15). Opponents of globalization believe this to be a very threatening development for several reasons. First of all, they point to the fact that the diffusion of industry from industrialised to industrialising economies takes place very rapidly and also includes advanced technologies like electronics and technologically sophisticated industries. The industrialized world has become dependent on these sophisticated industries, which are moving to southern industrializing economies, thus intensifying

competition. Opponents of globalization fear that, if these industrializing economies cannot improve their lot in a market-oriented global economy, "they will surely develop the weaponry with which to destroy that economy" (Gilpin, R.: ibid., p. 40). Secondly, critics of globalization blame multinational corporations for accelerating the diffusion of sophisticated technologies in that they try to increase their international competitiveness by combining cheap labor of the South with the advanced manufacturing techniques of the North. Thirdly, the challenge this shift in manufacturing poses has been aggravated by the magnitude of the problem. Since the end of the Cold War, hundreds of millions of low-wage workers have entered the world labor pool, a thing that never happened before. Moreover, these new entrants are willing to forgo the welfare and health standards that Western workers demand (Gilpin, R.: ibid., pp. 37–38). European governments that take this observation seriously would have to reconsider the constraints they have imposed on their university education systems. Some European governments seem to realize this. For example, the Dutch government of 1994–1998 launched a national action program, of which tax reductions for employers for the costs of training their employees, equalling €114 million, were an essential part (Oosterbeek, H.: Waarom de Fiscus zich niet met Scholing moet Bemoeien, in: Dalen, H. van en Kalshoven, F., (eds.): ibid., pp. 66–67).

125. Frank, S.: ibid., pp. 66–67.
126. Research revealed that 42% of American workers feel exhausted by the end of the day (Gates, J.: ibid., p. 155).
127. Rifkin, J.: ibid.
128. Peter Drucker in: Rifkin, J.: ibid., p. 12.
129. Gilpin gives figures that show that, in 1960, the manufacturing sector in the United States accounted for 27% of GDP, a figure that had decreased to 15% by 1998. Consequently, the United States lost 2.6 million manufacturing jobs over the period 1980–1998 (Buchanan, P. J.: ibid., p. 13). As a consequence of the transformation into a service society, three-quarters of the American and Canadian workforces were employed in services at the end of the 20th century. The United States alone created (net) 44 million jobs, particularly in services and government, during the period 1972–1992 (Buchanan, P. J.: ibid., p. 37), a development which leaves the rest of the industrialized world far behind (Gilpin, R.: ibid., p. 33). Nevertheless, regarding the Netherlands, only 20% of the working population now works in industry, of which only half is really producing (Berenschot BV: ibid., p. 161).
130. Rifkin, J.: ibid., p. 291. For the production of services, the author expects a near-workerless era by the 2050s. He fears that the knowledge sectors in society can only partly absorb superfluous labor which, consequently, will mean that hundreds of millions of people will be permanently jobless through the combined effect of globalization and automation.
131. Reich, R. B.: *The Future of Success*, ibid.
132. Mittelman, J. H.: ibid., p. 16.
133. Gilpin, R.: ibid., pp. 31–32.
134. In this respect, Reich distinguishes between "geeks" and "shrinks," representing two different talents and ways of perceiving the world. The "geeks" are the ones who take pleasure in exploring and developing new possibilities, i.e., artists, inventors, designers, engineers, financial wizards, scientists, writers, and

musicians. Complementary to them are the "shrinks," i.e., those who can identify opportunities in the marketplace for what consumers might want to have, to see, or to experience. They also know how to deliver these opportunities. These two, "geeks" and "shrinks," will be the boosters of the New Economy.

135. According to Hofstede, all jobs that are so predictable that they can be automated will disappear in the future. What will remain are those jobs that, by their nature, are not suitable for automation. Firstly, these are jobs that have to do with giving sense to the lives of individuals and society, and with determining human and societal objectives. These jobs include top management functions in politics and corporate business. Secondly, Hofstede distinguishes creative jobs like inventing new things, followed by testing them according to criteria with respect to their usefulness, beauty, and ethical aspects. Thirdly, there is a wide range of jobs that cannot be automated and that relate to things like safety, surveillance, defense, and maintenance. Finally, many jobs will remain in which human contact has a central position, i.e., managing, keeping people company, listening to them, supporting them materially and mentally, and motivating them to learn. Though computers can be used as tools in these jobs, they will never be able to replace humans, according to Hofstede (Hofstede, G.: ibid., pp. 138–139).
136. In 1967, Bell wrote that the average time between the development of a technological innovation and the recognition of its commercial opportunities decreased from 30 years between 1880 and 1919 to 16 between 1919 and 1945, and then to 9 years between 1945 and 1967. Since then, this time has further decreased to months rather than years for the most advanced technological products like computers and software (Fukuyama, F.: *The End of History and the Last Man*, ibid., p. 117).
137. Reich, R. B.: *The Future of Success*, ibid., p. 98.
138. In this respect, Fukuyama mentions that, in the 19th century, four out of five Americans were their own master. They did not participate in any bureaucratic organization. In the beginning of the 1990s, this ratio was one out of ten (Fukuyama, F.: *The End of History and the Last Man*, ibid., p. 102). Moreover, this absorption potential is also determined by the number of people who can afford the products that Reich's domains will deliver.
139. Frank, S.: ibid., pp. 70–71.
140. Frank, S.: ibid., p. 68.
141. Frank, S.: ibid., p. 65.
142. Evans, Ph. and Wurster, Th. S.: ibid., chapter 10.
143. Evans, Ph. and Wurster, Th. S.: ibid., p. 210.
144. Leadbeater, C.: ibid., pp. 220–226.
145. Evans, Ph. and Wurtster, Th. S.: ibid., p. 221.
146. Hutton, W.: *The State We're In*, Vintage Books, 1995, pp. 106–108.

Chapter 5

1. See: Saltman, R. B. and Figueras, J., (eds.): *European Health Care Reform: Analysis of Current Strategies*, World Health Organization, Regional Office for Europe, Copenhagen, 1997, pp. 39–42.

2. Houtepen and Ter Meulen, quoted in Saltman, R. B. and Dubois, H. F. W.: The Historical and Social Base of Social Health Insurance Systems, in: Saltman, R. B., Busse, R., Figueras, J., (eds.): *Social Health Insurance Systems in Western Europe*, European Observatory on Health Systems and Policies Series, Open University Press, 2004, p. 27.
3. Saltman, R. B. and Dubois, H. F. W.: ibid., chapter 2.
4. Scrivens, E.: *Quality, Risk and Control in Health Care*, Open University Press, 2005, p. 2.
5. Mechanic, D.: *Politics, Medicine, and Social Science*, John Wiley & Sons, 1974, p. 1.
6. Saltman and Figueras add two other dilemmas. Firstly, they note the fact that physicians are simultaneously suppliers of services (to patients) and demanders of services (from hospital staff). Secondly, they note the fact that, once the solidarity principle has been accepted, substantial cross-subsidies from sick to healthy, from rich to poor, and from young to old, cannot be prevented.
7. Evans, R. G., et al., (eds.): *Why are Some People Healthy and Others Not? The Determinants of Health of Populations*, Aldine de Gruyter, New York, 1994. A well-known example, demonstrating the limited contribution of medicine to the improved health of the population in the 19th century, was provided by McKeown (McKeown, T.: *The Role of Medicine*, Princeton University Press, 1979). Also see: White, K.: *An Introduction to the Sociology of Health and Illness*, SAGE Publications, 2002, and Wilkinson, R. G.: ibid. Furthermore, see: Benzeval, M., et al. (eds.): ibid; Graham, H., (ed.): ibid.
8. Wilkinson, R. G.: ibid., p. 67.
9. Figueras, J., Saltman, R. B., Busse, R., and Dubois, H. F. W.: Patterns of Performance in Social Health Insurance Systems, in: Saltman, R. B., Busse, R., Figueras, J., (eds.): ibid., p. 83.
10. See: Lock, K.: Opportunities for Inter-Sectoral Health Improvement in New Member-States—The Case for Health Impact Assessment, in: McKee, M., MacLehose, L., and Nolte, E., (eds.): *Health Policy and European Union Enlargement*, European Observatory on Health Systems and Policies Series, Open University Press, 2004, pp. 225–239.
11. Jones, A. and Rice, N.: Using Longitudinal Data to Investigate Socioeconomic Inequality in Health, in: Smith, P. C., Ginelly, L., Sculpher, M., (eds.): *Health Policy and Economics: Opportunities and Challenges*, Open University Press, 2005, p. 89.
12. Their activities in health care have been described by many authors. See, for example, (1) Beek, H. H.: *De Geestesgestoorde in de Middeleeuwen: Beeld en Bemoeienis*, Haarlem, 1969, and (2) Goerke, H.: *Arzt und Heilkunde: 3000 Jahre Medizin.* Vom Asklepiospriester zum Klinikarzt, Callwey, 1984.
13. See section 1.2.1. A similar approach can be found in De Vos (Vos, P. de: Hoe Gezond is de Europese Gezondheidspolitiek? in: Materne, L., et al., ibid., pp. 17–22).
14. Juffermans, P.: *Staat en Gezondheidszorg in Nederland*, SUN, Nijmegen, 1982, chapter 2. In this book, I do not follow Juffermans, who, based on the ideas of American economist Stevenson, limits the health care domain to the professional activities of doctors, nurses, physiotherapists, et cetera. This approach ignores the fact that developments in the health care process are highly determined by other players. I will go into this in chapter six.

15. I define a health care system as a legal and organizational framework, directed at producing, distributing, managing, regulating, supervising, coordinating, and controlling health care activities in order to realize defined social health care values.
16. In prosperous times, when health care systems are amply financed, interested parties are more ready to agree. In these circumstances, they can play a zero-plus game with each party getting its own share of an ever-growing pie.
17. I refer to the 15 members of the European Union prior to May 2004.
18. In a two-party-system like in the United Kingdom, Thatcher was able to implement fundamental changes in the NHS which, after their introduction, were soon modified. Clinton tried to introduce a health care system, which would have included the many uninsured Americans. He did not succeed.
19. For incrementalism, see, Braybrooke, D. and Lindblom, C. E.: ibid. Walt has summarized the characteristics of incrementalism in five points: (1) a close connection between the objectives and the means of implementation; (2) a small number of alternatives, which differ only marginally from existing policies; (3) only the most important consequences of the alternatives are considered; (4) policy options on which policy makers agree are implemented, irrespective of whether these options would result in optimal outcomes; and (5) the focus is on small changes for the short-term to existing policies, without considering major future changes (Walt, G.: ibid., pp. 48–49).
20. It seems that Dutch politicians are increasingly trying to bypass the departmental bureaucratic hierarchy to obtain the information they believe to be necessary to fulfil their parliamentary tasks (Nieuwenkamp, R.: *De Prijs van het Politieke Primaat: Wederzijds Vertrouwen en Loyaliteit in de Verhouding tussen Bewindspersonen en Ambtelijke Top*, Eburon, Delft, 2001).
21. Busse, R., Saltman, R. B., and Dubois, H. F. W.: Organization and Financing of Social Health Insurance Systems: Current Status and recent Policy Developments, in: Saltman, R. B., Busse, R., Figueras, J., (eds.), ibid., p. 74.
22. See: Busse, R., Saltman, R. B., and Dubois, H. F. W., (eds.): ibid., pp. 58–60.
23. American research from 1987 revealed that 91% of the respondents agreed that "everybody should have the right to the best possible healthcare—as good as a millionaire gets" (in: Kuttner, R.: *Everything for Sale*, ibid., p. 116). Comparable research from 1995 for Finland delivered a result of 95%.
24. Scheerder, R. L. J. M. and Schrijvers, A. J. P.: Health Care Policy Making against an OECD Background, in: Schrijvers, A. J. P., (ed.): *Health and Health Care in the Netherlands: A Critical Self-Assessment by Dutch Experts in the Medical and Health Sciences*, De Tijdstroom, Utrecht, 1997, p. 248.
25. See section 3.2.2.
26. Donaldson, C. and Gerard, K.: *Economics of Health Care Financing: The Visible Hand; Economic Issues in Health Care*, MacMillan, 1993, chapter 2.
27. Ludmerer, K. M.: *Time to Heal: American Medical Education from the Turn of the Century to the Era of Managed Care*, Oxford University Press, 1999, p. 122.
28. Ludmerer, K. M.: ibid., p. 119.
29. Ludmerer, K. M.: ibid.
30. Glied, S.: *Chronic Condition: Why Health Reform Fails*, Harvard University Press, 1997, p. 25.
31. Glied, S.: ibid., p. 140.

32. Moreover, it is uncertain whether this large number refers to people who cannot afford the insurance premium. In this respect, American research from 1987 found that only 37% of uninsured people had investigated the possibility of health insurance, and only 2.5% were ever denied coverage or offered limited coverage because of health conditions (Glied, S.: ibid., p. 140).
33. As for regulating the health care market in the United States, Maynard and Dixon refer to the so-called Jackson Hole group of academics who tried to set up a regulatory framework for a competitive health care market. The group identified six causes of market failure in the United States: (1) *cost-unconscious demand*, with providers and insurers not having an incentive to economize; (2) *biased risk selection as a source of profit*, which leads to providers' garnering profits by product differentiation and cream-skimming; (3) *market segmentation to minimize price competition*, resulting in large numbers of benefit packages, thus making comparison and choice-making very difficult; (4) *lack of information on outcomes relative to cost*, causing little outcome measurement; (5) *little choice for members of small groups*, consequently offering people belonging to these groups hardly any opportunities to choose from different health care plans; and (6) *perverse public subsidies*, with tax breaks benefitting rich employees. Countering these market failures would demand extensive government regulation, including (1) *universal access*, which would ensure that every citizen has access to at least a minimum benefit package; (2) *choice of packages*, particularly directed at members of small groups; and (3) *national regulation* by standard-setting boards that would have to ensure uniform definitions and standards of performance. The Jackson Hole proposals were not accepted, however (Maynard, A. and Dixon, A.: Private Health Insurance and Medical Savings Accounts: Theory and Experience, in: Mossialos, E., Dixon, A., Figueras, J., Kutzin, J., (eds.): *Funding Health Care: Options for Europe*, European Observatory on Health Care Systems Series, Open University Press, 2002, pp. 112–114).
34. Based on: Donaldson, C. and Gerard, K.: ibid., chapter 3.
35. It is worth mentioning that research has shown that more privately oriented health care systems appear to have higher costs of administration (Donaldson, C. and Gerard, K.: ibid., p. 30).
36. For more examples, see: Donaldson, C. and Gerard, K.: ibid., p. 34 and 89.
37. For more examples, see: Donaldson, C. and Gerard, K.: ibid., p. 34.
38. *The Guardian*, 17 May 1996.
39. Hayman, H.: The Nation's Health, in: Radice, G., (ed.): *What Needs to Change? New Visions for Britain*, HarperCollins Publishers, 1996, p. 164.
40. Hayman, H.: ibid., p. 165.
41. White, S. and Stancombe, J.: *Clinical Judgement in the Health and Welfare Professions: Extend the Evidence Base*, Open University Press, 2003, p. 26.
42. Saltman, R. B.: A Conceptual Overview of Recent Health Care Reforms, in: *European Journal of Public Health*, volume 4, 1994, no. 4, p. 290.
43. Kuttner, R.: *Everything for Sale*, ibid., p. 19.
44. Saltman, R. B. and Figueras, J., (eds.): ibid., p. 40.
45. Kuttner, R.: *Everything for Sale*, ibid., p. 19.
46. In this respect, I refer to the Dunning Committee in the Netherlands, which in 1992 advised the government on what types of health care should be included

in the coverage package. In one of the appendices to the report, in vitro fertilisation (IVF) was mentioned as an example of the discussions within the committee. It shows that even this committee could not decide whether IVF should be considered a health care intervention.

47. Sandier, S., Paris, V., and Polton, D.: Health Care Systems in Transition: France, 2004, *European Observatory on Health Systems and Policies*, Thomson, S. and Mossialos, E., (eds.), WHO Regional Office for Europe, Copenhagen, 2004, p. 40.
48. New, B. and Le Grand, J.: *Rationing in the NHS: Principles and Pragmatism*, King's Fund, 1996, p. 43.
49. Walt, G.: ibid., p. 49.
50. See: Saltman, R. B.: Assessing Social Health Insurance Systems: Present and Future Policy Issues, in: Saltman, R. B., Busse, R., Figueras, J., (eds.): ibid., pp. 145–149.
51. Schut, F. T.: *Competition in the Dutch Health Care Sector*, Erasmus University, Rotterdam, 1995, pp. 39–40.
52. Schut, F. T.: ibid., p. 86.
53. Referring to the situation in the Netherlands, Van Doorslaer shows moderate optimism. To him, more market-like operation is inevitable if the Dutch want to improve health services delivery. Such a development does not necessarily detract from solidarity. On the contrary; if principles of financing are based on individuals' capacity to pay taxes through a solidarity-based collection of premiums, and health services are delivered according to need via standardized distribution payments among insurers, income- and risk-solidarity might even increase (Doorslaer, E. K. A.: *Gezondheidzorg tussen Marx en Markt*, inaugural lecture, Erasmus University, Rotterdam, 1998, pp. 23–24). I do not share Van Doorslaer's optimism. It is precisely the idea of income-related premiums that, over the past 18 years, has not attained political agreement. This also applies to the system reforms of 2006 for which policy tricks were necessary to get them accepted.
54. Brommels, M.: Contracting and Political Boards in Planned Markets, in: Saltman, R. B. and Otter, C. von, (eds.): *Implementing Planned Markets in Health Care: Balancing Social and Economic Responsibility*, Open University Press, 1995, p. 106.
55. Deppe, H-U.: *Zur sozialen Anatomie des Gesundheitssystems: Neoliberalismus und Gesundheitspolitik in Deutschland,* Verlag für Akademische Schriften, Frankfurt, 2000, p. 20.
56. Thus said Alan Maynard at the Ecosanté Conference in respect of the British government (Paris, November 1995).
57. According to Nigel Lawson in an interview, in: Deakin, N.: ibid., p. 144.
58. Illich, I.: *Medical Nemesis* (Dutch Translation), Het Wereldvenster, Baarn, 1975, p. 93.
59. Raad voor de Volksgezondheid en Zorg: Technologische Innovatie in de Zorgsector, Zoetermeer, 2001, p. 50.
60. Gevaerts, P. O. H.: De Patientenorganisaties, in: Lens, P. and Kahn, Ph. S., (eds.): *Over de Schreef: Over Functioneren en Disfunctioneren van Artsen*, uitgeverij Van der Wees, Utrecht, 2001, p. 377.
61. Trappenburg, M.: *Gezondheidszorg en Democratie*, inaugural lecture, Erasmus University, Rotterdam, 2005, p. 9.

62. Verkaar, E. A. M. J.: *Strategisch Gedrag van Kategorale Patientenorganisaties*, dissertation, Rotterdam, 1991.
63. Attempts in the Netherlands to reach consensus on a change of policy after the Dekker report failed for this reason (Björkman, J. M. and Okma, K. G. H.: Restructuring Health Care Systems in the Netherlands: Institutional Heritage of Dutch Health Policy Reforms, in: Altenstetter, Ch. and Björkman, J. W., (eds.): ibid., pp. 101–103).
64. Raffel, M. W.: Dominant Issues: Convergence, Decentralization, Competition, Health Services, in: Raffel, M. W., (ed.): ibid., p. 302.
65. Dent, M.: ibid., p. 101.
66. Durieux, P., et al.: The "Natural History" of the Introduction and Development of the First Lithotripter in France, Paper for the EEC workshop on regulatory mechanisms concerning medical technology, London, 22–25 April, 1986.
67. Stocking, B., (ed.): *Expensive Health Technologies: Regulatory and Administrative Mechanisms in Europe*, Oxford University Press, 1988, p. 175.
68. Gooijer, W. J. de: Over Zorggestuurde Vraag en Vraaggestuurde Zorg, in: Dijkstra, G. S. A., Meer, F. M. van der and Rutgers, M. R., (eds.): *Het Belang van de Publieke Zaak*, Eburon, 2003, pp. 137–138.
69. Based on an interview with the surgeon who performed the operation.
70. Wildner, M., Exter, A. P. den, and Kraan, W. G. M. van der: The Changing Role of the Individual in Social Health Insurance Systems, in: Saltman, R. B., Busse, R., Figueras, J., (eds.): ibid., p. 252.
71. In this respect, the American philosopher Daniels, for example, delineates the characteristics which a health care system needs to possess in order for it to be called a just system. In such a system, the responsibility of the state is limited to providing individual citizens a fair equality of opportunity to species-typical normal functioning. Negative deviations from the norm cause health care needs, which have to be distinguished from health care preferences. Where treatment can restore health, the health care need at issue constitutes a legitimate claim for care as a moral right. Services regarding health care preferences, as well as those which do not result in restoration of equal opportunity (care for the mentally retarded, for example), do not belong in the health care domain. In short: according to Daniels, health care needs "are concerned with maintaining, restoring, or compensating normal species functioning" (in: Vathorst, S. van de: ibid., pp. 34 and 37).
72. http://www.un.org, 20 December 2003.
73. This followed from the establishment of the United Nations in 1945, after the demise of the League of Nations of 1919, and constituted a second attempt to promote international cooperation and to achieve peace and security.
74. Out of gratitude to several (observer) members of the Subcommittee on Economics and Planning of the European Hospital and Health Care Federation, the staff of the Latvian School of Public Health, as well as the Bulgarian Association of Hospital Managers, I will give some examples. In Article 22, paragraph 1 of the amended Dutch Constitution of 1983, it says that the government has to take measures to promote public health. Promoting, in this respect, also includes protection, which, in turn, means that the government may not impair its citizens' health. In addition to legislation, promoting includes formulating and executing health (care) policies, as well as administering the necessary organizations. Article 11 of the Constitution of Luxem-

bourg of May 1948 promises the citizens of this duchy that the law will organize social security, health protection, and industrial peace, while guaranteeing the rights of labor unions. The Constitution of Greece of 1975 entitles persons suffering from incurable bodily or mental ailments to special care by the state. Moreover, the Greek constitution promises that the state will take care of its citizens' health, and that it will adopt special measures for the protection of the young, the elderly, and the disabled. The Belgian Constitution of 1994 states in Article 23 that each citizen is entitled to a dignified existence. Social security and health protection, as well as social, medical, and judicial assistance, are among the items assumed to contribute to that dignified existence. The French Constitution of 1946 guarantees in Article 11 of its preamble that each French citizen, particularly children, mothers, and retired workers, should enjoy health protection, social security, industrial peace, and leisure time. Moreover, the French constitution promises those citizens who, for physical, mental, or economic reasons, as well as for reasons of age, cannot participate in the employment process, the means to be able to enjoy a dignified life. In Great Britain, "the NHS is based upon the principle that there should be a comprehensive range of publicly provided services designed to help the individual stay healthy and to provide effective and appropriate treatment and care where necessary while making the best use of available resources" (*Social Welfare in Britain*, COI-reference pamphlet 1989, p. 1. Legislation in 1948 and 1977 set out the requirements to provide a comprehensive health service). Sweden has special legislation, enacted in 1992, regarding health and medical services, as well as health and medical personnel. Furthermore, supervision, duties, and disciplinary sanctions are all laid down in legal regulations (Ministry of Health and Social Affairs: *Swedish Legislation on Health and Medical Services and Health and Medical Personnel*, March 1997). Finally, Article 70 of the German legislation on social affairs provides that the citizens of Germany are equally entitled to effectively and efficiently delivered medical care according to their needs (in German it reads: "Die Krankenkassen und die Leistungserbringer haben eine bedarfsgerechte und gleichmässige dem allgemein anerkannten Stand der medizinische Erkenntnisse entsprechende Versorgung der Versicherten zu gewährleisten. Die Versorgung der Versicherten muss ausreichend und zweckmässig sein, darf das Mass des Notwendigen nicht überschreiten und muss wirtschaftlich erbracht werden.").

The European Union as of May 2004 was enlarged by a number of countries which were under communist rule until the beginning of the 1990s, and it is interesting to review some of the constitutions of these countries. For Hungary, the government had to arrange an adjustment of the constitution of 1949 "in order to facilitate a peaceful political transition to a constitutional state, establish a multiparty system, parliamentary democracy and social market economy" (Article 1 of Act XXXI of 1989; effective as of 23 October 1989). The consequences of that adjustment for the government's responsibility regarding its citizens' health is, first of all, set out in Article 35g, which reads that "the Government shall define the State system of social welfare and health care services, and ensure sufficient funds for such services" (Article 22, paragraph 1 of Act XXXI of 1989). Furthermore, Article 70d, part 1 states that "everyone living in the territory of the Republic of Hungary has the right to the highest possible level of physical and mental health" (Article 34 of Act XXXI of 1989), and part 2 of the same Article promises that "the Republic of Hungary shall implement this right through institutions of labor safety and health care, through the organization of medical care and the opportunities for regular physical activity, as well as through the protection of the urban and natural environment" (Article 47, paragraph 2, of Act XL of 1990; effective as of June 1990). In Bulgaria, the Constitution of the People's Republic of Bulgaria of 1947 guaranteed the citizens the right to health care in Article 81, which stipulates that the state would look after its citizens' health by organizing health care services and institutions, and by disseminating health education. This constitution was abrogated in 1999 and replaced by the Constitution of the Republic of Bulgaria. In this subsequent constitution, the government's responsibility regarding health is set out in Articles 43 and 47. Part 3 of the latter article states that every citizen is entitled to medical care free of charge, whereas Article 43 deals with the financial aspects regarding this entitlement. Finally, Chapter VIII of the Latvian Constitution deals with fundamental human rights. In this respect, the state not only promises in Article 111 to protect human health, but also guarantees a basic level of medical assistance for everyone. In addition to this, Article 15 of this constitution states that local governments have to ensure access to health care as well as to promote a healthy lifes-tyle.

75. Meij, A. W. H. en Zimmeren, E. van, ibid.
76. See www.usembassy.nl. (2003)
77. Cliteur, P.: ibid., p. 101.
78. Wildner, M., Exter, A. P. den, and Kraan, W. G. M. van der: ibid., p. 257.
79. Commissie van de Europese Gemeenschappen: *Communautaire Samenwerking op het Gebied van de Volksgezondheid: Mededeling van de Commissie aan de Raad*, COM(84) 502 def., Brussels, 18 September 1984.
80. In this respect, recent research in the Netherlands showed that almost half of all respondents were prepared to pay a higher health insurance premium in order to maintain the principle of solidarity (Bongers, I. M. B., Weert, C. M. C. van, Vis, C. M., Garretsen, H. F. L. and Das, M.: *Kwaliteit en Kwantiteit van de Gezondheidszorg en Actuele Beleidsontwikkelingen in de Gezondheidszorg in 2005: Nederlanders aan het Woord*, Universiteit van Tilburg, 2005, p. 44).
81. Asperen, G. M. van: Jouw Geld of mijn Leven, in: Jacobs, F. C. L. M. en Wal, G. A. van der, (eds.): *Medische Schaarste en het Menselijk Tekort*, Baarn, 1988, p. 54.
82. Decker, N.: Cross-Border Cooperation and Free Movement of Patients: The Different Viewpoints, in: *Free Movement and Cross-Border Cooperation in Europe: The Role of Hospitals & Practical Experiences in Hospitals*, Proceedings of the HOPE Conference and Workshop, Luxembourg, June 2003, p. 62.
83. Here, formulations may differ between countries. For the Netherlands, for example, the constitutional formulation regarding health is an item of the basic law that provides the foundation of universal social rights and entitlements, which are legally formulated in the Sick Fund Law and the Law on Exceptional Medical Expenses. Conversely, Italy has formulated the right to health and health care almost as an individual item of basic rights (Hermans, H. E. G. M. and France, G.: Beperkingen aan het Recht op Gezondheidszorg:

Realisering Zorgaanspraken in Nederland en Italië, in: *Sociaal Recht*, 1998–2, pp. 47–54).

84. Commission of the European Communities: Communication from the Commission to the Council, the European Parliament, the Economic and Social Committee and the Committee of the Regions on the Health Strategy of the European Community: Proposal for a Decision of the European Parliament and of the Council, adopting a programme of Community Action in the Field of Public Health (2001–2006), COM (2000) 285 final, Brussels, 16.5.2000, p. 8.
85. Friedman, E.: Because Someone Has To Be Responsible: Duty and Dilemma for the American Hospital, in: Friedman, E., (ed.): *Making Choices: Ethical Issues for Health Care Professionals*, American Hospital Association, 1986, pp. 79–84.
86. Commissie van de Europese Gemeenschappen: Mededeling van de Commissie aan de Raad, het Europees Parlement, het Economisch en Sociaal Comité en het Comité van de Regio's. De Toekomst van de Gezondheidszorg en de Ouderenzorg: de Toegankelijkheid, de Kwaliteit en de Betaalbaarheid waarborgen, ibid., p. 4.
87. Kam, F. de en Nypels, F.: *Tijdbom*, Amsterdam/Antwerpen, 1995, p. 22.
88. Kam, F. de en Nypels, F.: ibid., pp. 16–17.
89. By the late 1980s, around 28 million Americans were AARP members. The organization employed 1,300 staff members—(Pierson, P.: The New Politics of the Welfare State, in: Pierson, Chr. and Castles, F., (eds.): ibid., p. 311).
90. Becker, H.: De *Toekomst van de verloren Generatie*, Amsterdam, 1997, p. 74.
91. Komter, A. E., et al.: *Het Cement van de Samenleving: Een Verkennende Studie naar Solidariteit en Cohesie*, Amsterdam University Press, 2000, chapter 5.
92. Komter, A. E., et al.: ibid., p. 80.
93. Wittenberg, R., Sandhu, B., and Knapp, M.: Funding Long-Term Care: The Public and Private Options, in: Mossialos, E., Dixon, A., Figueras, J., Kutzin, J., (eds.): ibid., pp. 246–247.
94. Kam, F. de and Nypels, F.: ibid., p. 21.
95. Rifkin, J.: *The European Dream*, ibid., p. 254.
96. Dykstra opposes the idea that the growing number of elderly people is responsible for the increasing costs of health care. To him, the determining factors are increasing labor costs and the use of new technologies. However, Dykstra misses several points here. First of all, in contrast to some 25 years ago, almost 60% of nursing days in general hospitals are consumed by people over 65 years old. Secondly, new technologies and developments in the pharmaceutical industry contribute enormously to the aging of the population (in: Komter, A. E., et al.: ibid., p. 80).
97. Kam, F. de and Nypels, F.: ibid.
98. Fairlamb, D.: ibid.
99. Ours, J. van: Schaarste op de Arbeidsmarkt: nou én? in: Dalen, H. van and Kalshoven, F., (eds.), ibid., p. 111.
100. Judt, T.: ibid., p. 105.
101. Bovenberg, L: Nieuwe Spelregels voor een Nieuwe Levensloop, in: Dalen, H. van and Kalshoven, F., (eds.), ibid., pp. 71–72.
102. In this respect, in has been calculated for the United States that it took 4.8 working-age adults to fund health care for one person over 65 years of age in 1993. By 2030, when the last baby boomers will have retired, there will

only be 2.8 working-age adults to pay for the health care costs of each person over 65, which may be partly compensated by the fact that post-baby boomers will have fewer children under 19 to support (Glied, S.: ibid., p. 136).
103. Kam, F. de and Nypels, F.: ibid., p. 129.
104. McKee, M., Healy, J., Edwards, N., and Harrison, A.: Pressures for Change, in: McKee, M. and Healy, J., (eds.): *Hospitals in a Changing Europe,* European Observatory on Health Care Systems Series, Open University Press, 2002, p. 39
105. Mossialos, E. and Le Grand, J.: Cost Containment in the EU: An Overview, in: Mossialos, E. and Le Grand, J., (eds.): ibid., pp. 55–56.
106. Bleichrodt, H. Het Dilemma van de Minister van Volksgezondheid, in: Dalen, H. van and Kalshoven, F., (eds.), ibid., pp. 201–211.
107. *De Volkskrant*, 10 June 2005.
108. Jochemsen, H.: The Practice and Legalisation of Euthanasia in the Netherlands, in: *Hospital: Official Journal of the European Association of Hospital Managers*, Volume 5, Issue 6/2003, pp. 18–20.
109. I am grateful to Prof. K. Schutyser from the University of Leuven, Belgium, for providing this information.
110. Jochemsen, H.: ibid., p. 20.
111. Ansieau, G.: Belgium: One Year after the Decriminalisation of Euthanasia, in: *Hospital: Official Journal of the European Association of Hospital Managers*, Volume 5, Issue 6/2003, p. 23.
112. Ansieau, G.: ibid., p. 23.
113. Gross, N.: Active Assisted Dying (Euthanasia) in Europe: Where are We Heading? in: *Hospital: Official Journal of the European Association of Hospital Managers*, Volume 5, Issue 6/2003, p. 22.
114. Gross, N.: ibid., p. 22.
115. Commission of the European Communities: Report from the Commission to the Council, the European Parliament and the Economic and Social Committee on the Integration of Health Protection Requirements in Community Policies, ibid., p. 33.
116. Bardoux, Chr.: European Group on Ethics: Opinion on Genetic Testing in the Workplace, in: *Hospital: Official Journal of the European Association of Hospital Managers*, Volume 5, Issue 5/2003, p. 18.
117. Herten, L. van and Gunning-Schepers, L. J.: Historical Perspectives on European Health and Policy, in: Marinker, M., (ed.): ibid., p. 28.
118. Anselm, R. and Ley, F.: Between Euphoria and Disillusion: What do Clinical Ethical Committees Achieve? in: *Hospital: Official Journal of the European Association of Hospital Managers*, Volume 5, Issue 5/2003, p. 20.
119. May, A. T.: Ethics as a Measure of Quality, in: *Hospital: Official Journal of the European Association of Hospital Managers*, Volume 5, Issue 5/2003, p. 17.
120. Kölking, H.: Building Blocs of an Institutional Ethic: The Development of Medical-Ethical Competence among Doctors and Nurses, in: *Hospital: Official Journal of the European Association of Hospital Managers*, Volume 5, Issue 5/2003, p. 15.
121. Health Council of the Netherlands: *The Future of Our Selves*, ibid., p. 64.
122. Health Council of the Netherlands: *The Future of Our Selves*, ibid., p. 81.
123. Health Council of the Netherlands: *The Future of Our Selves*, ibid., p. 85.

124. Coulter, A. and Magee, H., (eds.): *The European Patient of the Future*, Open University Press, 2004, p. 124.
125. Dijn, H. de: Technology in Health Care: A Philosophical Ethical Appraisal, in: Gastmans, Chr., (ed.): ibid., p. 20.
126. Dijn, H. de: ibid., p. 16.

Chapter 6

1. An alternative approach involves distinguishing between *primary*, *secondary*, and *tertiary* care.
2. Gooijer, W. J. de, Siem Tjam, F., and Stott, G.: *Hospital and Institutional Care: An Approach to a Generic Delineation*, WHO, WHO/EIP/OSD/00.3, Geneva, 2000.
3. In this respect, Tronto distinguishes between four phases of care: (a) caring about, (b) taking care of, (c) care-giving, and (d) care-receiving. The focus in the diagram is on (c). (Widdershoven, G.: Technology and Care: From Opposition to Integration, in: Gastmans, Chr., (ed.): *Between Technology and Humanity: The Impact of Technology on Health Care Ethics*, Leuven University Press, 2002, p. 41).
4. See, for example, Payer, L.: *Medicine and Culture: Varieties of Treatment in the United States, England, West Germany, and France*, Henry Holt and Company, New York, 1998.
5. Payer, L.: ibid., p. 26.
6. Payer, L.: ibid., p. 108.
7. Payer, L.: ibid., p. 101.
8. Payer, L.: ibid., p. 33.
9. Payer, L.: ibid., p. 54. Also, see: Pols, A.: Buiten Proportie: Opschudding over de Siliconen Borstprothese, in: Everdingen, J. J. E. van, (ed.): ibid., pp. 195–203.
10. Payer, L.: ibid., p. 78.
11. Payer, L.: ibid., p. 78.
12. Payer, L.: ibid., p. 121.
13. Payer, L.: ibid., p. 125.
14. Mechanic, D.: ibid., p. 38.
15. Mossialos, E. and Le Grand, J.: *Cost Containment in the EU: An Overview*, ibid., p. 35.
16. Malleson refers to research in the city of New York, showing how arbitrarily doctors diagnose the need for a tonsillectomy (Malleson, A.: *Need Your Doctor Be So Useless?* (Dutch Translation), Het Spectrum, 1974, p. 14).
17. Research has shown that the effects of different types of psychotherapy are often rather limited, due to non-specific factors like the relation between the therapist and the client and the large variability in the natural course of disorders (Health Council of the Netherlands: *The Future of Our Selves*, The Hague, Health Council of the Netherlands, 2002, publication no. 2002/13, p. 49).
18. Apart from the examples given, Everdingen, et al. argue that medicine is not free from fashionable trends, giving several examples from gynecology and neurology (Everdingen, J. J. E. van, (ed.): ibid., p. 69).

19. Lasch, C.: ibid., pp. 207 and 211. Giving examples of a patient who "abruptly" broke off analysis after the 1,172nd session and a patient who remained in analysis for 11 years, Lasch concludes that psychoanalytic therapies in their classic form cost too much, last too long, and demand too much intellectual sophistication from the patient.
20. Health Council of the Netherlands: ibid., p. 84.
21. Kahn, H. and Wiener, A. J.: ibid., pp. 59–65.
22. Banta, H.: *An Approach to the Social Control of Hospital Technologies*, WHO/SHS/CC/95.2, SHS Paper number 10, WHO, 1995, p. 1.
23. Newhouse and Cutler (1996), in: *Raad voor de Volksgezondheid en Zorg: Technologische Innovatie in de Zorgsector*, ibid., pp. 47–48.
24. See for this aspect of the developments in health care: Fanu, J. le: *The Rise and Fall of Modern Medicine*, Abacus Books, 2004.
25. Fanu, J. le: ibid., p. 142.
26. Fanu, J. le: ibid., chapters 1–4.
27. Fanu, J. le: ibid., p. 138.
28. A known example, in this respect, was Barry Marshall, an Australian doctor who discovered a cure for peptic ulcers (Fanu, J. le: ibid., chapter 12).
29. Fanu, J. le: ibid., p. 157.
30. Freidson, E.: *Profession of Medicine: A Study of the Sociology of Applied Knowledge*, Harper & Row, Publishers, 1970, p. 5. Also see: Boer, J. de: *Paradoxen in de Geneeskunde*, Erasmus-lezing, Rotterdam, 1985, pp. 3–4.
31. Fanu, J. le: ibid., part 1, chapter 1.
32. Corrected for inflation, during the 20 years following the Second World War, the total dollar amount invested in medical research increased 15-fold (Ludmerer, K. M.: ibid., p. 142).
33. Fanu, J. le: ibid., p. 192.
34. Fanu, J. le: ibid., part 1, chapter 2.
35. Fanu, J. le: ibid., p. 216.
36. Fanu, J. le: ibid., part 1, chapter 4.
37. Fanu, J. le: ibid., p. 219.
38. Fanu, J. le: ibid., pp. 237–238.
39. Ludmerer, K. M.: ibid., p. xix.
40. Sparrow, M.: ibid., p. viii.
41. PriceWaterhouseCoopers: *Health Cast Tactics: A Blueprint for the Future*, the Health Cast 2010 Series, 2002, p. 52.
42. Here, the Council expects business process redesign to contribute to improvements (Raad voor de Volksgezondheid en Zorg: *Technologische Innovatie in de Zorgsector*, ibid., chapter 3).
43. Gann, B.: Enabling Patient Access and Expertise, in: Dean, K., (ed.): *Connected Health: Essays from Health Innovators*, Cisco Systems, undated, p. 9.
44. Raad voor de Volksgezondheid en Zorg: *Technologische Innovatie in de Zorgsector*, ibid., p. 6.
45. Gann, B.: ibid., p. 10–11. The "digital divide" may exclude the poor, the homeless, refugees and ethnic minorities. Figures from the United Kingdom from 2000 confirm that internet users tend to be young, affluent, and employed; 48% are under 35 years old, and only 11% are over 55 years old.

46. See: Beolchi, L., (ed.): *Telemedicine Glossary*, fifth edition, 2003, Working Document, European Commission, Brussels, September 2003.
47. Health Council of The Netherlands: *The Future of Our Selves*, ibid.
48. Fanu, J. le: ibid., p. 243. The "Age of Optimism" ended around the late 1970s.
49. Fanu, J. le: ibid., part 2.
50. Fanu. J. le: ibid., p. 262.
51. With, of course, the vaccine against hepatitis B and the "triple therapy" for the treatment of AIDS being important exceptions Fanu, J. le: ibid., p. 249.
52. Fanu, J. le: ibid., p. 253.
53. Fanu, J. le: ibid., p. 260.
54. Fanu, J. le: ibid., part 3.
55. Fanu, J. le: ibid., p. 271.
56. Mitchell refers to the launching of 525,000 new products in Europe over a period of 13 months during the 1990s. Research showed, however, that only 2.2% could be classified as innovative, with 76.7% being, in fact, line extensions (Michell, A.: ibid., p. 44).
57. A few examples are (1) Parker, J. E. S.: *The Economics of Innovation: The National and Multinational Enterprise in Technological Change*, Longman, 1974; (2) Rogers, E. M. and Shoemaker, F.: *Communication of Innovation:. A Cross-Cultural Approach*, New York, 1971; (3) Schon, D. A.: *Technology and Change: The Impact of Invention and Innovation on American Social and Economic Development*, New York, 1967; (4) Baudet, H.: *Over Acceptatie van Innovaties*, Amsterdam, 1970; (5) Twiss, B.: *Managing Technological Innovation*, London, 1974.
58. Parker, J. E. S.: ibid., p. 123.
59. McKinlay, J. B.: From 'Promising Report' to 'Standard Procedure': Seven Stages in the Career of a Medical Innovation, in: McKinlay, J. B., (ed.): *Technology and the Future of Health Care*, Milbank Reader 8, the MIT Press, 1982, pp. 233–270. Notes 60–65 are all based on McKinlay.
60. These media may employ special reporters who devote special columns to the developments in health care. Also, they may get their information through direct contact with researchers. Characteristic of this reporting is that it is mostly limited to positive results. Going into these reports in more detail may reveal that methodological criteria are rarely met and that failures are not reported. In particular, when medical journals report on coming innovations, this may influence important parties in the next stage of the diffusion process.
61. Professionals may, for different reasons, decide to adopt the innovation. They may be responding to peer pressure, they may see it as an opportunity to perform better, they may want to be judged as being up-to-date, or they may really want to be able to respond to their clients' needs. Some more suspicious commentators consider personal financial gain as the motivation for physicians' adoption of an innovation. To me, it seems very doubtful, however, whether this is the primary motivation for the majority of physicians. It seems to me that in adopting an innovation, physicians and their associations primarily believe that they will be more effective, humane, scientific, or whatever. As for hospitals, its administrators may adopt the innovation for reasons of efficiency, because of pressure from the medical staff, or because they just want to improve the hospital's reputation. Furthermore, a hospital's affiliation with a medical school may be a reason for early adoption. Such an affiliation may

result in an influential boost for the innovation, particularly when the new technology is included in the educational curriculum and is endorsed by influential trainers and respected medical institutions. On the other hand, being included in the curriculum, the innovation may prove very difficult to remove from the training programme when, after all, it does not fulfill its promises, the reason for this being that medical professionals can be very reluctant in changing practices once they have been taught one.

62. Such a demand, however, does not occur in a vacuum. It is mobilized by professional interest groups that are already committed to the innovation. This acceptance is instrumental to the further advancement of the career of the innovation. It may be used by manufacturers, medical professionals, and hospitals to legitimate their association with the innovation. It may also be used as a reason for its expansion. When, finally, the innovation is endorsed and supported by the state and underwritten by third parties, one can say that it is about to become an element of regular medical practice. For the achievement of this objective, McKinlay distinguishes between two mutually supportive activities. The first one, the *indirect* method, involves lobbying public officials, so-called expert testimony before legislative committees, and campaign contributions to potentially supportive individuals and parties. The second activity, the *direct* method, is meant to mobilize support for the innovation among community or interest groups. They, in turn, can pressure the state to support the particular innovation. Through these two methods, the state is persuaded to accept the promising but yet-to-be-tested innovation. Consequently, for governments, there are no other options left than to go along with the promoters of the innovation. Their compliance, however, is not based on reliable evidence on the added value of the innovation, but on the basis of some combination of professional, organizational, and public pressure. It must be emphasized that at this highly public third stage in its career, the innovation usually remains without formal evaluation. The innovation is simply there as a result of the claims of manufacturers, the opinions of researchers, enthusiast professionals and trainers, and public demand. Nevertheless, when the innovation has gone through this stage in the diffusion process, the point of no return has been reached. When, afterwards, governments have second thoughts about their compliance, seeking to determine whether the step taken was the correct one, research more often than not shows, according to McKinlay, that the step was in the wrong direction.
63. As for these observational studies, several characteristics can be distinguished. Firstly, they may follow from the wish governments have to evaluate the innovation's effectiveness, after it has received general endorsement. Mostly, these studies are retrospective case reports or follow-up investigations which are limited to selected patients who were treated with help of the innovation. Secondly, interested parties from the foregoing stages (manufacturers, medical professionals, hospitals) are often the ones to initiate and to conduct these observational studies, thus having an interest in positive outcomes. Therefore, the objectivity of these studies can be questioned. Thirdly, these observational studies usually suffer from methodological limitations. The sample size may be inadequate, the study may be limited to specific groups of patients or problems, there may not be an appropriate comparison group, or one may use subjective outcomes only. Fourthly, observational studies seldom add much

knowledge concerning the effectiveness of the innovation in relation to the problem it is designed to assist. "In view of these and other limitations it is difficult to determine from most observational reports whether the innovation is actually effective and whether some observed outcome may with certainty be attributed to it," according to McKinlay (McKinlay, J. B., (ed.): ibid., p. 248). Nevertheless, public support remains strong, with governments and third parties underwriting most of its costs. To question the innovation's effectiveness or desirability raises hostility towards the one who dares to make the suggestion.

64. As for the objections, McKinlay distinguishes between legitimate and illegitimate ones. Legitimate objections spring from genuine concern. The others, being the majority, are directed at making proper evaluations virtually impossible, so that the innovation is protected from potentially incriminating results. Here, ethical and legal arguments are used to prevent an RCT from being conducted. Besides, there are other problems, such as the high costs of an RCT, the qualifications of those involved in the sponsoring and conducting of the trial, as well as arguments regarding the appropriateness of certain interventions and situations and the way an RCT can alter individual clinicians' behavior. In coping with, and recognizing the legitimacy of, these objections, the RCT's design is often adjusted to the criticism. These adjustments boil down to making methodological allowances and reconsidering sample criteria. Consequently, the researcher is forced by circumstances to depart form the ideal textbook design. This obviously affects the reliability of an RCT's outcomes. Ironically, these outcomes are next used to discredit the entire RCT by those who objected the RCT from the beginning. However, without methodological accommodations, the RCT would never have been permitted in the first place. If the results of an RCT do show an innovation to be effective, this, of course, is used immediately by the innovation's proponents, thus advancing its career.
65. In particular, professional journals which show the courage to publish negative RCT results may be attacked by write-in campaigns from parties committed to the innovation, thus creating the impression that the opposition is not as intense as it may seem. Furthermore, disquieting RCT findings may be moderated by "invited experts," who try to reconcile contradictory findings with their clinical experience. Another method is that parties who have an interest in advancing the innovation's career constitute a special committee to evaluate the RCT results with the objective of disqualifying the outcomes. In the event that such a committee reviews "data," they mostly are from the above-mentioned methodologically defective observational studies. According to McKinlay, "the issue of double standards is perhaps most evident during the sixth stage. The many defective observational studies conducted up to this point seldom receive adequate methodological and statistical scrutiny, whereas RCTs are subject to the most stringent criticism, employing standards that are almost never involved during the earlier stages. Questions are raised and motivations challenged that, again, are seldom raised during earlier stages." (McKinlay, J. B., (ed.): ibid., p. 256). Given all this, "it is reasonable to argue that the success of an innovation has little to do with its intrinsic worth [. . .] but is dependent on the power of the interest groups that sponsor and maintain it, despite the absence or inadequacy of empirical support" (McKinlay, J. B., (ed.): ibid., p. 257).

66. McKinlay, J. B., (ed.): ibid., p. 258.
67. Steering Committee on Future Health Scenarios: *Anticipating and Assessing Health Care Technology*, Volume 2, *Future Technological Changes*, Kluwer Academic Publishers, 1988, p. 5.
68. Popta, S. van: *De Gemende Economische Orde en de Christelijk-Sociale Geachte*, Kampen, 1974, p. 5.
69. Jennet, B.: *High Technology Medicine: Benefits and Burdens*, Oxford University Press, 1986, p. 14.
70. Ludmerer, K. M.: ibid., p. 269.
71. Gooijer, W. J. de: De Planning van Dure Medische Apparatuur in het Europa van 1992, *ZM-Magazine*, jaargang 5, nummer 11, November 1989, pp. 11–19.
72. Sargentini, A., Marino, F., and Bravar, D.: Medical Technology in Italy, in: Stocking, B., (ed.): ibid., p. 137.
73. Tsouros, A. D.: Medical Technology in Greece, in: Stocking, B., (ed.): ibid., p. 128.
74. Sissouras, A., Karokis, A. and Mossialos, E.: Health Care and Cost Containment in Greece, in: Mossialos, E. and Le Grand, J., (eds.): ibid., p. 387.
75. Held, H.: Medical Technology in the Federal Republic of Germany, in: Stocking, B. (ed.): ibid., p. 118.
76. *Deutsches Ärzteblatt*, 85, Heft 31/32, 8 August 1988, Seite B-1250.
77. *Deutsches Ärzteblatt*, 85, Heft 31/32, 8 August 1988, Seite B-1250.
78. Gress, S., Niebuhr, D., Rothgang, H., Wasem, J.: Benefit Decisions in German Social Health Insurance, in: Stoltzfus Jost, T., (ed.): *Health Care Coverage Determinations: An International Comparative Study*, Open University Press, 2005, p. 125.
79. Pereira, J., Campos, A. C. de, Ramos, F., Simões, J., and Reis, V.: Health Care Reform and Cost Containment in Portugal, in: Mossialos, E. and Le Grand, J., (eds.): ibid., p. 648.
80. Buxton, M. J.: Heart Transplantation in the UK: The Decision-Making Context of an Economic Evaluation, in: Stocking, B., (ed.): ibid., pp. 44–45.
81. Buxton, M. J.: ibid., p. 43.
82. Hughes, J.: Health Expenditure and Cost Containment in Ireland, in: Mossialos, E. and Le Grand, J., (eds.): ibid., p. 506.
83. Stocking, B. (ed.): ibid.
84. One of these departments had just moved to a brand-new and well-equipped building.
85. Lancry, P-J. and Sandier, S.: Twenty Years of Cures for the French Health Care System, in: Mossialos, E. and Le Grand, J., (eds.): ibid., p. 456.
86. Crainich, D. and Closon, M-C.: Cost Containment and Health Care Reform in Belgium, in: Mossialos, E. and Le Grand, J., (eds.): ibid., p. 259.
87. Ministry of Social Affairs and Health: *Social Security and Health Care in Finland*, the Finnish Government Printing Centre, 1991.
88. Hindori, M.: *Health Sector Reform in Suriname: Draft White Paper*, Ministry of Health/Inter-American Development Bank, Paramaribo, November, 2002, p. 18.
89. Standing Committee of the Hospitals of the European Union (HOPE): Newsletter No. 7 January 2004.
90. McKee, M., MacLehose, L., and Nolte, E.: Health and Enlargement, in: McKee, N., MacLehose, L. and Nolte, E., (eds.): *Health Policy and European Union*

Enlargement, European Observatory on Health Systems and Policies Studies, Oxford University Press, 2004, p. 3.
91. Jansen van Galen, J.: ibid., pp. 93 and 184.
92. Wanless, D.: *Securing our Future Health: Taking a Long-Term View; Interim Report*, The Public Enquiry Unit, HM Treasury, November, 2001, p. 5.
93. See note 23 of chapter five, which shows, for that matter, that Americans do not think differently.
94. Cyert, R. M. and March, J. G.: ibid.
95. For an analysis regarding the Netherlands in this respect, see: Wetenschappelijke Raad voor het Regeringsbeleid: *Bewijzen van Goede Dienstverlening*, Amsterdam University Press, 2004, pp. 81–83.
96. Wanless, D.: ibid., p. 51.

Chapter 7

1. Roscam Abbing, H. D. C.: Wetgeving binnen de Europese Unie, in: Lens, P. and Kahn, Ph. S., (eds.): ibid., pp. 67–81.
2. Dubois, C.-A. and McKee, M.: Health and Health Care in the Candidate Countries to the European Union: Common Challenges, Different Circumstances, Diverse Policies, in: McKee, M., MacLahose, L., Nolte, E., (eds.): ibid., p. 45.
3. Field, in: Krukemayer, H.: *Vergleichende Systemanalyse des Krankenhauswesens in OECD-Ländern*, Bremen, 1985, p. 30.
4. OECD: *The Reform of Health Care: A Comparative Analyses of Seven OECD Countries*, Health Policy Studies, No. 2, Paris, 1992, pp. 19–29.
5. In: Materne, L., et al.: ibid.
6. For example Groot, L. M. J., in: Stocking, B., (ed.): ibid., chapter 1.
7. Dent, M.: *Remodelling Hospitals and Health Professions in Europe: Medicine, Nursing and the State*, Palgrave, 2003, p. 85.
8. Commissie van de Europese Gemeenschappen: Mededeling van de Commissie aan de Raad, het Europees Parlement, het Economisch en Sociaal Comité en het Comité van de Regio's. *De Toekomst van de Gezondheidszorg en de Ouderenzorg: de Toegankelijkheid, de Kwaliteit en de Betaalbaarheid waarborgen*, COM(2001) 723 definitief, Brussels, 5 December 2001, p. 11.
9. Appleby, J.: *Financing Health Care in the 1990s*, Open University Press, 1993, pp. 46–47.
10. For the different methods of financing health care, see: Mossialos E., Dixon, A., Figueras, J., Kutzin, J., (eds.): ibid.
11. Fattore, G.: Cost Containment and Reforms in the Italian National Health Service, in: Mossialos, E. and Le Grand, J., (eds.): ibid., p. 513.
12. European Parliament, Directorate General for Research: *Health Care Systems in the EU: A Comparative Study*, Working Paper, Public Health and Consumer Protection Series, SACO 101/rev. EN, November 1998, p. 5.
13. Illustrative for the staggering differences is the first chapter of Mossialos and Le Grand's Health Care and Cost Containment in the European Union (Mossialos, E. and Le Grand, J., (eds.): ibid., chapter 1).
14. In this respect, see: Saltman, R. B., Busse, R., Figueras, J., (eds.): ibid.

15. Jakubowski, E. and Hess, R.: The Market for Physicians, in: McKee, M., MacLehose, L., Nolte, E., (eds.), ibid., p. 141.
16. Saltman, R. B. and Figueras, J.: ibid., p. 9.
17. Theofilatou, M. A.: ibid., p. 174.
18. Commission of the European Communities: Report from the Commission to the Council, the European Parliament and the Economic and Social Committee on the Integration of Health Protection Requirements in Community Policies, COM (95) 196 final, Brussels, 29 May 1995.
19. In this respect, the Commission's 1993 Green Paper on European Policy reveals that 8,000 Europeans die annually due to accidents at their work place. Throughout the Community, 10 million workers suffer an industrial accident or occupational disease every year (Commission of the European Communities. Directorate-General for Employment, Industrial Relations and Social Affairs: *European Social Policy: Options for the Union*, Green Paper, COM (93) 551, Brussels, 17 November 1993, p. 65).
20. European Commission: *The Internal Market and Health Services.* Report of the High Level Committee on Health, 17 December 2001, p. 19).
21. European Health Management Association: *The European Union and Health Services—The Impact of the Single European Market on Member States; Summary of a Report to the European Commission's Directorate General for Research*, Dublin, May 2001, p. 7. EHMA's report was part of the European Commission's BIOMED2 program. It identified 233 regulations, directives, decisions, recommendations, and ECJ rulings issued between 1958 and 1988 which had the potential to affect member states' health systems. Of these regulations, almost two-thirds emanated from political decision-making and more than one-third from rulings of the European Court of Justice.
22. Marinker, M., (ed.): *Health Targets in Europe: Polity, Progress and Promise*, BMJ Books, 2002.
23. Commissie van de Europese Gemeenschappen: *Kostenbewaking bij de Planning en Organisatie van de Gezondheidszorg*. Werkdocument van de Commissie, COM (84) 1652 def., Brussels, 25 October 1984, p. 1.
24. Commissie van de Europese Gemeenschappen: *Communautaire Samenwerking op het Gebied van de Volksgezondheid.* Mededeling van de Commissie aan de Raad, COM(84) 502 def., Brussels, 18 September 1984, p. 11.
25. European Parliament, Directorate General for Research: *Health Care Systems in the EU: A Comparative Study*, Working Paper, Public Health and Consumer Protection Series, ibid., p. 5.
26. Commission of the European Communities: *Commission Communication on the Framework for Action in the Field of Public Health*, COM (93) 559 final, Brussels, 24 November 1993, p. 4.
27. Commission of the European Communities: *Commission Communication on the Framework for Action in the Field of Public Health*, ibid., p. 14.
28. Commission of the European Communities: Report from the Commission to the Council, the European Parliament and the Economic and Social Committee on the Integration of Health Protection Requirements in Community Policies, ibid., pp. 21–24.
29. Commission of the European Communities: Report from the Commission to the Council, the European Parliament and the Economic and Social

Committee on the Integration of Health Protection Requirements in Community Policies, ibid., p. 35.
30. Commission of the European Communities: *Communication from the Commission concerning a Community Action Programme on Health Monitoring in the Context of the Framework for Action in the Field of Public* Health, COM(95) 449 final, Brussels, 16 October 1995.
31. Commission of the European Communities: *The Future of Social Protection: A Framework for a European Debate*. Communication from the Commission, COM (95) 466 final, Brussels, 31 October 1995, p. 12.
32. Commissie van de Europese Gemeenschappen: Mededeling van de Commissie. *Modernisering en Verbetering van de Sociale Bescherming in de Europese Unie*, COM(97) 102 def., Brussels, 12 March 1997, p. 25.
33. Commission of the European Communities: *Communication from the Commission to the Council, the European Parliament, the Economic and Social Committee and the Committee of the Regions on the Health Strategy of the European Community. Proposal for a Decision of the European Parliament and of the Council adopting a Programme of Community Action in the Field of Public Health* (2001–2006), ibid. (2000) 285 final, Brussels, 16 May 2000, pp. 2, 3, 8, 10, 11.
34. European Parliament: Texts adopted at the Sitting of Thursday, 16 November 2000, provisional edition PE 297.763.
35. Commissie van de Europese Gemeenschappen: Mededeling van de Commissie aan de Raad, het Europees Parlement, het Economisch en Sociaal Comité en het Comité van de Regio's. *De Toekomst van de Gezondheidszorg en de Ouderenzorg: de Toegankelijkheid, de Kwaliteit en de Betaalbaarheid waarborgen*, ibid., p. 12.
36. McKee, M., Rosenmöller, M., MacLehose, L. and Zajac, M.: The Process of Enlargement, in: McKee, M., MacLehose, L., Nolte, E., (eds.): ibid., p. 14.
37. European Commission, Health & Consumer Protection Directorate-General: *The Internal Market and Health Services*. Report of the High Level Committee on Health, 17.12.2001, pp. 25–26.
38. Byrne, D.: The European Role in Patient Mobility, in: *Free Movement and Cross-Border Cooperation in Europe: The Role of Hospitals and Practical Experiences in Hospitals*, ibid., p. 29.
39. In 1996, the European Parliament had already requested the European Commission to submit a proposal regarding a European health card. Such a card would not only have to carry information regarding the civil status of its holder, but also information on his or her health condition, as well as social and health insurance data. As for the history of a European Health card, one can distinguish three phases: (a) 1978–1986, a period of good intentions mainly, because technically the card was not feasible yet; (b) 1986 to the beginning of the 1990s, a period during which some countries started to experiment with the idea of a health card, accompanied by technological research at European level; and (c) the period which started around the mid-1990s. Since then, the technology has been available, but it still has to overcome political obstacles. (Europees Parlement. Zittingsdocumenten: *Verslag over de Europesegezondheidskaart*, 26 March 1996).
40. Schemken, H-W.: Cross-Border Cooperation and Free Movement of Patients: the Point of View of the Financial Bodies, in: *Free Movement and Cross-Border*

Cooperation in Europe: The Role of Hospitals and Practical Experiences in Hospitals, ibid., p. 73.

41. Dehaye, J. C.: Interreg III Projects: French-Belgian Health Observatory (O.F.B.S.), Wallonia, Lorraine, Luxumbourg EEIG Luxlorsan, in: *Free Movement and Cross-Border Cooperation in Europe: The Role of Hospitals and Practical Experiences in Hospitals*, ibid., p. 93.
42. European Commission: *High Level Process of Reflection on Patient Mobility and Healthcare Developments in the European Union*, p. 4. The public health programme was adopted by the European Parliament and the Council of Ministers on the 23 September 2002 with the following general objectives (a) health information, (b) rapid reaction to health threats, and (c) health promotion.
43. In this respect, see: Theofilatou, M. A.: ibid., p. 28.
44. Gibis, B., Koch-Wulkan, P., and Bultman, J.: Shifting Criteria for Benefit Decisions in Social Health Insurance Systems, in: Saltman, R. B., Busse, R., Figueras, J., (eds.), ibid., p. 198.
45. McKee, M., MacLehose, L., and Albreht, T.: Free Movement of Patients, in: McKee, M., MacLehose, L., Nolte, E. (eds.), ibid., p. 168.
46. See: Standing Committee of the Hospitals of the European Union (HOPE): *Hospitals and Emergency Care in the European Union*, Leuven, undated.
47. Hermans, B. and Brouwer, W.: *Quality Issues on Cross-border Care: A Literature Search*, Rotterdam/Utrecht, June 2003, p. 43, www.ehma.org.
48. Zajac, M.: Free Movement of Health Professionals: The Polish Experience, in: McKee, M., MacLehose, L., Nolte, E., (eds.), ibid., p. 119.
49. It shows that the United Kingdom is the biggest importer of doctors, mainly due to the fact that English is the most internationally used language. In 1998, a total of 411 German doctors moved to the United Kingdom. For Greece their number was 291, followed by 200 from Italy and Ireland. In the same year, 219 doctors, mainly from Italy and Germany, emigrated to Greece.
50. Four projects of cross-border cooperation involve more than two national borders. An example in the cross-border cooperation in the south of the Netherlands with Belgium and German institutions.
51. Harant, Ph.: Hospital Cooperation in Border Regions in Europe, in: *Free Movement and Cross-Border Cooperation in Europe: The Role of Hospitals and Practical Experiences in Hospitals*, Proceeding of the HOPE Conference and Workshop, Luxembourg, June 2003, pp. 34–37.
52. Next to this, Hermans and Brouwer identify a number of problems which may seriously obstruct cross-border relations. They are (a) lack of funding, (b) lack of consistency and compatibility between different EU funding programs, (c) differences in administrative competences, (d) different tiers of government, (e) lack of experience, as well as language barriers and low prioritizing by authorities. In: Hermans, H. E. G. M. and Brouwer, W.: ibid., p. 83.
53. Scheres, J.: Cross-Border Health Care in the EU Region Meuse-Rhine: Pilot for Europe? in: *Free Movement and Cross-Border Cooperation in Europe: The Role of Hospitals and Practical Experiences*, ibid., pp. 40–42.
54. Weirauch, B.: Cross-Border Cooperation and Free Choice of Health Care for Patients from Various Viewpoints, in: *Free Movement and Cross-Border*

Cooperation in Europe: the Role of Hospitals and Practical Experiences in Hospitals, ibid., p. 59.
55. NVZ nieuws, jaargang 2003, No. 15, 16 April 2003.
56. An excellent overview of the health policy problems which have to be dealt with as a consequence of enlargement has been provided by McKee et al. (McKee, M., MacLehose, L., Nolte, E., (eds.): ibid.).
57. McKee, M., Rosenmöller, M., and Zajac, M.: ibid., p. 8.
58. McKee, M., Adany, R., and MacLehose, L.: Health Status and Trends in Candidate Countries, in: McKee, M., MacLehose, L., Nolte, E., (eds.): ibid., chapter 3.
59. McKee, M., Rosenmöller, M., MacLehose, L., and Zajac, M.: ibid., pp. 14–17.
60. McKee, M., Rosenmöller, M., MacLehose, L., and Zajac, M.: ibid., pp. 19–20.
61. Wright-Reid, A., McKee, M., and MacLehose, L.: Closing the Gap: Health and Safety, in: McKee, M., MacLehose, L., Nolte, E., (eds.): ibid., p. 180. In this respect, the World Bank estimates that two-thirds "of occupationally determined loss of healthy life years could be prevented by occupational health and safety programmes" (Wright-Reid, A., McKee, M., and MacLehose, L.: ibid., p. 180).
62. MacLehose, L., Coker, R., and McKee, M.: Communicable Disease Control: Detecting and Managing Communicable Disease Outbreaks across Borders, in: McKee. M., MacLehose, L., Nolte, E., (eds.): ibid., chapter 13.
63. Gilmore, A. B., Österberg, E., Heloma, A., Zatonski, W., Delcheva, E., and McKee, M.: Free Trade versus the Protection of Health: The Examples of Alcohol and Tobacco, in: McKee, M., MacLehose, L., Nolte, E., (eds.): ibid., p. 220.
64. Kanavos, P.: European Pharmaceutical Policy and Implications for Current Member States and Candidate Countries, in: McKee, M., MacLehose, L., Nolte, E., (eds.): ibid., pp. 240–264.
65. Hofmarcher, M. M. and Durand-Zaleski, I.: Contracting and Paying Providers in Social Health Insurance Systems in: Saltman, R. B., Busse, R., Figueras, J., (eds.): ibid., p. 220.
66. See: (1) Nicholas, S.: The Challenges of the Free Movement of Health Professionals; (2) Zajac, M.: ibid., and (3) Jakubowski, E. and Hess, R.: ibid. All three papers can be found in: McKee, M., MacLehose, L., Nolte, E., (eds.), ibid., chapters 7, 8, and 9.
67. McKee, M., MacLehose, L., and Albreht, T.: ibid., p. 169, table 11.1.
68. Dubois, C.-A. and McKee, M.: Health and Health Care in the Candidate Countries to the European Union: Common Challenges, Different Circumstances, Diverse Policies, in: McKee, M., MacLehorse, L., Nolte, E., (eds.): ibid., chapter 4.
69. Dubois, C.-A. and McKee, M.: ibid., p. 49.
70. Kanavos, P.: ibid., p. 261.

Chapter 8

1. See chapter 6, reference 39.
2. Nevertheless, when in 1978 I applied for the position of CEO in an acute hospital in the middle of the Netherlands, it appeared that out of the board of seven supervisors, six were ministers of religion.

3. OECD: *New Directions in Health Care Policy*, Health Policy Studies No. 7, OECD, Paris 1995, table 4, p. 12.
4. Banta, D.: ibid., p. 5.
5. NZR: Sectie Psychiatrische Instituten. Rapport van de Subwerkgroep LIT, ingesteld door de werkgroep fase II/III van het tripartite overleg, March 1975, appendix.
6. As for the position of the medical establishment in society, there is much difference between the developments in the United States, on the one hand, and those in the countries of the European Union, on the other.
7. See for this history: Ludmerer, K. M.: ibid.
8. Ludmerer, K. M.: ibid., p. 24.
9. Ludmerer, K. M.: ibid., p. 38.
10. Fanu, J. le: ibid., p. 191.
11. Fanu, J. le: ibid., p. 192.
12. Fanu, J. le: ibid., p. 192.
13. Ludmerer, K. M.: ibid., pp. 141–142.
14. Ludmerer, K. M.: ibid., p. 151.
15. Ludmerer, K. M.: ibid., p. 197.
16. Ludmerer, K. M.: ibid., p. 212, table 7.
17. Ludmerer, K. M.: ibid., p. 180.
18. Ludmerer, K. M.: ibid., p. 69.
19. For a brief summary of medical progress during the first decades after the Second World War see: Healy, J. and McKee, M.: The Evolution of Hospital Systems, in: McKee, M., Healy, J., (eds.): ibid., p. 17.
20. Ludmerer, K. M.: ibid., p. 279.
21. The Panama Canal, for example, probably would not have been completed without the elimination of yellow fever (Ludmerer, K. M.: ibid., p. 23).
22. Ludmerer, K. M.: ibid., pp. 23 and 279.
23. Ludmerer, K. M.: ibid., p. 38.
24. As for test-ordering, research in the 1970s showed that 25% of the average hospital bill was for laboratory and radiological studies. Yet only 5% of laboratory information was actually used in treatment and diagnosis (Ludmerer, K. M.: ibid., p. 324).
25. Freidson, E.: ibid., pp. 22–23.
26. Ludmerer, K. M.: ibid., p. 187.
27. Fanu, J. le: ibid., p. 253.
28. Fanu, J. le: ibid., p. 261.
29. Mechanic, D.: ibid., p. 40.
30. Fanu, J, le: ibid., p. 271.
31. Fanu, J. le: ibid., p. 252.
32. OECD Health Data 2003, third edition.
33. Ludmerer, K. M.: ibid., p. 210.
34. Fanu, J. le: ibid., p. 257.
35. Ludmerer, K. M.: ibid., pp. 222 and 228.
36. Dranove, D.: *The Economic Evolution of American Health Care: From Marcus Welby to Managed Care*, Princeton University Press, 2000, p. 49.
37. Fanu, J. le: ibid., p. 202.
38. Nevertheless, there were millions of Americans who, though not entitled to Medicaid, could not pay for private insurance. Happily therefore, although

many charitable patients had become private patients, charitable care did not disappear (Ludmerer, K. M.: ibid., p. 267).

39. Over the period 1968–1978, the number of traineeships awarded by the American National Institute of Health to doctors wishing to undertake postdoctoral research decreased from 3,000 to 1,500 (Fanu, J. le: ibid., p. 244).
40. Ludmerer, K. M.: ibid., p. 227.
41. Ludmerer, K. M.: ibid., p. 332.
42. Ludmerer, K. M.: ibid., p. 365.
43. Ludmerer, K. M.: ibid., p. 348.
44. Ludmerer, K. M.: ibid., p. 119.
45. Ludmerer, K. M.: ibid., p. 340.
46. Ludmerer, K. M.: ibid., p. 327.
47. Ludmerer, K. M.: ibid., p. 333.
48. Dranove, D.: ibid., p. 47.
49. Ludmerer, K. M.: ibid., p. 278. Characteristic of this arrogant behavior is what the Association of Medical Colleges declared, testifying before Congress in 1969: "It is interesting to speculate about the medical advances which might have occurred in the past decade if a sum equal to that invested in space exploration had been spent on health research" (Ludmerer, K. M.: ibid., p. 147).
50. Ludmerer, K. M.: ibid., p. 337.
51. Ludmerer, K. M.: ibid., pp. 286–287.
52. Mossialos, E. and Le Grand, J.: ibid., p. 57, table 1.16. According to this table, the exceptions are Belgium (99%), Germany (92.2%), Spain (99.3%), France (99.5%), the Netherlands (74.1%), and Austria (99%).
53. Financiële Overzichten Gezondheidszorg 1977–1983.
54. In this respect, research among Dutch citizens showed that over the period 1966–1985 "good health" had become by far the highest priority, climbing from 36 to 58, compared to "marriage" from 34 to 15, "family life" from 8 to 12, and "religion" from 16 to 5 (Sociaal en Cultureel Planbureau: *Sociaal en Cultureel Rapport 1996*). The researchers conclude that this trend applies for the whole of Western Europe (Sociaal en Cultureel Planbureau: *Sociaal en Cultureel Rapport 1994*, Rijswijk, 1994, p. 502).
55. Ludmerer, K. M.: ibid., p. 227.
56. Policies of corporatism were not limited to health care. Many countries of the EU in those days suffered from policy divisions along departmental lines (Trappenburg, M.: ibid., pp. 6–7).
57. Theurl, E.: Health Expenditure and Cost Control in Austria, in: Mossialos, E. and Le Grand, J., (eds.): ibid., p. 608.
58. O'Neill, P.: *Health Crisis 2000*, WHO Regional Office for Europe, Copenhagen, 1983, p. 15.
59. From: *Measuring Health Care, 1960–1983*, OECD, Paris, 1985. Portugal has been left out, since there were only figures available for 1975 and 1980.
60. See: Kanavos, P. and Yfantopoulos, J.: Cost Containment and Health Expenditure in the EU: A Macroeconomic Perspective, in: Mossialos, E. and Le Grand, J., (eds.): ibid., pp. 155–196. For a critical view regarding international comparisons, see: Turner, A.: *Just Capital: The Liberal Economy*, Pan Books, 2002, chapter 4.
61. I realize that this says nothing about the distribution of GDP and health care expenditure among citizens.

62. Mossialos and Le Grand rightfully argue that "international comparisons are only as good as the data on which they are based" (Mossialos, E. and Le Grand, J., (eds.): ibid., pp. 42–46).
63. Mossialos, E. and Le Grand, J.: Cost Containment in the EU: An Overview, in: Mossialos, E. and Le Grand, J., (eds.): ibid., p. 46.
64. Mosseveld, C. J. P. M. van: *International Comparison of Health Care Expenditure: Existing Frameworks, Innovations and Data Use*, Voorburg, 2003, p. XXII.
65. All figures in US$ PPP. GDP figures do not account for the informal economy or the informal health care sector, which, particularly in the southern countries of the European Union, is probably considerable (Mossialos, E., Dixon, A., Figueras, J., Kutzin, J., (eds.): ibid., p. 8).
66. From, respectively, the OECD Health Data 2002 and the OECD publication: *Social Expenditure 1960–1980: Problems of Growth and Control*, OECD Social Policy Studies, 1985. It should be noted that in the latter publication, quite a number of figures are OECD estimates. GDP figures, measured in US$ PPP, were taken from the OECD's *Quick Query* (OECD Health Data 2002, 29 April 2004). In the OECD's overview on social expenditure 1960–1980, health care refers to "expenditure on hospitals, clinics and medical, dental and paramedical practitioners, public health, medicaments, protheses, medical equipment and appliances or other prescribed health-related products, and applied research and experimental development related to health and medical delivery systems." Expenditure on education (in the second graph of this chapter) includes "pre-primary, primary, secondary, tertiary, education affairs and services and subsidiary services to education." Social security in the second graph of this chapter relates, first of all, to pensions (expenditure on old-age, disability, or survivors' benefits, other than for government employees, and government employee pensions). Furthermore, it includes unemployment compensation (expenditure on social insurance and other government schemes to individuals to compensate for loss of income due to unemployment), as well as expenditure on sickness, maternity or temporary disablement benefits, family and child allowances, other social assistance, and welfare affairs and services.
67. It has to be taken into account that the inflation rate during this period had a considerable influence on the slope of the lines.
68. Goodin, R. E., Heady, B., Muffels, R., and Dirven, H-J.: The Real Worlds of Welfare Capitalism, in: Pierson, Chr. and Castles, F., (eds.); ibid., p. 182.
69. Baumol, W. J.: Macro-economics of Unbalanced Growth. The Autonomy of Workers Crisis, in: *American Economic Review*, Volume 57, no. 3, 1967.
70. Sociaal en Cultureel Planbureau: *Sociaal en Cultureel Rapport 1996*, Rijswijk, 1996, p. 467.
71. Sociaal en Cultureel Planbureau: *Sociaal en Cultureel Rapport 1994*, ibid.: p. 502.
72. Sociaal en Cultureel Planbureau: *Sociaal en Cultureel Rapport 1996*, ibid., p. 469.
73. Mossialos and Le Grand observe that most of the "new" highly priced pharmaceutical products are not significant innovations (Mossialos, E. and Le Grand, J.: ibid., p. 61).
74. Fanu, J. le: ibid., part two. Also see section 6.2.1.
75. Fanu, J. le: ibid., p. 272.

76. Fanu, J. le: ibid., p. 373.
77. Fanu, J. le: ibid., pp. 348–349.
78. Fanu, J. le: ibid., p. 343.
79. Fanu, J. le: ibid., p. 373 and 381.
80. Fanu, J. le: ibid., part three, chapter 1.
81. Fanu, J. le: ibid., p. 395.
82. Fanu, J. le: ibid., pp. 394–395.
83. Fanu, J. le: ibid., p. 398.
84. Coulter, A. and Magee, H., (eds.): ibid., p. 64.
85. Coulter, A. and Magee, H., (eds.): ibid., p. 145.
86. Honoré, C.: ibid., p. 119.
87. Coulter, A. and Magee, H., (eds.): ibid., p. 41.
88. Honoré, C.: ibid., p. 120.
89. Wheen, F.: ibid., p. 133.
90. Illich, I.: ibid.
91. The term *iatrogeneses* refers to the consequences of medical treatment which may inevitably involve unwanted and damaging side effects. The Dutch physician Tempelaar distinguishes between five damaging causes of medical intervention: (1) taking risks, (2) unexpected complications, (3) too few interventions, (4) too many interventions, and (5) wrong interventions (in: Boer, J. de: ibid., p. 13).
92. Comparable American criticism was published three years later in a report from 20 prominent physicians, economists, and politicians. In this report, it was concluded that despite tremendous success in health care, people's health had not improved significantly (Boer, J. de: ibid., p. 4).
93. Tempelaar, A. F.: Disfunctioneren als Iatrogene Factor, in: Lens, P. and Kahn, Ph. S., (eds.): ibid., p. 232.
94. Foudraine, J.: *Wie is van Hout? Een Gang door de Psychiatrie*, Ambo boeken, Baarn, 1971.
95. Foudraine, J.: *Oorspronkelijk Gezicht: Een Gang naar Huis*, Ambo boeken, Baarn, 1979, p. 30.
96. Malleson, A.: *Need Your Doctor Be So Useless?* (Dutch Translation), Het Spectrum, 1974.
97. Taylor, R.: *Medicine Out of Control* (Dutch Translation), De Tijdstroom, Lochem, 1983.
98. Ludmerer, K. M.: ibid., p. 279.
99. O'Neill, P.: ibid., in particular pp. ix, 2, and 6.
100. O'Neill, P.: ibid., p. 42.
101. Ludmerer, K. M.: ibid., p. 280.
102. Freidson, E.: ibid., p. 73.
103. Ensor, T. and Duran-Moreno, A.: Corruption as a Challenge to Effective Regulation in the Health Sector, in: Saltman, R. B., Busse, R., Mossialos, E., (eds.): *Regulating Entrepreneurial Behaviour in European Health Care Systems*, Open University Press, 2003, p. 112.
104. Sparrow, M. K.: ibid.
105. Glied, S.: ibid., p. 38.
106. Ensor, T. and Duran-Moreno, A.: ibid., p. 109.
107. Ensor, T. and Duran-Moreno, A.: ibid., p. 113.
108. Ensor, T. and Duran-Moreno, A.: ibid., chapter five.

109. Department of Health: *Countering Fraud in the NHS*, London, October 1998.
110. Bos, M. A. J. M.: Fraudeonderzoek en Fraudebestrijding, in: Lens, P. and Kahn, Ph. S., (eds.): ibid., pp. 137–152.
111. *Resultaten Inventarisatie Fraudebeleid 2003*, Zorgverzekeraars Nederland.
112. European Observatory on Health Care Systems: *Health Care Systems in Transition*. Luxembourg 1999, WHO Regional Office for Europe, Copenhagen, 1999, p. 47.
113. European Healthcare Fraud & Corruption Conference: *Countering Healthcare Fraud and Corruption in Europe*, The European Healthcare Fraud and Corruption Declaration, AGIS 2004.

Chapter 9

1. I follow Saltman and Figueras, who define reform as "a process that involves sustained and profound institutional and structural change, led by government and seeking to attain a series of explicit policy objectives" (Saltman, R. B. and Figueras, J.: ibid., p. 3).
2. Much of the factual information in this chapter is from the European Observatory Reports "Health Care Systems in Transition," WHO Regional Office for Europe, Copenhagen. These reports cover the period 1999–2004, except for Greece (1996).
3. Altenstetter, Ch.: Health Policy-Making in Germany: Stability and Dynamics, in: Altenstetter, Ch. and Björkman, J. W., (eds.): ibid., pp. 143–144.
4. See: Scrivens, E.: ibid., chapter 2.
5. Plumptre and Graham define governance as "the process whereby, within accepted traditions and institutional frameworks, interests are articulated by different sectors of society, decisions are taken, and decision-makers are held to account" (Chinitz, D., Wismar, M., and Le Pen, C.: Governance and (Self-) Regulation in Social Health Insurance Systems, in: Saltman, R. B., Busse, R., Figueras J., (eds.): ibid., p. 156).
6. Scrivens, E.: ibid., p. 19. It has been suggested that the origins of modern corporate governance stem from the Watergate scandal in the United States (Scrivens, E.: ibid., p. 20).
7. Scrivens, E.: ibid., p. 18.
8. British Ministry of Health: *The New NHS: Modern-Dependable*, London, 1997.
9. British Ministry of Health: *The New NHS: Modern-Dependable*, ibid., pp. 48–49.
10. Omachonu, V. K.: *Total Quality and Productivity Management in Health Care Organizations*, Institute of Industrial Engineers, Georgia, 1991, pp. 77–78.
11. Hjortsberg, C. and Ghatnekar, O.: *Health Care Systems in Transition: Sweden 2001*, in: Rico, A., Wisbaum, W. and Cetani, T., (eds.): European Observatory on Health Systems, WHO Regional Office for Europe, Copenhagen, 2001, p. 54.
12. Hofmarcher, M. M. and Rack, H.: *Health Care Systems in Transition: Austria 2001*, in: Dixon, A., (ed.): European Observatory on Health Care Systems, WHO Regional Office for Europe, Copenhagen, 2001, p. 24.
13. Hofmarcher, M. M. and Rack, H.: ibid., p. 101.
14. Sandier, S., Paris, V., Polton, D.: ibid., p. 33.

15. Exter, A. den, Hermans, H., Dosljak, M., and Busse, R.: *Health Care Systems in Transition. Netherlands 2004*, in: Busse, R., Ginneken, E. van, Schreyögg, J., Wisbaum, W., (eds.): European Observatory on Health Care Systems, WHO Regional Office for Europe, Copenhagen, 2004, p. 22.
16. Exter, A. den, Hermans, H., Dosljak, M., and Busse, R.: ibid., p. 26.
17. Health Policy Monitor, international network for Health Policy & Reform, Bertelsmann Stiftung, survey, January 2003.
18. Examples are Italy, Spain, and Portugal.
19. European Observatory on Health Care Systems: *Health Care Systems in Transition*: United Kingdom 1999 WHO Regional Office for Europe, Copenhagen, 1999, p. 37.
20. Hofmarcher, M. M. and Rack, H.: ibid., p. 40.
21. Vallgärda, S. Krasnik, A., and Vrangbæk, K.: ibid., p. 79.
22. Järvelin, J.: *Health Care Systems in Transition: Finland 2002*, European Observatory on Health Care Systems, WHO Regional Office for Europe, Copenhagen, 2002, p. 27.
23. Bentes, M., Dias, C. M., Sakellarides, C., and Bankauskaite, V.: *Health Care Systems in Transition: Portugal 2004*, European Observatory on Health Care Systems, WHO Regional Office for Europe, p. 26.
24. Glied, S.: ibid., p. 48.
25. Wildner, M., Exter, A. P. den, and Kraan, W. G. M. van der: The Changing Role of the Individual in Social Health Insurance Systems, in: Saltman, R. B., Busse, R., Figueras, J., (eds.): ibid., p. 257.
26. Saltman, R. B. and Busse, R.: Balancing Regulation and Entrepreneurialism in Europe's Health Sector: Theory and Practice, in: Saltman, R. B., Busse, R., Mossialos, E., (eds.): *Regulating Entrepreneurial Behaviour in European Health Care Systems*, Open University Press, 2003, p. 47.
27. Legemaate, J.: Regelgeving in Nederland, in: Lens, P. and Kahn, Ph. S., (eds.): ibid., p. 63.
28. Scrivens, E.: Accreditation and the Regulation of Quality in Health Services, in: Saltman, R. B., Busse, R., Mossialos, E., (eds.): ibid., p. 95.
29. Crul, B. V. M.: De Media en de Disfunctionerende Dokter, in: Lens, P. and Kahn, Ph. S., (eds.): ibid., p. 470.
30. Most Swedish county councils have developed their own website to inform citizens about health matters, patients' rights, and the structure and organization of the health care system (Coulter, A. and Magee, H., (eds.): ibid., p. 147.
31. Coulter, A. and Magee, H., (eds.): ibid., p. 44.
32. Dranove, D.: ibid., p. 13.
33. Coulter, A. and Magee, H., (eds.): ibid., p. 46.
34. Hofmarcher, M. M. and Rack, H.: ibid., p. 19.
35. Coulter, A. and Magee, H., (eds.): ibid., p. 128.
36. Bentes, M., Dias, C. M., Sakellarides, C., and Bankauskaite, V.: ibid., pp. 31–32.
37. Mossialos, E. and Le Grand, J., (eds.): ibid., p. 33.
38. Vallgårda, S., Krasnik, A., and Vrangbæk, K.: ibid., p. 25.
39. Håkansson, S. and Nordling, S.: The Health System of Sweden, in: Raffel, M. W., (ed.), ibid., p. 205.
40. Hjortsberg, C. and Ghatnekar, O.: ibid., pp. 21–23.
41. Järvelin, J.: ibid., p. 28.

42. Bentes, M., Dias, C. M., Sakellarides, C., and Bankauskaite, V.: ibid., pp. 31–32.
43. García-Altés, A.: Health Care Coverage Determinations in Spain, in: Stoltzfus Jost, T., (ed.): ibid., p. 158.
44. García-Altés, A.: ibid., p. 160.
45. García-Altés, A.: ibid., p. 160.
46. Scrivens, E.: ibid., p. 1.
47. Scrivens, E.: ibid., p. 17
48. European Observatory on Health Care Systems: *Health Care Systems in Transition: United Kingdom 1999*, ibid., pp. 18–19.
49. Walshe, K.: *Regulating Health Care: A Prescription for Improvement?* Open University Press, 2003, p. 12.
50. Cookson, R., Goddard, M., and Gravelle, H.: Regulating Health Care Markets, in: Smith, P. C., Ginelly, L., Sculpher, M., (eds.): ibid., pp. 122–123.
51. European Observatory on Health Care Systems: *Health Care Systems in Transition: Germany 2000*, WHO Regional Office for Europe, Copenhagen, 2000.
52. Reid, T. R.: ibid., p. 159.
53. OECD: *Internal Markets in the Making: Health Systems in Canada, Iceland and the United Kingdom*, Health Policy Studies No. 6, OECD, Paris, 1995, p. 9.
54. OECD: *Internal Markets in the Making: Health Systems in Canada, Iceland and the United Kingdom*, ibid., p. 13.
55. OECD: *Internal Markets in the Making: Health Systems in Canada, Iceland and the United Kingdom*, ibid., pp. 9–27.
56. Hayman, H.: ibid., p. 164.
57. Blair, T.: *New Britain: My Vision of a Young Country*, London, 1996, p. 69.
58. Wheen, F.: ibid., p. 219.
59. Wheen, F.: ibid., p. 222.
60. The National Audit Office calculated that 35% of the savings were used to improve fund-holders' surgeries, 25% for surgeries' design, and 15% for medical instruments (National Audit Office: *General Practitioner: Fund-holding in England*, Report by the Comptroller and Auditor General, London, HMSO, HC 51, session 1994–5, 9 December 1994).
61. OECD: *Internal Markets in the Making: Health Systems in Canada, Iceland and the United Kingdom*, ibid., p. 22.
62. Donatoni, A., Rico, A., D'Ambrosio, M. G., Lo Scalzo, A., Orzella, L., Cicchetti, A., and Profili, S.: Health Care Systems in Transition: Italy 2001, in: Rico, A. and Cetani, T., (eds.): *European Observatory on Health Care Systems*, WHO Regional Office for Europe, Copenhagen, 2001, p. 32.
63. Donatoni, A., Rico, A., D'Ambrosio, M. G., Lo Scalzo, A., Orzella, L., Cicchetti, A., and Profili, S.: ibid., p. 93.
64. Bentes, M., Dias, C. M., Sakellarides, C., and Bankauskaite, V.: ibid., pp. 91–92.
65. Vallgårda, S., Krasnik, A., and Vrangbæk, K.: ibid., p. 81. Austria also outsourced these services in the late 1980s and early 1990s (Hofmarcher, M. M. and Rack, H.: ibid., p. 102).
66. Hjortsberg, C. and Ghatnekar, O.: ibid., pp. 86–88.
67. Hjortsberg, C. and Ghatnekar, O.: ibid., p. 19.
68. European Observatory on Health Care Systems: *Health Care Systems in Transition: Spain 2000*, ibid., pp. 106–109.
69. Exter, A. den, Hermans, H., Dosljak, M., Busse, R.: ibid., p. 114.
70. Sandier, S., Paris, V., Polton, D.: ibid., p. 118.

71. For the Netherlands see: Exter, A. den, Hermans, H., Dosljak, M., and Busse, O.: ibid., pp. 124–125.
72. Johson, H. T. and Kaplan, R. S.: *Relevance Lost: The Rise and Fall of Management Accounting*, Harvard Business School Press, 1987, p. 260.
73. Johson, H. Y. and Kaplan, R. S.: ibid., p. 155.
74. OECD: *New Directions in Health Care Policy*, Health Policy Studies No. 7, OECD, Paris, 1995, p. 60.
75. Greiner, W. and Schulenburg, J-M Graf v. d.: The Health System of Germany, in: Raffel, M. W., (ed.), ibid., p. 88.
76. Sandier, S., Paris, V., Polton, D.: ibid., pp. 70–73.
77. Hofmarcher, M. M. and Rack, H.: ibid., p. 62.
78. World Health Organization: *Health Care Systems in Transition: Greece 1996*, WHO Regional Office for Europe, 1996, p. 13.
79. García-Altés, A.: ibid., p. 160.
80. European Observatory on Health Care Systems: *Health Care Systems in Transition: United Kingdom 1999*, ibid., p. 68.
81. Boelens, E. and Schreuder, R. F.: *Platform Privatisering in de Gezondheidszorg: Terreinverkenning en Aandachtspunten voor Beleid*, Health Management Forum, 1999, chapter 3.
82. In this respect, 1999 research among 2,400 people living in Stockholm showed that 25% of the respondents thought that they had to wait too long to be able to see their general practitioner. A similar result came out of national research among 3,200 Swedes one year later. The number of people who thought their waiting time to see a doctor had become unacceptably long doubled between 1994 and 1999 (Coulter, A. and Magee, H., (eds.): ibid., p. 136).
83. College Bouw Ziekenhuisvoorzieningen: *Signaleringsrapport het zelfstandig Behandelcentrum: van noodzakelijk Kwaad tot nuttig Goed?*, Voorstel voor een nieuw Beoordelingskader, Utrecht, 2003.
84. Brief van de minister van Volksgezondheid, Welzijn en Sport aan de Voorzitter van de Tweede Kamer der Staten-Generaal, de dato 31 maart 2003 (kenmerk: CZ/IZ-2369484).
85. In: Edwards, P., Shaoul, J., Stafford, A., Arblaster, L.: *Evaluating the Operation of PFI in Roads and Hospitals*, the Association of Chartered Certified Accountants, London, 2004, p. 15.
86. In fact, there are at least seven types of PPS, being (1) Design and Construct; (2) Operate and Maintain; (3) Design, Build, Operate; (4) Build, Own, Operate, Transfer; (5) Build, Own, Operate; (6) Lease, Own, Operate; and (7) Alliance (College Bouw Ziekenhuisvoorzieningen: Publiek Private Samenwerking in de Gezondheidszorg. Een vergelijkende Studie, Signaleringsrapport, Rapportnummer 568, Utrecht, 2004, pp. 4–5).
87. Under Private Finance Initiatives, "the public sector procures a capital asset and non-core services from the private sector on a long-term contract, typically at least 30 years, in return for an annual payment" (Edwards, P., Shaoul, J., Stafford, A., Arblaster, L.: ibid., p. 7).
88. Edwards, P., Shaoul, J., Stafford, A., Arblaster, L.: ibid., p. 8.
89. Edwards, P., Shaoul, J., Stafford, A., Arblaster, L.: ibid., p. 135.
90. Busse, R., Grinten, T. van der, and Svensson, P.-G.: Regulating Entrepreneurial Behaviour in Hospitals: Theory and Practice, in: Saltman, R. B., Busse, R., Mossialos, E., (eds.): ibid., p. 137.

91. Edwards, P., Shaoul, J., Stafford, A., Arblaster, L.: ibid., p. 173.
92. Edwards, P., Shaoul, J., Stafford, A., Arblaster, L.: ibid., p. 174.
93. College Bouw Ziekenhuisvoorzieningen: *Publiek Private Samenwerking in de Gezondheidszorg. Een vergelijkende Studie*, Signaleringsrapport, Rapportnummer 568, Utrecht, 2004, p. VI.
94. Edwards, P., Shaoul, J., Stafford, A., Arblaster, L.: ibid., p. 144.
95. Bentes, M., Dias, C. M., Sakellarides, C., and Bankauskaite, V.: ibid., pp. 38–39.
96. European Observatory on Health Care Systems: *Health Care Systems in Transition: Spain, 2000*, ibid., p. 119.
97. Donatini, A., Rico, A., D'Ambrosio, M. G., Lo Scalzo, A., Orzella, L., Cicchetti, A., and Profili, S.: ibid., pp. 44–45.
98. A similar survey of 1993 showed that 55% of the respondents argued that the sickness funds should pay for everything, with 41% excluding coverage for certain diseases (*European Observatory on Health Care Systems*: Health Care Systems in Transition: Germany, 2000, ibid., p. 44).
99. New, B. and Le Grand, J.: *Rationing in the NHS: Principles & Pragmatism*, King's Fund, London, 1996, p. 17.
100. The Netherlands did so by organizing a public debate after the Dunning report was released in 1992. The British government encouraged health authorities to involve the general public in decisions about rationing and priority-setting. At the local level, the British applied numerous methods for eliciting the public's view, including population surveys, public meetings, citizens' juries, et cetera (The European Observatory on Health Care Systems: *Health Care System in Transition: United Kingdom 1999*, ibid., p. 39).
101. European Observatory on Health Care Systems: *Health Care Systems in Transition: United Kingdom*, 1999, ibid., p. 35.
102. In Italy, the second National Health Plan (1998–2000) stressed the need to define such a package, but to date there has been little progress in this respect. Discussions in Portugal about defining a basic package have not yet resulted in decisions.
103. Järvelin, J.: ibid., p. 33.
104. Hjortsberg, C. and Ghatnekar, O.: ibid., pp. 27–28.
105. Gezondheidsraad: *Grenzen van de Gezondheidszorg*, Den Haag, 1986.
106. Government Committee on Choices in Health Care: Choices in Health Care, Ministry of Welfare, Health and Cultural Activities, Rijswijk, the Netherlands, 1992.
107. The European Observatory on Health Care Systems: *Health Care System in Transition: United Kingdom, 1999*, ibid., p. 40.
108. In: Standing Committee of the Hospitals of the European Union. Subcommittee on Economics and Planning: *Hospitals and Health Care Rationing*, Leuven, September 2000, p. 5.
109. New, B. and Le grand, J.: ibid.
110. Wille, E., (ed.): *Rationierung im Gesundheitswesen und ihre Alternativen*, Nomos Verlagsgesellschaft, Baden-Baden, 2003.
111. New, B. and Le Grand, J.: ibid., p. 21.
112. Standing Committee of the Hospitals of the European Union. Subcommittee on Economics and Planning: *Hospital and Health Care Rationing*, ibid., p. 12.
113. Berg and Van der Grinten distinguish between four types of strategy: (1) the introduction of health technology assessment, (2) assessment of the basic

package, (3) the use of waiting lists, and (4) stimulating appropriate use of health care (Berg, M. and Grinten, T. van der: The Netherlands, in: Ham, Ch. and Glenn, R., (eds.): *Reasonable Rationing: International Experience of Priority Setting in Health Care*, Open University Press, 2003, p. 119).

114. As an example: The United Kingdom has a National Institute of Clinical Excellence (NICE) to evaluate drugs and technologies, which provides a mechanism to control their introduction and to support equity of access. Furthermore, Banta reports on several initiatives regarding technology assessment, coordinated through an international network (Banta, D.: ibid).
115. European Observatory on Health Care Systems: *Health Care Systems in Transition: Luxembourg, 1999*, ibid., p. 49.
116. European Observatory on Health Care Systems: *Health Care Systems in Transition: Belgium, 2000*, pp. 59–61.
117. Donatini, A., Rico, A., D'Ambrosio, M. G., Lo Scalzo, A., Orzella, L., Cicchetti, A., and Profili, S.: ibid., pp. 81–82.
118. European Observatory on Health Care Systems: *Health Care Systems in Transition: Spain*, ibid., p. 99.
119. Stoltzfus Jost, T.: What Can We Learn From Our Country Studies? in: Stoltzfus Jost, T., (ed.): ibid., p. 240.
120. European Observatory on Health Care Systems: *Health Care Systems in Transition: United Kingdom, 1999*, WHO Regional Office for Europe, p. 83.
121. Nevertheless, since its inception, the program has allocated around £40 million to some 180 assessment projects. The program was devolved to a large number of local commissioners, physicians, and hospital managers.
122. Newdick, Ch.: Evaluating New Health Technology in the English National Health Service, in: Stoltzfus Jost, T., (ed.): ibid., p. 88.
123. Newdick, Ch.: ibid., p. 93.
124. In addition to NICE, the United Kingdom has a counterpart for social care with the establishment of the Social Care Institute for Excellence in 2001 (Scrivens, E.: ibid., p. 27).
125. Gibis, B., Koch-Wulkan, P., and Bultman, J.: Shifting Criteria for Benefit Decisions in Social Health Insurance Systems, in: Saltman, R. B., Busse, R., Figueras, J., (eds.): ibid., p. 193.
126. For a detailed description, see: Carino, T., and Rutten, F.: Health Care Coverage in the Netherlands: The Dutch Drug Reimbursement Scheme (GVS), in: Stoltzfus Jost, T., (ed.): ibid., chapter 6.
127. Carino, T. and Rutten, F.: ibid., p. 137.
128. Carino, T. and Rutten, F.: ibid., p. 138.
129. Vallgårda, S., Krasnik, A., and Vrangbæk, K.: ibid., p. 69.
130. Stoltzfus Jost, T., (ed.): ibid.
131. Raad voor de Volksgezondheid en Zorg: *Technologische Innovatie in de Zorgsector*, ibid., p. 72.
132. Bentes, M., Dias, C. M., Sakellarides, C., and Bankauskaite, V.: ibid., p. 72.
133. Stoltzfus Jost, T., (ed.): ibid., p. 254.
134. Carino, T. and Rutten, F.: ibid., p. 141.
135. Nederlandse Zorgfederatie: *Gezondheidszorg in Tel 4*, Utrecht, 1996, p. 193.
136. See for example: Nederlandse Zorgfederatie: *Gezondheidszorg in Tel 6*, Utrecht, 1998.
137. Vallgärda, S., Krasnik, A., and Vrangbæk, K.: ibid., p. 80.

138. Bentes, M., Dias, C. M., Sakellarides, C., and Bankauskaite, V.: ibid., pp. 62–64.
139. Hjortsberg, C. and Ghatnekar, O.: ibid., p. 81.
140. European Observatory on Health Care Systems: *Health Care Systems in Transition: United Kingdom, 1999*, ibid., pp. 36–38.
141. Ham, Ch. and Coulter, A.: International Experience of Rationing, in: Ham, Ch. and Robert, G., (eds.): ibid., p. 8.
142. Appleby, J.: ibid., p. 135.
143. Berg, M. and Grinten, T. van der: ibid., p. 130.
144. Vallgårda, S., Krasnik, A., and Vrangbæk, K.: ibid., pp. 83–84.
145. Sandier, S., Paris, V., and Polton, D.: ibid., p. 65.
146. Sandier, S., Paris, V., and Polton, D.: ibid., p. 128.
147. European Observatory on Health Care Systems: *Health Care Systems in Transition: Belgium, 2000*, ibid., pp. 75–77.
148. Järvelin, J.: ibid., p. 27.
149. Donatini, A., Rico, A., D'Ambrosio, M. G., Lo Scalzo, A., Orzella, L., Cicchetti, A., and Profili, S.: ibid., pp. 102–103.
150. European Observatory on Health Care Systems: *Health Care Systems in Transition: United Kingdom, 1999*, ibid., p. 23.
151. European Observatory on Health Care Systems: *Health Care Systems in Transition: United Kingdom, 1999*, ibid., pp. 25 and 27.
152. European Observatory on Health Care Systems: *Health Care Systems in Transition: United Kingdom, 1999*, ibid., p. 28.
153. European Observatory on Health Care Systems: *Health Care Systems in Transition: United Kingdom, 1999*, ibid., p. 30.
154. White, S. and Stancombe, J.: *Clinical Judgement in the Health and Welfare Professions: Extending the Evidence Base*, Open University Press, 2003, p. 25.
155. Gunning-Schepers, L. J.: Verkleining van sociaal-economische Gezondheidsverschillen vanuit de Zorg: bestuurlijke en politieke implicaties, in: Stronks, K. and Hulshof, J., (eds.): *De Kloof verkleinen. Theorie en Praktijk van de Strijd tegen sociaal-economische Gezondheidsverschillen*, Van Gorcum, 2001, p. 132.
156. White, S. and Stancombe, J.: ibid., p. viii.
157. White, S. and Stancombe, J.: ibid., p. 20.
158. White, S. and Stancombe, J.: ibid., p. ix.
159. White, S. and Stancimbe, J.: ibid., p. 17.
160. Glied, S.: ibid., p. 72
161. Mossialos and Le Grand present a threefold classification of cost-containment measures: budget shifting, budget setting, and direct and indirect controls (Mossialos, E. and Le Grand, J.: ibid., p. 62).
162. Hofmarcher, M. M. and Durand-Zaleski, I.: Contracting and Paying Providers in Social Health Insurance Systems, in: Saltmans, R. B., Busse, R., Figueras, J., (eds.): ibid., p. 220.
163. Consequently, the number of drug prescriptions fell by 11% in 1994.
164. The drug expenditure budget in Italy was exceeded by 8.7%, 11.6%, and 16.5% in 1998, 1999, and 2000, respectively.
165. Reference-pricing is only useful if products are interchangeable because they have similar therapeutical effects or produce similar outcomes (Mossialos, E. and Mrazek, M.: Entrepreneurial Behaviour in Pharmaceutical Markets and

the Effects of Regulation, in: Saltman, R. B., Busse, R., Mossialos, E., (eds.): ibid., p. 155).

166. For patients, reference-pricing had two effects. Firstly, reference-priced drugs were without copayments, and secondly, copayments were charged when patients chose non-reference-priced drugs.
167. Reference-pricing came under threat in 1999 when a German court ruled that price-setting by the sickness funds (the price-setters) violated European Union cartel regulations.
168. Mossialos, E. and Mrazek, M.: ibid., p. 155.
169. Belgium has generic drugs available for only about 40 products. These generics are furthermore only between 15% and 20% cheaper.
170. Mossialos, E. and Le Grand, J., (eds.): ibid., p. 500.
171. As of the first of January 2004, another 200 items were taken off the list of reimbursable drugs.
172. Other figures are the United Kingdom, 117 in 1997; Denmark, 145 in 1999; France, 117 in 2000, Portugal, 130. in 1998; Austria, 139 in 1997; and Sweden, no less than 197 in 1997.
173. Angell, M.: ibid., p. 219. President Clinton gave it a try with his plans for the establishment of a price-review board for drugs, but did not succeed (Greider, K.: *The Big Fix: How the Pharmaceutical Industry Rips Off American Consumers*, Public Affairs, New York, 2003, p. 168).
174. Greider, K.: ibid., p. 1.
175. Angell, M.: ibid., p. xii.
176. Angell, M.: ibid., p. 198.
177. In the 1999–2000 election cycle, \$85 million was contributed, of which \$20 million was in direct contributions; the rest was "soft money" (Angell, M.: ibid., p. 200).
178. According to a 2003 PhRMA report (the Association of Pharmaceutical Research and Manufacturers of America), spending for fiscal influence in 2004 was budgeted at \$150 million, of which \$73 million would be spent at the federal level and \$49 million at state levels (Angell, M.: ibid., p. 214).
179. Angell, M.: ibid., p. 139.
180. Angell, M.: ibid., p. 3. On the contrary, the share of prescription drugs remained fairly static during the period 1960–1980.
181. Coulter, A. and Magee, H., (eds.): ibid., p. 45.
182. Research from 1999 showed that 94% of health information magazines handed out by general practitioners in Berlin came from the pharmaceutical industry. In addition to this, the industry supplied 84% of the magazines that were available in the waiting rooms. People, in general, mistrusted this information, however (Coulter, A., and Magee, H., (eds.): ibid., p. 43).
183. Angell, M.: ibid., p. 10.
184. Huffington, A.: ibid., p. 121.
185. Angell, M.: ibid., p. 11.
186. All in all, about half of the larger drug companies are based in Europe (Angell, M.: *The Truth about the Drug Companies: How They Deceive Us and What To Do About It*, Random House, 2004, p. xvii).
187. Angell, M.: ibid., pp. 12–13.
188. Angell, M.: ibid.

189. According to Mossialos and Mrazek, 20 of the leading American pharmaceutical industries spent between 11% and 21% on research and development in 1997 (Mossialos, E. and Mrazek, M.: ibid., p. 147).
190. Other sources mention an amount of $500 million, while assuming that it takes between seven and ten years to bring a new chemical entity to the market (Mossialos, E. and Mrazek: ibid., p. 147).
191. Angell, M.: ibid., p. 65.
192. Angell, M.: ibid., p. 143.
193. Angell, M.: ibid., pp. 54–55. Mossialos and Mrazek mention a decrease in new chemical entities introduced on the world market from 100 in 1963 to 37 in 1998 (Mossialos, E. and Mrazek, M.: ibid., p. 148).
194. Greider, K.: ibid., p. 29.
195. Angell, M.: ibid., p. xviii.
196. Mossialos, E. and Mrazek, M.: ibid., p. 149.
197. Angell, M.: ibid., pp. 30–31.
198. Angell, M.: ibid., p. 86.
199. The former CEO of Bristol-Myers Squibb received almost $75 million in 2001, plus a similar amount of stock options. His colleague from Wyeth received a salary of $40 million, plus the same amount in stock options. Unexercised stock options held by the CEOs of the ten large American drug companies were valued on average to be $52 million in 2001 (Angell, M.: ibid., pp. 12 and 49).
200. Angell, M.: ibid., p. 92.
201. Huffington, A.: ibid., pp. 138–139.
202. Greider, K.: ibid., p. 171.
203. Angell, M.: ibid., pp. 235–236.
204. Greider, K.: ibid., p. 17.
205. *De Volkskrant*, 6 December 2004.
206. Even considerably higher than commercial banking, with 13.5% (Angell, M.: ibid., p. 11).
207. Regarding this, see, for example: (1) Lichtenberg, F. R.: The Economic and Human Impact of New Drugs, in: *Journal of Clinical Psychiatry*, 2003, 64 (supplement 17), pp. 15–18; and (2) Goudriaan, R.: Recepten voor Extramuralisering van de Zorg, in: *Economisch-Statistische Berichten*, 26 November 2004, pp. 572–575.
208. Lichtenberg, F. R.: Availability of New drugs and Americans' Ability to Work, in: *JOEM*, volume 47, no. 4, April 2005, pp. 373–380.
209. *Der Spiegel*, February 2003, p. 73.
210. There are considerable historic differences between countries as regards the importance of cost-sharing. Some countries had already meaningful cost-sharing at the beginning of the period at issue; in other countries the phenomenon was negligible.
211. European Observatory on Health Care Systems: *Health Care Systems in Transition: Belgium 2000*, WHO Regional Office for Europe, Copenhagen, 2000, p. 23.
212. Crainich, D. and Closon, M.-C.: Cost Containment and Health Care Reform in Belgium, in: Mossialos, E. and Le Grand, J., (eds.): ibid., p. 254.
213. Donatini, A., Rico, A., D'Ambrosio, M. G., Lo Scalzo, A., Orzella, L., Cicchetti, A., and Profili, S.: ibid., p. 46.

214. European Observatory on Health Care Systems: *Health Care Systems in Transition: Germany, 2000*, ibid., p. 47.
215. Hofmarcher, M. M. and Rack, H.: ibid., p. 35.
216. Appleby, J.: ibid., p. 144.
217. European Observatory on Health Care Systems: *Health Care Systems in Transition, United Kingdom, 1999*, ibid., p. 41.
218. European Observatory on Health Care Systems: *Health Care Systems in Transition: Belgium, 2000*, ibid., pp. 25–26.
219. European Observatory on Health Care Systems: *Health Care Systems in Transition: United Kingdom, 1999*, ibid., p. 43.
220. Sandier, S., Paris, V., Polton, D.: ibid., pp. 44–45 (figure 4).
221. Hjortsberg, C. and Ghatnekar, O.: ibid., p. 30.
222. Vallgårda, S., Krasnik, A., and Vrangbæk, K.: ibid., p. 31.
223. Bentes, M., Dias, C. M., Sakellarides, C., and Bankauskaite, V.: ibid., p. 37.
224. Hofmarcher, M. M. and Rack, H.: ibid., pp. 37–38
225. Bentes, M., Dias, C. M., Sakellarides, C., and Bankauskaite, V.: ibid., p. 37
226. Evans, G.: Financing Health Care: Taxation and the Alternatives, in: Mossialos, E., Dixon, A., Figueras, J., Kutzin, J.: ibid., p. 47.
227. European Observatory on Health Care Systems: *Health Care Systems in Transition: Belgium, 2000*, ibid., p. 25.
228. European Observatory on Health Care Systems: *Health Care Systems in Transition: United Kingdom, 1999*, ibid., p. 44.
229. Donatini, A., Rico, A., D'Ambrosio, M. G., Lo Scalzo, A., Orzella, L., Cicchetti, A., and Profili, S.: ibid., p. 49.
230. Vallgårda, S., Krasnik, A., and Vrangbæk, K.: ibid., p. 31.
231. Hjortsberg, C. and Ghatnekar, O.: ibid., p. 30.
232. Donatini, A., Rico, A., D'Ambrosio, M. G., Lo Scalzo, A., Orzella, L., Cicchetti, A., and Profili, S.: ibid., pp. 85–87.
233. Järvellin, J.: ibid., p. 76.
234. European Observatory on Health Care Systems: *Health Care Systems in Transition: Luxembourg, 1999*, ibid., p. 51.
235. Maarse, J. A. M.: The Health System of the Netherlands, in: Raffel, M. W., (ed.), ibid., p. 144.
236. Wiley, M. M.: Hospital Budgeting and Financing using DRGs, in: Roger-France, F. H., Moor, G. de, Hofdijk, J., Jenkins, L., (eds.): *Diagnosis Related Groups in Europe*, ISBN 90-73045-01-0, Gent, 1989, p. 59.
237. According to Altenstetter and Björkman, ideas on managed care stem "from an oxymoronic mating of two major 'faiths' of the contemporary era: the virtues of the market as a mechanism to allocate costs as well as benefits efficiently; and the virtues of the directive state to 'guide' those allocations through efficacious regulation" (Altenstetter, Chr. and Björkman, J. W., (eds.): ibid., p. 7).
238. In 2002, 80% of employees were covered through managed care plans (Maynard, A. and Dixon, A.: ibid., p. 118).
239. In the year 2000, there were over 500 American HMOs with more than 60 million enrolees, while over 80% of the American population took part in some managed care plan (Dranove, D.: ibid., 67).
240. Furthermore, tens of millions of Americans had looser forms of managed care, such as preferred provider organizations and discounted fee-for-service (Ludmerer, K. M.: ibid., p. 353).

241. Rodwin, V.: The Rise of Managed Care in the United State: Lessons for French Health Policy, in: Altenstetter, Chr. and Björkman, J. W., (eds.): ibid., p. 16.
242. Feuerstein G. and Kuhlmann, E.: Der Rationierungsdiskurs: Eine Einleitung, in: Feuerstein, G. and Kuhlmann, E., (eds.): ibid., p. 3.
243. Dranove, D.: ibid., p. 8.
244. Dranove, D.: ibid., p. 62.
245. Ludmerer, K. M.: ibid., p. 351.
246. Mossialos, E. and Thomson, S. M. S.: Voluntary Health Insurance in the European Union, in: Mossialos, E., Dixon, A., Figueras, J., Kutzin, J., (eds.): ibid., p. 143.
247. Bentes, M., Dias, C. M., Sakellarides, C., and Bankauskaite, V.: ibid., p. 81.
248. European Observatory on Health Care Systems: *Health Care Systems in Transition: Spain, 2000*, ibid., p. 109.
249. Järvellin, J.: ibid., p. 77.
250. European Observatory on Health Care Systems: *Health Care Systems in Transition: Belgium, 2000*, ibid., p. 70.
251. Hughes, J.: Health Expenditure and Cost Containment in Ireland, in: Mossialos, E. and Le Grand, J., (eds.): ibid., p. 489.
252. Exter, A. den, Hermans, H., Dosljak, M., and Busse, R.: ibid., pp. 108–109.
253. Dranove, D.: ibid., p. 52.
254. Dranove, D.: ibid., pp. 103–104.
255. Contracts may be (1) block contracts, (2) cost-and-volume contracts, or (3) per-case contracts. Block contracts couple finances to a range of services for citizens of a defined region. Cost-and-volume contracts specify the number of treatments or cases that a provider will deliver at an agreed price, whereas per-case contracts define medical activity and expenditure at the level of an individual patient. The last type of contract causes considerable transaction costs. In practice, the British contracting system resulted in a new type of contract called the "sophisticated block" contract, which comes down to implementing a certain margin (floor or ceiling) in the contract (European Observatory on Health Care Systems: *Health Care Systems in Transition: United Kingdom, 1999*, ibid., p. 89).
256. Until now, health insurers in the Netherlands have been in a weak position as regards negotiating the price of DBCs, since hospitals are not obliged to give insurers an insight into how a DBCs price has been calculated. It is a matter of "take it or leave it." Leaving it would mean that insurers would have to find an other hospital with lower DBC prices.
257. Sandier, S., Paris, V., Polton, D.: ibid., p. 108.
258. European Observatory on Health Care Systems: *Health Care Systems in Transition: Spain, 2000*, ibid., p. 108.

Chapter 10

1. Crainich, D. and Closon, M.-C.: Cost Containment and Health Care Reform in Belgium, in: Mossialos, E. and Le Grand, J., (eds.): ibid., p. 219.
2. Christiansen, T., Enemark, U., Clausen, J., and Poulsen, P.: Health Care and Cost Containment in Denmark, in: Mossialos, E. and Le Grand, J., (eds.): ibid., p. 289.

3. Hughes, J.: ibid., p. 487.
4. *De Volkskrant*, 16 September 2005.
5. Le Fanu: ibid., p. xviii.
6. In this respect, Louckx correctly observes that this is a simplistic view of moral hazard. To him, moral hazard involves a complex interaction of different factors. It is not correct to assume that patients necessarily consume more health care if cost-sharing is left out, and neither does cost-sharing automatically result in a lesser use of health services (Louckx, F.: Patient Cost-Sharing and Access to Care, in: Mackenbach, J. and Bakker, M., (eds.): *Reducing Inequalities in Health: A European Perspective*, Routledge, 2002, pp. 191–192).
7. Mossialos, E. and Le Grand, J.: ibid., p. 63.
8. Mossialos, E. and Le Grand: ibid., pp. 82–83.
9. Mossialos, E. and Le Grand, J., (eds.): ibid., p. 454.
10. Donatini, A., Rico, A., D'Ambrosio, M. M., Lo Scalzo, A., Orzella, L., Cicchetti, A., and Profili, S.: ibid., pp. 46–47.
11. European Observatory on Health Care Systems: *Health Care Systems in Transition: Spain, 2000*, ibid., p. 114.
12. Coulter, A. and Magee, H.: ibid., p. 120.
13. Vallgårda, S., Krasnik, A., and Vrangbæk, K.: ibid., p. 30.
14. Mossialos, E. and Le Grand: ibid., p. 83.
15. Hughes, J.: ibid., p. 500.
16. Robinson, R.: User Charges for Health Care, in: Mossialos, E., Dixon, A., Figueras, J., Kutzin, J., (eds.): ibid., p. 181.
17. OECD: *The Reform of Health Care Systems: A Review of Seventeen OECD Countries*, ibid., p. 261.
18. Exter, A. den, Hermans, H., Dosljak, M., and Busse, R.: ibid., p. 48.
19. Busse, R. and Howorth, Ch.: Cost Containment in Germany, in: Mossialos, E. and Le Grand, J., (eds.): ibid., p. 324.
20. Lancry, P.-J. and Sandier, S.: Twenty Years of Cures for the French Health Care System, in: Mossialos, E. and Le Grand, J., (eds.): ibid., p. 449.
21. Saltman, R. B. and Figueras, J.: ibid., p. 100.
22. Sandier, S., Paris, V., and Polton, D.: ibid., pp. 40–41.
23. European Observatory on Health Care Systems: *Health Care Systems in Transition: Germany, 2000*, ibid., pp. 48–49.
24. Sissouras, A., Karokis, A., and Mossialos, E.: Health Care and Cost Containment in Greece, in: Mossialos, E. and Le Grand, J. (eds.): ibid., p. 379.
25. Pereira, J., Campos, A. C. de, Ramos, F., Simões, J., and Reis, V.: Health Care Reform and Cost Containment in Portugal, in: Mossialos, E. and Le Grand, J., (eds.): ibid., p. 655.
26. Theurl, E.: ibid., pp. 623–624.
27. Mossialos, E. and Dixon, A.: Funding Health Care: An Introduction in: Mossialos, E., Dixon, A., Figueras, J., Kutzin, J., (eds.): ibid., p. 23.
28. Fattore, G.: Cost Containment and Reforms in the Italian National Health Service, in: Mossialos, E. and Le Grand, J., (eds.), ibid., p. 522.
29. Fattore, G.: Cost Containment and Health Care Reforms in the British NHS, in: Mossialos, E. and Le Grand, J., (eds.): ibid., p. 740.
30. Robinson, R.: User Charges for Health Care, in: Mossialos, E. and Le Grand, J., (eds.): ibid., p. 178.

31. In this respect, it should be taken into account that the much-quoted Rand Corporation research, showing consumers' moral hazard, gave the 6,000 individuals a choice out of five individual insurance plans, covering the same services and reimbursing the providers for the full amount they charged. The only difference among the plans was copayments. Four plans had copayments which ranged from 25% to 95% of the medical bill, up to a maximum of $1,000 out-of-pocket payment per individual per year. Copayments could be very high, therefore. No wonder the Rand experiment proved "moral hazard," showing that those who had all their care for free would incur 30% higher medical costs (Dranove, D.: ibid., pp. 30–31).
32. Mossialos, E. and Le Grand, J.: ibid., p. 64.
33. Järvelin, J.: ibid., p. 37.
34. European Observatory on Health Care Systems: *Health Care Systems in Transition: United Kingdom, 1999*, ibid., p. 42.
35. Hjortsberg, C. and Ghatnekar, O.: ibid., p. 69.
36. OECD: *The Reform of Health Care Systems: A Review of Seventeen OECD Countries*, ibid., p. 200.
37. Saltman, R. B. and Figueras, J.: ibid., p. 79. Louckx points to two other ways of controlling the demand side: prevention and information (Louckx, F.: ibid., p. 189).
38. Raad voor de Volksgezondheid en Zorg: *Gepaste Zorg*, Zoetermeer, 2004, pp. 9 and 24.
39. Saltman, R. B. and Figueras, J.: ibid., p. 100.
40. Robinson, R.: ibid., p. 181.
41. Mossialos, E. and Le Grand, J.: ibid., p. 83.
42. Mossialos, E. and Dixon, A.: Funding Health Care in Europe: Weighing up the Options, in: Mossialos, E., Dixon, A., Figueras, J., Kutzin, J., (eds.): ibid., p. 283.
43. Figueras, J., Saltman, R. B., Busse, R., and Dubois, H. F. W.: Patterns and Performance in Social Health Insurance Systems, in: Saltman, R. B., Busse, R., Figueras, J., (eds.): ibid., p. 112.
44. Robinson, R.: ibid., p. 178.
45. Coulter, A. and Magee, H.: ibid., p. 139.
46. Paterson, I. and Judge, K.: Equality of Access to Healthcare, in: Mackenbach, J. and Bakker, M., (eds.): *Reducing Inequalities in Health: A European Perspective*, Routledge, 2002, p. 172.
47. European Observatory on Health Care Systems: *Health Care Systems in Transition: Germany, 2000*, ibid., p. 113.
48. Berg, M. and Grinten, T. van der: ibid., pp. 133–134.
49. For an extensive discourse on rationing in health care see: Feuerstein, G. and Kuhlmann, E., (eds.): *Rationierung im Gesundheitswesen*, Ullstein Medical, 1998.
50. Feuerstein, G. and Kuhlmann, E., (eds.): ibid., p. 195.
51. Rodwin, V. G.: The Rise of Managed Care in the United States: Lessons for French Health Policy, in: Altenstetter, Ch. and Björkman, J. M., (eds.): ibid., p. 51.
52. Sandier, S., Paris, V., and Polton, D.: ibid., p. 41.
53. Written information received via Mr. Paul Robinson and Mr. John Scannell from the Irish Department of Health and Children. Other reasons for not taking voluntary health insurance were (a) people had a medical card, (b)

people were satisfied with public health services, (c) disposition of medical care, and (d) people had not thought about it.

54. Casasnovas, G. L. I.: Health Care and Cost Containment in Spain, in: Mossialos, E. and Le Grand, J., (eds.): ibid., p. 430.
55. Ziekenfondsraad: *Tweede Evaluatie Beperking Aanspraak Tandheelkunde per 1 januari 1995*, Amstelveen, publikatienummer 1996/707, p. 8.
56. Mossialos, E. and Thomson, S. M. S.: Voluntary Health Insurance in the European Union, in: Mossialos, E., Dixon, A., Figueras, J., Kutzin, J., (eds.): ibid., p. 153.
57. Mackenbach, J. P.: Hoe kan de Gezondheidszorg bijdragen aan het verkleinen van social-economische Gezondheidsverschillen? in: Stronks, K. and Hulshof, J., (eds.): ibid., p. 114.
58. European Observatory on Health Care Systems: *Health Care Systems in Transition: United Kingdom, 1999*, ibid., p. 44.
59. Donatini, A., Rico, A., D'Ambrosio, M. M., Lo Scalzo, A., Orzella, L., Cicchetti, A., and Profili, S.: ibid., p. 63.
60. Mossialos, E. and Thomson, S. M. S.: ibid., p. 153.
61. Colombo, F. and Tapay, N.: *Private Health Insurance in Ireland: A Case Study*, OECD Working Paper No. 10, Directorate for Employment, Labour and Social Affairs, Paris, February 2004, p. 4.
62. Mossialos, E. and Thomson, S. M. S.: ibid., pp. 148–149.
63. Jones, A. and Rice, N.: ibid., pp. 89–90.
64. European Observatory on Health Care Systems: *Health Care Systems in Transition: United Kingdom, 1999*, ibid., p. 25.
65. European Observatory on Health Care Systems: *Health Care Systems in Transition: United Kingdom, 1999*, ibid., p. 60.
66. Vallgårda, S., Krasnik, A., and Vrangbæk, K.: ibid., p. 9.
67. Donatini, A., Rico, A., D'Ambrosio, M. M., Lo Scalzo, A., Orzella, L., Cicchetti, A., and Profili, S.: ibid., p. 107.
68. Hjortsberg, C. and Ghatnekar, O.: ibid., p. 78.
69. Coulter, A. and Magee, H., (eds.): ibid., pp. 139–140.
70. Coulter, A. and Magee, H., (eds.): ibid., p. 132.
71. Sandier, S., Paris, V., and Polton, D.: ibid., p. 119.
72. See for the accumulative effects regarding elderly people in the Netherlands: Sociaal en Cultureel Planbureau: *Rapportage Ouderen 1996*, Rijswijk, 1997, chapter 6.
73. Therefore there are people who prefer to speak of healthy public policy instead of health policy. In this regard, see, for example: Marmor, T. R. and Boyum, D.: Medical Care and Public Policy: The Benefits and Burdens of Asking Fundamental Questions, in: Gunning-Schepers, L. J., Kronjee, G. J., Spasoff, R. A., (eds.): *Fundamental Questions about the Future of Health Care*, Netherlands Scientific Council for Government Policy, The Hague, 1996, pp. 89–103.
74. Engbersen, G., Vrooman, J. C., and Snel, E.: *Arm Nederland: Het eerste Jaarrapport Armoede en Sociale Uitsluiting*, the Hague, 1996, pp. 110–111.
75. Algemeen Verslag over de Armoede (General Report on Poverty), on instructions from the Minister of Social Integration, compiled by the King Baudouin Foundation in cooperation with ATD Fourth World Belgium and the Association of Belgian Cities and Municipalities, Social Welfare Department, 1995, pp. 120–153.

76. "L'hôpital et l'access et l'exclusion aux soins des plus démunis," in: *Revue Hospitalière de France*, no. 6, Novembre/Décembre, 1995, pp. 628–635.
77. For example, see (1) Kam, F. de: Keuzes in de Zorg, in: *Economisch-Statistische Berichten*, 31 August 1994, p. 766; (2) Saltman, R. B.: A Conceptual Overview of Recent Health Care Reforms, in: *European Journal of Public Health*, volume 4, 1994, no. 4, pp. 287–293.
78. Congress of Local and Regional Authorities of Europe, Strasbourg, 8–9 February 1996.
79. International Association of Mutual Insurance Companies, Brussels, 13–14 June 1996.
80. Interuniversity Centre for Social Science and Methodology, Groningen, 26–28 June 1996.
81. European Social Services Conference, London, 3–4 July 1996.
82. In this connection, see: Donovan, J. and Coast, J.: Public Preferences in Priority Setting: Unresolved Issues, in: Malek, M., (ed.): *Priority Setting in Health Care*, West Sussex, 1994, pp. 32–43.
83. Quoted in: Poorthuis, F.: Is de Gezondheidszorg te duur? in: *Intermediair*, volume 46, 13 November 1987, p. 7.
84. *Staatscourant*, 18 May 1995.
85. *Nieuwe Noordhollandse Courant*, 13 March 1996.
86. *Nieuwe Noordhollandse Courant*, 27 March 1996.
87. *NRC/Handelsblad*, 21 June 1996.
88. Paterson, I. and Judge, K.: Equality of Access to Health Care, in: Mackenbach, J. and Bakker, M., (eds.): ibid., p. 171.
89. Figueras, J., Saltman, R. B., Busse, R., and Dubois, H. F. W.: Patterns and Performance in Social Health Insurance Systems, in: Saltman, R. B., Busse, R., Figueras, J., (eds.): ibid., p. 115.
90. Coulter, A. and Magee, H.: Key Issues for European Patients, in: Coulter, A. and Magee, H., (eds.): ibid., pp. 233–235.
91. Walshe, K.: ibid., p. 9.
92. Walshe, K.: ibid., p. 77.
93. Walshe, K.: ibid., p. 65.
94. Walshe, K.: ibid., p. 227.
95. Walshe, K.: ibid., pp. 101–102.
96. Walshe, K.: ibid., p. 228.
97. Ludmerer, K. M.: ibid., p. 277.
98. Walshe, K.: ibid., p. 57.
99. OECD: *New Directions in Health Policy*, ibid., p. 34.
100. Walshe, K.: ibid., p. 127.
101. Walshe, K.: ibid., p. 151.
102. Walshe, K.: ibid., pp. 152–153.
103. Bentes, M., Dias, C. M., Sakellarides, C., and Bankauskaite, V.: ibid., pp. 30–31.
104. Vallgårda, S., Krasnik, A., and Vrangbæk, K.: ibid., pp. 21–24.
105. In: Trappenburg, M.: ibid., pp. 21–22.
106. European Observatory on Health Care Systems: *Health Care Systems in Transition: Belgium, 2000*, ibid., pp. 16–17.
107. Saltman, R. B. and Busse, R.: ibid., p. 4.
108. Glied, S.: ibid., pp. 38–39.
109. In this respect, Glied argues that there is evidence that tends to rebut Baumol's hypothesis to medicine. Following Baumol, he would have predicted a widen-

ing gap between medical and other prices in a period of rapid productivity growth. In the 1980s, however, when industrial productivity increases were minimal, medical prices grew relatively more quickly than they had in the 1960s. The 1980s, however, was also the time when, through the introduction of important new health care technologies, health care became a curing industry (Glied, S.: ibid., p. 107).

110. Secretary of State for Health: *The New NHS: Modern—Dependable*, ibid., p. 75.
111. Ministerie van Volksgezondheid, Welzijn en Sport: *Minder Regels, Meer Zorg, Eindrapport van de Commissie Terugdringing Administratieve Lasten Zorgsector*, Den Haag, 2002.
112. Walshe, K.: ibid., p. 77.
113. Walshe, K.: ibid., p. 8.
114. Dranove, D.: ibid., p. 110.
115. Walburg, J. A.: *Uitkomstenmanagement in de Gezondheidszorg: Het Opbouwen van Lerende Teams in Zorgorganisaties*, Elsevier Gezondheidszorg, hoofdstuk 3. Also see: Dranove, D.: ibid., pp. 144–146.
116. There is some evidence on the relation between processes and outcomes. A Harvard study found that substandard processes were responsible for more than one-fourth of all adverse inpatient events, whereas another study concluded that patients suffered fewer inpatient complications when their physicians followed clinical guidelines (Dranove, D.: ibid., p. 145).
117. Weggeman, M.: *Leidinggeven aan Professionals: Het Verzilveren van Creativiteit*, Kluwer Bedrijfswetenschappen, 1993, p. 17.
118. Dranove, D.: ibid., p. 83.
119. Dranove, D.: ibid., p. 101.
120. Walshe, K.: ibid., p. 160.
121. Walshe, K.: ibid., p. 161.
122. Dranove, D.: ibid., p. 137.
123. Dranove, D.: ibid., p. 93.
124. In this respect, see: Walburg, J. A.: ibid.
125. Dranove, D.: ibid., pp. 87–89.
126. Dranove, D.: ibid., p. 65.
127. Dranove, D.: ibid., p. 53.
128. The Dutch government, for example, carried through an absolute salary cut of 3% for all civil servants and health care personnel in January 1984, and medical specialists agreed to a decrease in the tariffs for medical interventions in mid-1985.
129. Dranove, D.: ibid., p. 114.
130. Cookson, R., Goddard, M., and Gravelle, H.: ibid., pp. 131–132.
131. Dranove, D.: ibid., chapter 6.
132. Dranove, D.: ibid., p. 159.
133. Ludmerer, K. M.: ibid., p. 350.
134. Now that the Dutch have introduced their variant of DBCs, the Dutch Health Care Inspectorate requires hospitals to set up a system of 28 performance indicators. The software each hospital will have to buy to comply with this demand will cost more than €200,000 per hospital.
135. Marmor, Th. R.: Global Health Policy Reform: Mythology or Learning Opportunity, in: Altenstetter, Ch. and Björkman, J. W., (eds.): ibid., p. 350.

136. In this respect, see: Castles, F. G.: *The Future of the Welfare State: Crisis Myths and Crisis Realities*, Oxford University Press, 2004.
137. Glied, S.: ibid., pp. 84–85.
138. In this respect, see: Sparrow, M. K.: ibid., p. 35.
139. Wasem, J., Greß, S., and Okma, K. G. H.: The Role of Private Health Insurance in Social Health Insurance Countries, in: Saltman, R. B., Busse, R., Figueras, J., (eds.): ibid., p. 236.
140. In: Saltman, R. B.: Assessing Social Health Insurance Systems: Present and Future Policy Issues, in: Saltman, R. B., Busse, R., Figueras, J., (eds.): ibid., p. 145.
141. See: Saltman, R. B.: Assessing Social Health Insurance Systems: Present and Future Policy Issues, ibid., pp. 145–150.
142. Feuerstein, G. and Kuhlmann, E., (eds.): ibid., p. 24.
143. Trappenburg, M.: ibid., p. 26.
144. Bongers, I. M. B., Weert, C. M. C. van, Vis, C. M., Garretsen, H. F. L., and Das, M.: *Kwaliteit en Kwantiteit van de Gezondheidszorg en actuele Beleidsontwikkelingen in de Gezondheidszorg in 2005: Nederlanders aan het Woord*, Universiteit van Tilburg, 2005.
145. Health Care 2000: *UK Health and Healthcare Services: Challenges and Policy Options*, London, 1995, pp. 4–5.
146. Hofmarcher, M. M.: *Cross-Section Analysis of Health Spending with Special Regard to Trends in Austria*, Institute for Advanced Studies, Vienna, Economic Series, No. 70, 1999, p. 1.
147. Turner, A.: ibid., p. 95.
148. Evans, R. G. and Stoddart, G. L.: Producing Health, Consuming Health Care, in: Evans, R. G., Barer, M. L., Marmor, Th. R., (eds.): ibid. pp. 36–37.
149. Information received via personal communication with M. Boereboom from the Ministry of Health, Welfare and Sports (RIVM, demographic projection 2000–2020).
150. Böhlke, R., Söhnle, N., and Viering, S.: *Gesundheitsversorgung 2020. Konzentriert. Marktorientiert. Saniert*, Ernst & Young, Frankfurt am Main, 2005.
151. Vathorst, S. van der: ibid., p. 9.
152. The term is from: Schrijvers, A. J. P.: *Een Kathedraal van Zorg*, ibid.
153. The term is from: Turner, A.: ibid., p. 97.
154. Turner, A.: ibid., p. 96.

Chapter 11

1. As said in the first chapter, moving to the left or to the right side of the continuum is a matter of normative economics, because it involves ethical and value judgments. My personal viewpoint is that people who, due to policies of moving to the right side of the continuum, are hampered from fulfilling a position in society, are threatened in their dignity. Likewise, unemployment for people who want to work can be considered as a lack of recognition of their usefulness to society. To me, we have a double problem of core values here. Firstly, increasing inequalities between people, leaving many behind, is not in accordance with the appropriate development of a civilized society. Secondly, increasing dissatisfaction with present-day liberal democratic capitalism may

encourage those who are left behind to "restart history." History has seen several examples of opportunistic politicians who succeeded in mobilizing dissatisfied masses. Concluding international treaties could be of help in this respect. As an indication that world politics, particularly the G8, takes this challenge seriously, the suggestion of the Commission on Global Governance to the United Nations to establish an Economic Security Council, which I suggest could be adapted into a Social-Economic Security Council, is certainly worth considering, not only as a sign of civilization but also from the perspective of the "self-interest of the privileged." There is reason, however, not to be too optimistic in this respect. Even now, the United Nations has a *central system* to which the General Assembly, the Security Council, and the Economic and Social Council (ECOSOC) belong. The latter is supposed to deal with specific economic and social problems without "the necessary powers to manage effectively" (Taylor, P.: The United Nations and International Order, in: Baylis, J. & Smith, S., (eds.): ibid., pp. 332–335). All the more so since international organizations like the IMF, the World Bank, the WTO, and the OECD (OECD: *Towards a New Global Age: Challenges and Opportunities*. Policy Report, OECD, Paris, 1997) appear to pursue neo-liberal policies worldwide.

2. Stiglitz, J.: *The Roaring Nineties*: ibid., p. xii.
3. Stiglitz, J.: *The Roaring Nineties*: ibid., p. 318.
4. Turner argues that privatization is not absolutely necessary for market liberalization, although in practice it is difficult for governments to own companies and resist subsidization at the same time (Turner, A.: ibid., p. 167).
5. Stiglitz, J.: *The Roaring Nineties*: ibid., p. 284.
6. Stiglitz, J.: *The Roaring Nineties*: ibid., p. 283.
7. Hertz, N.: ibid.: p. 57.
8. Hertz, N.: ibid.: p. 57.
9. Snel, E., Hoek, T. van der, and Chessa, T.: *Kinderen in Armoede: Opgroeien in de Marge van Nederland*, Van Gorcum, 2001, p. 72.
10. Commission on Social Justice: What is Social Justice? in: Pierson, Chr. and Castles, F., (eds.): ibid., p. 61.
11. Happily, there is a ray of hope, since, particularly at the American state level, there is a growing number of grassroots organizations which are exposing the outrageous behavior of the corporate/political combination to the detriment of the American people. Through their actions, these organizations try to send a message to the market about the importance of corporate responsibility and conduct. An increasing number of companies are moving away from conventional corporate accounting, trying to include social and environmental considerations (Huffington, A.: ibid., pp. 250–257).
12. Pilger, J.: *Hidden Agendas*, Vintage Books, 1999, p. 57.
13. Gates, J.: ibid.: p. 32. The figure of 80 million is based on the worldwide trend.
14. Pilger, J.: *Hidden Agendas*, ibid.: p. 104.
15. Legrain, Ph.: ibid.: p. 16.
16. Mestrum, F.: ibid.: p. 24.
17. Hutton, W.: *The State To Come*, Vintage Books, 1997, p. x.
18. Galbraith, J. K.: *The Culture of Contentment*, London, 1992, p. 170. Galbraith argues here that "Yet the possibility of an underclass revolt, deeply disturbing the contentment, exists and grows stronger. There have been outbreaks in the

past, notably the major inner-city riots of the latter 1960s, and there are several factors that might lead to a repetition."

19. Peterson, W. C.: ibid. Peterson says, "If slow economic growth and stagnant real wages continue for the rest of the century, it will take some extraordinary creative and political leadership to avoid an explosion" (p. 92).
20. Reich, R.: *The Work of Nations: A Blueprint for the Future*, London, 1993.
21. Lasch, C.: ibid., p. 85.
22. Soros observes that globalization did not cause this misery. To him, armed conflicts and oppressive and corrupt regimes are to blame for that. Therefore, while recognizing that globalization, as well as resulting in more interdependence between the countries of the world, has also increased the possibilities of internal problems in those (underdeveloped) countries, he suggests that next to the necessity of thinking out better regulations regarding the provision of collective goods (education, health care, environment, etc.), we should also find ways to improve political and social circumstances within separate countries (Soros, G.: *Soros on Globalization* (Dutch Translation), ibid.: pp. 31–32). In this respect, Scholte rightfully observes that globalization has not been the only force behind persistent and growing poverty, but that local social structures, national policies, natural calamities, and other forces have also been influential (Scholte, J. A.: *Globalization: A Critical Introduction*: ibid.: p. 217). Furthermore, Kupchan argues that the ongoing struggle between the United States and Islamic radicals is no proof of a clash of civilizations. To him, the root causes of disaffection within Islamic society and the resulting terrorism are the illegitimacy of governing regimes, clan and factional rivalries, income inequalities, poverty, and a sense of being left behind (Kupchan, C. A.: ibid., p. 70). Similarly, Lagendijk and Wiersma argue that in the longer term reducing poverty and underdevelopment, guaranteeing civil rights, combating cultural and religious contrasts, as well as the reconstruction of *failed states* and dispelling feelings of humiliation will be necessities for the prevention of terrorism (Lagendijk, J. and Wiersma, J. M.: *Na Mars komt Venus: Een Europees Antwoord op Bush*, uitgeverij Balans, 2004, p. 115).
23. Dawson, A. D.: ibid., p. 52.
24. Hertsgaard, M.: ibid., p. 21.
25. As an example, representatives of the urban poor of Southern Africa and Asia have organized themselves into Slack/Slum Dwellers International in 1996, whereas the Participation Resource Action Network has linked poor people across continents (Scholte, J. A.: *Globalization: A Critical Introduction*, ibid.: pp. 73–74).
26. Pilger, J.: *Hidden Agendas*, ibid.: p. 328.
27. Huntington, S. P.: *Who are We? America's Great Debate*, ibid., p. 315.
28. The state of Michigan alone already had many militia groups in the 1990s (Moore, M.: *Downsize This*: ibid.: pp. 13–14). It should be mentioned that the number of active militia movements had dwindled to 197 in 2000 (Huntington, S. P.: Who are we?, ibid., p. 315).
29. Mexico has its Zapatistas, and Italy its 150 "*centri sociali*," both organizations demanding local organization and self-determination.
30. Pilger, J.: *Hidden Agendas*: ibid.: p. 330.
31. As an example, the city of Ahmedabad in India has the Self-Employed Women's Association, campaigning to improve the life of its impoverished

members and representing more than 200,000 poor women. Moreover, in countries such as Peru, Mexico, Brazil, South Africa, and Nicaragua, women are campaigning for fair prices, rents, basic social needs, schools, health centers, and sanitation (Pilger, J.: *Hidden Agendas*: ibid., p. 536).

32. OECD: *The Reform of Health Care: A Comparative Analysis of Seven OECD Countries*, ibid., p. 16.
33. Pen, J.: Slechte Mensen, in: *Openbare Uitgaven*, 17 April 1985, pp. 38–40.
34. Polanyi, K.: ibid.: p. 250.
35. List, F.: *The National System of Political Economy*, Reprints of Economic Classics, August M. Kelley Publishers, New York, 1966, p. 166.
36. Kuttner, R.: *Everything for Sale*, ibid., p. 45.
37. Kuttner, R.: ibid., chapter 2.
38. Ormerod, P.: ibid., pp. 137 and 3.
39. Ormerod, P.: ibid., p. 76. Besides, in the long run we all die, according to Keynes.
40. Ormerod, P.: ibid., p. 109.
41. Ormerod, P.: pp. 109–110.
42. Ormerod, P.: ibid., p. 111.
43. As an example: Friedman is a strong supporter of completely free world trade. Nevertheless, he too has to take it for a fact that political decision-making regarding tariffs and subsidies is a serious impediment to completely free trade (Friedman, M. and Friedman, R.: ibid., chapter 2).
44. Ormerod, P.: ibid., p. 205.
45. Ormerod, P.: ibid., p. 75.
46. Layard, R.: *What Labour Can Do*, Warner Books, London, 1997, p. 83. China, for example, is among the countries with a very high economic growth rate, despite the fact that it had one government official for every 34 citizens in 1996. In Wilson's *China: The Big Tiger; A Nation Awakes*, we read: "The medieval Han emperors maintained only one official for every 8,000 people. The Tang doubled that, and the Qing emperors doubled it again. When Mao Zedong stormed into power in 1949, the ratio was one official to every 290 persons. Today, for all the Communists' efforts it stands about 1 to 34, an extraordinarily heavy concentration of talent in the work of bureaucracy. Beijing alone hosts two million of them—a quarter of the city's total population" (Wilson, D.: *China: The Big Tiger; A Nation Awakes*, London, 1996, p. 75).
47. Stiglitz, J.: *Whither Socialism?*, MIT Press, 1995, pp. 275–276.
48. Commission on Social Justice: ibid., p. 62.
49. Lewin, L.: *Self-Interest and Public Interest in Western Politics*, Oxford University Press, 1991, p. 112. According to the author, American voters are "sociotropic."
50. Orren, G. R.: Beyond Self-Interest, in: Reich, R. B., (ed.): *The Power of Public Ideas*, Harvard University Press, Cambridge, Massachusetts, 1990, p. 13.
51. Edgerton, R. B.: Traditional Beliefs and Practices. Are Some Better than Others? in: Harrison, L. E. and Huntington, S. P.: *Culture Matters: How Values Shape Human Progress*, Basic Books, 2000, p. 137.
52. With this paradigm, the author is attempting to bring about a synthesis between "factors that form society and personality, as well as factors that form markets and rational decision-making." With this in mind, he adjusts the main points of the neo-classical paradigm. In the first place, the underlying princi-

ple is that people strive after "morality" as well as "pleasure." Also, the supposition of rational decision-making is replaced by decision-making which is based primarily on values and feelings. Finally, the supposition of individual decision-making is replaced by decision-making which takes place in the context of "social collectivities" (Etzioni, A.: *The Moral Dimension: Towards a New Economics*, London/New York, 1988, pp. 3–5).

53. Etzioni, A.: *The Moral Dimension*, ibid., p. 9.
54. Regarding this, see: Handy, C.: *The Empty Raincoat*, ibid., p. 46.
55. Etzioni elaborates the concept of a responsive community in *The Spirit of Community*, culminating in a communitarian agenda: Etzioni, A.: *The Spirit of Community: Rights, Responsibilities and the Communitarian Agenda*, London, 1995.
56. Sen, A.: *Development as Freedom*, ibid., pp. 65–66.
57. Buchanan, P. J.: ibid., p. 176.
58. Wight, Jonathan, B.: ibid.
59. Smith, A.: *The Theory of Moral Sentiments*, Reprint, Oxford University Press, 1976, p. 9.
60. Etzioni, A.: *The Moral Dimension*, ibid., p. 22.
61. Hirsch, F.: ibid., p. 137.
62. Huffington, A.: ibid., p. 119.
63. The philosopher Van der Wal distinguishes between three levels of meaning regarding the solidarity principle. First, there is the descriptive level. This is "the actual realisation of solidarity [. . .] which exists between people and the resulting preparedness to share existence with others, in particular where the dark sides are involved" (author's translation). The second level, the analytical level of the solidarity principle, involves "the central notion of a theory of society" (author's translation). At the third level, solidarity is "a yardstick to promote the quality of interpersonal relationships" (author's translation): Wal, G. A. van der: Solidair, Hoe en Waarom? Over de Betekenis van Solidariteit bij de Bekostiging van de Gezondheidszorg, in: Jacobs, F. C. L. M. and Wal, G. A. van der, (eds.): *Medische Schaarste en het Menselijk Tekort*, Ambo, Baarn, 1988, pp. 85–87).
64. Sen, A.: *Welzijn, Vrijheid en Maatschappelijke Keuze. Opstellen over de Politieke Economie van het Pluralisme*, Amsterdam, 1995, p. 263.
65. Wetenschappelijke Raad voor het Regeringsbeleid: *Tweedeling in Perspectief*, Den Haag, 1996, pp. 140–141.
66. Kuttner, R.: *The End of Laissez-Faire: National Purpose and the Global Economy after the Cold War*, University of Pennsylvania Press, Philadelphia, 1992, p. 4.
67. Groen, J. F.: *Een Stem in het Publieke Domein: Een Onderzoek naar Documenten van Protestantse Kerken in Duitsland, Engeland en Nederland 1979–1994*, Amsterdam, 1979, pp. 48 and 50.
68. Etzioni, A.: *The Moral Dimension*, ibid., p. 63.
69. Ploug, N. and Kvist, J.: *Social Security in Europe: Development or Dismantlement*, The Hague, 1996, pp. 2–3.
70. Groen, J. F.: ibid., p. 70.
71. Etzioni, A.: *The Moral Dimension*, ibid., p. 77.
72. Hofstede, G.: ibid., pp. 102–103.
73. Scholte, J. A.: *Globalization: A Critical Introduction*, ibid., p. 39.

74. Barrez, D.: ibid., pp. 45–49.
75. Barrez, D.: ibid., pp. 56–57.
76. Lindert, P. H.: *Growing Public: Social Spending and Economic Growth since the Eighteenth Century*, Cambridge University Press, 2004.
77. Lindert, P. H.: ibid., pp. 17–18.
78. Turner, A.: ibid., p. 165.
79. Lindert, P. H.: ibid., p. 18.
80. Lindert, P. H.: ibid., pp. 306–307.
81. Lindert, P. H.: ibid., p. 29.
82. Castles, F. G.: *The Future of the Welfare State: Crisis Myths and Crisis Realities*, Oxford University Press, 2004, p. 15. Similarly, American research shows little or no effect of employer-provided insurance benefits on employment, whereas German research found that employment is not sensitive to the employer's contribution to the health insurance portion of the wage bill (Mossialos, E. and Dixon, A.: Funding Health Care in Europe: Weighing up the Options, in: Mossialos, E., Dixon, A., Figueras, J., Kutzin, J., (eds.): ibid., p. 287).
83. Pierson, P.: The New Politics of the Welfare State, in: Pierson, Chr. and Castles, F., (eds.): ibid., pp. 309–319.
84. Gough, I.: Social Welfare and Competitiveness, in: Pierson, Chr. and Castles, F., (eds.): ibid., p. 239.
85. Castles, F. G.: ibid., table 2.1, p. 25.
86. Aggregates of total public social expenditure as a percentage of GDP divided by the percentage of the dependent population, that is, the population aged 65 and over, plus the percentage of the civilian population registered as unemployed (Castles, F. G.: ibid., p. 36).
87. Castles, F. G.: ibid., table 2.4, p. 37.
88. Clayton, R. and Pontusson, J.: Welfare State Retrenchment Revisited, in: Pierson, Chr. and Castles, F., (eds.): ibid., pp. 320–334.
89. Castles, F. G.: ibid., p. 45.
90. Castles, F. G.: ibid., p. 39.
91. Rifkin, J.: *The European Dream*, ibid., p. 45. In 1970, labor productivity in the Netherlands was 75% of the American level. However, in 2000, Dutch laborers were 5% more productive than their American colleagues (Vries, B. de: ibid., p. 152).
92. Lindert, P. H.: ibid., p. 18.
93. In this respect, Rifkin points out that three-quarters of the difference in productivity levels between the USA and Europe is attributable to the fewer hours worked in Europe (Rifkin, J.: *The European Dream*, ibid., p. 48).
94. Castles, F. G.: ibid., p. 91.
95. Castles, F. G.: Social Expenditure in the 1990s: Data and Determinants, forthcoming in *Policy and Politics*, 33 (3), July 2005.
96. Forrester, V.: *L'horreur économique*, ibid., p. 109. This is the International Monetary Fund, which, like the World Bank, is part of the United Nations, but which nevertheless operates like the "self-righteous surgeons, skilfully removing the remnants of political control over market forces" (Castells, M.: *The Power of Identity*, ibid., p. 269). Meanwhile, these tax-free salaried surgeons saw their remuneration increase by 38% during the period 1992–1993, with a further budgeted increase of 22% for 1994 (Ormerod, P.: ibid., pp. 3 and 124).

97. Rifkin, J.: *The European Dream*, ibid., pp. 53–54.
98. *De Volkskrant*, 22 March 2005.
99. Swaan, A. de: Dutch Welfare in Europe XL, in: Gier, E. de, Swaan, A. de, & Ooijens, M., (eds.): ibid., pp. 7–8.
100. Calleo, D. P.: ibid., p. 295.
101. Calleo, D. P.: ibid., p. 296.
102. Thurow, L.: ibid., p. 111.
103. In this respect, see: Castles, F. G.: ibid., p. 92.
104. Calleo, D. P.: ibid., p. 208.
105. Kapteyn, P.: Zonder Openbaring verwildert het Volk—over de Grenzeloosheid van het Europese Integratieproces, in: Kaars Sijpesteijn, E. J., (ed.): ibid., p. 4.
106. Lindert's analysis is based on figures to 1995. Castles' figures go to 1998.
107. Hutton, W.: *The World We're In*, ibid., p. 183.
108. Scholte, J. A.: ibid., pp. 9 and 7.
109. Legrain, Ph.: ibid., p. 7.
110. Myrdal, G.: ibid., pp. 61–68.
111. As for the malfunctioning of democracy, four types of criticism can be distinguished. Firstly, it is argued that democracy has become a matter of cooperation between political, corporate, and professional elites. In this respect, Huffington speaks of "a toxic marriage of money and political influence" (Huffington, A.: ibid., p. 136), whereas Myrdal labels the close connection between business leaders, politicians, universities, and other social spheres as the power oligarchy (Myrdal, G.: ibid., p. 116). Consequently, democracy is no longer connected to ordinary people. This would explain why citizens of the developed world have hardly any appreciation left for their political system (Zakaria, F.: ibid., p. 20). They feel unheard and they no longer believe that governments work in their interests. Therefore, they turn away from politics. In this respect, an "alienation index" has even been developed. Since 1960, it shows a continuously decreasing spiral from 34% in the 1960s to 63% in the 1990s (Zakaria, F.: ibid., p. 151). The American political scholar Putnam calculated that, since the 1960s, active participation in public and social activities in the United States decreased by 40% (Zakaria, F.: ibid., p. 152). People have been turning away from politics for decades already, despite increasing average wealth and political stability. The latter makes the developments even more mysterious (Zakaria, F.: ibid., p. 153). Democracy, in theory an open and accessible system, is in reality controlled "by organised or rich and fanatic minorities who protect their short-term interests, while sacrificing the future" (author's translation) (Zakaria, F.: ibid., p. 240). And they are supported by an amazingly increasing number of lobbyists. In the United States, lobbyists, together with professional consultants, opinion leaders, and activists, all there in the name of democracy, have become a powerful elite which appears to be capable of undermining the work of the institutions of representative democracy (Zakaria, F.: ibid., p. 186), including the government itself, as all American presidents over the past decades have experienced (Zakaria, F.: ibid., p. 164). In the United States lobbying has become a $1.55 billion annual business, with 38 lobbyists for every member of congress. Many of these lobbyists have family ties with members of congress (Huffington, A.: ibid., pp. 78 and 91–96). The second type of criticism suggests what might be called an erosion of the *Trias Politica*, i.e., a clear distinction in society between legal, executive, and

judicial powers. Contrary to the situation in the 1960s and 1970s, nowadays "ordinary" citizens (a hairdresser, a businessman, a self-employed medical specialist, or what have you) are far less represented in parliament or in the other layers of democracies. In this respect, a recent publication regarding politics in the Netherlands is rather revealing. It shows that roughly two-thirds of Dutch politicians, whether at the national, the county, or the local level, are civil servants (Westerloo, G. van: ibid.). Civil servants, depending on the government for their income, are believed to have taken over. Together with politicians they are assumed to have created a closed political circuit with policy formulation, determination, execution, and control in their hands. This circuit is thought to represent a kind of aristocracy, a caste of professional administrators. In this small and closed world of its own, maintaining political coalitions has become sacrosanct. In these same coalitions evident political blunders of the ruling elite remain without consequences in a political "sorry culture." As a further consequence of this erosion of the *Trias Politica*, one can observe disappearing Weber-like hierarchical relations between those who determine policy (politicians) and those who have to execute the decisions in this respect (the bureaucracy). Politicians who try to re-establish these relations, pursuing the primacy of politics, experience worsening relations with leading bureaucrats (Nieuwenkamp, R.: ibid.) Contributing to this development is the fact that over the past few years, members of the cabinet, expecting a fresh wind, favor the appointment of outsiders to deal with their organizational and budgetary problems. The present Dutch Minister of Health appointed a top manager from the Dutch postal organization to consult on the running of Dutch hospitals. That country's Secretary of Health asked the manager of the Dutch Golden Tulip hotel chain to consult on the financing of nursing homes (*De Volkskrant*, 22 June 2005). Tony Blair hired a former British president of Coca Cola to consult on the running of British schools, and a former head of the British Confederation of Industries to review the functioning of hospitals (Daily Telegraph, 9 January 2002), whereas the Chancellor of the Exchequer hired a banker to report on the economic foundations of the NHS. Also, the Irish minister of health put his confidence in a banker by appointing him as the CEO for Irish health. In general, these days leading politicians show a reverence for so-called management gurus, and, consequently, running the state or government departments has become a growing market for management consultants. The Blair government's spending on consultants' fees, for example, rose by 25% during the fiscal years 1998–1999 and 1999–2000, and by 50% in the following year to £550 million (Wheen, F.: ibid., p. 57). One can wonder, therefore, who really rules: politicians or technocrats. Thirdly, politics is thought to be no longer based on the wish to pursue ideals regarding the design of society. Instead, it has more to do with a person's personal career path. It is good for your curriculum vitae to be able to mention that you are politically active. In the old days, a political appointment was a crown to one's career. These days it seems to be a springboard to become someone important. As the Dutch political scientist Rosenthal has formulated it: members of the Dutch parliament live *on* politics not *for* politics (Westerloo, G. van: ibid., p. 204). These characteristics together have led some to label Dutch politics as a perversion of democracy (Westerloo, G. van: ibid., p. 144). The fourth type of criticism has to do with the openness of democracy. This openness makes it very easy for interest groups to contact the political level. However, the more open a democracy is, the more it is accessible for money, lobbyists, and fanatics, which, in turn may result in a loss of status (Zakaria, F.: ibid., p. 155). To restore this situation, several authors suggest protecting the political institutions from easy access by citizens and interest groups. Political institutions should for certain periods be mandated to do the job which they are there for without having constantly to react to incidental interventions. This might be called a restoration of political authority (for example: Zakaria, F.: ibid.; Cliteur, P.: ibid.). It seems to me that the four types of criticism all apply to the present-day international political economy, with the corporate elite in a position of determining cultural hegemony (Antonio Gramsci in: Ellwood, W.: ibid., p. 70). In this respect, Ellwood remarks that corporate business, through a subtle public relations policy, through manipulation of the media, and through having friends in high places [i.e., politics], has succeeded in transforming neo-liberal ideas on the world economy into a generally accepted way of life (Ellwood, W.: ibid., p. 70). Formulating it this way refers to a powerful combination of the corporate and the political elite, which is the determining factor in today's international political economy. They hold on to each other, exchanging skills to their mutual benefit. Cabinet members hiring corporate managers to solve their organizational and budgetary problems, and corporate business hiring former political leaders in order to better be able to play the political game. As an example, shortly after having left office as Prime Minister, Margaret Thatcher was hired by (hedge fund) Tiger Management as an expert to attend five board meetings a year because of her "political insight and experience to help inform investment decisions" for a payment of £1 million a year (Wheen, F.: ibid., p. 264). Similarly, former Prime Minister Kok of the Netherlands was hired by one of the biggest banking/insurance companies shortly after his second term. Examples like these may lead ordinary citizens to conclude that politics is a closed-shop affair to which outsiders have no access. This assumption may be reinforced by politicians who, after having come to power, do not live up to the promises they made during election campaigns. This may explain why ordinary citizens, believing that they cannot change the course of things, turn away from politics.

112. Phillips, K.: ibid., pp. 149–150.
113. Lamy, S. L.: Neo-Realism and Neo-Liberalism, in: Baylis, J. and Smith, S., (eds.): ibid., p. 194.
114. Frankel, J.: ibid., p. 67.
115. Rodrik, D.: ibid., p. 2.
116. Gates, J.: ibid., p. xxxi.
117. Servan-Schreiber, J. J.: *Le Défi Américain* (Dutch Translation), Utrecht/Antwerpen, 1967.
118. Servan-Schreiber, J. J.: ibid., p. 48.
119. Servan-Schreiber, J. J.: ibid., p. 56.
120. Servan-Schreiber, J. J.: ibid., p. 122.
121. Servan-Schreiber, J. J.: ibid., pp. 18–19.
122. Servan-Schreiber's ideas have been contested heavily by Marxist economists like Ernest Mandel. To the latter, the innovation gap between the United States and Europe in those days was not a consequence of lagging mental and technological possibilities, but of the unavailability of capital to finance quick

innovation (Mandel, E.: *Die EWG und die Konkurrenz Europa-Amerika* (Dutch translation), Van Gennep, Amsterdam, 1969, p. 31).

123. Fukuyama, F.: *The End of History and the Last Man*, ibid., p. 126. It is eye-catching that the economic success of these countries was not realized at the expense of social justice. In Taiwan and South Korea, income inequality has decreased steadily during the past 25 years. In Taiwan, the highest paid 20% of the population earned 15 times as much as the lowest 20% in 1952, but this difference decreased to four and a half in 1980.
124. Nevertheless, also in 1967 it was predicted that China would become a powerful industrialized socialist state by the year 2001 (Suyin, H.: *China in the Year 2001* (Dutch Translation), Lemniscaat, Rotterdam, 1967, p. 223).
125. World Bank: *China 2020: Development Challenges in the New Century* (Washington D.C.: World Bank, 1997, p. 103, quoted in: Kupchan, C. A.: ibid., p. 63).
126. Meanwhile, Russia has been designated an official "partner" of NATO, complete with a NATO ambassador who takes part in NATO meetings (Reid, T. R.: ibid., p. 185).
127. Eyden, T. van der: ibid., p. 71.
128. Croft, S. et al.: ibid., p. 4.
129. Lagendijk, J. and Wiersma, J. M.: ibid., p. 118.
130. Calleo describes two other Pan-European models for an enlarged European Union, including Russia. Firstly, in bipolar Pan-Europe, the EU benefits from the collapse of communism. Countries which have been liberated from communism join the EU, except for Russia itself. The latter country is kept at arm's length, but receives compensatory aid and enjoys diplomatic respect. In the second model, i.e., a unified Pan-Europe, the East and the West of Europe create an integrated Eurasian system, which eventually includes Russia (Calleo, D. P.: ibid., pp. 343–353).
131. In the year 2000, the EU accounted for 24% of world trade in services, with the United States reaching 22%, and Japan no more than 8% (Rifkin, J.: *The European Dream*, ibid., p. 61).
132. The facts mentioned can be found in: Rifkin, J.: *The European Dream*, ibid.
133. Reid, T. R.: ibid., p. 115.
134. Reid, T. R.: ibid., pp. 113–114.
135. Reid, T. R.: ibid., p. 120.
136. Reid, T. R.: ibid., p. 124.
137. Rifkin, J.: *The European Dream*, ibid., p. 68.
138. Lagendijk, J. and Wiersma, J. M.: ibid., p. 67.
139. Lamy, P.: ibid. In 2003, after the start of the American action in Iraq 70% of Europeans wanted the EU to become a superpower, with more than 70% expecting this to happen (Reid, T. R.: ibid., p. 11).
140. Lagendijk, J. and Wiersma, J. M.: ibid., pp. 71 and 98. Judging from the (sub)titles of their books, apparently American authors also believe that the United States is the losing party. Rifkin's *The European Dream* has as the subtitle *How Europe's Vision of the Future is Quietly Eclipsing the American Dream*; Reid's *The United States of Europe* has *The New Superpower and the End of American Supremacy* as its subtitle, while Kupchan writes unrestrictedly on *The End of the American Era*.
141. In: Rifkin, J.: *The European Dream*, ibid., p. 201.
142. Rifkin: J.: *The European Dream*, ibid., p. 201.

143. Rifkin, J.: *The European Dream*, ibid., p. 208. It should be realized, however, that a positive attitude of citizens toward Europe does not necessarily mean an appreciation of EU politicians.
144. As for the latter, it is rather cheap to argue, like Ernest Mandel does, that the United States had its own (business) interests in helping the countries of Europe by creating markets, and preventing the European continent from being taken over completely by communism (Mandel, E.: ibid., p. 11). Of course American self-interest played a role here, but that leaves unaddressed the fact that the United States contributed tremendously to Europe's liberation and reconstruction, as well as to the preservation of its democracy (also see: Myrdal, G.: ibid., pp. 192–193).
145. These Europeans are supported, for that matter, by a range of American authors like Moore, Klein, Hertz, Pilger, Gates, Hertsgaard, et cetera (see the bibliography). A TimeEurope.com poll of 2003 showed that no less than 87% of Europeans believe that the United States "poses the greatest danger to world peace." Furthermore, a 2002 Gallup International poll reports that the population in 23 out of 33 countries believe American foreign policy to negatively influence their country (Rifkin, J.: *The European Dream*, ibid., p. 302).
146. Rifkin, J.: *The European Dream*, ibid., p. 3.
147. Calleo, D. P.: ibid., p. 128. To some, globalization *is* Americanization, because the American-led global economy "is the only game in town" (Kupchan, C. A.: ibid., p. 60). This game refers to a particular interpretation of the globalization process, promoted by Americans but at the same time disliked by non-Americans. Much of this dislike has to do with differences in cultural values and with the way Americans are trying to impose their neo-liberal views on the rest of the world. Their way of doing business may be perceived as insulting to indigenous practices. Authors like Huntington, Fukuyama, and Barber have warned about the resentment this may breed. There are even those who link the dreadful events of September 11, 2001, to the worldwide discontent with the way present-day American neo-liberal capitalism leaves many people behind, destroys their culture, ruins their environment, and rapes their dignity. To these people, the twin towers in New York were not mere buildings. They were destroyed "symbols of American capitalism" (Klein, N.: *Fences and Windows*, ibid., p. 235). Furthermore, Chomsky argues that the September 11 attacks were the reply of oppressed people from the Third World to centuries of American depredations (Berman, P.: *Terror and Liberalism*, W. W. Norton & Company, New York, 2003, p. 151). With several examples, he illustrates that, according to him, with good reason, in much of the world, the United States is regarded as "a leading terrorist state" (Chomsky, N.: *9–11*, Seven Stories Press, New York, 2002, p. 23). In line with this, a poll by *Time* magazine in the beginning of 2003 revealed that 80% of the respondents thought the United States to be the greatest threat to peace, compared to 7% to 8% for Iraq and North Korea (Barber, B. R.: *Fear's Empire*: ibid., p. 59). In this respect, it should be noted that the "war on terrorism" declared after September 11, except for its dreadfulness, is nothing new. Already in the 1950s, President Eisenhower and his staff had discussed the "campaign of hatred against us" in the Arab world. In the 1960s, President Kennedy ordered that "the terrors of the earth" must be visited upon Cuba, whereas in the 1980s President Reagan launched "a terrorist war" against Nicaragua. If we add to this the American support for

the Suharto regime in Indonesia, as well as American behavior regarding East Timor, Bush's plaintive words "why do they hate us" seem rather naïve. This is the same naïveté he demonstrated during his visit to Europe in 2001 when he spoke of "*My* NATO" (author's italics) (Barrez, D.: ibid., p. 182). The reason for hatred against the United States is simply the fact that the country "has generated so much violence to protect its economic interests" (Chomsky, N.: ibid., p. 116).

148. An illustration for this attitude is a declaration as recently as 1999 of the then American Secretary of Defense, that the Unites States "is committed to 'unilateral use of military power' to defend vital interests, which include 'ensuring uninhibited access to key markets, energy supplies, and strategic resources' and indeed anything that Washington might determine to be within its own jurisdiction" (Chomsky, N.: ibid., p. 111). The attacks of September 11, therefore, can also be interpreted as a sign that people are no longer prepared to accept American self-interested action. In line with this, Ritzer argues that the attacks on the World Trade Center "serve as a backdrop for a wide range of expressions of outrage against the United States (Ritzer, G.: *McDonaldization: The Reader*, Sage Publications Inc., 2002, pp. 186–187). However, statements like the one of the American Secretary of Defense are nothing new, in fact. Already in 1948, George Kennan, a US strategic planner, is known to have said: "We have 50% of the world's wealth but only 6.3% of its population. In this situation, our real job in the coming period [. . .] is to maintain this position of disparity. To do so, we have to dispense with all sentimentality [. . .], we should cease thinking about human rights, the raising of living standards and democratization" (Pilger, J.: *The New Rulers of the World*, Verso, New York, 2002, p. 98). The history of American interventions in the world delivers many examples which support this policy. In this respect, Grossman produced a list of 134 American interventions, covering 111 years between 1890 and 2001, with an average of 1.15 interventions per year. This average increased to 2.0 per year after the fall of the Berlin Wall. Furthermore, Galtung shows that the spatial patterns of the interventions changed drastically in the post-war period. Starting with East Asia (Korea, Vietnam, Indonesia, Iran), via Eastern Europe (less violent because of the presence of the Soviet Union), to Latin America (starting in Cuba and reaching most of the continent), and, finally, focused on West Asia (Palestine, Iran, Libya, Libanon, Syria, Iraq and Afghanistan). Although the argument for these interventions was always the defense of democracy, human rights, and freedom, they somehow always ended up in securing free trade markets (Sardar, Z. and Davies, M. W.: *Why do People Hate America?* Icon Books, 2002, pp. 67 and 71. Also Lagendijk and Wiersma point out that in the United States "values" and "interests" appear to coincide (Lagendijk, J. and Wiersma, J. M.: ibid., p. 30)). After all, if democracy, freedom, and human rights had been the motives for intervention, why, then, did the Americans support the Greek colonels, the Argentine generals, the shah of Persia, Pinochet of Chile, and Marcos of the Philippines? (Barber, B. R.: *Fear's Empire*, ibid., p. 130) Why did they assist in the removal of Mossadegh in Iran, Arbentz in Guatamala, and Allende in Chili? And why did they invade the Dominican Republic and Grenada?).

149. Barber, B. R.: *Fear's Empire*, ibid., p. 60.

150. The Marshall Plan, in this respect, was more than an expression of that alliance. It was also meant to be an instrument for the United States "to secure markets for its own products" and, at least partly, "a result of its own strategic interests."
151. Rifkin, J.: *The European Dream*, ibid., pp. 290–291. See for American neo-conservatism: Halper, S. and Clarke, J.: *America Alone: The Neo-Conservatives and the Global Order*, Cambridge University Press, 2004).
152. As for the latter, around 260,000 military staff are stationed in no less than 26 countries worldwide (Todd, E.: *Après l' empire: Essai sur la decomposition du système américain* (Dutch Translation), Prometheus, 2003, p. 114).
153. Legrain, Ph.: ibid., p. 11.
154. Firstly, despite the fact that in November 1999 the General Assembly of the United Nations passed a resolution with 163 countries in favor, saying that outer space should be reserved for peaceful purposes, the United States, together with Israel, abstained. Bush wanted to have a new defense missile operational in 2002, thus tearing up the 1972 arms control treaty with the Russians. Since Russia was no longer a threat, the new motive became the presence of so-called "rogue states." Publicly expressed concerns (Russia, China, Sri Lanka, and Canada) about the prospect of an arms race in space did not help. Secondly, the United States walked out on a landmine prohibition conference in Canada in 2000, saying that they still needed to lay mines in Korea. Consequently, a proposed treaty could not be realized. Thirdly, the United States wanted American soldiers, exclusively, to be exempted from trial by a proposed international criminal court. Here, Russia and China took the same position (Halper, S. and Clarke, ibid., p. 123). Finally, the United States withdrew from the Kyoto agreement directed at a reduction of carbon dioxide emissions. Each withdrawal is, according to Neale, an illustration of US determination to dominate the world (Neale, J.: ibid., chapter 7; also, Moore, M.: *Stupid White Men*, ibid., p. 183).
155. Chomsky, N.: ibid., p. 13.
156. A U.S. State Department poll of 1999 showed that 78% of Germans were positive about the United States. Shortly after the war on Iraq had started, this figure dropped to 38%. In France, only 37% of respondents were positive about the United States in 2004, down from 62% in 1999 (Reid, T. R.: ibid., p. 24).
157. Sardar, Z. and Davies, M. W.: ibid., p. 194. Furthermore, the American Hertsgaard observes that the Americans, only 14% of whom have a passport, hardly know anything about the rest of the world because they are neither interested nor taught to know. As an example: a 1995 test among high school students about to graduate revealed that more than half of them had never heard of the Cold War (Herstgaard, M.: ibid., p. 56). This also applies to over one-third of the members of Congress (Gates, J.: ibid., p. 193). In this respect, a poll in 2002 among Americans aged 18–24 revealed that 83% could not find Afghanistan on a map, whereas 85% and 69% could not identify Israel or the United Kingdom, respectively (Petras, K. and Petras, R.: *Unusually Stupid Americans: A Compendium of All-American Stupidity*, Villard, New York, 2003, p. 7).
158. Hertsgaard, M.: ibid., p. 196. This same self-esteem also explains the ease with which Bush managed to pass the Patriot Act of October 2001, turning 20 million non-American inhabitants into outlaws with a simple signature. The law, which intrudes on half of the American Constitutional rights, was accepted

by 98 votes to 1 in the Senate and opposed by only 66 out of 435 votes in the House of Representatives. Furthermore, opinion polls revealed that over 70% of the American population agreed (Hertsgaard, M.: ibid., pp. 52–54). Regarding American arrogance, it should be taken into account, however, that there is a difference between America and the Americans. They are not automatically the same. The American government, the military, and the official economic institutions are the ones who determine American policy. This makes the United States a country that is ruled by an elite, preaching democracy worldwide, but not living up to that for its own citizens. Consequently, most Americans do not vote. In a world ranking of developed capitalistic democracies regarding participation in elections, the country is positioned at number 114 (Hertsgaard, M.: ibid., p. 162). Americans feel alienated from the political system, which they rightfully believe to be in the hands of the rich and powerful. And if we add to this the American belief that open markets are an antidote to the terrorists' violent rejectionism and that we have to "fight terror with trade" (Klein, N.: *Fences and Windows*, ibid., p. 239), or, even stronger, that "you're either for free trade—or for Al-Quaeda" (a conclusion drawn by Palast from a speech delivered by Bush's "globalization czar" to a meeting of CEOs shortly after the events of September 11, in: Palast, G.: ibid., p. 165), it may well be that Fukuyama is completely wrong with his conclusion that we have reached the end of history. Instead, history may well be restarted. For Americans at large this will come as a surprise, not because they are morally corrupt, but because they simply are not informed. And it is unlikely that they will be informed objectively, since the highly monopolized press is part of the American establishment, which is courting the ruling American elite (Hertsgaard, M.: ibid., pp. 90–111). Since around the turn of the millennium, the global media market, through mergers, acquisitions, and joint ventures, has become dominated by ten trans-national corporations—Time Warner, Disney, Bertelsmann, Viacom, Tele-Communications Inc., News Corporation, Sony, Seagram's (formerly Universal), General Electric (formerly NBC), and Dutch Philips (formerly Polygram). This is in line with Hutton's observation that, for example, 57% of the *New York Times* and 52% of the *Washington Post* are "owned by institutional investors whose priority is shareholder value" (Hutton, W.: *The World We're In*, ibid., p. 176). Contributing to a one-sidedly informed American public is the fact that, in 2000, only six corporations accounted for 50% of media outlets, down from 50 in the mid-1970s (Gates, J.: ibid., p. xxi). In turn, this is in line with Neale's observation that the US media have to lie, because there is "a moral gulf between the ruling class and working America." If the truth were told, most Americans would be outraged, he assumes (Neale, J.: ibid., p. 173). According to Todd, this current American behavior cannot last much longer. The essence of his explanatory paradoxical model is that, if the rest of the world discovers the advantages of democracy and learns that it can do without the United States, the latter country will not only be inclined to lose its democratic principles, but will also discover that it cannot do without the rest of the world economically. The spread of liberal democracy and peace would be a threat to the United States. The country, because of its very high consumption level, is already very dependent on the rest of the world and has, therefore, an interest in a certain disorder in order to justify its political and military power (Todd, E.: ibid.).

159. Halper, S. and Clarke, J.: ibid., p. 10.
160. Hutton, W.: *The World We're In*, ibid., pp. 192–193.
161. In this regard, it is argued that the WTO lets the interests of the developed world prevail, that the developing world would not benefit from the WTO, that environmental damage caused by free trade would hardly be of concern to the WTO, and that labor terms would not be the WTO's business. As for the last point, one even argues that the WTO is worse than its predecessor, the ITO, since the Havana Charter of 1948 required members to "take fully into account the rights of workers under inter-governmental declarations, conventions and agreements" (Wilkinson, R.: *Multilateralism and the World Trade Organisation: The Architecture and Extension of International Trade Regulation*, Routledge, 2000, p. 158). Now, however, the only thing the WTO asks from its members is to conduct their commercial relations "with a view to raising standards of living, ensuring full employment and a large and steadily growing volume of real income and effective demand" (Wilkinson, R.: ibid., p. 58). This seems to be more rhetorical than substantial, given the fact that, contrary to the Havana Charter, the WTO has no formal relations with the International Labor Organization (ILO), nor does it want to have such relations. Moreover, the WTO managed to resist pressures from a number of members in this respect. France, for example, did not succeed in establishing a permanent working party between the ILO and the WTO (Jospin, L.: ibid., p. 38).
162. It is impossible to consider the World Bank, the IMF, and the WTO in a completely isolated way, because their activities are closely tied up with foreign policy of the developed world, especially American foreign policy, as is illustrated by the fact that, within the IMF, the ten most industrialized countries have over 50% of the votes, of which the United States has 18%.
163. Phillips, K.: ibid., p. 232.
164. Palast, G.: ibid., p. 155.
165. Phillips, K.: ibid., p. 230. Dornbusch from MIT simply states that the IMF is "a tool of the United States to pursue its policy off-shore" (Phillips, K.: ibid., p. 230), making developing countries their "desperate satellites" (Ellwood, W.: ibid., p. 55). Furthermore, the former secretary-general of the United Nations, Mr. Boutros-Boutros Ghali, observes that this global governance agency to which the IMF, the World Bank and the WTO belong "is now the sole property of a single power—the US—which, through intimidation, threats and the use of its veto manipulates the world body for the benefits of its own interests" (Sardar, Z. and Davies, M. W.: ibid., p. 69).
166. Regarding this, a 1994 study by Hufbauer and Elliot found that efforts to preserve jobs trough trade barriers cost, on average, $170,000 per job saved. In some industries, this was even $500,000 or more (Gilpin, R.: ibid., p. 91). However, the other side of the coin is that free trade has also its price. If workers in the developed world lose their jobs to workers in the developing world, they no longer pay income taxes, receive unemployment benefits and, eventually, welfare and food stamps if, out of desperation, they quit looking for a job (Buchanan, P. J.: ibid., p. 285). To this other side of the coin one should also add the medical and psychological costs of deteriorating working conditions like ulcers, colitis, hives and hand tremors (Kelly, C. M.: ibid., p. 108).

167. Gilpin, R.: ibid., p. 89. Chomsky holds the view that "free trade is imposed on the poor countries by the leaders of the world whose industries and commerce have long been amply protected" (Fox, J.: ibid., p. 7). Consequently, WTO regulation of international trade is not based on equality of rights, but on the dominance of the economically strong. All of this occurs, despite the fact that trade protection appears to be very costly, as discussed in note 165.
168. Bové, J. and Dufour, F.: ibid.
169. Legrain, Ph.: ibid., p. 180.
170. Huffington, A.: ibid., p. 143.
171. Reid, T. R.: ibid., p. 238.
172. Reid, T. R.: ibid., p. 237. The legislation at issue is the Foreign Sales Corporations and Extra-Territorial Income Exclusion Act, which provided a tax break to American firms that sell overseas.
173. Kupchan, C. A.: ibid., 156.
174. *De Telegraaf*, 1 June 2005.
175. Hertsgaard, M.: ibid., p. 80. Boeing received billions of dollars in research grants, and the Americans introduced the Buy American Act (Reid, T. R.: ibid., 135).
176. Wheen gives examples of American politicians (Wheen, F.: ibid., p. 169).
177. Hettne, B. and Söderbaum, F., in: Breslin, S., Hughes, Ch. W., Phillips, N., and Rosamond, B., (eds.): ibid., p. 41.
178. Legrain, Ph.: ibid., p. 99.
179. Rugman, A.: *The End of Globalisation*, Washington, 2000, p. 56.
180. Legrain, Ph.: ibid., p. 190.
181. Castells, M.: *The Rise of the Network Society*, ibid., p. 102.
182. Rugman, A.: ibid., p. 116.
183. Legrain, Ph.: ibid., p. 8.
184. Legrain, Ph.: ibid., p. 191.
185. Legrain, Ph.: ibid., p. 191.
186. Legrain, Ph.: ibid., p. 195. After September 11, 2001, ambitions were scaled back to a more modest deal with Central America.
187. Frankel and Rose in Legrain, Ph.: ibid., p. 191.
188. Wheen, F.: ibid., chapter 10.
189. The Commission on Global Governance: ibid., p. 288.
190. Bφås, M.: The Trade-Environment Nexus and the Potential of Regional Trade Institutions, in: Breslin, S., Hughes, Ch. W., Phillips, N., Rosamond, B., (eds.): ibid., p. 59.
191. Reid, T. R.: ibid., p. 99. The author gives several examples of American products which were forced to adjust to EU rules regarding labeling, manufacturing, design, and safety (Reid, T. R.: ibid., p. 232).
192. Rifkin, J.: *The European Dream*, ibid., p. 55. Also see: Rodrik: ibid., pp. 69–85.
193. Reid, T. R.: ibid., p. 158.
194. Reid, T. R.: ibid., pp. 5–6.
195. Reid, T. R.: ibid., pp. 148–149.
196. Calleo, D. P.: ibid., p. 245.
197. Calleo, D. P.: ibid., p. 239.
198. Calleo, D. P.: ibid., p. 245.
199. Kupchan, C. A.: ibid., pp. 28–29.

200. Of course, we do not know how the costs of health care would have had developed if reform measures had not been carried through.
201. Turner, A.: ibid., pp. 8 and 82.
202. Turner, A.: ibid., pp. 164–165.
203. Levine, A.: ibid., p. 4.

Chapter 12

1. It is argued that burn-out is caused by insufficient knowledge of the rapidly changing external environment and the way one has to deal with it. In short, burn-out is believed not to be a psychiatric illness but a problem of self-management (Bruijn, J. H. B. de: Burn-Out van Topmanagement en Topprofessionals, in: Lens, P. and Kahn, Ph. S., (eds.): *Over de Schreef. Over Functioneren en Disfunctioneren van Artsen*, Van der Wees uitgeverij, Utrecht, 2001, p. 97). The causes of burn-out among doctors are thought to lie in stress factors like an increasing workload, fear of making mistakes, conflicts, and decreasing autonomy as a consequence of governmental measures and budget cuts (Rooijen, A. P. N. van: Het Loopbaanbeleid van de KNMG, in: Lens, P. and Kahn, Ph. S., (eds.): ibid., p. 333).
2. As an example: in the United States, the number of administrative employees in hospitals, HMOs, and other provider organizations multiplied sixfold during the period from 1972 to the early 1990s, which is three times faster than medical employees (OECD: *New Directions in Health Care Policy*, ibid., p. 34).
3. Based on OECD sources.
4. Glied, S.: ibid., p. 31.
5. Ludmerer, K. M.: ibid., p. 123.
6. Here, Van Waarden compares the health care sector with a brewery, in: Schut, E.: *De Zorg is toch geen Markt? Laveren tussen Marktfalen en Overheidsfalen in de Gezondheidszorg*, inaugural lecture, Erasmus University, Rotterdam, 2003, p. 12.
7. Buchegger and Stöger quote examples from the Netherlands, where in 1997 around 6% of the total employed population worked in hospitals. The public health sector's share of total employment in the Federal Republic of Germany was just under 11% in 1995. For France, the figure was 8.3% in the same year (long-term care and assistance excluded), whereas Austria's figure was 9.7% in 2001. Finally, it has been calculated that health care in the city of Munich accounted for 13.6% of total employment (Buchegger, R. and Stöger, K.: *Health as a Growth Factor. A Comparative Analysis*, Standing Committee of the Hospitals of the European Union, Leuven, 2003, pp. 10–12).
8. Buchegger, R. and Stöger, K.: ibid., pp. 15 and 21.
9. Wanless, D.: ibid., p. 58.
10. The Director-General in the Year 2000 Reith Lecture (Marinker, M., (ed.): ibid., p. 179).
11. McKee, M.: Values, Beliefs, and Implications, in: Marinker, M., (ed.): ibid., p. 188.
12. Glied, S.: ibid., p. 195.
13. McKee, M.: ibid., p. 188.
14. Walshe, K.: ibid., p. 8.
15. Friedman, M. and Friedman, R.: ibid., chapter 2.

16. As for bureaucracy, it is fashionable these days to complain about the number of bureaucrats, their operational rigidities, their lack of practical insight and creativity, their slowness, and so on. Bureaucracy has a negative ring. Society would be better off without it, it is assumed. And, indeed, bureaucracy has grown enormously. As an example, the European Union's Commission establishment of administrative and related posts in 1998 already consisted of 16,344 permanent posts, including 1,903 assigned in translation and interpretation, and 750 temporary posts (Nugent, N., (ed.): ibid., p. 3). Nevertheless, some modification is appropriate. First of all, one has to realize that creating the welfare state not only demanded money, but also the setting up of adequate organizational structures. After all, how can a government fulfill its obligations to its citizens if it does not have the employees to do so? Often, this is associated with the negative connotations of the term *bureaucracy*. It seems only fair, however, to distinguish between the demand side, or the "citizen-over-state" bureaucracy, on the one hand, and the supply side, or the "state-rules-citizen" view, on the other (Mueller, D. C.: ibid., p. 344). The demand side of bureaucracy refers to the consequence of citizens who want their government to provide public goods and to eliminate externalities. It also requires a government large enough to execute the citizens' wishes regarding the redistribution of income and wealth. On the demand side, the government is executing "the will of the people." In this respect, Myrdal argues that the welfare state is an "organized state." In such a state, market operation is subjected to the rules imposed by the state or other governmental levels (Myrdal, G.: ibid., p. 170). The supply side of bureaucracy refers to bureaucratic power and fiscal illusion as inducers of government growth. Here, the preferences of the state are decisive, with bureaucrats and political leaders pursuing their personal interests. The daily practice of bureaucracy seems to be a reasonable mixture of both sides. Research in the mid-1980s among 12 OECD countries showed a dominant demand side in Sweden and the United Kingdom and a dominant supply side in Canada, France, and the United States, whereas both sides were of equal importance in Australia, Austria, Belgium, the former Federal Republic of Germany, Italy, the Netherlands, and Norway (Mueller, D. C.: ibid., pp. 344–345). Critics of bureaucracy should take these findings into account. Many bureaucrats exist as a consequence of the design of systems of political democracy. This is quite different from the gigantic number of bureaucrats that could be found in former communist countries. This, however, leaves aside the fact that supply-side bureaucracy was not meant to be. Furthermore, there is another reason to modify criticism of bureaucracy, because a lot of damage to society could be caused by a reduction in the number of bureaucrats that is mainly motivated by ideological arguments. If we follow Klein in this respect, the United States, after 20 years of reducing the number of bureaucrats, delivers a sad example with the events of September 11, 2001. To her, the public sector has become "America's Weakest Front," which became cynically clear after the dreadful events of that day. According to Klein, it is not a depleted weapons arsenal that makes the United States vulnerable, but "its starved, devalued and crumbling public sector." A lack of federal experts trained in bio-terrorism, insufficiently funded laboratories scrambling to keep up with the demands for tests, health departments closed on weekends with no staff on call, the only licensed American laboratory to produce the anthrax vaccine gone from the country, and the U.S.

Environmental Protection Agency years behind schedule in safeguarding the water supply against bio-terrorist attacks, are examples of "the rips and holes in the United States' public infrastructure" (Klein, N.: *Fences and Windows*, ibid., pp. 115–118). If Klein is right, the United States bureaucracy is out of balance. And apparently she *is* right, since after the events of September 11, 2001, the American federal bureaucracy has grown by over 1 million persons to 12 million. According to the Brookings Institute and the University of New York, the terrorists' attack on September 11, 2001, is a major reason for this development (*De Volkskrant*, 6 September 2003). Behind all this is an essential difference between the United States and the countries of the European Union. In the United States, there is an appeal to the government for more intervention in order to redress the excessive consequences of too much market operation (I use the word *excessive* because I do not understand how one can otherwise describe the fact that increasing the minimum wage by no less than 20%–25% was being proposed in manifestos for the presidential elections in November 1996 (*Nieuwe Noordhollandse Courant*, 8 May 1996; *NRC/Handelsblad*, 5 March 1996)). In the countries of the European Union, there is an appeal to the government for less intervention in market operations in order to improve the flexibility and efficiency of the system by stopping overregulation, overtaxation, and the alarmingly static socio-economic infrastructure known as Eurosclerosis (Kuttner, R.: *The End of Laissez-Faire*, ibid., p. 136). Or, in Bok's terms, "if European welfare programs put prosperity at risk by doing too much, America's social policies threaten to do the same by accomplishing too little. If overgenerous benefits in Europe prove difficult to roll back, America may have allowed its social problems to become so deeply rooted that they will be all but impossible to overcome" (Bok, D.: *The State of the Nation: Government and the Quest for a Better Society*, Harvard University Press, Cambridge Massachusetts, 1996, p. 399). Here, differences in the social-cultural history of the United States and Europe should be taken into account. Where, on the one hand, conservative Americans accepted the idea of Keynesian welfare states in Western Europe "as necessary anticommunist allies, not as ideological soul mates," it was, on the other hand, "hard to find European leaders who did not embrace the idea of a substantial welfare state and a degree of state involvement in the economy" (Kuttner, R.: *The End of Laissez-Faire*, ibid., pp. 17 and 53). In both cases, what is involved is finding a new balance. That always requires a subtle approach regarding the role of the government and, with that, the scale of government bureaucracies. It means, among other things, that the privatization of social legislation requires the government to continue to fulfill its political guarantee function unchallenged (See: Geelhoed, A.: "Maastricht en de Nederlandse Sociaal-Democratie," in: *Nederland en de Wereld*, het Zestiende Jaarboek voor het Democratisch Socialisme, Amsterdam, pp. 106–108). In other words: a government's public responsibility limits the scope of ideas like deregulation and privatization (Leenen, K. J. J.: *Recht op Zorg voor de Gezondheid*, April, 1997, ISBN 90-73923-05-0, p. 12). The role of governments could probably be less initiatory and regulatory, but they need to continue to condition, control, and correct in matters like good education, good medical facilities, a good social infrastructure and social cohesion. They need "to create a healthy framework for economic and social activity" (Alexander, R.: ibid., p. 5). Finding a new balance could mean both more market *and* more

government (in this regard, see an interview with the Dutch economist Van der Ploeg, in: *NRC/Handelsblad*, 2 November 1995).
17. Chinitz, D.: Good and Bad Health Sector Regulation: An Overview of the Public Policy Dilemmas, in: Saltman, R. B., Busse, R., Mossialos, E., (eds.): ibid., p. 69.
18. Walshe, K.: ibid., p. 156.
19. Walshe, K.: ibid., pp. 41–48.
20. Walshe, K.: ibid., p. 46.
21. Wetenschappelijke Raad voor het Regeringsbeleid: Bewijzen van goede Dienstverlening, ibid., p. 45.
22. Fukuyama, F.: *State Building*, ibid., p. 101.
23. Gordon, R.: *Great Medical Disasters*, Hutchinson & Co. Ltd, London, 1983, pp. 33 and 106.
24. Walshe, K.: ibid., p. 3.
25. Scrivens, E.: ibid., p. 5.
26. Conradi, M.: Medische Missers: Huisartsen, Fouten en Disfunctioneren, in: Lens, P. and Kahn, Ph. S., (eds.): ibid., p. 165.
27. According to the WHO, in: Scrivens, E.: ibid., p. 5.
28. Glied, S.: ibid., p. 69.
29. Even to Hippocrates, medicine was a trade or technique (Dunning, A. J.: De Ziekenhuiswereld en het Disfunctioneren, in: Lens, P. and Kahn, Ph. S., (eds.): ibid., p. 289.
30. Dranove, D.: ibid., p. 79.
31. Glied, S.: ibid., p. 69.
32. Dranove, D.: ibid., p. 79.
33. Glied, S.: ibid., p. 71.
34. OECD: *New Directions in Health Care Policy*, ibid., p. 35.
35. Evans, R. G., Barer, M. L., and Marmor, Th. R., (eds.): ibid., p. 39.
36. Evans, R. G., Barer, M. L., and Marmor, Th. R., (eds.): ibid., p. 38.
37. Evans, R. G., Barer, M. L., and Marmor, Th. R., (eds.): ibid., p. 39.
38. Eekhof, J. A. H. and Everdingen, J. J. E. van: Over Fouten Gesproken: Ook Communicatie Kent haar Fouten, in: Everdingen, J. J. E. van, (ed.): ibid., p. 89.
39. Mulcahy, L.: ibid., p. 98.
40. Mulcahy, L.: ibid., p. 94.
41. Tempelaar, A. F.: Disfunctioneren als Iatrogene Factor, in: Lens, P. and Kahn, Ph. S., (eds.): ibid., p. 240. Also see: Hensher, M. and Edwards, N.: The Hospital and the External Environment, in: McKee, M. and Healy, J., (eds.): ibid., p. 86.
42. Formal complaints about the British NHS increased by 11% between 1999–2000 and 2000–2001 (Mulcahy, L.: ibid., p. 66).
43. Dunning, A. J.: ibid., p. 290.
44. Legemate, J.: Regelgeving in Nederland, in: Lens, P. and Kahn, Ph. S., (eds.): ibid., p. 63.
45. Dunning, A. J.: ibid., p. 290.
46. Saltman and Busse have summarized the advantages and disadvantages of self-regulation. Regarding this, see: Saltman, R. B. and Busse, R.: ibid., p. 22.
47. Mulcahy, L.: ibid., p. 12.
48. Walshe, K.: ibid., p. 127.
49. Walshe, K.: ibid., pp. 128–129.

50. Dranove, D.: ibid., p. 80.
51. Mintzberg, H.: *The Structuring of Organizations: A Synthesis of the Research*, Prentice-Hall, 1979.
52. Mintzberg, H.: *The Structuring of Organizations: A Synthesis of the Research*, ibid., p. 352.
53. Uncertainty may be caused by the incomplete knowledge of the physician, by his or her inability to distinguish between personal ignorance and the scientific level of the trade, or by limitations in medical knowledge as such (Mulcahy, L.: ibid., p. 113).
54. An analysis of 67 health care mistakes in the Netherlands revealed that 78% were made during the phase of diagnosing (Conradi, M.: ibid., p. 167).
55. Arrow, K. J., in: Weggeman, M., ibid., p. 147.
56. Weggeman, M.: ibid., p. 13.
57. There are those who, in this respect, foresee a change in medical education. Regarding this, Miettinen distinguishes between the needs of future medical practitioners, on the one hand, and medical researchers and developers, on the other. Future medical practitioners will learn the requisite skills for executing normative care, either in primary care or in health care institutions. Researchers and developers will be found in academic settings, concentrating on the scientific subject-matters of specific areas of health care (Miettinen, O. S.: *Theory of Medicine: At the Core of Post-Flexnerian Education in Medicine?* inaugural lecture, Free University, Amsterdam, 1987). The latter group will probably continue to enjoy a certain professional autonomy. After all, scientific progress and innovation need some room to maneuvre. But the first group will become medical technicians who have to work according to instructions. This means, in fact, the end of their professional autonomy.
58. Koning, P. C. J. de, and Vries, P. G.: *Ketenvorming; Samen de Schouders eronder*, in: ZM-Magazine, May, 1998, pp. 16–21.
59. I mean managers at CEO level in hospitals.
60. Keuning, D. and Eppink, D. J.: *Management en Organisatie: Theorie en Toepassing*, H. E. Stenfert Kroese, 1986, chapter 2.
61. Covey, S. R., Merrill, A. R., and Merrill, R. R.: *First Things First*, Simon & Schuster, 1994, p. 245.
62. For more on hospital management, see: Hensher, M. and Edwards, N.: ibid., pp. 83–99.
63. Busse, R., Grinten T. van der, and Svensson, P.-G.: ibid., p. 140.
64. I suggest that older health care managers who have experienced "the heat of the battle" would be qualified for this position.
65. Regarding balancing regulation and entrepreneurialism, see: Saltman, R. B. and Busse, R.: ibid., chapter 1.
66. Forder, J.: Regulating Entrepreneurial Behaviour in Social Care, in: Satman, R. B., Busse, R., Mossialos, E., (eds.): ibid., p. 165.

Epilogue

1. Friedman, Th. L.: ibid., pp. 437–440.
2. In the Netherlands, for example, relocating industrial activities to low-wage countries did not, on balance, result in a loss of jobs over the past ten years. In

contrast, almost 1,000,000 full-time equivalent new jobs have been created during this period (Vries, B. de: ibid., p. 38).

3. Vries, B. de: ibid., p. 151.
4. The predicted salary increase for 2006 for the countries of the European Union is 2%, with upward peaks of 5.5% and 5.0% for Lithuania and Estonia, respectively (De Volkskrant, 3 October 2005).
5. De Volkskrant, 3 October 2005.
6. Borghuis-Lub, T. L., Bruine, M. de, and Lapré, R. M.: Gezondheidszorg geordend: *Een Kwartet Scenario's. Scenariorapport opgesteld in opdracht van de Stichting Toekomstscenario's Gezondheidszorg,* Insituut Beleid en Management Gezondheidszorg, Erasmus Universiteit, Rotterdam, 1994.

Bibliography

Abercombie, N. and Wade, A., (eds.): *Social Change in Contemporary Britain*, Polity Press, Cambridge, 1992

Abrams, F.: *Below the Breadline: Living on the Minimum Wage*, Profile Books, London, 2002

Albert, M.: *Capitalism versus Capitalism* (Dutch Translation), Uitgeverij Contact, Amsterdam, 1992

Alexander, R.: *The Voice of the People: A Constitution for Tomorrow*, Weidenfeld & Nicolson, London, 1997

Altenstetter, C. and Warner Björkman, J., (eds.): *Health Policy Reform, National Variations and Globalization*, MacMillan Press Ltd, London, 1997

Andersen, T. M., Moene, K. O., and Sandmo, A., (eds.): *The Future of the Welfare State*, Blackwell Publishers, Cambridge, 1995

Angell, M.: *The Truth About the Drug Companies. How They Deceive Us and What To Do About It*, Random House, New York, 2004

Anselm, R. and Ley, F.: *Between Euphoria and Disillusion. What Do Clinical Ethical Committees Achieve*? in: Hospital. Official Journal of the European Association of Hospital Managers, Volume 5, Issue 5/2003, pp. 20–21

Ansieau, G.: Belgium: *One Year after the Decriminalisation of Euthanasia*, in: Hospital. Official Journal of the European Association of Hospital Managers, Issue 6/2003, p. 23–26

Appleby, J.: *Financing Health Care in the 1990s*, Open University Press, Buckingham, 1993

Arts, B.: *The Political Influence of Global NGO's. Case Studies on the Climate and Biodiversity Conventions*, International Books, Utrecht, 1998

Axford, B.: *The Global System. Economics, Politics and Culture*, Polity Press, Cambridge, 1995

Banning, W.: *Karl Marx. Leven, Leer en Betekenis*, Aula Boeken, Utrecht/Antwerpen, 1960

Banta, D.: *An Approach to the Social Control of Hospital Technologies*, WHO Paper number 10, WHO/SHS/CC/95.2, WHO, Geneva, 1995

Barber, B. R.: *Jihad versus McWorld. How Globalism and Tribalism Are Reshaping the World*, Ballantine Books, New York, 1995

Barber, B.: *Fear's Empire. War, Terrorism and Democracy* (Dutch Translation), Ambo/Manteau, Antwerpen, 2003

Bardoux, Chr.: European Group on Ethics: *Opinion on Genetic Testing in the Workplace*, in: Hospital. Official Journal of the European Association of Hospital Managers, Volume 5, Issue 5/2003, p. 18
Barrez, D.: *De Antwoorden van het Antiglobalisme. Van Seattle tot Porto Alegre*, Mets and Schilt, Amsterdam, 2001
Baumol, W. J.: *Macro-economics of Unbalanced Growth. The Autonomy of Workers Crisis*, in: American Economic Review, Volume 57, number 3, 1967
Baylis, J. and Smith, S., (eds.): *The Globalization of World Politics. An Introduction to International Relations*, second edition, Oxford University Press, Oxford, 2001
Beck, U.: *What is Globalization?* Polity Press, Cambridge, 2001
Becker, H.: *De Toekomst van de verloren Generatie*, Meulenhoff, Amsterdam, 1997
Becker, U.: *Europese Democratieën. Vrijheid, Gelijkheid, Solidariteit en Soevereiniteit in Praktijk*, Het Spinhuis, Amsterdam, 1999
Beek, H. H.: *De Geestesgestoorde in de Middeleeuwen. Beeld en Bemoeienis*, De Toorts/G. F. Callenbach, Haarlem/Nijkerk, 1969
Beigbeder, F.: *99 Francs* (Dutch Translation), De Geus, Breda, 2000
Bendiner, B.: *International Labour Affairs. The World Trade Unions and the Multinational Companies*, Clarendon Press, Oxford, 1987
Benzeval, M., Judge, K., and Whitehead, M., (eds.): *Tackling Inequalities in Health. An Agenda for Action*, King's Fund, London, 1995
Beolchi, L. (ed.): *Telemedicine Glossary*, 5th Edition, 2003 Working Document. Glossary of Concepts, Technologies, Standards and Users, European Commission, Brussels, September, 2003
Berg, C. A. van den and Albeda, W., (eds.): *100 Jaar Verantwoordelijkheid. Verleden, Heden en Toekomst van Christelijk-Sociaal Denken*, Kok, Kampen, 1991
Bergsma, S.: *De Vermaatschappelijking van de Onderneming*, Kluwer, Deventer, 1965
Berman, P.: *Terror and Liberalism*, W. W. Norton & Company, New York, 2003
Blair, T.: *New Britain. My Vision of a Young Country*, Fourth Estate, London, 1996
Boelens, E. and Schreuder, R. F.: *Platform Privatisering in de Gezondheidszorg. Terreinverkenning en Aandachtspunten voor Beleid*, Health Management Forum, Zoetermeer, 1999
Boer, J. de: *Paradoxen in de Geneeskunde*, Erasmus-lecture, Rotterdam, 1985
Böhlke, R., Söhnle, N., and Viering, S.: *Gesundheitsversorgung 2020. Konzentriert. Marktorientiert, Saniert*, Ernst & Young, Frankfurt am Main, 2005
Bok, D.: *The State of the Nation. Government and the Quest for a Better Society*, Harvard University Press, Cambridge, Massachusetts, 1996
Bongers, I. M. B., Weert, C. M. C. van, Vis, C. M., Garretsen, H. F. L., and Das, M.: *Kwaliteit en Kwantiteit van de Gezondheidszorg en actuele Beleidsontwikkelingen in de Gezondheidszorg in 2005: Nederlanders aan het Woord*, Universiteit van Tilburg, 2005
Borghuis-Lub, T. L., Bruine, M. de, and Lapré, R. M.: *Gezondheidszorg geordend. Een Kwartet Scenario's. Scenariorapport opgesteld in opdracht van de Stichting Toekomstscenario's Gezondheidszorg*, Instituut Beleid en Management Gezondheidszorg, Rotterdam, 1994
Bové, J. and Dufour, F.: *The World is Not for Sale. Farmers against Junk Food*, Verso, London, 2001
Braybrooke, D. and Lindblom, C.: *A Strategy of Decision. Policy Evaluation as a Social Process*, The Free Press, New York, 1970

Breslin, S., Hughes, Ch. W., Phillips, N., and Rosamond, B.: *New Regionalism in the Global Political Economy*, Routledge, London, 2002
British Ministry of Health: *The New NHS. Modern-Dependable*, NHS, London, 1997
Bronk, R.: *Progress and the Invisible Hand. The Philosophy and Economics of Human Advance*, Little, Brown and Company, London, 1998
Buchanan, P. J.: *The Great Betrayal. How American Sovereignty and Social Justice Are Being Sacrificed to the Gods of the Global Economy*, Little, Brown and Company, Boston, 1998
Buchegger, R. and Stöger, K.: *Health as a Growth Factor. A Comparative Analysis*, Standing Committee of the Hospitals of the European Union, Leuven, 2003
Burton-Jones, A.: *Knowledge Capitalism*, Oxford University Press, Oxford, 1999
Busch, G. K.: *The Political Role of International Trades Unions*, MacMillan Press, London, 1983
Calleo, D. P.: *Rethinking Europe's Future*, Princeton University Press, Princeton, 2001
Cameron, S.: *The Cheating Classes. How Britain's Elite Abuse their Power*, Simon and Schuster, London, 2002
Carew, A.: *Democracy and Government in European Trade Unions*, Allen and Unwin Ltd., London, 1976
Castells, M.: *End of Millennium. The Information Age: Economy, Society and Culture*, Volume 3, Blackwell Publishers, Oxford, 1998
Castells, M.: *The Power of Identity. The Information Age: Economy, Society and Culture*, Volume 2, Blackwell Publishers, Oxford, 1997
Castells, M.: *The Rise of the Network Society. The Information Age: Economy, Society and Culture*, Volume 1, Blackwell Publishers, Oxford, 1996
Castles, F. G.: *The Future of the Welfare State. Crisis Myths and Crisis Realities*, Oxford University Press, Oxford, 2004
Centraal Planbureau: *Scanning the Future. A Long-Term Scenario of the World Economy*, 1900–2015, SDU Publishers, Den Haag, 1992
Chalmers Johnson: *Blowback. The Costs and Consequences of American Empire*, Little, Brown and Company, London, 2002
Chomsky, N.: *9–11*, Seven Stories Press, New York, 2002
Cini, M. and McGowan, L.: *Competition Policy in the European Union*, MacMillan Press Ltd., London, 1998
Cliteur, P.: *Tegen de Decadentie. De Democratische Rechtstaat in Verval*, De Arbeiderspers, Amsterdam/Antwerpen, 2004-03-17
College Bouw Ziekenhuisvoorzieningen: *Publiek Private Samenwerking in de Gezondheidszorg. Een vergelijkende Studie*, Signaleringsrapport, Rapportnummer 568, CBZ, Utrecht, 2004
College Bouw Ziekenhuisvoorzieningen: *Signaleringsrapport Het zelfstandig Behandelcentrum: van noodzakelijk Kwaad tot nuttig Goed?* Voorstel voor een nieuw Beoordelingskader, Signaleringsrapport, CBZ, Utrecht, 2003
Colombo, F. and Tapay, N.: Private Health Insurance in Ireland: A Case Study, OECD Health Working Paper No. 10, Directorate for Employment, Labour and Social Affairs, OECD, Paris, February, 2004
Commissie van de Europese Gemeenschappen: *Communautaire Samenwerking op het Gebied van de Volksgezondheid*. Mededeling van de Commissie aan de Raad, COM(84) 502 def., Brussel, 18 September, 1984

Commissie van de Europese Gemeenschappen: *De Toekomst van de Gezondheidszorg en de Ouderenzorg: de Toegankelijkheid, de Kwaliteit en de Betaalbaarheid waarborgen*. Mededeling van de Commissie aan de Raad, het Europees Parlement, het Economisch en Sociaal Comité en het Comité van de Regio's, COM(2001) 723 definitief, Brussel, 05.12.2001

Commissie van de Europese Gemeenschappen: *Kostenbewaking bij de Planning en Organisatie van de Gezondheidszorg*. Werkdocument van de Commissie, COM(84) 1652 def., Brussel, 25 October, 1984

Commission of the European Communities: *The Commission and Non-Governmental Organisations: Building a Stronger Partnership*. Commission Discussion Paper COM(2000), 11 final, Brussels, 18.1.2000

Commission of the European Communities: *Commission Communication on the Framework for Action in the Field of Public Health*, COM(93) 559 final, Brussels, 24 November, 1993

Commission of the European Communities: *Communication from the Commission concerning a Community Action Programme on Health Monitoring in the Context of the Framework for Action in the Field of Public Health*, COM(95) 449 final, Brussels, 16.10.1995

Commission of the European Communities: *European Social Policy. Options for the Union*, Green Paper, Consultative Document by Mr. Flynn, 17 November, 1993, Com (93) 551, Directorate-General for Employment, Industrial Relations and Social Affairs

Commission of the European Communities: *European Social Policy. Options for the Union*. Consultative Document. Green Paper Communication by Mr. Flynn COM(93) 551, Brussels, 17 November, 1993

Commission of the European Communities: *Growth, Competitiveness, Employment. The Challenges and Ways forward into the 21st Century*, White Book (Dutch Translation), Brussels, 1994

Commission of the European Communities: *Proposal for a Decision of the European Parliament and the Council, adopting a Programme of Community Action in the Field of Public Health*. Communication of the Commission to the Council, the European Parliament, the Economic and Social Committee and the Committee of the Regions on the Health Strategy of the European Community. (2001–2006). COM(2000) 285 final, Brussels, 16.5.2000

Commission of the European Communities: *Report from the Commission to the Council, the European Parliament and the Economic and Social Committee on the Integration of Health Protection Requirements in Community Policies*, COM(95) 196 final, Brussels, 29.5.1995

Commission of the European Communities: *The Future of Social Protection: a Framework for a European Debate*. Communication from the Commission, COM(95) 466 final, Brussels, 31.10.1995

Commission on Global Governance: *Our Global Neighborhood*, Oxford University Press, Oxford, 1996

Corbett, R.: *The Treaty of Maastricht*, Longman Group, United Kingdom, 1993

Coulter, A. and Magee, H., (eds.): *The European Patient of the Future*, Open University Press, Maidenhead, 2004

Council of Churches for Britain and Ireland: *Unemployment and the Future of Work. An Enquiry for the Churches*, Inter-Church House, London, 1997

Covey, S. R., Merrill, A. R., and Merrill, R. R.: *First Things First*, Simon & Schuster, New York, 1994

Cowles, M. G., Caporaso, J., and Risse, Th., (eds.): *Transforming Europe. Europeanization and Domestic Change*, Cornell University Press, New York, 2001
Croft, S., Redmond, J., Wyn Rees, G., and Webber, M.: *The Enlargement of Europe*, Manchester University Press, Manchester, 1999
Cyert, R. M. and March, J. G.: *A Behavioral Theory of the Firm*, Prentice Hall, New Jersey, 1963
Dalen, H. van and Kalshoven, F., (eds.): *Meesters van de Welvaart. Topeconomen over Nederland*, Uitgeverij Balans, Amsterdam, 2002
Daly, H. E.: *Beyond Growth. The Economics of Sustainable Development*, Beacon Press, Boston, 1996
Dawson, A. D.: *The Two Faces of Economics*, Longman, New York, 1996
Deakin, N.: *The Politics of Welfare. Continuities and Change*, Simon & Schuster, New York, 1994
Dean, K. (ed.): *Connected Health. Essays from Health Innovators*, Cisco Systems, undated
Delsen, L.: *Exit Poldermodel? Sociaal-Economische Ontwikkelingen in Nederland*, second edition, Van Gorcum, Assen, 2001
Dent, M.: *Remodelling Hospitals and Health Professions in Europe. Medicine, Nursing and the State*, Palgrave MacMillan, New York, 2003
Deppe, H. -U.: *Zur sozialen Anatomie des Gesundheitssystems. Neoliberalismus und Gesundheitspolitik in Deutschland, Verlag für Akademische Schriften*, Frankfurt, 2000
Dijkstra, G. S. A., Meer, F. M., and Rutgers, M. R., (eds.): *Het Belang van de Publieke Zaak. Beschouwingen over Bestuurskunde en Openbaar Bestuur*, Eburon, Delft, 2003
Doel, J. van den: *Konvergentie en Evolutie*, Van Gorcum, Assen, 1971
Donaldson, C. and Gerard, K.: *Economics of Health Care Financing. The Visible Hand, Economic Issues in Health Care*, MacMillan Press, London, 1993
Donatini, A., Rico, A., D'Ambrosio, M. G., Lo Scalzo, A., Orzella, L., Cicchetti, A., and Profili, S.: *Health Care Systems in Transition: Italy, 2001*, European Observatory on Health Care Systems (Rico, A. and Cetani, T., [eds.]), WHO, Copenhagen, 2001
Doorslaer, E. K. A. van: *Gezondheidszorg tussen Marx en Markt*, inaugural lecture, Erasmus University, Rotterdam, 1998
Dranove, D.: *The Economic Evolution of American Health Care. From Marcus Welby to Managed Care*, Princeton University Press, Princeton, 2000
Drucker, P.: *Management Challenges for the 21st Century*, Harper Collins Publishers, New York, 1999
Dunkerley, D., Hodgson, L., Konopacki, S., Spybey, T., and Thompson, A.: *Changing Europe. Identities, Nations and Citizens*, Routledge, London, 2002
Dyson, K.: *The Politics of the Euro-Zone. Stability or Breakdown?* Oxford University Press, Oxford, 2000
Edwards, P., Shaoul, J., Stafford, A., and Arblaster, L.: *Evaluating the Operation of PFI in Roads and Hospitals*, The Association of Chartered Certified Accountants, London, 2004
Ehrenreich, B.: *Nickel and Dimes. Undercover in Low-Wage USA*, Granta Books, London, 2002
Einerhand, M., Kerklaan, M., Metz, H., Siegelaer, E., and Vliegenthart, M.: *Sociale Zekerheid. Stelsels en Regelingen in enkele Europese Landen*, VUGA Uitgeverij, Den Haag, 1995

Ellwood, W.: *The No-Nonsense Guide to Globalization* (Dutch Translation), Lemniscaat, Rotterdam, 2003

Engbersen, G., Vrooman, J. C., and Snel, E.: *Arm Nederland. Het eerste Jaarrapport Armoede en Sociale Uitsluiting*, VUGA Uitgeverij, The Hague, 1996

Entzinger, H. and Meer, J. van der, (eds.): *Grenzeloze Solidariteit. Naar een Migratiebestendige Verzorgingsstaat*, De Balie, Amsterdam, 2004

Esping-Anderson, G., (ed.): *Welfare States in Transition. National Adaptations in Global Economics*, SAGE Publications, London, 1997

Etzioni, A.: *The Moral Dimension. Toward a New Economics*, The Free Press, New York, 1990

Etzioni, A.: *The New Golden Rule. Community and Morality in a Democratic Society*, Profile Books, London, 1997

Etzioni, A.: *The Spirit of Community. Rights, Responsibilities and the Communitarian Agenda*, Fontana Press, London, 1995

Eucken, W.: *Die Grundlagen der Nationalökonomie, Achte Auflage*, Springer-Verlag, Berlin, 1965

European Commission. Health & Consumer Protection Directorate-General: *The Internal Market and Health Services.* Report of the High Level Committee on Health, Brussels, 17.12.2001

European Commission: *High Level Process of Reflection on Patient Mobility and Healthcare Developments in the European Union*, Brussels, 8 December, 2003

European Health Management Association: *The European Union and Health Services—The Impact of the Single European Market on Member States.* Summary of a Report to the European Commission, Dublin, May 2001

European Observatory on Health Care Systems: *Health Care Systems in Transition: Portugal, 2004*, WHO, Copenhagen, 2004

European Observatory on Health Care Systems: *Health Care Systems in Transition: Luxembourg, 1999*, WHO, Copenhagen, 1999

European Observatory on Health Care Systems: *Health Care Systems in Transition: Belgium, 2000*, WHO, Copenhagen, 2000

European Observatory on Health Care Systems: *Health Care Systems in Transition: United Kingdom, 1999*, WHO, Copenhagen, 1999

European Observatory on Health Care Systems: *Health Care Systems in Transition: Spain, 2000*, WHO, Copenhagen, 2000

European Observatory on Health Care Systems: *Health Care Systems in Transition: Germany, 2000*, WHO, Copenhagen, 2000

European Parliament. Directorate General for Research: *Health Care Systems in the EU. A Comparative Study*, Working Paper, Public Health and Consumer Protection Series, SACO 101/rev. EN, 11-1998

Europees Parlement. Zittingsdocumenten: *Verslag over de Europese Gezondheidskaart*, 26 maart, 1996, A4-0091/96

Evans, Ph. and Wurster, Th. S.: *Blown to Bits. How the Economics of Information Trans-forms Strategy* (Dutch Translation), Uitgeverij Business Contact, Amsterdam/Antwerpen, 2002

Evans, R. G., Barer, M. L., and Marmor, Th. R., (eds.): *Why Are Some People Healthy and Others Not? The Determinants of Health of Populations*, Aldine de Gruyter, New York, 1994

Everdingen, J. J. E. van, (ed.): *Smetten op de witte Jas*, Belvédère/Boom, 1993

Exter, A. den, Hermans, H., Dosljak, M., and Busse, R.: *Health Care Systems in Transition: The Netherlands, 2004*, European Observatory on Health Care Systems (Busse, R., Ginneken, E. van, Schreyögg, J., and Wisbaum, W., [eds.]), WHO, Copenhagen, 2004
Feigenbaum, H., Henig, J., and Hamnet, Chr.: *Shrinking the State. The Political Underpinnings of Privatisation*, Cambridge University Press, Cambridge, 1999
Feuerstein, G. and Kuhlmann, E., (eds.): *Rationierung im Gesundheitswesen*, Ullstein Medical, Wiesbaden, 1998
Filer, R. K., Hamermesh, D. S., and Rees, A. E.: *The Economics of Work and Pay*, sixth Edition, Harper Collins, New York, 1996
Forrester, V.: *L'horreur économique* (Dutch Translation), Ambo, Amsterdam, 1997
Forrester, V.: *Une étrange Dictature* (Dutch Translation), Rainbow Pocketboeken, Amsterdam, 2001
Foudraine, J.: *Oorspronkelijk Gezicht. Een Gang naar Huis*, Ambo, Baarn, 1979
Foudraine, J.: *Wie is van Hout? Een Gang door de Psychiatrie*, Ambo, Baarn, 1971
Fox, J.: *Chomsky and Globalization*, Icon Books, Cambridge, 2001
Frank, R. H. and Cook, Ph. J.: *The Winner-Take-All Society. Why the Few at the Top Get So Much More Than the Rest of Us*, Penguin Books, New York, 1995
Frank, S.: *Having None of It. Women, Men and the Future of Work*, Granta Books, London, 1999
Freidson, E.: *Profession of Medicine. A Study of the Sociology of Applied Knowledge*, Harper & Row Publishers, New York, 1970
Friedman, E., (ed.): *Making Choices. Ethical Issues for Health Care Professionals*, American Hospital Association, 1986
Friedman, M. and Friedman, R.: *Free to Choose. The Classic Inquiry into the Relationship between Freedom and Economics*, Harvest Book, Harcourt, Inc., San Diego, 1990
Friedman, Th. L.: *The Lexus and the Olive Tree. Understanding Globalization*, Anchor Books, New York, 2000
Fukuyama, F.: *The End of History and the Last Man* (Dutch Translation), 4th edition, Olympus, Amsterdam, 1999
Fukuyama, F.: *The Great Disruption. Human Nature and the Reconstruction of Social Order* (Dutch Translation), Uitgeverij Contact, Amsterdam/Antwerpen, 1999
Fukyama, F.: *State Building. Governance and World Order in the Twenty-First Century*, Profile Books, 2004
Fukuyama, F.: *Trust. The Social Virtues & the Creation of Posperity*, The Free Press, New York, 1995
Galan, C. de: *De Invloed van de Vakvereniging op Loonshoogte en Werkgelegenheid*, H. E. Stenfert Kroese N. V., Leiden, 1958
Galbraith, J. K.: *The Affluent Society*, Houghton Mifflin, Boston, 1958
Galbraith, J. K.: *The Culture of Contentment*, Penguin Books, London, 1992
Galbraith, J. K.: *A Journey through Economic Time. A Firsthand View* (Dutch Translation), Sesam, Baarn, 1995
Gastmans, Chr., (ed.): *Between Technology and Humanity. The Impact of Technology on Health Care Ethics*, Leuven University Press, Leuven, 2002
Gates, J.: *Democracy at Risk. Rescuing Main Street from Wall Street*, Perseus Publishing, Cambridge, Massachusetts, 2001

Geelhoed, A.: *"Maastricht" en de Nederlandse Sociaal-Democratie*, in: Nederland en de Wereld, Zestiende Jaarboek voor het Democratisch-Socialisme, Amsterdam, 1995

Geleijnse, L., Vrooman, J. C., and Muffels, R. J. A.: *Tussen Ministelsel en Participatiemodel. Een verkennende Studie naar Stelselvarianten in de Sociale Zekerheid*, Sociaal en Cultureel Planbureau, Rijswijk, 1993

Gezondheidsraad: *Grenzen van de Gezondheidszorg*, Gezondheidsraad, Den Haag, 1986

Gier, E. de, Swaan, A. de, and Ooijens, M., (eds.): *Dutch Welfare Reform in an Expanding Europe. The Neighbours' View*, Het Spinhuis, Amsterdam, 2004

Gilpin, R.: *The Challenge of Global Capitalism. The World Economy in the 21st Century*, Princeton University Press, Princeton, 2000

Glied, S.: *Chronic Condition. Why Health Reform Fails*, Harvard University Press, Cambridge, Massachusetts, 1997

Goerke, H.: *Arzt und Heilkunde. 3000 Jahre Medizin. Vom Asklepiospriester zum Klinikarzt*, Callwey, München, 1984

Goodman, A. and Webb, S.: *For Richer, for Poorer. The Changing Distribution of Income in the United Kingdom*, 1961–91, The Institute of Fiscal Studies, London, 1994

Gooijer, W. J. de, Siem Tjam, F., and Stott, G.: *Hospital and Institutional Care. An Approach to a Generic Classification*, WHO, WHO/EIP/OSD/00.3, Geneva, 2000

Gooijer, W. J. de: *Beheersing van Technologische Vernieuwing*, Samsom Uitgeverij, Alphen a/d Rijn, 1976

Gooijer, W. J. de: *De Planning van Dure Medische Apparatuur in het Europa van 1992*, in: *ZM-Magazine*, jaargang 5, nummer 11, November 1989, pp. 11–19

Gooijer, W. J. de: *On Solidarity in Changing Health Care Systems. Europe in Search of a New Balance*, inaugural lecture, Standing Committee of the Hospitals of the European Union, Leuven, 1996

Gooijer, W. J. de: *Ziekenhuismanagement als Afstemmings-en Structureringsprobleem. Historie en Perspectief*, inaugural lecture, Van Gorcum, Assen/Maastricht, 1988

Goudswaard, K. P.: Sociale Covergentie, inaugural lecture, Leiden, 1996

Goudzwaard, B., Laeyendecker, L., Lange, H. M. de, Thung, M. A., Tieleman, H. J., and Wezel, J. van: *Een Gezonde Economie? Maatschappelijke Dimensies van het Economisch Handelen*, Uitgeverij Kok, Kampen, 1994

Graham, H., (ed.): *Understanding Health Inequalities*, Open University Press, Maidenhead, England, 2003

Gray, J.: *False Dawn. The Delusions of Global Capitalism*, Granta Books, London, 1999

Green, D. G.: *From Welfare State to Civil Society. Towards Welfare that Works in New Zealand*, New Zealand Business Roundtable, Wellington, 1996

Greider, K.: *The Big Fix. How the Pharmaceutical Industry Rips Off American Consumers*, Public Affairs, New York, 2003

Groen, J. F.: *Een Stem in het Publieke Domein. Een Onderzoek naar Documenten van Protestantse Kerken in Duitsland, Engeland en Nederland, 1979–1994*, Hagé-Uitgeverij, Amsterdam, 1997

Gross, N.: *Active Assisted Dying (Euthanasia) in Europe. Where Are We Heading?* in: Hospital. Official Journal of the European Association of Hospital Managers, Volume 5, Issue 6/2003, pp. 20–22

Gunning-Schepers, L. J., Kronjee, G. J., and Spasoff, R. A.: *Fundamental Questions about the Future of Health Care, Netherlands Scientific Council for Government Policy*, The Hague, 1996
Haas, B. de and Lotringen, C. van: *Mister Euro. Een Biografie van Wim Duisenberg*, Business Contact/Het Financiële Dagblad, 2005
Halper, S. and Clarke, J.: *America Alone. The Neo-Conservatives and the Global Order*, Cambridge University Press, Cambridge, 2004
Ham, C. and Robert, G.: *Reasonable Rationing. International Experience of Priority Setting in Health Care*, Open University Press, Maidenhead, 2003
Handy, C.: *The Empty Raincoat* (Dutch Translation), Arrow, Amsterdam/Antwerpen, 1994
Handy, C.: *Beyond Certainty. The Changing World of Organisations*, Arrow Business Books, London, 1996
Hansen, J. D., (ed.): *European Integration. An Economic Perspective*, Oxford University Press, Oxford, 2001
Harrison, L. E. and Huntington, S. P.: *Culture Matters. How Values Shape Human Progress*, Basic Books, New York, 2000
Hartog, F.: *Economische Stelsels*, Wolters Noordhoff, Groningen, 1970
Hartog, F.: *Overheid en Economisch Leven*, Samsom, Alphen a/d Rijn, 1965
Hay, C.: *Re-Stating Social and Political Change*, Open University Press, Buckingham, 1996
Hayek, F. A.: *The Road to Serfdom*, University of Chicago Press, Chicago, 1994
Healthcare 2000: *UK Health and Healthcare Services. Challenges and Policy Options*, NHS, London, 1995
Health Council of the Netherlands: *The Future of Our Selves,* Health Council of the Netherlands, publication no. 2002/13, The Hague, 2002
Held, D. (ed.): *A Globalizing World? Culture, Economics, Politics*, Routledge, London, 2000
Held, D., McGrew, A., Goldblatt, D., and Perraton, J.: *Global Transformations. Politics, Economics and Culture*, Polity Press, Cambridge, 1999
Held, D. and McGrew, A.: *Globalization/Anti-Globalization*, Blackwell Publishers, Polity Press, Cambridge, 2002
Hermans, B. and Brouwer, W.: *Quality Issues on Cross-Border Care: A Literature Search*, Rotterdam/Utrecht, June 2003, www.ehma.org
Hermans, H. E. G. M. and France, G.: *Beperking van het Recht op Gezondheidszorg: Realisering van Zorgaanspraken in Nederland en Italië*, in: Sociaal Recht, 1998–2, pp. 47–54
Hertsgaard, M.: *The Eagle's Shadow* (Dutch Translation), Cossee, Amsterdam, 2002
Hertz, N.: *The Silent Takeover—Global Capitalism and the Death of Democracy* (Dutch Translation), Uitgeverij Contact, Amsterdam/Antwerpen, 2002
Hirsch, F.: *Social Limits to Growth*, Routledge, London, 1995
Hitiris, Th.: *European Union Economics*, 4th edition, Prentice Hall, London, 1998
Hjortsberg, C. and Ghatnekar, O.: *Health Care Systems in Transition: Sweden, 2001*, European Observatory on Health Care Systems (Rico, A., Wisbaum, W., and Cetani, T. [eds.]), WHO, Copenhagen, 2001
Hofmarcher, M. M.: *Cross-Section Analysis of Health Spending with special Regard to Trends in Austria*, Insitute for Advanced Studies, Vienna, Economic Series, No. 70, Vienna, 1999

Hofmarcher, M. M. and Rack, H.: *Health Care Systems in Transition: Austria, 2001*, European Observatory on Health Care Systems (Dixon, A., [ed.]), WHO, Copenhagen, 2001
Hofstede, G.: *Culture and Organizations. Software of the Mind* (Dutch Translation), Uitgeverij Contact, Amsterdam, 2002
Honoré, C.: *In Praise of Slow: How a Worldwide Movement is Challenging the Cult of Speed* (Dutch Translation), Lemniscaat, Rotterdam, 2004
Hoogerwerf, A.: *Politiek als Evenwichtskunst*, Samsom/Tjeenk Willink, Alphen a/d Rijn, 1995
Huffington, A.: *Pigs at the Trough. How Corporate Greed and Political Corruption are Undermining America*, Crown Publishers, New York, 2003
Huntington, S. P.: *The Clash of Civilizations and the Remaking of the World Order*, Simon & Schuster, New York, 1996
Huntington, S. P.: *Who Are We? America's Great Debate*, Free Press, London, 2005
Hutton, W. and Giddens, A.: *On the Edge. Living with Global Capitalism*, Jonathan Cape, London, 2000
Hutton, W.: *The State to Come*, Vintage Books, London, 1997
Hutton, W.: *The State We're In*, Vintage Books, London, 1995
Hutton, W.: *The World We're In*, Little Brown, London, 2002
Illich, I.: *Medical Nemesis* (Dutch Translation), Het Wereldvenster, Baarn, 1975
Independent Commission on Population and the Quality of Life: *Caring for the Future*, Oxford University Press, Oxford, 1996
Jacobs, F. C. L. M. and Wal, G. A., (eds.): *Medische Schaarste en het Menselijk Tekort*, Ambo, Baarn, 1988
Jallade, J.-P., (ed.): *The Crisis of Redistribution in European Welfare States*, Trentham Books, Stoke-on-Trent, 1988
Jansen van Galen, J.: *Het Suriname-Syndroom. De PvdA tussen Den Haag en Paramaribo*, Bert Bakker/Wiardi Beckman Stichting, Amsterdam, 2001
Järvelin, J.: *Health Care Systems in Transition: Finland, 2002*, European Observatory on Health Care Systems (Rico, A. and Cetani, T., [eds.]), WHO, Copenhagen, 2002
Jennet, B.: *High Technology Medicine. Benefits and Burdens*, Oxford University Press, Oxford, 1986
Jochemsen, H.: *The Practice and Legalisation of Euthanasia in the Netherlands*, in: *Hospital.* Official Journal of the European Association of Hospital Managers, Volume 5, Issue 6/2003, pp. 18–20
Johson, H. T. and Kaplan, R. S.: *Relevance Lost. The Rise and Fall of Management Accounting*, Harvard Business School Press, Boston Massachusetts, 1987
Jones, L. J.: *The Social Context of Health and Health Work*, MacMillan, London, 1994
Judt, T.: *A Grand Illusion. An Essay on Europe* (Dutch Translation), Erven Bijleveld, Utrecht, 1997
Juffermans, P.: *Staat en Gezondheidszorg in Nederland*, SUN, Nijmegen, 1982
Kaars Sijpesteijn, E. J., (ed.): *Het Volk en Europa. Grenzen aan Europa*, Vereniging Democratisch Europa, Amsterdam, 2004
Kahn, H. and Wiener, A. J.: *The Year 2000. A Framework for Speculation on the next Thirty-Three Years*, MacMillan, New York, 1967
Kalma, P.: *De Illusie van de "Democratische Staat,"* WBS-cahier, Kluwer, 1982
Kam, F. de and Nypels, F.: *Tijdbom*, Uitgeverij Contact, Amsterdam/Antwerpen, 1995

Kaplan, R. B.: *The Coming Anarchy. Shattering the Dreams of the Post Cold War*, Random House, New York, 2000
Kapstein, E. B.: *Sharing the Wealth. Workers and the World Economy*, Norton and Company, New York, 1999
Kelly, C. M.: *Class War in America. How Economic and Political Conservatives are Exploiting Low- and Middle-Class Americans*, Fithian Press, Santa Barbara, California, 2000
Keuning, D. and Eppink, D. J.: *Management en Organisatie. Theorie en Toepassing*, H. E. Stenfert Kroese, Leiden/Antwerpen, 1986
Keynes, J. M.: *The General Theory of Employment, Interest and Money*, The Easton Press, Collector's Edition, The Easton Press, Norwalk, Connecticut, 1995
Kirschen, E. S., Benard, J., Besters, H., Blackaby, F., Eckstein, O., Faaland, J., Hartog, F., Morissens, L., and Tosco, E.: *Economic Policy in our Time.* Vols. I, II and III, second edition, North-Holland Publishing Company, Amsterdam, 1964
Kleerekoper, S.: *De Fictie van het Algemeen Belang*, Kluwer, Deventer/Antwerpen, 1963
Klein, N.: *Fences and Windows. Dispatches from the Front Lines of the Globalization Debate*, Picador USA, New York, 2002
Klein, N.: *No Logo*, Flamingo Books, London, 2001
Koekkoek, A. K., (ed.): *De Grondwet. Een systematisch en artikelsgewijs Commentaar*, derde druk, Tjeenk Willink, Deventer, 2002
Kölking, H.: *Building Blocs of an Institutional Ethic: The Development of Medical-Ethical Competence among Doctors and Nurses*, in: Hospital. Official Journal of the European Association of Hospital Managers, Volume 5, Issue 5/2003, p. 15
Kolnaar, A. H. H. J.: *Sociale Zekerheid en Verantwoordelijkheid. Een Discussienota voor de CDA-werkgroep Sociale Zekerheid*, The Hague, 1992
Komter, A. E., Burgers, J., and Engbersen, G.: *Het Cement van de Samenleving. Een verkennende Studie naar Solidariteit en Cohesie*, Amsterdam University Press, Amsterdam, 2000
Koning, P. C. J. de, and Vries, P. G. de: *Ketenvorming; Samen de Schouders eronder*, in: ZM-Magazine, May, 1998, pp. 16–21.
Koning Boudewijn Stichting en Vereniging van Belgische Steden en Gemeenten: *Algemeen Verslag over de Armoede, in opdracht van de minister van sociale integratie*, 1995
Krugman, P.: *The Return of Depression Economics*, Allen Lane/Penguin Press, London, 1999
Krukemayer, H.: *Vergleichende Systemanalyse des Krankenhauswesens in den OECD-Ländern*, Verlag H. M. Hauschild, Bremen, 1985
Kupchan, C. A.: *The End of the American Era. U.S. Foreign Policy and the Geopolitics of the Twenty-First Century*, Vintage Books, New York, 2002
Kuttner, R.: *Everything for Sale. The Virtues and Limits of Markets*, The University of Chicago Press, Chicago, 1999
Kuttner, R.: *The End of Laissez-Faire. National Purpose and the Global Economy after the Cold War*, University of Pennsylvania Press, 1992
Lagendijk, J. and Wiersma, J. M.: *Na Mars komt Venus. Een Europees Antwoord op Bush*, Uitgeverij Balans, 2004
Lamy, P.: *L'Éurope en première ligne* (Dutch Translation), Lemniscaat, Rotterdam, 2004

Landes, D. S.: *The Wealth and Poverty of Nations. Why Some Are So Rich and Some So Poor* (Dutch Translation), Het Spectrum, Utrecht, 1998

Lasch, C.: *The Revolt of the Elites and the Betrayal of Democracy*, W. W. Norton & Company, New York, 1995

Layard, R.: *What Labour Can Do*, Warner Books, London, 1997

Leadbeater, C.: *Up the Down Escalator. Why the Global Pessimists Are Wrong*, Viking Books, London, 2002

Leenen, H. J. J.: *Recht op Zorg voor de Gezondheid*, preliminary report, April, 1997, ISBN 90-73923-05-0

Le Fanu, J.: *The Rise and Fall of Modern Medicinc*, Abacus, London, 2004

Legrain, Ph.: *Open World:/The Truth about Globalisation*, Abacus, London, 2002

Leibfried, S. and Pierson, P., (eds.): *European Social Policy. Between Fragmentation and Integration*, The Brookings Institution, Washington DC, 1995

Leijnse, F.: *Verzorgingsstaat. Last of Lust?* inaugural lecture, Erasmus university, Rotterdam, 1994

Lens, P. and Kahn, Ph., (eds.): *Over de Schreef*, Van der Wees Uitgeverij, Utrecht, 2001

Levine, A.: *The American Ideology. A Critique*, Routledge, New York, 2004

Levine, M.: *A Branded World. Adventures in Public Relations and the Creation of Superbrands*, John Wiley & Sons, Inc., New Jersey, 2003

Levitt, A.: *Take on the Street. What Wall Street and Corporate America Don't Want You To Know. What You Can Do To Fight Back*, Pantheon Books, New York, 2002

Lewin, L.: *Self-Interest and Public Interest in Western Politics*, Oxford University Press, Oxford, 1991

Lindert, P. H.: *Growing Public. Social Spending and Economic Growth since the Eighteenth Century*, Cambridge University Press, Cambridge, 2004

List, F.: *The National System of Political Economy.* Augustus M. Kelley Publishers. Reprints of Economic Classics, New York, 1966

Loney, M., Boswell, D., and Clarke, J., (eds.): *Social Policy & Social Welfare*, Open University Press, Philadelphia, 1993

Loo, H. van der and Reijen, W. van: *Paradoxen van Modernisering*, Coutinho, Bussum, 1997

Lubbers, E.: *Battling Big Business* (Dutch Translation), Uitgeverij Fagel, Amsterdam, 2002

Ludmerer, K. M.: *Time To Heal. American medical Education form the Turn of the Century to the Era of Managed Care*, Oxford University Press, New York, 1999

Luttwak, E.: *Turbo Capitalism. Winners and Losers in the Global Economy*, Weidenfield & Nicolson, London, 1998

Mackenbach, J. and Bakker, M., (eds.): *Reducing Inequalities in Health. A European Perspective*, Routledge, London, 2002

Malek, M., (ed.): *Priority Setting in Health Care*, John Wiley & Sons, Chichester, 1994

Malleson, A.: *Need your Doctor Be So Useless?* (Dutch Translation), Het Spectrum, Utrecht/Antwerpen, 1974

Mandel, E.: *Die EWG und die Konkurrenz Europa—Amerika* (Dutch Translation), Van Gennep, Amsterdam, 1969

Marinker, M.: *Health Targets in Europe. Polity, Progress and Promise*, BMJ Books, London, 2002

Materne, L., Vos, P. de, Vandepitte, M., Belder, B. de, Tavernier, Ph., Russell, R., and Manuel, E. S.: *Globalisering en Gezondheid. Een Alternatief voor Commercialis-*

ering en Privatisering, Marxistische Studies, nr. 58, EPO, Brussel, April–June, 2002

May, A. T.: *Ethics as a Measure of Quality*, in: Hospital. Official Journal of the European Association of Hospital Managers, Volume 5, Issue, 5/2003, p. 16–17

McCloskey, D. N.: *The Vices of Economists—The Virtues of the Bourgeoisie* (Dutch Translation), Amsterdam University Press, Amsterdam, 1997

McIntosh, A.: *Soil and Soul. People versus Corporate Power*, Aurum Press, London, 2002

McKee, M., MacLehose, L., and Nolte, E., (eds.): *Health Policy and European Union Enlargement*, European Observatory on Health Systems and Policies Series, Open University Press, Maidenhead, England, 2004

McKee, M. and Healy, J., (eds.): *Hospitals in a Changing Europe*, European Observatory on Health Care Systems Series, Open University Press, Buckingham, 2002

McKeown, T.: *The Role of Medicine*, Princeton University Press, 2002

McKinlay, J. B., (ed.): *Technology and the Future of Health Care*, A Milbank Reader 8, MIT Press, Cambridge, Massachusetts, 1982

Meadows, D. L.: *The Limits to Growth.* A Report for the Club of Rome Project (Dutch Translation), Uitgeverij Het Spectrum, Utrecht/Antwerpen, 1972

Mechanic, D.: *Politics, Medicine, and Social Science*, John Wiley & Sons, New York, 1974

Meij, A. W. H. en Zimmeren, E. van: *Ontwerp-Verdrag tot Vaststelling van een Grondwet voor Europa*, Europocket, supplement bij de 13e druk, Kluwer, Deventer, 2003

Meijer, G.: *Neo-Liberalisme. Neoliberalen over Economische Orde en Economische Theorie*, Van Gorcum, Assen/Maastricht, 1988

Mestrum, F.: *Globalisering en Armoede. Over het Nut van Armoede in de Nieuwe Wereldorde*, EPO, Berchem, 2000

Michel, F., (ed.): Jospin, L.: *My Vision of Europe and Globalization*; Lamy, P. and Pisani-Ferry, J.: *The Europe We Want*, Polity Press, Cambridge, 2002

Miegel, M.: *Die deformierte Gesellschaft. Wie die Deutschen ihre Wirklichkeit verdrängen*, Propyläen, Berlin, 2002

Miettinen, O. S.: *Theory of Medicine: At the Core of Post-Flexnerian Education in Medicine?* inaugural lecture, Free University, Amsterdam, 1987

Ministerie van Volksgezondheid, Welzijn en Sport: *Choices in Health Care* (Dunning Committee), VWS, Rijswijk, 1991

Ministerie van Volksgezondheid, Welzijn en Sport: *Minder Regels, meer Zorg*, Eindrapport van de Commissie Terugdringing administratieve Lasten in de Zorgsector, VWS, Den Haag, 2002

Mintzberg, H.: *The Structuring of Organizations. A Synthesis of the Research*, Prentice-Hall, New York, 1979

Mishan, E. J.: *The Costs of Economic Growth* (Dutch Translation), Het Spectrum, Utrecht/Antwerpen, 1971

Mitchell, M.: *Right Side Up. Building Brands in the Age of the Organized Consumer*, HarperCollinsBusiness, London, 2002

Mittelman, J. H.: *The Globalization Syndrome. Transformation and Resistance*, Princeton University Press, Princeton, 2000

Moore, M.: *Downsize This. Random Threats From an Unarmed American*, Pan Books, New York, 2003

Moore, M.: *Stupid White Men ... and Other Sorry Excuses for the State and the Nation* (Dutch Translation), Uitgeverij De Arbeiderspers, Amsterdam/Antwerpen, 2003
Mosseveld, C. J. P. M. van: *International Comparison of Health Care Data. Existing Frameworks, Innovations and Data Use*, dissertation, ISBN 903572688 X, Statistics Netherlands, Voorburg, 2003
Mossialos, E. and Le Grand, J., (eds.): *Health Care and Cost Containment in the European Union*, Ashgate, Aldershot, England, 1999
Mossialos, E., Dixon, A., Figueras, J., and Kutzin, J., (eds.): *Funding Health Care: Options for Europe*, European Observatory on Health Care Systems Series, Open University Press, Buckingham, 2002
Mulcahy, L.: *Disputing Doctors. The Socio-Legal Dynamics of Complaints about Medical Care*, Open University Press, Maidenhead, 2003
Mueller, D. C.: *Public Choice II.* A Revised Edition of *Public Choice,* Cambridge University Press, Cambridge, 1995
Myrdal, G.: *Beyond the Welfare State* (Dutch Translation), N. V. De Arbeiderspers, Amsterdam, 1963
Neale, J.: *You are G8, We Are 6 Billion. The Truth Behind the Genoa Protests*, Vision Paperbacks, London, 2002
Nederlandse Zorgfederatie: *Gezondheidszorg in Tel*, NZf, Utrecht, 1996
Nederlandse Zorgfederatie: *Gezondheidszorg in Tel*, NZf, Utrecht, 1998
Nelsen, B. F. and Stubb, A., (eds.): *The European Union. Readings on the Theory and Practice of European Integration*, second edition, Palgrave, New York, 1998
New, B. and Le Grand, J.: *Rationing in the NHS. Principles and Pragmatism*, King's Fund, London, 1996
Nieuwenkamp, R.: *De Prijs van het politieke Primaat. Wederzijds Vertrouwen en Loyaliteit in de Verhouding tussen Bewindspersonen en ambtelijke Top*, Eburon, Delft, 2001
Nugent, N., (ed.): *At the Heart of the Union. Studies of the European Commission*, 2nd edition, MacMillan Press Ltd., London, 2000
Nye, J. S. and Donahue, J. D., (eds.): *Governance in a Globalizing World*, Brookings Institution Press, Washington D.C., 2000
O'Rourke, K. H. and Williamson, J. G.: *Globalization and History. The Evolution of a Nineteenth-Century Atlantic Economy*, MIT Press, Boston, Massachusetts, 2000
OECD: *Internal Markets in the Making. Health Systems in Canada, Iceland and the United Kingdom*. Health Policy Studies No. 6, OECD, Paris, 1995
OECD: *Measuring Health Care, 1960–1983*, OECD, Paris, 1985
OECD: *New Directions in Health Care Policy*, Health Policy Studies No. 7, OECD, Paris, 1995
OECD: OECD *Health Systems. Facts and Trends 1960–1991*, Health Policy Studies No. 3, Volume I, Paris, 1993
OECD: OECD *Health Systems. The Socio-Economic Environment. Statistical References*, Health Policy Studies No. 3, Volume II, OECD Paris, 1993
OECD: *The OECD Jobs Study. Facts, Analysis, Strategies*, OECD, Paris, 1994
OECD: *The Reform of Health Care Systems. A Review of Seventeen OECD Countries*, OECD, Paris, 1994
OECD: *The Reform of Health Care. A Comparative Analysis of Seven OECD Countries*, Health Policy Studies, No. 2, OECD, Paris, 1992

OECD: *Towards a New Global Age. Challenges and Opportunities*. Policy Report, OECD, Paris, 1997
Offe, C.: *Contradictions of the Welfare State*, Keane, (ed.), MIT Press, Cambridge, Massachusetts, 1993
Omachonu, V. K.: *Total Quality and Productivity Management in Health Care Organizations*, Institute of Industrial Engineers Norcross, Georgia, 1991
O'Neill, P.: *Health Crisis 2000*, WHO Regional Office for Europe, Copenhagen, 1983
Ormerod, P.: *The Death of Economics*, Faber and Faber, London, 1994
Owen Smith, E., (ed.): *Trade Unions in the Developed Economies*, Croom Helm, London, 1981
Palast, G.: *The Best Democracy Money Can Buy*, Robinson, London, 2003
Parker, J. E. S.: *The Economics of Innovation. The National and Multinational Enterprise in Technological Change*, Longman, 1974
Payer, L.: *Medicine and Culture. Varieties of Treatment in the United States, England, West Germany, and France*, Henry Holt and Company, New York, 1998
Pen, J.: *Harmonie en Conflict*, De Bezige Bij, Amsterdam, 1962
Peterson, W. C.: *Silent Depression. Twenty-Five Years of Wage Squeeze and Middle-Class Decline*, Norton and Company, New York, 1995
Petras, K. and Petras, R.: *Unusually Stupid Americans. A Compendium of All-American Stupidity*, Villard, New York, 2003
Phillips, K.: *Wealth and Democracy. A Political History of the American Rich*, Broadway Books, New York, 2002
Pierre, J. and Guy Peters, B.: *Governance, Politics and the State*, MacMillan Press Ltd., London, 2000
Pierson, C. and Castles, F. G., (eds.): *The Welfare State Reader*, Polity Press, Cambridge, 2003
Pilger, J.: *Hidden Agendas*, Vintage Books, London, 1999
Pilger, J.: *The New Rulers of the World*, Verso, New York, 2002
Ploeg, R. van der: *Ik geloof in Europa. Agenda voor een sterker, veiliger en democratischer Europa*, Bert Bakker, Amsterdam, 2004
Ploug, N. and Kvist, J.: *Social Security in Europe. Development or Dismantlement?* Kluwer Law International, The Hague, 1996
Polanyi, K.: *The Great Transformation. The Political and Economic Origins of our Time*, Beacan Press, Boston, 1957
Popta, S. van: *De Gemengde Economische Orde en de Christelijk-Sociale Gedachte*, Kok, Kampen, 1974
Popta, S. van: *Inhalen en Voorbijstreven. Het Hoe en Waarom van de Sovjet-Economie*, dissertation, University Press, Rotterdam, 1971
PriceWaterhouseCoopers: *HealthCast Tactics: A Blueprint for the Future*, The Health Cast 2010 Series, PriceWaterhouseCoopers, 2002
Raad voor de Volksgezondheid en Zorg: *Europa en de Gezondheidszorg*, Zoetermeer, 1999
Raad voor de Volksgezondheid en Zorg: *Patiënt en Internet*, Zoetermeer, 2000
Raad voor de Volksgezondheid en Zorg: *Technologische Innovatie in de Zorgsector*, Zoetermeer, 2001
Raad voor de Volksgezondheid en Zorg: *E-Health in Zicht*, Zoetermeer, 2002
Raad voor de Volksgezondheid en Zorg: *Gepaste Zorg*, Zoetermeer, 2004

Radice, G., (ed.): *What Needs to Change? New Visions for Britain*, Harper Collins Publishers, London, 1996

Raffel, M. W., (ed.): *Health Care and Reform in Industrialized Countries*, The Pennsylvania State University Press, Pennsylvania, 1997

Raphael, D. D. and MacFie, A. F., (eds.): Adam Smith. *The Theory of Moral Sentiments*, Liberty Fund, Indianapolis, 1982

Reich, C. A.: *Opposing the System*, Crown Publishers Inc., New York, 1995

Reich, R. B.: *The Future of Success. Working and Living in the New Economy*, Vintage Books, New York, 2000

Reich, R. B.: *The Work of Nations. A Blueprint for the Future*, Simon & Schuster, London, 1993

Reich, R. B., (ed.): *The Power of Public Ideas*, Harvard University Press, Cambridge, Massachusetts, 1990

Reid, T. R.: *The United States of Europe. The New Superpower and the End of American Supremacy*, Penguin Press, New York, 2004

Rifkin, J.: *The End of Work. The Decline of the Global Labor Force and the Dawn of the Post-Market Era*, G. P. Putnam's Sons, New York, 1996

Rifkin, J.: *The European Dream. How Europe's Vision of the Future is Quietly Eclipsing the American Dream*, Tarcher/Penguin, New York, 2004

Ritter, S. and Rivers Pitt, W.: *War on Iraq. What Team Bush Doesn't Want You to Know*, Profile Books, London, 2002

Ritzer, G.: *McDonaldization. The Reader*, Pine Forge Press, Thousand Oaks, California, 2002

Rodrik, D.: *Has Globalization Gone Too Far?* Institute for International Economics, Washington D.C., 1997

Roger-France, F. H., Moor, G. de, Hofdijk, J., and Jenkins, L., (eds.): *Diagnosis Related Groups in Europe*, EFMI-Working Conference '89, ISBN 90-73045-01-0, Gent, 1989

Rugman, A.: *The End of Globalisation*, Random House, Washington, 2000

Ruigrok, W. and Tulder, R. van: *The Logic of International Restructuring*, Routledge, London, 1995

Rupert, M. and Smith, H., (eds.): *Historical Materialism and Globalization*, Routledge, London, 2002

Saltman, R. B. and Figueras, J., (eds.): *European Health Care Reform. Analysis of Current Strategies*, WHO Regional Office for Europe, Copenhagen, 1997

Saltman, R. B. and Otter, C. von, (eds.): *Implementing planned Markets in Health Care. Balancing Social and Economic Responsibility*, Open University Press, Buckingham, 1995

Saltman, R. B., Busse, R., and Mossialos, E., (eds.): *Regulating Entrepreneurial Behaviour in European Health Care Systems*, Open University Press, Buckingham, 2003

Saltman, R. B., Busse, R., and Figueras, J., (eds.): *Social Health Insurance Systems in Western* Europe, European Observatory on Health Systems and Policies Series, Open University Press, Maidenhead, 2004

Samuelson, P. A. and Nordhaus, W. D.: *Economics.* International Edition, McGraw-Hill Inc., New York, 1995

Sandier, S., Paris, V., and Polton, D.: *Health Care Systems in Transition: France, 2004.* European Observatory on Health Care Systems (Thomson, S. and Mossialos, E., [eds.]), WHO, Copenhagen, 2004

Sardar, Z. and Davies, M. W.: *Why Do People hate America*, Icon Books, Cambridge, 2002
Saul, J. R.: *The Unconscious Civilization*, Penguin Books, London, 1997
Scambler, G.: *Health and Social Change. A Critical Theory*, Open University Press, Buckingham, 2002
Schlosser, E.: *Fast Food Nation. What the All-American Meal Is Doing to the World*, Penguin Books, London, 2002
Scholte, J. A.: *Globalization. A Critical Introduction*, Palgrave, New York, 2002
Schrijvers, A. J. P., (ed.): *Health and Health Care in the Netherlands. A critical Self-Assessment by Dutch Experts in the Medical and Health Sciences*, De Tijdstroom, Utrecht, 1997
Schrijvers, A. J. P.: *Een Kathedraal van Zorg*, De Tijdstroom, Utrecht, 1994
Schumpeter, J. A.: *Capitalism, Socialism and Democracy* (Dutch Translation), Sterrenserie 9, De Boer/Brand, Hilversum, 1963
Schut, F. T.: Competition in the Dutch Health Care Sector, dissertation, Erasmus University, Rotterdam, 1995
Schut, F. T.: *De Zorg is toch geen Markt? Laveren tussen Marktfalen en Overheidsfalen in de Gezondheidszorg*, inaugural lecture, Erasmus University, Rotterdam, 2003
Schuyt, K. and Veen, R. van der, (eds.): *De Verdeelde Samenleving. Een Inleiding in de Ontwikkeling van de Nederlandse Verzorgingsstaat*, Stenfert Kroese, Houten, 1995
Scrivens, E.: Quality, *Risk and Control in Health Care*, Open University Press, Maidenhead, 2005
Seedhouse, D., (ed.): *Reforming Health Care. The Philosophy and Practice of International Health Reform*, Wiley & Sons, Chichester, 1995
Self, P.: *Rolling Back the Market. Economic Dogma and Political Choice*, MacMillan Press Ltd., London, 2000
Sen, A.: *Development as Freedom* (Dutch Translation), Uitgeverij Contact, Amsterdam/Antwerpen, 2000
Sen, A.: *Welzijn, Vrijheid en Maatschappelijke Keuze. Opstellen over de Politieke Economie van het Pluralisme*, Van Gennip, Amsterdam, 1995
Sennett, R.: *The Corrosion of Character. The Personal Consequences of Work in the New Capitalism*, W. W. Norton and Company, New York, 1998
Servan-Schreiber, J. J.: *Le Défi Américain* (Dutch Translation), A. W. Bruna en Zoon, Utrecht/Antwerpen, 1967
Shipler, D. K.: *The Working Poor. Invisible in America*, Alfred A. Knopf, New York, 2004
Smith, A.: *An Inquiry into the Nature and the Causes of the Wealth of Nations*, collector's edition, the Easton Press, Norwalk, Connecticut, 1991
Smith, P. C., Ginelly, L., and Sculpher, M., (eds.): *Health Policy and Economics. Opportunities and Challenges*, Open University Press, Berkshire, 2005
Snel, E., Hoek, T. van der, and Chessa, T.: *Kinderen in Armoede. Opgroeien in de Marge van Nederland*, Van Gorcum, Assen, 2001
Sociaal Economische Raad: *Sociale Dimensie Europa*, 1992, Den Haag, 1990
Sociaal en Cultureel Planbureau: *Sociaal en Cultureel Rapport 1994*, Rijswijk, 1994
Sociaal en Cultureel Planbureau: *Sociaal en Cultureel Rapport 1996*, Rijswijk, 1996
Sociaal en Cultureel Planbureau: *Rapportage Ouderen 1996*, Rijswijk, 1996

Soros, G.: *George Soros on Globalization* (Dutch Translation), Uitgeverij Contact, Amsterdam/Antwerpen, 2002

Soros, G.: *The Crisis of Global Capitalism. Open Society Endangered*, Little, Brown and Company, London, 1998

Sparrow, M. K.: *License To Steal. How Fraud Bleeds America's Health Care System*, updated edition, Westview Press, Boulder, Colorado, 2000

Spicker, P.: *Social Policy. Themes and Approaches*, Prentice Hall, London, 1995

Springer, B.: *The Social Dimension of 1992. Europe Faces a New EC*, Praeger, New York, 1992

Standing Committee of the Hospitals of the European Union (HOPE)/Entente des Hôpitaux Luxembourgois (EHL): *Free Movement and Cross-Border Cooperation in Europe: the Role of Hospitals & practical Experiences in Hospitals*, Proceedings of the HOPE Conference and Workshop, Luxembourg, June 2003

Standing Committee of the Hospitals of the European Union. Sub-Committee on Coordination: *Measures to Reduce Surgical Waiting Lists*, Leuven, 1998

Standing Committee of the Hospitals of the European Union. Subcommittee on Economics and Planning: *Hospital and Health Care Rationing*, Leuven, 2000

Steering Committee on Future Health Scenarios: *Anticipating and Assessing Health Care Technology*, Volume 2, Future Technological Changes, Kluwer, 1988

Stiglitz, J.: *Globalization and its Discontents* (Dutch Translation), Uitgeverij Het Spectrum, Utrecht, 2002

Stiglitz, J.: *The Roaring Nineties. Seeds of Destruction*, Allen Lane, London, 2003

Stiglitz, J.: *Whither Socialism?* MIT Press, Cambridge, Massachusetts, 1995

Stocking, B. and Morrison, L.: *The Image and the Reality. A Case-Study of the Impacts of Medical Technology*, Oxford University Press, Oxford, 1978

Stocking, B., (ed.): *Expensive Health Technologies. Regulatory and Administrative Mechanisms in Europe*, Oxford University Press, Oxford, 1988

Stoltzfus Jost, T., (ed.): *Health Care Coverage Determinations. An International Comparative Study*, Open University Press, Maidenhead, 2005

Stronks, K. and en Hulshof, J., (eds.): *De Kloof verkleinen. Theorie en Praktijk van de Strijd tegen sociaal-economische Gezondheidsverschillen*, Van Gorcum, Assen/Maastricht, 2001

Swaan, A. de: *Zorg en de Staat. Welzijn, Onderwijs en Gezondheidszorg in Europa en de Verenigde Staten in de Nieuwe Tijd*, Bert Bakker, Amsterdam, 1993

Taylor, R.: *Medicine out of Control* (Dutch Translation), De Tijdstroom, Lochem, 1983

Tawney, R. H.: *Religion and the Rise of Capitalism*, Pelican Books, 1964

The Group of Lisbon (Petrella, R., chairman): *Limits to Competition*, VUBPRESS, Brussels, 1994

Theofilatou, M. A.: *The Emerging Health Agenda. The Health Policy of the European Community*, dissertation, Maastricht University, Maastricht, 2000

Thurow, L. C.: *Head to Head. The Coming Economic Battle among Japan, Europe and America*, Warner Books, New York, 1993

Thurow, L. C.: *The Future of Capitalism*, Nicholas Brealy Publishing, London, 1996

Todd, E.: *Après l'empire. Essai sur la décomposition du système américain* (Dutch Translation), Prometheus, Amsterdam, 2003

Tomlins, Chr. L.: *The State and the Unions. Labor Relations, Law, and the Organized Labor Movement in America, 1880–1960*, Cambridge University Press, Cambridge, 1985

Toren, J. P. van den and Vos, P. J., (eds.): *Overleeft het Rijnlandse Model? Perspectief op Arbeidsverhoudingen I*, Nationaal Vakbondsmuseum/Stichting Beheer IISG, 1997

Toren, J. P. van den: *Van Loonslaaf tot Bedrijfsgenoot. 100 Jaar Christelijk-Sociaal Denken, Medezeggenschap en Sociale Zekerheid*, Kok, Kampen, 1991

Trappenburg, M.: *Gezondheidszorg en Democratie*, inaugurele rede, Erasmus University, Rotterdam, 2005

Trouw Dossier 31: *Europa. Paradijs of Puinhoop?* Rainbow Pockets, Trouw, Amsterdam, 2004

Turner, A.: *Just Capital. The Liberal Economy*, Pan Books, London, 2002

Twist, M. W. J. van, Boer, M. C. den, Mil, B. P. A. van, and Geut, L.: *Beelden van* Bestuur. Berenschot Trendstudie, Uitgeverij Lemma, Utrecht, 2002

United Nations Research Institute for Social Development: *States of Disarray. The Social Effects of Globalization*, UNRISD, London, 1995

Urwin, D. W.: *A Political History of Western Europe since 1945*, fifth edition, Longman, London, 1997

Vallgårda, S., Krasnik, A., and Vrangbæk, K.: *Health Care Systems in Transition: Denmark, 2001*, (Thomson, S. and Mossialos, E. [eds.], WHO. Regional Office for Europe, Copenhagen, 2001

Vathorst, S. van de: *Your Money or My Life. Justice, Solidarity and Responsibility in Dutch Health Care*, dissertation, Free University of Amsterdam, 2001

Vries, B. de: *Overmoed en Onbehagen. Het Hervormingskabinet-Balkenende*, Bert Bakker, Amsterdam, 2005

Vroonhoven, L. van: *De Al-Ene Mens. Op Zoek naar het Individu*, Damon, Budel, 1999

Walburg, J. A.: *Uitkomstenmanagement in de Gezondheidszorg. Het Opbouwen van Lerende Teams in Zorgorganisaties*, Elsevier Gezondheidszorg, Maarssen, 2003

Walshe, K.: *Regulating Health Care. A Prescription for Improvement?* Open University Press, Maidenhead, 2003

Walt, G.: *Health Policy. An Introduction to Process and Power*, Witwatersrand University Press, Witwatersrand, 1994

Wanless, D.: *Securing Our Future Health: Taking a Long-Term View*, The Public Enquiry Unit, HM Treasury, London, November, 2001

Weber, M.: *The Protestant Ethic and the Spirit of Capitalism*, Routledge Classics, London, 2002

Weggeman, M.: *Leidinggeven aan Professionals. Het Verzilveren van Creativiteit*, Kluwer Bedrijfswetenschappen, 1993

Weiss, L.: *The Myth of the Powerless State. Governing the Economy in a Global Era*, Polity Press, Cambridge, 1998

Went, R.: *Grenzen aan Globalisering?* Het Spinhuis, Amsterdam, 1996

Werner, K. and Weiss, H.: *Schwarzbuch Markenfirmen* (Dutch Translation), Elmar, Rijswijk, 2002

Westerloo, G. van: *Niet spreken met de Bestuurder*, De Bezige Bij, Amsterdam, 2004

Wetenschappelijke Raad voor het Regeringsbeleid: *Bewijzen van goede Dienstverlening*, Amsterdam University Press, Amsterdam, 2004

Wetenschappelijke Raad voor het Regeringsbeleid: *Tweedeling in Perspectief*, Sdu Uitgeverij, Den Haag, 1996

Wheen, F.: *How Mumbo-Jumbo Conquered the World*, Harper Perennial, 2004

White, K.: *An Introduction to the Sociology of Health and Illness*, SAGE Publications, 2002

White, S. and Stancombe, J.: *Clinical Judgement in the Health and Welfare Professions. Extending the Evidence Base*, Open University Press, Maidenhead, 2003

Wight, J. B.: *Saving Adam Smith. A Tale of Wealth, Transformation and Virtue*, Prentice-Hall, Inc., New Jersey, 2002

Wilkinson, G. R.: *Unhealthy Societies. The Afflictions of Inequality*, Routledge, London, 1996

Wilkinson, R.: *Multilateralism and the World Trade Organisation. The Architecture and Extension of International Trade Regulation*, Routledge, London, 2000

Wille, E., (ed.): *Rationierung im Gesundheitswesen und ihre Alternativen*, Nomos Verlagsgesellschaft, Baden-Baden, 2003

Wilson, D.: China. *The Big Tiger. A Nation awakes*, Abacus Books, London, 1996

Wilterdink, N.: *Ongelijkheid en Interdependentie. Ontwikkelingen in Welstandsverhoudingen*, inaugurele rede, Groningen, 1993

Windmuller, J. P., et al.: *Collective Bargaining in Industrialised Market Economies: A Reappraisal*, International Labour Office, Geneva, 1987

World Health Organization. Regional Office for Europe: *Health Care Systems in Transition: Greece, 1996*, WHO, Copenhagen, 1996

Wright, M.: *Transnational Corporations, Trade Unions and Industrial Relations*, University of Sydney, Faculty of Economics, University of Sydney, 1981

Yergin, D. and Stanislaw, J.: *The Commanding Heights. The Battle between Government and the Marketplace that is Remaking the Modern World*, Simon & Schuster, New York, 1998

Zakaria, F.: *The Future of Freedom. Illiberal Democracy at Home and Abroad* (Dutch Translation), Uitgeverij Contact, Amsterdam/Antwerpen, 2003

Ziekenfondsraad: *Tweede Evaluatie Beperking Aanspraak Tandheelkunde per 1 januari 1995*. Amstelveen, publikatienummer 1996/707

Zijlstra, J.: *Economische Orde en Economische Politiek*, Stenfert Kroese, Leiden, 1956

Zonneveld, M.: *Kermis in de Politiek. Waarom de Nederlandse Kiezer op Drift raakte*, Van Gennep, Amsterdam, 2002

Zuthem, H. J. van: *De Geloofwaardigheid van onze Economische Orde*, Kok, Kampen, 1969

Zuthem, H. J. van: *Verantwoord Bestaan*, Agora/Kok, Kampen, 1993

Index

n after page numbers indicate an endnote

MIX
Papier aus verantwortungsvollen Quellen
Paper from responsible sources
FSC® C105338

If you have any concerns about our products,
you can contact us on
ProductSafety@springernature.com

In case Publisher is established outside the EU,
the EU authorized representative is:
Springer Nature Customer Service Center GmbH
Europaplatz 3, 69115 Heidelberg, Germany

Printed by Libri Plureos GmbH
in Hamburg, Germany